Preoperative Assessment

Derek Dillane • Barry A. Finegan
Editors

Preoperative Assessment

A Case-Based Approach

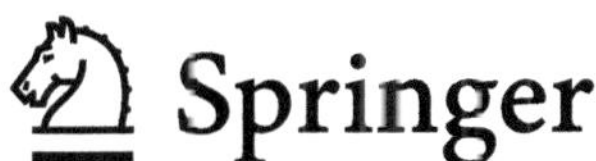
Springer

Editors
Derek Dillane
Department of Anesthesiology and Pain Medicine
University of Alberta
Edmonton, AB
Canada

Barry A. Finegan
Department of Anesthesiology and Pain Medicine
University of Alberta
Edmonton, AB
Canada

ISBN 978-3-030-58841-0   ISBN 978-3-030-58842-7 (eBook)
https://doi.org/10.1007/978-3-030-58842-7

This Springer imprint is published by the registered company Springer Nature Switzerland AG
The registered company address is: Gewerbestrasse 11, 6330 Cham, Switzerland

Foreword

The long-established goal of preoperative management of the elective surgical patient is identification, assessment, and reduction of perioperative risk. This may involve *de novo* diagnosis of an unrelated condition (e.g., sleep apnea); management of a disease process related to a preexisting condition (e.g., anemia); assessment and treatment optimization of a chronic medical condition (e.g., poorly controlled diabetes mellitus); or preemptive mitigation of postoperative issues that increase morbidity (e.g., pain management planning, nausea, and vomiting prophylaxis). Increasingly, there is a recognition that prehabilitation – a multidisciplinary endeavor aimed at enhancing physical, medical, nutritional, and mental well-being prior to surgical intervention – may offer an opportunity to not only decrease risk but also reduce recovery time, and by extension cost of care.

This targeted, concise, and comprehensive book provides a case-based approach to preoperative optimization. Each chapter starts with a clinical vignette followed by a question-and-answer style investigation of the relevant issues. The concept is to provide the reader with a brief update of the current thinking on the medical diagnosis and highlight key issues that need to be addressed preoperatively. This excellent book contains the authors' thoughts on how such patients could be managed in the clinic and, as such, is not prescriptive but written to inform the reader of current medical management suggestions and to provoke thoughtful assessment of the patient in that context. Most of the chapters were written by Drs Dillane and Finegan and, as such, there is a uniformity to the structure and content of the book.

The growing incidence of comorbidities in the surgical population such as obesity, frailty, diabetes mellitus, and cardiovascular disease is challenging in the context of a demand for shorter postoperative stays or ambulatory surgery. To this end, the editors and authors of this perceptive text provide judicious guidance based on a comprehensive analysis of current evidence. Everyone would benefit from reading this book.

Frances Chung
Professor, Department of Anesthesiology and Pain Medicine
University of Toronto, ResMed Research Chair of Anesthesiology
Sleep, and Periop Medicine at University Health Network
Toronto, ON, Canada

Krembil Research Institute
Toronto, ON, Canada

Toronto Western Hospital, University Health Network
Toronto, ON, Canada

Preface

The past decade has seen renewed interest in preoperative optimization as a result of the shift towards an outcomes-based prudential model of perioperative care. Both Enhanced Recovery After Surgery and Perioperative Surgical Home programs identify the value of timely patient optimization strategies for improving postoperative outcome. This is good news for those of us who identify as perioperative physicians. While technically proficient surgery performed under skillfully delivered anesthesia is a necessary condition for a successful outcome, the long-term impact of multidisciplinary preoperative intervention is becoming increasingly evident.

This book provides a case-based approach to preoperative evaluation and optimization. Preoperative assessment, at its core, aims to improve patient care and safety, enhance the efficient use of resources, and diminish patient concerns by comprehensively addressing any harbored fears. There are surprisingly few resources for the physician who works in this capacity and this is the first case-based approach to the subject.

The book is organized into parts according to body system and each part consists of chapters delineating a specific disorder. The vast majority of cases deal with elective surgical patients. There is a miscellaneous part with a number of chapters dealing with increasingly relevant topics such as surgery in the chronic opioid user and management of the frail patient. The dilemmas encountered are authentic, sometimes contentious, and sure to resonate with many readers. We hope this approach will be both entertaining and edifying. Our aim is to provide the structure and information necessary to successfully evaluate the patient who presents for preoperative optimization. We are not internists and periodically throughout the text we identify situations where it would be prudent to seek specialist advice. Our overall goal in this context is to enable the reader to identify the at-risk patient and participate fluently in subsequent multidisciplinary care.

Each chapter starts with a clinical vignette followed by a question-and-answer style investigation of the relevant issues. These questions attempt to address commonly encountered clinical dilemmas where opinion often differs between, and occasionally within, medical subspecialties, for example, whether to bridge the chronically anticoagulated patient. Rather than limit the discussion only to matters of direct relevance to each case, we expand the conversation to provide a broad overview of each topic. A case-based approach is an ideal format for preoperative evaluation – a conversational yet informed and evidence-based appraisal of the literature infused with the authors' experience. We believe the book can be browsed in a cursory manner or used as a reference in the preadmission clinic.

One of the challenges we faced over the 3-year process of writing this book relates to the protean nature of best evidence and related guidelines. This is especially relevant when one considers the practicality and utility of point of care digital resources. Why write a textbook when parts of it may already be obsolete on publication? Our hope is that, in addition to serving as a stand-alone reference in itself, the book provides a series of jumping off points to other more fluid resources, if required.

We are grateful to our contributing authors for their expertise in helping us write this book. They have been generous in allowing us to revise the manuscript in an attempt to achieve accuracy and consistency. We thank our colleagues for identifying many of the interesting cases that appear throughout the text. We wish to express our gratitude to Ms. Katherine Kreilkamp (Developmental Editor, Springer Nature) for her guidance and encouragement on every step of this journey. We also thank Gregory Sutorius, Senior Editor, Clinical Medicine, Springer Nature, for his support and patience. Finally, and most importantly, we wish to acknowledge our patients who consented to share their stories in this format.

Edmonton, AB, Canada Derek Dillane
Edmonton, AB, Canada Barry A. Finegan

Laboratory Test Reference Values

Laboratory Test	Reference Range SI units	Conventional Units
Albumin (serum)	35–50 g/L	3.5–5.0 g/dL
Alkaline phosphatase	30–130 U/L	30–130 U/L
Bilirubin total (serum)	3–22 µmol/L	0.2–1.3 mg/dL
Calcium (serum)		
Total	2.10–2.60 mmol/L	8.4–10.6 mg/dL
Ionized	1.15–1.35 mmol/L	4.6–5.1 mg/dL
Cholesterol (serum)	<5.2 mmol/L	<200 mg/dL
Cortisol (plasma) 8 AM	170–635 nmol/L	3–15 µg/dL
Cortisol (plasma) 4 PM	82–413 nmol/L	0.6–1.2 mg/dL
Creatinine (serum)	50–110 µmol/L	0.6–1.2 mg/dL
Erythrocytes (RBC)		
Males	4.6–6.2 × 1012/L	4.6–6.2 million/mm^3
Females	4.2–5.4 × 1012/L	4.2–5.4 million/mm^3
Ferritin (serum)	20–200 µg/L	20–200 ng/mL
Glucose (fasting) (plasma or serum)	3.9–6.1 mmol/L	70–110 mg/dL
Growth hormone (serum) fasting	0–10 µg/L	0–10 ng/mL
Hematocrit		
Males	0.40–0.54	40–54%
Females	0.37–0.47	37–47%
Hemoglobin (Hb)		
Males	140–180 g/L	14.0–18.0 g/dL
Females	120–160 g/L	12.0–16.0 g/dL
High density lipoproteins (HDL)	>0.91 mmol/L	>35 mg/dL
Iron (serum) - Males	13–31 µmol/L	75–175 µg/dL
Iron (serum) - Females	5–29 µmol/L	28–162 µg/dL
Iron binding capacity (serum) (TIBC)	45–73 µmol/L	250–410 µg/dL
Leukocytes - Total	3.5–12.0 × 10^9/L	3500–12,000/mm^3
Low density lipoproteins (LDL)	<3.4 mmol/L	<130 mg/dL
Magnesium (Serum)	0.65–1.05 mmol/L	1.3–2.1 mg/dL
Mean corpuscular volume (MCV)	76–100 fL	76–100 µm^3
Osmolality (serum)	285–295 mmol/kg	285–295 mOsm/kg
Parathyroid hormone (PTH)	1.4–6.8 pmol/L	13.2–64.1 pg/mL
Platelet count	150–400 × 10^9/L	150,000–400,000/mm^3
Potassium (serum)	3.5–5.1 mmol/L	3.5–5.1 mEq/L
Reticulocytes	25–75 × 10^9/L	25,000–75,000/mm^3
Sodium (serum)	135–145 mmol/L	135–145 mEq/L
Testosterone		
Males	9.5–30 nmol/L	275–875 ng/dL
Females	0.8–2.6 nmol/L	23–75 ng/dL
Thyroid-stimulating hormone (TSH) (serum)	0.4–4.8 mIU/L	0.4–4.8 mIU/L
Thyroxine (T4), total (serum)	66–155 nmol/L	5–12 µg/dL

Laboratory Test	Reference Range SI units	Conventional Units
Thyroxine (T4), free (serum)	9–23 pmol/L	1.0–2.1 ng/dL
Triiodothyronine (T3), free (serum)	3.5–6.5 pmol/L	2.4–5.0 pg/mL
Transaminase (serum)		
AST (SGOT)	7–40 IU/L	7–40 IU/L
ALT (SGPT)	5–35 IU/L	5–35 mU/mL

Common laboratory tests with reference ranges in SI and conventional units. Reference ranges may differ slightly from those provided in individual chapters. Adapted from the recommendations of the Royal College of Physicians and Surgeons of Canada. Some additions and modifications have been made

Contents

Editors (and Authors)

Derek Dillane, MB BCh, BAO, MMedSci, FCARCSI Department of Anesthesiology & Pain Medicine, University of Alberta, Edmonton, AB, Canada

Barry A. Finegan, MB BCh, BAO, FRCPC Department of Anesthesiology & Pain Medicine, University of Alberta, Edmonton, AB, Canada

Contributors

Chris Douglas, RN Acute Pain Service, University of Alberta Hospital, Edmonton, AB, Canada

Susan Halliday, MB ChB, BSc Med Sci, FRCA, FRCPC Department of Anesthesiology & Pain Medicine, University of Alberta Hospital, Edmonton, AB, Canada

Michael J. Jacka, MD, MSc, MBA Department of Anesthesiology & Pain Medicine/ Department of Critical Care, University of Alberta, Edmonton, AB, Canada

Stephanie Keeling, MD, MSc, FRCPC Division of Rheumatology, Department of Medicine, University of Alberta, Edmonton, AB, Canada

Rachel G. Khadaroo, MD, PHD, FRCSC, FACS Department of Surgery, University of Alberta, Edmonton, AB, Canada

Jalal A. Nanji, MD, FRCPC University of Alberta Faculty of Medicine and Dentistry, Department of Anesthesiology and Pain Medicine, Royal Alexandra Hospital DTC OR, Edmonton, AB, Canada

Lora B. Pencheva, BSc, MB ChB, FANZCA Department of Anaesthesia & Pain Medicine, Middlemore Hospital, Auckland, New Zealand

Surita Sidhu, MD, FRCP(C), FASE Department of Anesthesiology & Pain Medicine, Perioperative Echocardiography, Mazankowski Alberta Heart Institute, University of Alberta, Edmonton, AB, Canada

Ryan Snelgrove, MD, FRCSC Department of Surgery, University of Alberta, Edmonton, AB, Canada

Ciaran Twomey, MB BCh, BAO, FCARCSI Department of Anesthesiology & Pain Medicine, University of Alberta Hospital, Edmonton, AB, Canada

Stephen Young, MB CHb, FANZCA Department of Anaesthesia, Hawke's Bay Fallen Soldiers' Memorial Hospital, Hastings, New Zealand

Preoperative Assessment and Optimization

1

Derek Dillane and Barry A. Finegan

On October 13, 1804, Seishu Hanaoka performed a mastectomy in Hirayama, Japan [1]. This is considered by many to be the first operation under general anesthesia, predating by 42 years the first public demonstration of ether administration by Henry Thomas Green Morton. Hanaoka did not record his anesthesia technique. However, his student, Gendai Kamada, documented his use of a mixture of herbal extracts, Mafutsuto, in *Mafutsuto-Ron*, the first extant anesthesia textbook. Written in 1839, *Mafutsuto-Ron* is ten pages long and covers six topics beginning with preoperative assessment, on which Gendai Kamada reports the following:

> ...we perform six peri-anesthesia diagnoses, of which three are performed before the administration of the Mafutsuto. Performing these diagnoses in detail is the most important process in the administration of Mafutsuto. Pre-administration diagnoses are made to assess whether the use of Mafutsuto is appropriate for a patient, and there are three major conditions for which the Mafutsuto is contraindicated; (1) if a patient is frail with pale face and wasted limbs, frequently feverish and having low appetite, or not showing rise and fall of ki of the yingyang [ki means spirit]; (2) if a patient does not readily regain strength after a hemorrhagic event, or is feeling an epigastric fullness, coughing, and experiences shortness of breath upon exertion; (3) if a patient feels a strong palpitation, frequently yawns, experiences a heartburn, or vomits. The patient should be assessed carefully for the presence of any of the above three conditions, and then Mafutsuto can be used. If any of those conditions is present, the patient should receive a treatment for it first, and Mafutsuto can be administered upon its resolution. Even if a patient is young and naturally sturdy, the presence of above-mentioned conditions merits a prior treatment [1].

Almost two centuries ago, at the advent of general anesthesia, preoperative assessment and optimization were recognized as being indispensable for achieving a successful surgical outcome. Remarkably, in the foregoing, we can also identify elements which have only recently gained widespread traction in contemporary practice, e.g., frailty, conditioning, nutrition, and psychological prehabilitation [2]. Yet despite this prescient endorsement, many questions remain unanswered regarding preoperative evaluation. What is its effect on postoperative outcome? When should it be performed? Which discipline is best placed to perform the assessment? What format should evaluation take – which patients need to be seen in person?

In a thought-provoking and erudite account of their implementation of a multidisciplinary preoperative clinic, Aronson and colleagues accentuate a perennial barrier to meritorious preoperative care – a predilection to accept, and adapt to, the medical condition of the patient in close proximity to the surgery date [3]. However, evidence is beginning to emerge from Enhanced Recovery After Surgery and Perioperative Surgical Home programs for an association between optimization of modifiable comorbidities and surgical outcome [4, 5]. Thus far the data has not been granular enough to assign an improvement in outcome solely to preoperative optimization. This paucity of evidence can engender a culture of reluctance to postpone surgery for preoperative optimization. For instance, it may be challenging to defer surgery for optimization of diabetes control in a patient with a markedly elevated HbA1c value without disrupting patient and surgeon expectations. Without evidence demonstrating an association with outcome, such delays may only be accepted when day-of-surgery cancellations are anticipated.

The cultural intransigence to timely preoperative assessment is understandable when patients have to travel long distances for tertiary care. However, advances in telemedicine, which permit early triage and risk stratification, should obviate the need for the eleventh hour visit to the anesthesia preadmission clinic (PAC). To guarantee success, remotely delivered healthcare requires robust algorithms for identification of high-risk patients. The foundational elements of such care pathways can be found throughout this textbook, e.g., the Revised Cardiac Risk Index [6], the STOP-Bang Score [7], the Duke Activity Status Index [8], and the Clinical Frailty Scale [9], to name but a few.

D. Dillane (✉) · B. A. Finegan
Department of Anesthesiology & Pain Medicine, University of Alberta, Edmonton, AB, Canada

D. Dillane, B. A. Finegan (eds.), *Preoperative Assessment*, https://doi.org/10.1007/978-3-030-58842-7_1

These assertions also hold true for non-operating room anesthesia. Patients undergoing procedures in the endoscopy, interventional radiology, and cardiac physiology suites are not exempt from having significant comorbidities. It is not unusual for these patients to undergo their first, and only, preprocedure assessment immediately prior to induction. It is doubtful that a meaningful evaluation, as stipulated by the American Society of Anesthesiologists Practice Advisory for Preanesthesia Evaluation, can be performed in these circumstances [10].

The traditional PAC has long been the domain of the anesthesiologist. Even though there is reason to believe the model to be superannuated, there is still ample justification for the anesthesiologist to be at the center of the organization. As someone who understands the interplay between patient comorbidity, surgery, and anesthesia, in addition to having an established expertise in acute and chronic pain, and critical care medicine, there are few better qualified. However, an integrative approach with engagement of the entire perioperative team is necessary. This calls call upon resources not widespread in PACs, e.g., smoking cessation programs, exercise and conditioning clinics, nutrition and frailty assessment, psychological evaluation, and pain counseling, in addition to more established medical disciplines.

Patients with significant medical comorbidities, previously denied surgery, are now considered surgical candidates as a result of advances in surgery and minimally invasive techniques. A formal visit to a brick-and-mortar PAC will not be required for many patients. However, it is important that high-risk patients or patients undergoing high-risk surgeries are identified in a timely manner for optimization using measured and systematic evidence-based approaches. To borrow from the wisdom of Gendai Kamada, sometimes this may also be advisable for the apparently young and naturally sturdy patient.

References

1. Dote K, Ikemune K, Desaki Y, Yorozuya T, Makino H. Mafutsuto-Ron: the first anesthesia textbook in the world. Bibliographic review and English translation. J Anesth Hist. 2015;1(4):102–10.
2. Levett DZH, Grimmett C. Psychological factors, prehabilitation and surgical outcomes: evidence and future directions. Anaesthesia. 2019;74(Suppl 1):36–42.
3. Aronson S, Murray S, Martin G, Blitz J, Crittenden T, Lipkin ME, et al. Roadmap for transforming preoperative assessment to preoperative optimization. Anesth Analg. 2020;130(4):811–9.
4. Vetter TR, Barman J, Hunter JM Jr, Jones KA, Pittet JF. The effect of implementation of preoperative and postoperative care elements of a perioperative surgical home model on outcomes in patients undergoing hip arthroplasty or knee arthroplasty. Anesth Analg. 2017;124(5):1450–8.
5. Miller TE, Thacker JK, White WD, Mantyh C, Migaly J, Jin J, et al. Reduced length of hospital stay in colorectal surgery after implementation of an enhanced recovery protocol. Anesth Analg. 2014;118(5):1052–61.
6. Lee TH, Marcantonio ER, Mangione CM, Thomas EJ, Polanczyk CA, Cook EF, et al. Derivation and prospective validation of a simple index for prediction of cardiac risk of major noncardiac surgery. Circulation. 1999;100(10):1043–9.
7. Chung F, Yegneswaran B, Liao P, Chung SA, Vairavanathan S, Islam S, et al. STOP questionnaire: a tool to screen patients for obstructive sleep apnea. Anesthesiology. 2008;108(5):812–21.
8. Hlatky MA, Boineau RE, Higginbotham MB, Lee KL, Mark DB, Califf RM, et al. A brief self-administered questionnaire to determine functional capacity (the Duke Activity Status Index). Am J Cardiol. 1989;64(10):651–4.
9. Rockwood K, Song X, MacKnight C, Bergman H, Hogan DB, McDowell I, et al. A global clinical measure of fitness and frailty in elderly people. CMAJ. 2005;173(5):489–95.
10. Committee on Standards and Practice Parameters, Apfelbaum JL, Connis RT, Nickinovich DG; American Society of Anesthesiologists Task Force on Preanesthesia Evaluation, Pasternak LR, Arens JF, Caplan RA, Connis RT, Fleisher LA, Flowerdew R, et al. Practice advisory for preanesthesia evaluation: an updated report by the American Society of Anesthesiologists Task Force on Preanesthesia Evaluation. Anesthesiology. 2012;116(3):522–538.

Part I

Cardiac

The Cardiac Patient Undergoing Noncardiac Surgery

2

Derek Dillane

A preoperative consultation was requested on a 64-year-old male prior to radical cystectomy and ileal conduit formation. Three weeks previously he had been diagnosed with acute myocardial infarction (MI) type 2 (peak troponin I 5.6 μg/L) resulting in congestive cardiac failure, acute respiratory failure, acute exacerbation of chronic kidney injury, and acute liver injury. He had a background of type 2 diabetes, diabetic nephropathy, hyperlipidemia, hypertension, COPD, and obesity with a BMI of 39.2. Obstructive sleep apnea was suspected but undiagnosed. He had quit smoking over 20 years prior to this presentation. The acute coronary syndrome was treated with intravenous heparin anticoagulation and dual anti-platelet therapy (aspirin and clopidogrel).This resulted in frank hematuria. Computed tomography (CT) scan revealed a large 8 cm bladder mass with proximal left hydroureteronephrosis, small external iliac chain lymph nodes, and retroperitoneal lymph nodes. Dual anti-platelet therapy and heparinization were discontinued. A bladder tumor biopsy obtained at transurethral resection of bladder tumor revealed a high-grade muscle invasive urothelial cell carcinoma. Due to poor renal function, he was not a candidate for chemotherapy, and external beam radiotherapy was deemed to be a suboptimal approach compared to cystectomy.

Medications: Amlodipine, atorvastatin, ezetimibe, salbutamol, metoprolol, insulin glargine, insulin lispro, and isosorbide mononitrate.

Physical Examination: An obese, functionally limited gentleman with a heart rate of 86, blood pressure 169/77, and respiratory rate 18. Cardiac examination showed an A-wave dominant JVP 2 cm above the sternal angle, normal 1st and 2nd heart sounds, and no extra sounds or murmurs. Abdominal examination was normal except for the presence of a left nephrostomy tube placed after diagnosis of proximal left hydroureteronephrosis.

Investigations: Laboratory tests can be seen in Table 2.1. *Electrocardiograms (ECGs) from the time of presentation with acute MI and 3 weeks later at preoperative assessment can be seen in* Figs. 2.1 and 2.2. *Echocardiogram performed at the time of diagnosis of MI showed left ventricular ejection fraction 55–60%, no regional wall motion abnormalities, normal right ventricular function, mild mitral regurgitation, and normal diastolic function.*

Table 2.1 Laboratory values at preadmission clinic visit

Test	Result	Reference range (units)
Sodium	137	134–146 (mmol/L)
Potassium	4.4	3.6–5.0 (mmol/L)
Urea	21.5	2.8–7.5 (mmol/L)
Creatinine	314	50–120 (μmol/L)
Estimated GFR	17	>59 (mL/min/1.73m^2)
Ionized Ca^{2+}	1.09	1.10–1.35 (mmol/L)
Magnesium	0.70	0.65–1.05 (mmol/L)
Chloride	104	98–108 (mmol/L)
Albumin	36	33–48 (g/L)
Alkaline phosphatase	239	30–130 (U/L)
ALT	56	<50 (U/L)
AST	44	<40 (U/L)
Bilirubin	9	<20 (μmol/L)
HbA1c	10.0	4.3–6.1 (%)
Hemoglobin	99	140–175 (g/L)
Hematocrit	0.312	0.420–0.520 (L/L)
Platelet count	213	145–400 (×10^9/L)
WBC count	6.8	4.0–10.0 (×10^9/L)
PTT	30	27–39 (s)
INR	1.1	0.8–1.2
Troponin I	<0.10	<0.15 (ug/L)
BNP	464	<100 (pg/mL) heart failure unlikely

GFR Glomerular filtration rate, *ALT* alanine aminotransferase, *AST* aspartate aminotransferase, *WBC* white blood cell count, *PTT* partial thromboplastin time, *INR* international normalized ratio, *BNP* brain natriuretic peptide

D. Dillane (✉)
Department of Anesthesiology & Pain Medicine, University of Alberta, Edmonton, AB, Canada

D. Dillane, B. A. Finegan (eds.), *Preoperative Assessment*, https://doi.org/10.1007/978-3-030-58842-7_2

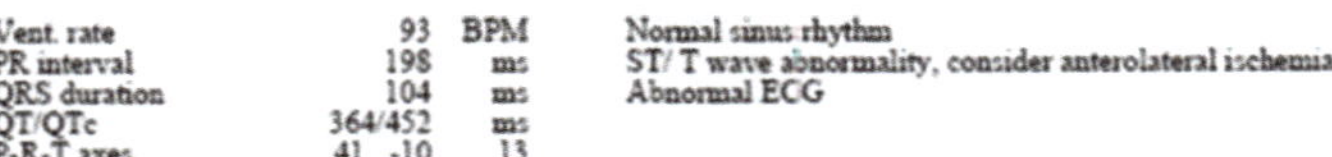

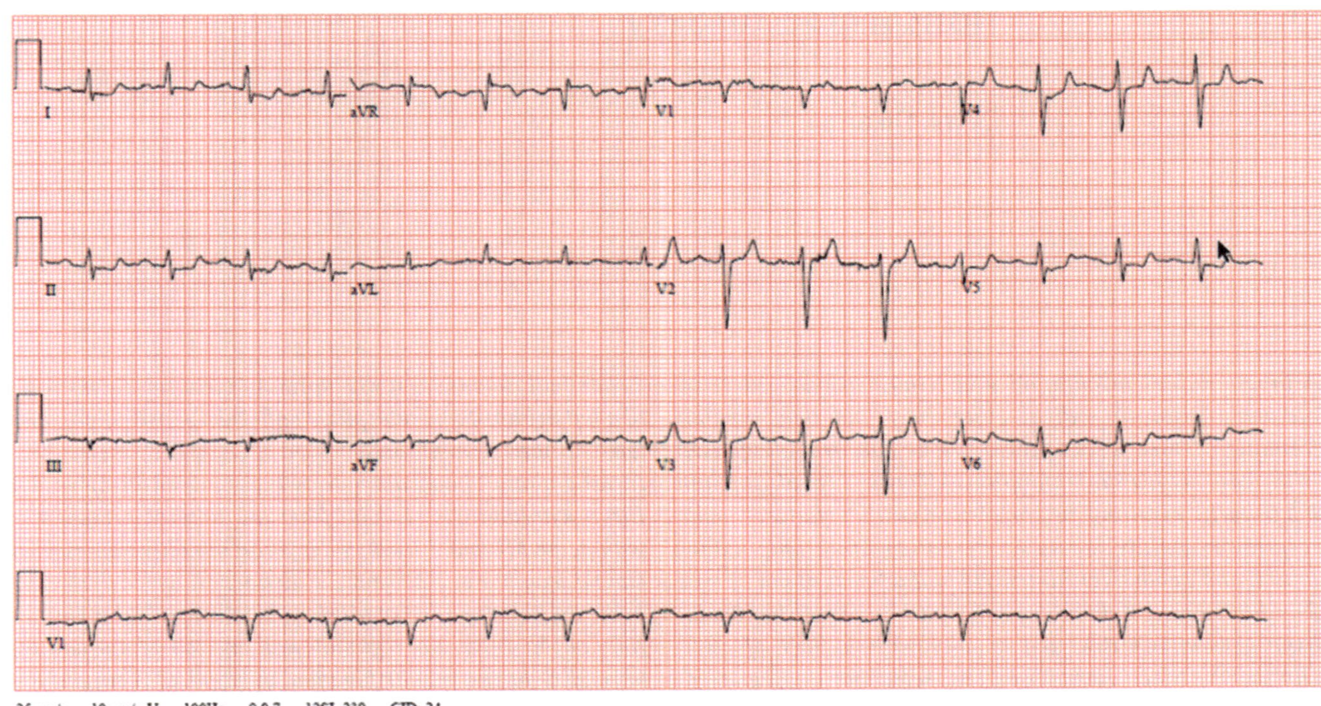

Fig. 2.1 Electrocardiogram at time of diagnosis of myocardial infarction type II showing lateral ST depression with aVR ST elevation

How Long Should Noncardiac Surgery Be Delayed Following Acute Myocardial Infarction?

The American College of Cardiology and American Heart Association (ACC/AHA) recommend avoidance of surgery for 60 days after acute MI [1]. This is partly based on a large retrospective study of 563,842 patients with recent MI having hip surgery, cholecystectomy, elective abdominal aortic aneurysm repair, or lower limb amputation [2]. The rate of postoperative MI decreased significantly as the interval between preoperative MI and surgery increased (0–30 days = 32.8%; 31–60 days = 18.7%; 61–90 days = 8.4%; and 91–180 days = 5.9%). The 30-day mortality rate associated with postoperative MI decreased in a similar fashion (0–30 days = 14.2%; 31–60 days = 11.5%; 61–90 days = 10.5%; and 91–180 days = 9.9%). It is worth noting that the elevated postoperative mortality risk when undergoing surgery 6 months after MI (9.9%) is greater than the 30-day mortality after acute coronary syndrome (ACS) from all causes by a factor of 2–3 [3]. In patients undergoing surgery after recent MI, revascularization by percutaneous coronary intervention (PCI)/stenting or coronary artery bypass surgery has been shown to improve postoperative infarction, and 30-day and 1-year mortality rate by at least 50% [4]. However, citing a lack of extensive evidence, the ACC/AHA recommend against routine coronary revascularization before noncardiac surgery outside of the current practice guidelines for coronary artery bypass grafting (CABG) and PCI [1].

What Is the Difference Between Type 1 and Type 2 Myocardial Infarction?

Type 1 MI is a spontaneous MI in the setting of atherothrombotic coronary artery disease. Type 1 MI is what we usually consider a traditional MI. It is usually secondary to plaque rupture or erosion.

Type 2 MI is due to a mismatch between myocardial oxygen supply and demand. Coronary artery disease may be present, but it is not the primary cause. Common underlying etiological causes include coronary artery dissection, spasm, emboli, anemia, arrhythmias, and hypotension [5]. The key diagnostic features of type 2 MI are an elevated and changing troponin, clinical features not consistent with type 1 MI, presence of clinical conditions known to disrupt oxygen supply/demand, e.g., tachycardia, and absence of causes indicating other nonischemic causes of raised troponin, e.g., myocarditis [5].

What Is Acute Coronary Syndrome?

"Acute coronary syndrome" is an umbrella term for myocardial infarction (STEMI or NSTEMI) and unstable angina. It is a medical emergency and necessitates referral to a cardiologist for evaluation and treatment that may include revascularization and subsequent initiation of antiplatelet therapy.

What Complications Is the Patient with Ischemic Heart Disease Subject to in the Perioperative Period?

- Perioperative MI
- Cardiac failure
- Cardiac arrest
- Arrhythmia
- Stroke
- Death

What Are the Characteristic Features of Perioperative Myocardial Infarction?

Unlike spontaneously occurring MIs, it is quite usual for the patient experiencing a perioperative MI to be asymptomatic [6]. In a study of 2546 patients at increased cardiovascular risk undergoing noncardiac surgery, only 6% of patients with postoperative MI reported chest pain (the incidence of postoperative MI was 16%) [7]. Because the typical symptoms of myocardial ischemia are not exhibited, the diagnosis is easily missed. Perioperative MI has a poor prognosis: despite its asymptomatic nature, 30-day mortality (10%) may be higher than that associated with non-postoperative MI (30-day mortality for NSTEMI and STEMI is approximately 2% and 2–10%, respectively [8–10]. The highest risk of death is in the first 48 postoperative hours. Because of the silent nature of postoperative ischemia, routine monitoring of troponin level is recommended in at-risk patients for the first 72 postoperative hours [7, 11, 12].

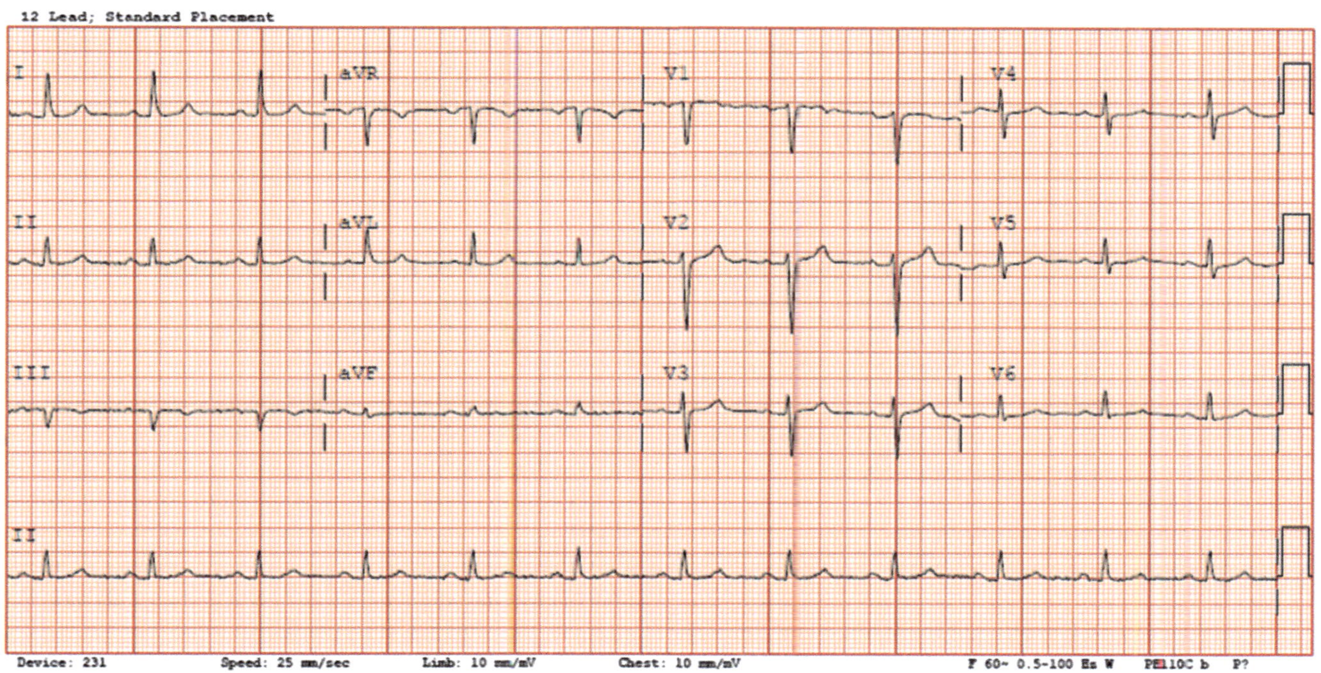

Fig. 2.2 Normal electrocardiogram at preoperative assessment

What Is Myocardial Injury After Noncardiac Surgery (MINS)?

Myocardial injury after noncardiac surgery (MINS) is defined as prognostically relevant myocardial injury due to ischemia occurring within 30 days of noncardiac surgery. Diagnosis is made in the presence of elevated troponin with or without ischemic symptoms or ECG changes [12, 13]. MINS is common with a reported incidence of up to 18% and is associated with a high 30-day mortality rate (4.1%) [11].

Describe a General Approach to Evaluation of a Patient with a History of Acute Coronary Syndrome Who Is Scheduled to Undergo Noncardiac Surgery?

History and physical examination should focus on symptoms and signs of cardiac disease in addition to comorbidities which increase perioperative cardiac risk. In the case outlined above, several such risk factors are present, i.e., cardiac failure, hypertension, hyperlipidemia, diabetes requiring insulin for control, COPD, chronic renal impairment, and possible OSA. The patient's functional status is elucidated; this is discussed in further detail below.

The algorithmic approach taken by the ACC/AHA for perioperative cardiac assessment for coronary artery disease is a good place to start (Fig. 2.3) [1]. This stepwise strategy has a number of critical junctures:

- Has the patient had an ST elevation MI (STEMI) or a non-ST elevation MI (NSTEMI), and if so, was this a recent occurrence? Is ongoing unstable angina a concern?
- What is the estimated risk of a major adverse coronary event (MACE)?
- When is it appropriate to order further investigations, e.g., exercise or pharmacological stress testing, echocardiography or angiography?
- What is the patient's functional capacity, and how does it relate to decision-making with regard to further investigations?
- When should revascularization be considered preoperatively?

These themes will be explored in the following series of questions.

Having Decided That Our Patient Has Established Coronary Artery Disease, How Do We Negotiate Step 2 of the ACC/AHA?

This patient's surgery, though time-sensitive, is not an emergency. There is time for further evaluation. In this case, the patient can be referred to a cardiologist for optimization according to what the ACC/AHA refer to as "guideline-directed medical therapy" for STEMI and NSTEMI [14, 15].

How Is the Risk of a Major Cardiovascular Complication Estimated Prior to Surgery?

A number of risk-prediction tools, e.g., Revised Cardiac Risk Index (RCRI) [16] and the American College of Surgeons (ACS) National Surgical Quality Improvement Program (NSQIP) Surgical Risk Calculator [17–19] (Tables 2.2, 2.3 and 2.4), are used to estimate the risk of non-fatal perioperative MI or cardiovascular death (together, non-fatal perioperative MI and cardiovascular death occasionally form a composite end-point in clinical trials, referred to as major adverse cardiovascular event [MACE]) [1]. The ACS NSQIP is a web-based universal risk calculator that is predictive for 18 disparate complications, including MI and cardiac arrest. A separate risk calculator, the American College of Surgeons Myocardial Infarction and Cardiac Arrest Calculator (ACS MICA), looks specifically at perioperative cardiac events. All risk-prediction tools incorporate elements of risk related to patient history in combination with surgical complexity. Level B evidence (data derived from a single randomized trial or nonrandomized studies) suggests that patients found to be at low risk of MACE do not benefit from further investigations prior to elective surgery [20, 21].

Revised Cardiac Risk Index or NSQIP Surgical Risk Calculator—Which Is Better for Assessing Perioperative Risk?

Both scores have their proponents and detractors. Critics of ACS NSQIP and MICA maintain that they likely underestimate cardiac risk because patients in contributing studies did not undergo perioperative troponin testing. Similarly, neither NSQIP risk calculator has undergone external validation in a study that systematically monitored troponin measurements after noncardiac surgery [19]. In contrast, the RCRI has been externally validated, and its predictive value was found to be significant in all types of elective noncardiac surgery except

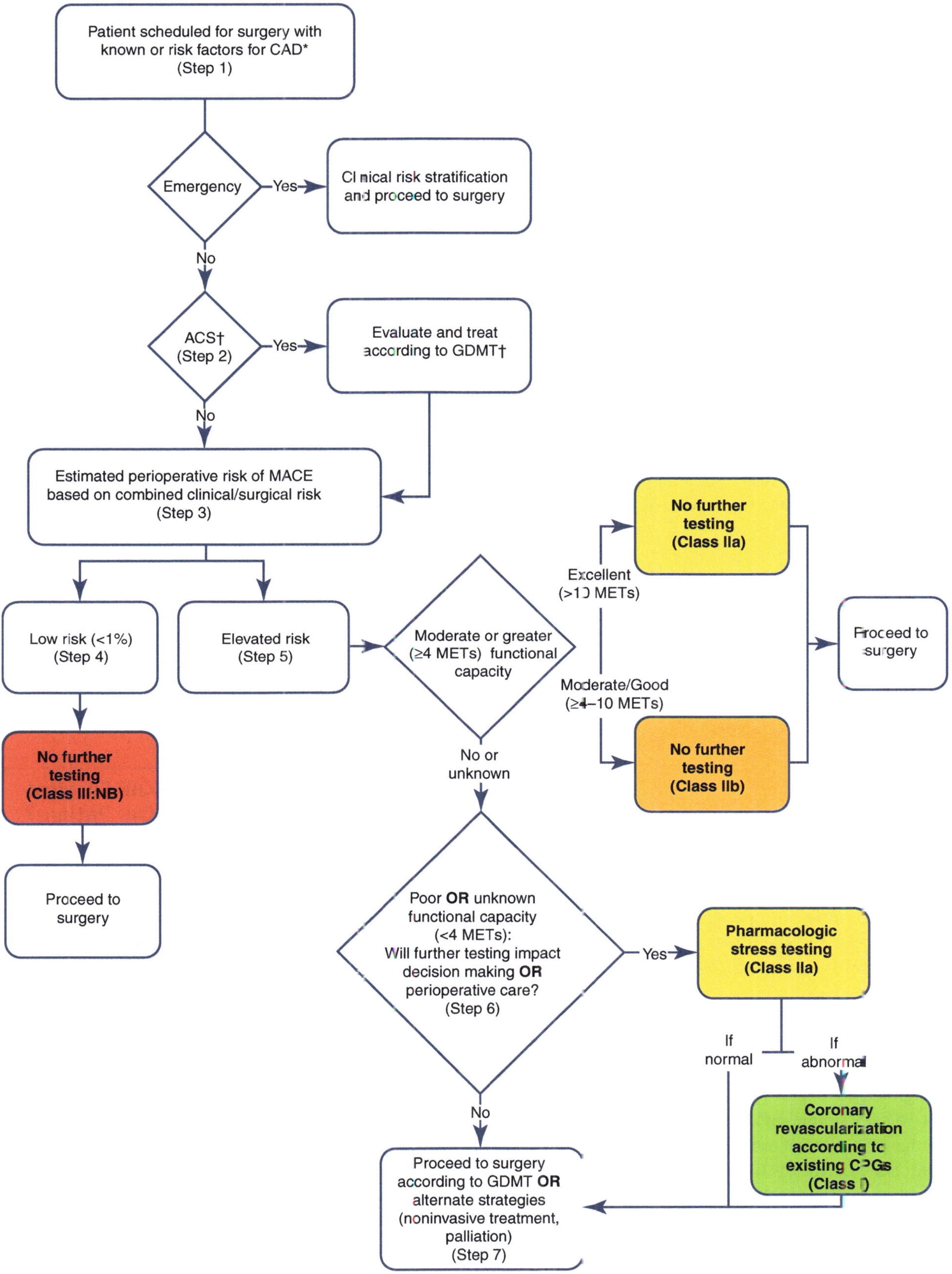

Fig. 2.3 AHA/ACC stepwise approach to perioperative assessment in the patient with known or suspected coronary artery disease. Color-coded classes of recommendation based on the level of supporting scientific evidence from clinical trials and other reports; Class I = Benefit >>> Risk; Class IIa = Benefit >> Risk; Class IIb = Benefit ≥ Risk; Class III: NB = No Benefit. ACS = acute coronary syndrome; CAD = coronary artery disease; CPG = clinical practice guideline; MACE = major adverse cardiac event; MET = metabolic equivalent; GDMT = guideline-directed medical therapy. (From Fleisher et al. [1], with permission from Elsevier)

Table 2.2 Revised Cardiac Risk Index (RCRI) score calculation (From Duceppe et al. [19], with permission from Elsevier)

Variable	Points
History of ischemic heart disease[a]	1
History of congestive heart failure[b]	1
History of cerebrovascular disease[c]	1
Use of insulin therapy for diabetes	1
Preoperative serum creatinine >177 μmol/(>2.0 mg/dL)	1
High-risk surgery[d]	1

[a]History of myocardial infarction, positive exercise test, current complaint of ischemic chest pain or nitrate use, electrocardiogram with pathological Q waves; patients with previous revascularization procedure meet criteria if they have such findings after coronary artery bypass or percutaneous coronary intervention (PCI)
[b]History of heart failure, pulmonary edema, or paroxysmal nocturnal dyspnea; an S3 gallop or bilateral rales on physical examination; chest radiograph showing pulmonary vascular redistribution
[c]Previous stroke or transient ischemic attack (TIA)
[d]Intraperitoneal, intrathoracic, or suprainguinal vascular surgery

Table 2.3 Revised Cardiac Risk Index (RCRI) score and corresponding risk of myocardial infarction, cardiac arrest, or 30-day mortality after noncardiac surgery[a] (From Duceppe et al. [19], with permission from Elsevier)

Total RCRI Points	Risk estimate (%)	95% CI for the risk estimate
0	3.9	2.8%–5.4%
1	6.0	4.9%–7.4%
2	10.1	8.1%–12.6%
≥3	15.0	11.1%–20.0%

[a]On the basis of high-quality external validation studies
CI Confidence interval

Table 2.4 Variables and possible answers for American College of Surgeons (ACS) National Surgical Quality Improvement Program (NSQIP) Surgical Risk Calculator (https://riskcalculator.facs.org/RiskCalculator/)

Variable	Possible answers
Surgical procedure	Multiple surgeries recognized
Age group	<65 / 65-74 / 75-84 / >85 years
Sex	Male/Female
Functional status	Independent/Partially dependent/Totally
Emergency case	Yes/No
ASA class	I–V
Steroid use for chronic condition	Yes/No
Ascites within 30 days of surgery	Yes/No
Systemic sepsis within 48 h prior to surgery	None/SIRS/Sepsis/Septic shock
Ventilator dependent	Yes/No
Disseminated cancer	Yes/No
Diabetes	No/Oral/Insulin
Hypertension requiring medication	Yes/No
Congestive heart failure in 30 days prior	Yes/No
Dyspnea	No/With moderate exertion/With rest
Current smoker within 1 year	Yes/No
History of severe COPD	Yes/No
Dialysis	Yes/No
Acute renal failure	Yes/No
BMI calculation	

ASA American Society of Anesthesiologists, *SIRS* systemic inflammatory response syndrome, *COPD* chronic obstructive pulmonary disease, *BMI* body mass index

for abdominal aortic aneurysm repair [16]. A further criticism of the NSQIP calculators relates to the definition of MI in the studies used to derive the NSQIP risk indices, which included only STEMIs or a large increase in troponin (>3 times normal) that occurred in symptomatic patients. As we saw earlier, most postoperative infarcts tend to be of the NSTEMI variety and silent [6]. Advocates for both NSQIP risk calculators point to the large patient numbers and multicenter methodology used in their development: over 200,000 patients from more than 250 hospitals for ACS MICA and over 1.4 million patients from 393 hospitals for ACS NSQIP [22]. The RCRI was developed from a prospective single-center cohort of 4315 patients [16]. In summary, the RCRI is a simple and easy-to-use risk prediction tool, while the ACS NSQIP provides a more detailed and wider ranging assessment of risk, beyond cardiovascular risk, which takes specific surgical procedures into account. There is no evidence that one is clearly superior.

What Do the RCRI and the NSQIP Surgical Risk Calculator Tell Us About Our Patient?

He has an RCRI score of 5 (all parameters are present except history of cerebrovascular disease). This gives him a 15% risk estimate for MI, cardiac arrest, or death within 30 days of surgery [19]. According to the NSQIP surgical risk calculator, he has a 5.6% risk of MI or cardiac arrest up to 30 days after surgery.

Having Established That the Patient Is at Risk for a Major Cardiac Complication, What Are the Next Steps in Assessment?

The next step in the evaluation of the high-risk patient is determination of functional capacity. The long-established metabolic equivalent of task (MET) score is frequently used for this (Table 2.5). The Duke Activity Status Index (DASI) is a self-assessment tool consisting of 12 questions relating to activities of daily living which appears to be a more objective measure of functional capacity (Table 2.6) [21, 23]. It has been shown to be a better predictor of death or MI within 30 days of major elective noncardiac surgery [24]. A finding of poor functional capacity warrants pharmacological stress testing (myocardial perfusion imaging or dobutamine stress echocardiography) if surgery is not urgent and the patient is a willing and appropriate candidate for revascularization. In other words, we must be reasonably certain that stress testing will change our approach to perioperative care. Patients who are at increased cardiac risk with unknown functional capacity may proceed to exercise stress testing if, similarly, it will alter preoperative optimization. Routine exercise stress testing is *not* beneficial for patients undergoing low-risk surgery or for patients deemed to be low risk for MACE.

Table 2.5 Metabolic equivalent (MET) score for subjective assessment of functional ability

Physical activity	MET score
Watching television	1
Light housework, e.g., cooking, ironing, washing dishes	2–3
Walking, slow stroll	2–3
Walking upstairs	4–5
Snow shoveling	5
Mowing lawn	5–7
Jogging	7
Playing soccer	10

Table 2.6 Duke Activity Status Index (From Hlatky et al. with permission from Elsevier) [23]

Item	Activity	Yes
1	Can you take care of yourself (eating, dressing, bathing, or using the toilet)?	2.75
2	Can you walk indoors such as around the house?	1.75
3	Can you walk a block or two on level ground?	2.75
4	Can you climb a flight of stairs or walk uphill?	5.50
5	Can you run a short distance?	8.00
6	Can you do light work around the house like dusting or washing dishes?	2.70
7	Can you do moderate work around the house like vacuuming, sweeping floors, or carrying in groceries?	3.50
8	Can you do heavy work around the house like scrubbing floors or lifting and moving heavy furniture?	8.00
9	Can you do yard work like raking leaves, weeding, or pushing a power mower?	4.50
10	Can you have sexual relations?	5.25
11	Can you participate in moderate recreational activities like golf, bowling, dancing, tennis doubles, or throwing a baseball or football?	6.00
12	Can you participate in strenuous sports like swimming, tennis singles, football, basketball, or skiing?	7.50

Is Echocardiographic Assessment of Left Ventricular Function of Benefit?

There appears to be little value in performing preoperative echocardiography in a non-discriminatory manner in cardiac patients. ACC/AHA recommend against routine preoperative echocardiographic assessment of LV function except for investigation of dyspnea of unknown origin, worsening dyspnea in the heart failure patient, and reassessment of LV function in clinically stable patients with previously documented LV dysfunction who have not been assessed within the past year [1]. The Canadian Cardiovascular Society recommends against performing resting echocardiography to enhance perioperative cardiac risk estimation. The two exceptions to this are clinical evidence of an undiagnosed severe obstructive intracardiac abnormality (e.g., aortic stenosis, mitral stenosis, hypertrophic obstructive cardiomyopathy) or severe pulmonary hypertension [19].

Which Noninvasive Imaging Technique—Stress Radionuclide Myocardial Perfusion Imaging or Stress Echocardiography—Is Preferable?

Practical or logistical concerns often dictate which noninvasive stress imaging test in performed, e.g., local availability, expertise, patient body habitus (precluding adequate echocardiography views), and cost. Both imaging techniques have similar diagnostic accuracy. A single meta-analysis demonstrated that stress myocardial perfusion imaging using single-photon emission computed tomography (SPECT) and stress echocardiography had similar sensitivities but stress echocardiography had higher specificity for detection of coronary artery disease [25, 26]. Both myocardial perfusion imaging and stress echocardiography had better discriminatory capabilities than exercise stress testing [25].

When Is Preoperative Angiography Indicated?

The indications for angiography before surgery are similar to those in a nonsurgical setting, i.e., high-risk features seen on noninvasive imaging. Examples include a strongly positive exercise stress test, imaging study suggestive of a significant amount of viable myocardium at risk, and multiple reversible defects.

What Are the Indications for Revascularization in the High-Risk Cardiac Patient Awaiting Noncardiac Surgery?

Recommendations for revascularization are the same as those for all patients with coronary artery disease, i.e., there are no RCTs which demonstrate perioperative benefit from revascularization [1, 27]. Indications for coronary revascularization (including the specific indications for CABG versus PCI) are beyond the scope of this book, but the decision to proceed is generally based upon the location and severity of the lesion, e.g., significant left main coronary artery disease, the number of diseased arteries, and the presence of left ventricular dysfunction. It should be borne in mind that patients undergoing PCI will need to have surgery deferred while on antiplatelet therapy.

For How Long Should Surgery Be Postponed in a Patient Who Has Undergone Coronary Artery Stenting?

Premature discontinuation of dual antiplatelet therapy (DAPT) in PCI patients can lead to stent thrombosis, MI, and death. General recommendations for DAPT are extensively reviewed in the 2016 ACC/AHA Guideline Focused Update on Duration of Dual Antiplatelet Therapy in Patients with Coronary Artery Disease [28] and the 2018 Canadian Cardiovascular Society/Canadian Association of Interventional Cardiology Focused Update of the Guidelines for the Use of Antiplatelet Therapy [29].

Patients with ACS who have undergone PCI with bare metal stent (BMS) or drug-eluting stent (DES) will require DAPT with aspirin and an ADP receptor antagonist, e.g., clopidogrel, ticagrelor, or prasugrel, for at least 12 months. According to the more recently updated Canadian guidelines, patients who have elective PCI in the absence of ACS will require DAPT for 6 months in the form of aspirin and clopidogrel, if not at high risk of bleeding. If risk of bleeding is high, DAPT is required for 1 month with BMS and 3 months for DES [29]. This is an evolving area as stent morphology and therapeutics are constantly being amended with one goal being to reduce the duration of DAPT.

Patients with a stent requiring elective noncardiac surgery should be evaluated bearing in mind the following considerations: urgency of surgery, risk of bleeding related to antiplatelet therapy, stent thrombosis in the absence of antiplatelet therapy, and type of stent, i.e., BMS versus DES. Each patient should be managed on a case-by-case basis in consultation with the patient's interventional cardiologist. Recommendations in general are based on low-quality evidence. Canadian and US guidelines are provided in Table 2.7 [10] and Fig. 2.4 [1, 19, 28].

Table 2.7 Canadian Cardiovascular Society Recommendations for interrupting discontinuation of dual antiplatelet therapy (DAPT) in patients with percutaneous coronary intervention PCI stenting requiring noncardiac surgery [10]

PCI stent	Delay surgery	Perioperative ASA	Perioperative ADP receptor antagonist	Restart DAPT after surgery
Bare metal	At least 1 month	Continue when possible	Hold clopidogrel for 5–7 days and prasugrel for 7–10 days preoperatively	As soon as deemed safe by surgeon
Drug-eluting	At least 3 months. If surgery is semi-urgent, delay for 1 month if possible	Continue when possible	Hold clopidogrel for 5–7 days and prasugrel for 7–10 days preoperatively	As soon as deemed safe by surgeon

ACS in Our Patient Was Treated with Intravenous Heparinization and DAPT. If He Had Not Experienced Frank Hematuria, For How Long Should DAPT Have Been Continued?

Patients with medically managed ACS who are not revascularized are treated with DAPT for at least 12 months if bleeding complications do not occur.

How Can Perioperative Cardiac Risk Be Medically Modified?

The question of whether to initiate pharmacological agents or to maintain those on which the patient is already established is an ever-changing domain. A summary of current recommendations from the ACC/AHA and Canadian Cardiovascular Society is presented in Table 2.8 [1, 10].

Should This Patient Have BNP Measured Preoperatively as a Screening Measure for Postoperative Myocardial Injury?

The Canadian Cardiovascular Society recommends measuring BNP before noncardiac surgery when RCRI ≥ 1, if the patient is 65 years or older or is 45–64 years with significant cardiovascular disease [19]. Patients with preoperative BNP >92 pg/mL should have daily pos-

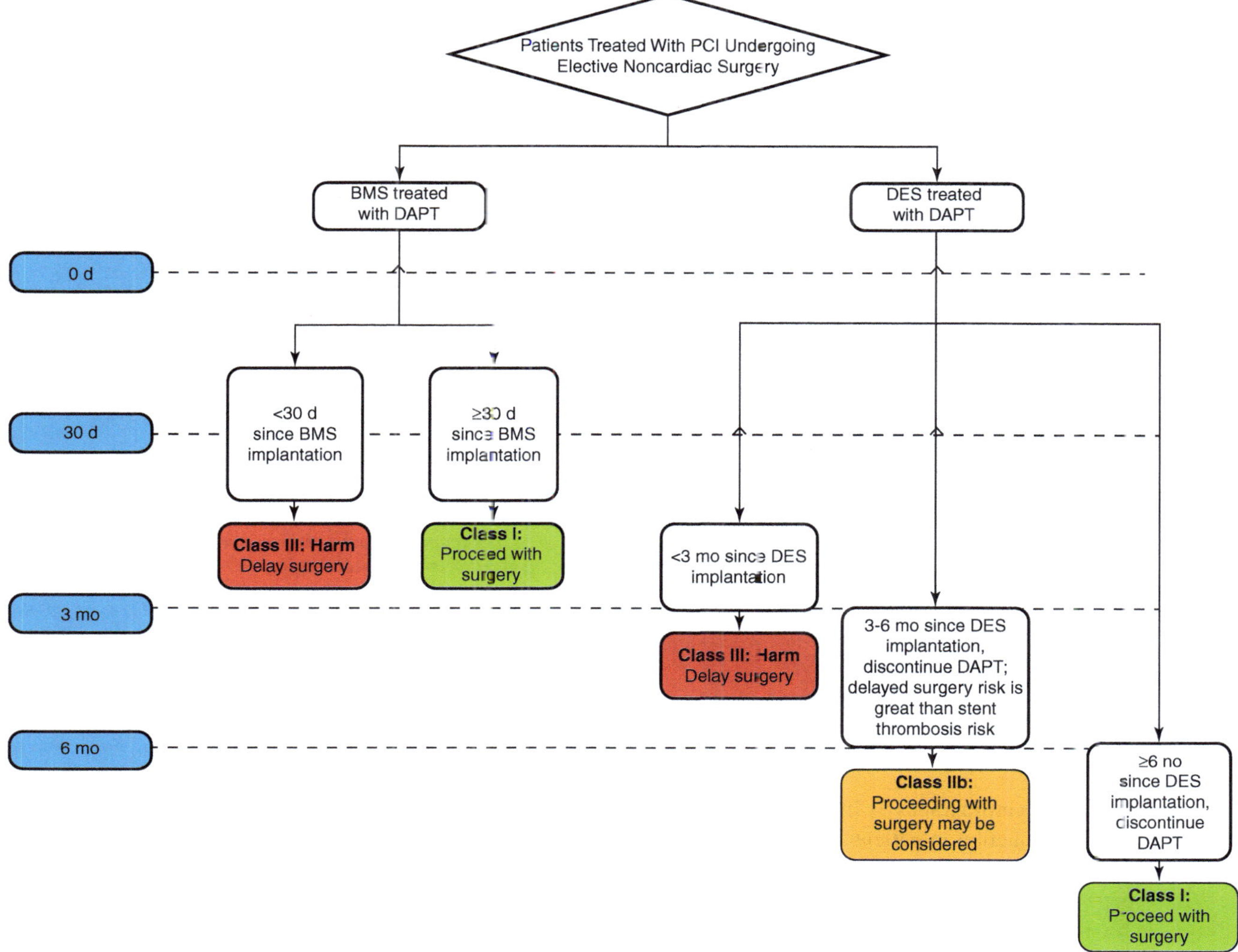

Fig. 2.4 ACC/AHA algorithm for discontinuation of dual antiplatelet therapy perioperatively. Classes of recommendation are color-coded. Perioperative continuation of aspirin is advised though it is noted that this recommendation is based on expert opinion (From Levine et al. [28], with permission from Elsevier)

toperative troponin measurement for 48–72 hours to detect silent ischemia. However, considering our patient had a recent episode of ACS with congestive cardiac failure and a recent BNP value of 464, it is of doubtful value. In this case, daily postoperative troponin measurement is indicated regardless.

The patient was reviewed by a cardiologist on the same day as the preoperative consultation. A decision was made against performing coronary angiography due to the presence of severe chronic kidney disease and the knowledge that DAPT would be required if any intervention deemed necessary. A recommendation was made to recommence aspirin therapy preoperatively if the bleeding risk was acceptable to the urology team, which it was. Two weeks after the above consult, the patient underwent a radical cystoprostatectomy, bilateral pelvic lymph node resection, and ileal conduit urinary diversion. He was admitted to a surgical step-down unit for the first 48 postoperative hours. He had normal daily troponin measurements for 3 consecutive days after surgery. He was discharged home on postoperative day 10.

True/False Questions

1. (a) Elective surgery should be deferred for at least 6 months after acute myocardial infarction.
   (b) By definition, myocardial injury after noncardiac surgery occurs within 30 days of surgery.
   (c) Most perioperative myocardial infarcts are symptomatic.
   (d) Revised Cardiac Risk Index (RCRI) is a superior perioperative cardiac risk prediction tool when compared with the American College of Surgeons National Surgical Quality Improvement Program (ACS NSQIP).
   (e) RCRI uses patient functional capacity as a variable when calculating perioperative cardiac risk.

Table 2.8 Comparison of American College of Cardiology (ACC)/American Heart Association (AHA) and Canadian Cardiovascular Society (CCS) recommendations for initiation and/or continuation of pharmacological agents for perioperative cardiac risk reduction [1, 10]

	ACC/AHA	CCS
Beta-blockers	Continue in patients using chronic beta-blockade. May be reasonable to begin in patients with intermediate-/high-risk ischemia or in patients with 3 or more RCRI risk factors. Beta-blockade should not be started the day before or the day of surgery	Continue in patients using chronic beta-blockade. Practical limitations cited for starting beta-blockade days or weeks before surgery. Beta-blockade should not be started within 24 h of surgery due to the risk of death and nonfatal stroke
ACE inhibitors/ARBs	Continuation perioperatively is reasonable. If held before surgery, should be restarted as soon as is clinically feasible	Recommend withholding ACE inhibitors/ARBs starting 24 h before surgery (strong recommendation; low-quality evidence)
Statins	Should be continued for patients using statins long term. Perioperative initiation is reasonable for vascular surgery patients and possibly patients with a clinical indication for statins having high-risk surgery	Evidence too weak to recommend initiation for reduction of perioperative cardiac risk. Should be continued in patients on long-term statin therapy
Calcium channel blockers	No recommendation. It is noted that a large-scale trial is required to define the value of calcium channel blockade and that those with substantial negative inotropic effects (e.g., verapamil, diltiazem) may precipitate or worsen heart failure	Recommend against preoperative initiation for prevention of perioperative cardiac events (low-quality evidence noted)
Antiplatelet agents	Continue aspirin if possible in PCI patient population. No benefit to initiating or continuing aspirin in non-PCI patients unless the risk of ischemia outweighs the bleeding risk. Management is case-by-case and interdisciplinary	Recommend against initiation or continuation of aspirin to prevent perioperative cardiac events unless the patient has had recent PCI with stenting
Alpha-2 agonists	Of no benefit and not recommended for prevention of perioperative cardiac events	Recommend against preoperative initiation for prevention of perioperative events

RCRI Revised cardiac risk index, *ACE* angiotensin-converting enzyme, *ARBs* angiotensin receptor blockers, *PCI* percutaneous coronary intervention

2. (a) Resting echocardiography is indicated to assess left ventricular function in patients with poor functional capacity.
   (b) Preoperative angiography is routinely recommended in high-risk cardiac patients preoperatively.
   (c) Recommendations for revascularization in the high-risk cardiac patient before noncardiac surgery are the same as those for all patients with coronary artery disease.
   (d) Disruption of dual antiplatelet therapy less than 30 days after PCI and bare metal stent placement has been shown to be harmful.
   (e) Aspirin should be continued perioperatively in patients who have had recent PCI and stent placement regardless of whether the stent is of the bare metal or drug eluting variety.

References

1. Fleisher LA, Fleischmann KE, Auerbach AD, Barnason SA, Beckman JA, Bozkurt B, et al. 2014 ACC/AHA guideline on perioperative cardiovascular evaluation and management of patients undergoing noncardiac surgery: a report of the American College of Cardiology/American Heart Association Task Force on practice guidelines. J Am Coll Cardiol. 2014;64(22):e77–137.
2. Livhits M, Ko CY, Leonardi MJ, Zingmond DS, Gibbons MM, de Virgilio C. Risk of surgery following recent myocardial infarction. Ann Surg. 2011;253(5):857–64.
3. Roe MT, Messenger JC, Weintraub WS, Cannon CP, Fonarow GC, Dai D, et al. Treatments, trends, and outcomes of acute myocardial infarction and percutaneous coronary intervention. J Am Coll Cardiol. 2010;56(4):254–63.
4. Livhits M, Gibbons MM, de Virgilio C, O'Connell JB, Leonardi MJ, Ko CY, et al. Coronary revascularization after myocardial infarction can reduce risks of noncardiac surgery. J Am Coll Surg. 2011;212(6):1018–26.
5. Collinson P, Lindahl B. Diagnosing type 2 myocardial infarction: American College of Cardiology; Latest in Cardiology; Expert Analysis. 2016. https://www.acc.org/latest-in-cardiology/articles/2016/05/18/13/58/diagnosing-type-2-myocardial-infarction. Accessed 6 Jul 2019.
6. Devereaux PJ, Xavier D, Pogue J, Guyatt G, Sigamani A, Garutti I, et al. Characteristics and short-term prognosis of perioperative myocardial infarction in patients undergoing noncardiac surgery: a cohort study. Ann Intern Med. 2011;154(8):523–8.
7. Puelacher C, Lurati Buse G, Seeberger D, Sazgary L, Marbot S, Lampart A, et al. Perioperative myocardial injury after noncardiac surgery: incidence, mortality, and characterization. Circulation. 2018;137(12):1221–32.
8. Puymirat E, Taldir G, Aissaoui N, Lemesle G, Lorgis L, Cuisset T, et al. Use of invasive strategy in non-ST-segment elevation myocardial infarction is a major determinant of improved long-term survival: FAST-MI (French Registry of Acute Coronary Syndrome). JACC Cardiovasc Interv. 2012;5(9):893–902.
9. Cannon CP, Weintraub WS, Demopoulos LA, Vicari R, Frey MJ, Lakkis N, et al. Comparison of early invasive and conservative strategies in patients with unstable coronary syndromes treated

with the glycoprotein IIb/IIIa inhibitor tirofiban. N Engl J Med. 2001;344(25):1879–87.
10. Bagai A, Lu D, Lucas J, Goyal A, Herzog CA, Wang TY, et al. Temporal trends in utilization of cardiac therapies and outcomes for myocardial infarction by degree of chronic kidney disease: a report from the NCDR Chest Pain-MI Registry. J Am Heart Assoc. 2018;7(24):e010394.
11. Writing Committee for the VSI, Devereaux PJ, Biccard BM, Sigamani A, Xavier D, Chan MTV, et al. Association of postoperative high-sensitivity troponin levels with myocardial injury and 30-day mortality among patients undergoing noncardiac surgery. JAMA. 2017;317(16):1642–51.
12. Botto F, Alonso-Coello P, Chan MT, Villar JC, Xavier D, Srinathan S, et al. Myocardial injury after noncardiac surgery: a large, international, prospective cohort study establishing diagnostic criteria, characteristics, predictors, and 30-day outcomes. Anesthesiology. 2014;120(3):564–78.
13. Modha K, Johnson KM, Kuperman E, Grant PJ, Slawski B, Pfeifer K, et al. Perioperative cardiovascular medicine: 5 questions for 2018. Cleve Clin J Med. 2018;85(11):853–9.
14. Fihn SD, Gardin JM, Abrams J, Berra K, Blankenship JC, Dallas AP, et al. 2012 ACCF/AHA/ACP/AATS/PCNA/SCAI/STS guideline for the diagnosis and management of patients with stable ischemic heart disease: a report of the American College of Cardiology Foundation/American Heart Association task force on practice guidelines, and the American College of Physicians, American Association for Thoracic Surgery, Preventive Cardiovascular Nurses Association, Society for Cardiovascular Angiography and Interventions, and Society of Thoracic Surgeons. Circulation. 2012;126(25):e354–471.
15. Jneid H, Anderson JL, Wright RS, Adams CD, Bridges CR, Casey DE Jr, et al. 2012 ACCF/AHA focused update of the guideline for the management of patients with unstable angina/non-ST-elevation myocardial infarction (updating the 2007 guideline and replacing the 2011 focused update): a report of the American College of Cardiology Foundation/American Heart Association Task Force on Practice Guidelines. J Am Coll Cardiol. 2012;60(7):645–81.
16. Lee TH, Marcantonio ER, Mangione CM, Thomas EJ, Polanczyk CA, Cook EF, et al. Derivation and prospective validation of a simple index for prediction of cardiac risk of major noncardiac surgery. Circulation. 1999;100(10):1043–9.
17. American College of Surgeons. ACS NSQIP surgical risk calculator. 2020. Available from: https://riskcalculator.facs.org/RiskCalculator/index.jsp.
18. Gupta PK, Gupta H, Sundaram A, Kaushik M, Fang X, Miller WJ, et al. Development and validation of a risk calculator for prediction of cardiac risk after surgery. Circulation. 2011;124(4):381–7.
19. Duceppe E, Parlow J, MacDonald P, Lyons K, McMullen M, Srinathan S, et al. Canadian cardiovascular society guidelines on perioperative cardiac risk assessment and management for patients who undergo noncardiac surgery. Can J Cardiol. 2017;33(1):17–32.
20. Jordan SW, Mioton LM, Smetona J, Aggarwal A, Wang E, Dumanian GA, et al. Resident involvement and plastic surgery outcomes: an analysis of 10,356 patients from the American College of Surgeons National Surgical Quality Improvement Program database. Plast Reconstr Surg. 2013;131(4):763–73.
21. Schein OD, Katz J, Bass EB, Tielsch JM, Lubomski LH, Feldman MA, et al. The value of routine preoperative medical testing before cataract surgery. Study of Medical Testing for Cataract Surgery. N Engl J Med. 2000;342(3):168–75.
22. Bose S, Sonny A. PRO: American college of surgeons national surgical quality improvement program risk calculators should be preferred over the revised cardiac risk index for perioperative risk stratification. J Cardiothorac Vasc Anesth. 2018;32(5):2417–9.
23. Hlatky MA, Boineau RE, Higginbotham MB, Lee KL, Mark DB, Califf RM, et al. A brief self-administered questionnaire to determine functional capacity (the Duke Activity Status Index). Am J Cardiol. 1989;64(10):651–4.
24. Wijeysundera DN, Pearse RM, Shulman MA, Abbott TEF, Torres E, Ambosta A, et al. Assessment of functional capacity before major non-cardiac surgery: an international, prospective cohort study. Lancet. 2018;391(10140):2631–40.
25. Fleischmann KE, Hunink MG, Kuntz KM, Douglas PS. Exercise echocardiography or exercise SPECT imaging? A meta-analysis of diagnostic test performance. JAMA. 1998;280(10):913–20.
26. Garber AM, Solomon NA. Cost-effectiveness of alternative test strategies for the diagnosis of coronary artery disease. Ann Intern Med. 1999;130(9):719–28.
27. McFalls EO, Ward HB, Moritz TE, Goldman S, Krupski WC, Littooy F, et al. Coronary-artery revascularization before elective major vascular surgery. N Engl J Med. 2004;351(27):2795–804.
28. Levine GN, Bates ER, Bittl JA, Brindis RG, Fihn SD, Fleisher LA, et al. 2016 ACC/AHA Guideline Focused Update on Duration of Dual Antiplatelet Therapy in Patients With Coronary Artery Disease: A Report of the American College of Cardiology/American Heart Association Task Force on Clinical Practice Guidelines. J Am Coll Cardiol. 2016;68(10):1082–115.
29. Mehta SR, Bainey KR, Cantor WJ, Lordkipanidze M, Marquis-Gravel G, Robinson SD, et al. 2018 Canadian cardiovascular society/Canadian association of interventional cardiology focused update of the guidelines for the use of antiplatelet therapy. Can J Cardiol. 2018;34(3):214–33.

The Adult Congenital Cardiac Patient for Noncardiac Surgery

3

Surita Sidhu

A 20-year-old man presents for laparoscopic cholecystectomy for acute cholecystitis. He has a history of tricuspid atresia (Fig. 3.1) *palliated with a right Blalock-Taussig (BT) shunt at birth* (Fig. 3.2), *a corrective superior vena cava to right pulmonary artery anastomosis (bidirectional Glenn shunt) procedure with ligation of the BT shunt at age 6 months* (Fig. 3.3), *and an extracardiac conduit from the inferior vena cava to right pulmonary artery (Fontan completion) at age 3* (Fig. 3.4).

In addition to several failed attempts at ablative procedures for supraventricular tachycardia, this patient has developed severe atrioventricular valvular regurgitation of the systemic ventricle and has a residual extracardiac conduit fenestration with a right to left shunt. He has developed failing Fontan physiology, with significantly reduced exercise tolerance in the last 6 months, and was recently listed for cardiac transplantation when he developed cholecystitis

Medications: Warfarin 2 mg PO QD, diltiazem 60 mg PO QD, furosemide 80 mg PO QD.

His dose of diltiazem was recently halved to 60 mg due to his worsening fatigue and presyncopal episodes. He is currently functioning at NYHA II-III. He developed symptoms consistent with acute cholecystitis 3 days ago, and the diagnosis was confirmed both clinically and with ultrasound.

Physical Examination: BP 95/60. HR 100 NSR. SaO2 90%. HT: 175 cm. WT: 70 kg. He has a loud pansystolic murmur, clubbing, and bilateral pitting edema to his shins.

Investigations: Hemoglobin 170 g/L, platelet count 150 × 10^9/L, white cell count 18 × 10^9/L, and an INR of 3.0. Creatinine is 150 μmol/L with a GFR of 40 mL/min/1.73 m^2. The transplant workup revealed normal liver function tests although mild hepatic fibrosis was noted on abdominal computed tomography (CT). An echocardiogram revealed the presence of severe systemic atrioventricular valvular regurgitation and a systemic ventricular ejection fraction of 30%. Recent cardiac catheterization revealed a central venous/Fontan pressure of 24 mmHg, pulmonary artery pressure of 40/20 mmHg, and left ventricular end diastolic pressure of 18 mmHg.

What Are the Physiologic Effects of a Fontan Procedure?

The Fontan procedure is generally used in patients who have univentricular physiology such as hypoplastic left heart, tricuspid atresia, or a double inlet left ventricle. A Fontan shunt bypasses the right ventricle and provides passive, non-pulsatile flow from the superior vena cava and inferior vena cava (IVC) to the pulmonary arteries [1]. Pulmonary blood flow is dependent on the difference between the central venous pressure (CVP) and the pulmonary venous atrium or transpulmonary gradient (TPG). In terms of hemodynamic goals, it is reasonable to strive for a CVP of 10–15 and TPG of 5–10 mmHg [2].

What Are Some of the Systemic Complications in the Patient with Failing Fontan Physiology?

- CARDIAC - Eventually pulmonary vascular resistance (PVR) increases, and it becomes difficult to maintain cardiac output. Patients may develop systolic and diastolic dysfunction of the systemic ventricle, atrioventricular valve regurgitation, pulmonary hypertension, and significant arrhythmias. As the systemic ventricular end-diastolic pressure rises, the common atrial pressure will also rise, and in turn, a higher CVP will be required to

S. Sidhu (✉)
Department of Anesthesiology & Pain Medicine, Perioperative Echocardiography, Mazankowski Alberta Heart Institute, University of Alberta, Edmonton, AB, Canada
e-mail: surita@ualberta.ca

D. Dillane, B. A. Finegan (eds.), *Preoperative Assessment*, https://doi.org/10.1007/978-3-030-58842-7_3

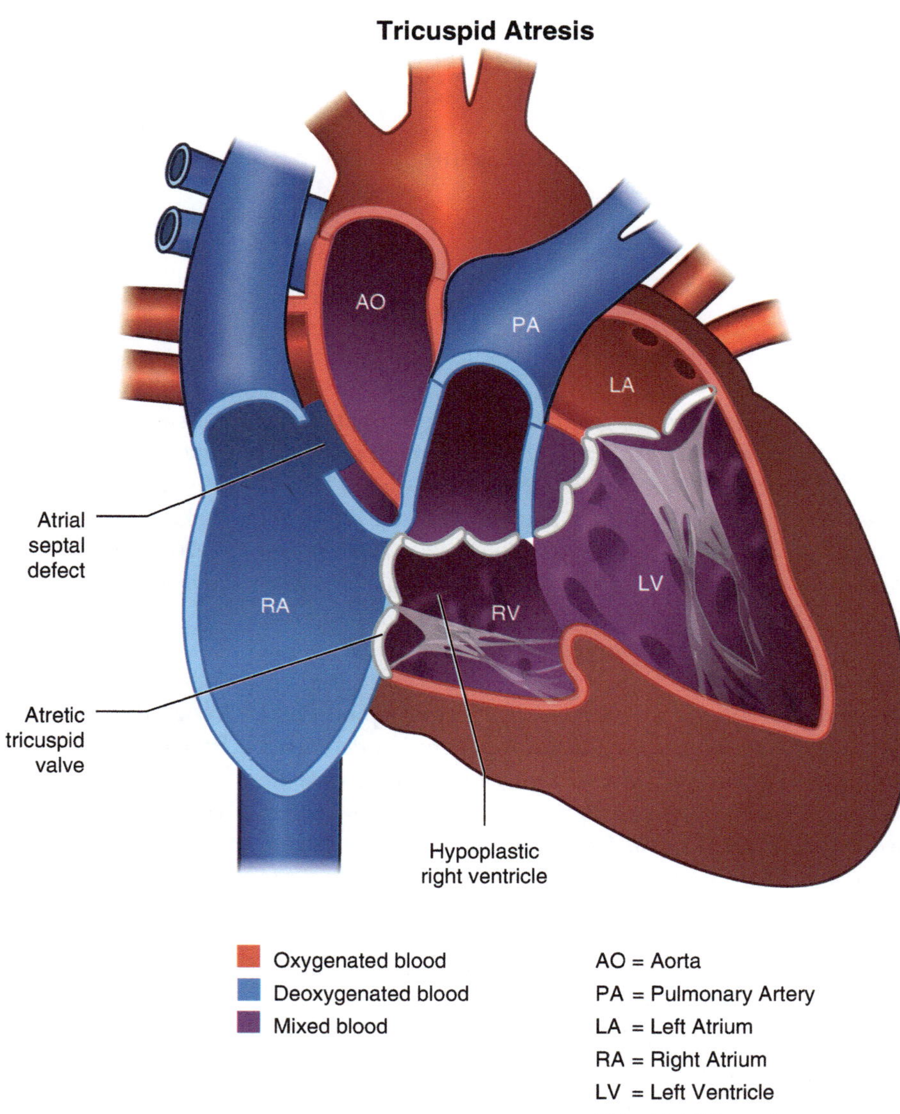

Fig. 3.1 Tricuspid atresia with a hypoplastic right ventricle (RV), atrial septal defect (ASD), and ventricular septal defect (VSD)

maintain cardiac output (CO) [3]. Increased risk of arrhythmias and conduction abnormalities such as SVT or sinoatrial node dysfunction is often due to atrial scarring, dilation, and hypertrophy [4].

- RESPIRATORY - Plastic Plastic bronchitis, restrictive lung disease, and/or reduced aerobic capacity due to nonpulsatile pulmonary flow and limited ability to augment pulmonary flow and pressure [5].
- HEPATIC - Chronic elevations in CVP and decreased CO may result in Fontan-associated liver disease (FALD), elevated transaminases, cirrhosis, as well as factor loss, hypoalbuminemia, and hypogammaglobulinemia from protein-losing enteropathy (PLE). Therefore, the patient's coagulation status may range from pro(thromboembolic) to anticoagulated [1].
- RENAL - Hypoalbuminemia may also increase the risk of perioperative renal dysfunction [6].
- HEMATOLOGIC - From a hematological standpoint, patients may develop erythrocytosis secondary to chronic hypoxemia. Hyperviscosity may be exacerbated in the setting of dehydration or fasting preoperatively. Transfusion triggers in cyanotic patients may need to be altered to maintain tissue oxygenation. A hematocrit >0.55 may falsely elevate the INR. Adult congenital heart disease patients may also develop acquired von Willebrand disease.
- NEUROLOGIC - Developmental delay or cognitive impairment may also present a challenge. Patient anxiety is a common feature in those transitioning from pediatric to adult care.

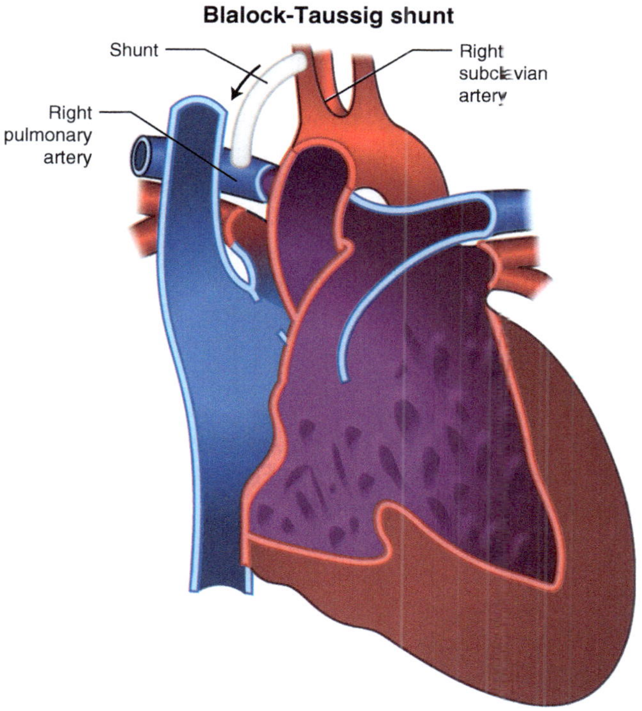

Fig. 3.2 Blalock-Taussig shunt connecting right subclavian artery to right pulmonary artery (RPA)

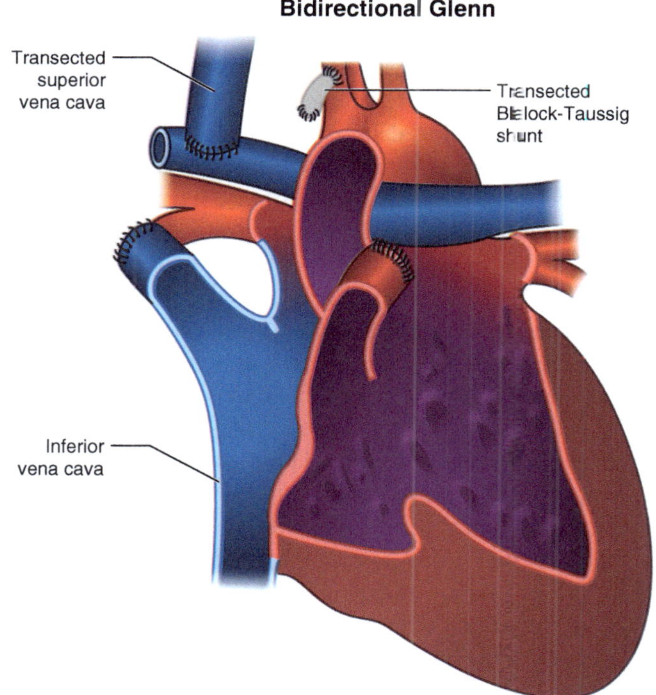

Fig. 3.3 Glenn shunt or bidirectional cavopulmonary anastomosis in a patient with a prior BT shunt. Both the BT shunt and superior vena cava (SVC) are transected. The SVC is anastomosed to the pulmonary circulation via the right pulmonary artery (RPA). The inferior vena cava (IVC) drains into the systemic circulation via the atrial septal defect (ASD) or tricuspid valve (TV)

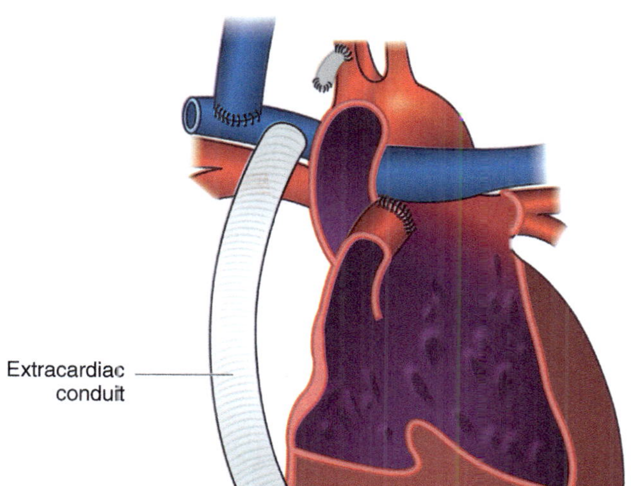

Fig. 3.4 Fontan completion with extracardiac conduit from inferior vena cava (IVC) to right pulmonary artery (RPA)

- AIRWAY - Securing the airway may present an issue if there is a history of subglottic stenosis secondary to prior prolonged intubation or an associated syndrome such as trisomy 21, DiGeorge, or Cornelia de Lange. The possibility of tracheomalacia should also be considered if dilated pulmonary arteries compress the trachea. Prior coarctation/aortic arch repair may cause recurrent laryngeal nerve dysfunction.

How Should This Patient Be Evaluated Preoperatively?

- Preoperative evaluation should involve interdisciplinary collaboration with the attending surgeon, adult congenital cardiologist, cardiac anesthesiologist, adult congenital cardiac surgeon, and electrophysiologist Moderate- or high-risk lesions (Table 3.1) [6] are ideally managed at a center with expertise for advanced monitoring and management [7].
- Detailed knowledge is required of the native congenital cardiac lesion and prior palliative and reparative interventions [8].
  - Identify specific anatomical repairs and any residual hemodynamic issues.
  - Establish whether prior procedures may affect proposed sites for peripheral/central venous/arterial or extracorporeal membrane oxygenation (ECMO) access.

Table 3.1 Classification of perioperative risk classification for patients with congenital heart disease undergoing noncardiac surgery (From Warnes et al. [6], with permission Elsevier)

High risk
Pulmonary hypertension, primary or secondary
Cyanotic congenital heart disease
New York Heart Association Class III or IV
Severe systemic ventricular dysfunction (ejection fraction less than 35%)
Severe left-sided heart obstructive lesions
Moderate risk
Prosthetic valve or conduit
Intracardiac shunt
Moderate left-sided heart obstruction
Moderate systemic ventricular dysfunction

  - Review imaging of upper/lower limb vessels to assess size and patency.
- Establish current cardiopulmonary reserve.
  - Review investigations including cardiopulmonary testing (VO_2 max studies), echocardiography, cardiac catheterization, MRI, and CT/CT angiography.
  - Evaluate arrhythmia control, implanted devices such as pacemakers or automated implantable cardioverter-defibrillators, and perioperative management in conjunction with an electrophysiologist.
- Consider the proposed surgical procedure and potential hemodynamic effects, including potential for increased bleeding in the setting of elevated venous pressure.

What Factors May Influence Planning for Sites of Invasive Monitoring?

- Prior BT shunt – this surgical connection between the ipsilateral subclavian and pulmonary arteries may result in absent pulses or unreliable monitoring on the shunt side. Invasive arterial access should be planned for the opposite side or in the lower limbs if bilateral BT shunts have been placed.
- Prior coarctation repair – any residual aortic coarctation may result in upper extremity (UE) hypertension and lower extremity (LE) hypotension. Both UE and LE should be monitored to assess perfusion.
- Prior need for peripheral or central cannulation – as noted earlier, peripheral venous and arterial vessel patency should be assessed. If placement of a bicaval dual lumen catheter into the internal jugular vein is required for central venovenous ECMO, the anatomy and patency of this vessel should also be established.

What Perioperative Hemodynamic Goals Should Be Taken into Consideration when Preparing for Noncardiac Surgery in the Patient with Failing Fontan Physiology?

The patient with failing Fontan physiology requires careful consideration of choice of anesthetic technique including local, regional, neuraxial, or general anesthesia, agents, pressor/inotrope management, and ventilator mode. As high preload is essential for the maintenance of cardiac output in the failing Fontan patient, spontaneous ventilation is preferred as positive pressure ventilation may dramatically decrease preload.

Are There Any Other Preoperative Considerations Specific to Fontan Patients for Noncardiac Surgery?

- These patients should be scheduled as first case of the day to minimize fluid shifts due to fasting and to ensure that adequate assistance is available if required. Chronic medications are usually continued and may include pulmonary vasodilators, endothelin receptor antagonists, and calcium channel blockers. Angiotensin-converting enzyme inhibitors, angiotensin II receptor blockers, and diuretics are the exception. Anticoagulants and antiplatelet agents should be coordinated by the multidisciplinary team, and bridging is generally required [9].
- Premedication with benzodiazepines may benefit uncooperative patients, and ketamine may be warranted for those with developmental delay.
- Bubble-free precautions including meticulous line de-airing as well as use of in-line air filters are warranted to avoid paradoxical embolism in the setting of intra-/extracardiac shunts. Fontan patients with venovenous collaterals are at increased risk of shunting.
- Endocarditis prophylaxis should be considered.
- Transcutaneous defibrillator pads should be applied during the perioperative period and the use of electrocautery discussed with the attending surgeon.
- Both positive pressure ventilation and the institution of pneumoperitoneum during laparoscopy may significantly impair systemic venous return to the Fontan circulation and adversely affect cardiac output [10]. Carbon dioxide (CO_2) insufflation pressures should be limited to less than 10–12 cmH_2O. Failing Fontan right to left shunt exacerbation may occur if PVR is increased by the physiologic effects of establishing a pneumoperitonuem. These include atelectasis secondary to increased intra-abdominal pressure, decreased preload, and hypercarbia secondary to CO_2 absorption.

What Monitoring Modalities Do You Envisage Using for This Procedure?

- End-tidal CO_2 may not accurately reflect arterial CO_2 as intra-/extracardiac shunts reduce pulmonary blood flow and CO_2 exchange. For this reason, invasive arterial monitoring allows for repeated blood sampling.
- Central venous access is indicated for the high-risk patient undergoing major surgery or who may have challenging vascular access. Removal as soon as possible in the post-operative period will decrease the thrombotic risk. Anatomical reasons preclude the use of a pulmonary artery catheter in many patients with adult congenital disease.
- Transesophageal echocardiography can be invaluable for perioperative management.
- Cerebral oximetry may indirectly reflect the CO_2.
- 4-Band electroencephalography may aid in monitoring depth of anesthesia given the variability of pulmonary blood flow and alveolar/blood transmission of volatile agents.

Is a Neuraxial Technique Appropriate for This Case?

The successful and safe use of epidural anesthesia has been described for laparoscopic cholecystectomy in patients with severe COPD [11]. However, neuraxial blockade should be avoided or utilized with extreme caution as the failing Fontan patient may not tolerate the reduction in systemic vascular resistance (SVR) associated with a sympathectomy. If epidural anesthesia is utilized, invasive arterial monitoring is warranted for beat-to-beat blood pressure monitoring as well as to guide intravascular volume administration. Careful titration of the epidural anesthetic is necessary.

The Patient Is Curious About What to Expect in the Early Recovery Period. What Factors Should Be Taken into Consideration When Counseling Him?

- Fontan patients benefit from immediate postoperative extubation, especially if pulmonary hypertension is present. Airway reactivity and coughing should be minimized to decrease the sympathetic response to extubation.
- Patients should be carefully monitored in the post-anesthesia care unit. Even partial airway obstruction with hypoxia and/or hypercarbia may increase PVR.
- Sympathetic stressors such as pain and anxiety should be aggressively managed.
- A period of controlled ventilation in an intensive care unit setting may be warranted.

Can This Procedure Be Performed on an Ambulatory Basis?

Young patients with Fontan physiology may undergo minor surgical procedures on an outpatient basis with appropriate preoperative workup. Minimum discharge criteria have been outlined in Table 3.2 [12].

This patient has a right to left intracardiac shunt through a fenestration in the extracardiac conduit, resulting in cyanosis. Paradoxical embolism may occur – aggressive de-airing of all lines is essential, and air filters should be considered. In addition, it is critical to maintain systemic vascular resistance (SVR) while avoiding to increase PVR. This includes avoiding hypoxia, hypercarbia, metabolic acidosis, hypothermia, and sympathetic surges. The choice and dose of induction and maintenance agents should minimize reductions in SVR. Both central venous and arterial invasive monitoring will likely be required to maintain the balance between SVR and PVR. The use of vasopressin versus *phenylephrine to maintain SVR offers the advantage of avoiding a concomitant rise in PVR. The clinical indicators of failing Fontan physiology in this particular patient warrant postoperative in-patient monitoring* [6].

True/False Questions

1. Which of the following is not considered a high-risk congenital cardiac lesion in a patient coming for a non-cardiac surgical procedure?
   (a) Systemic ventricular function of less than 35%.
   (b) Pulmonary hypertension.
   (c) Intracardiac shunt.
   (d) Cyanotic disease.
   (e) Severe left-sided obstructive lesion.
2. Which of the following is not a palliation treatment method for congenital heart disease?
   (a) Blalock-Taussig shunt.
   (b) Glenn shunt.
   (c) Pulmonary artery banding.
   (d) Norwood procedure.
   (e) Closure of atrial septal defect.

Table 3.2 Discharge criteria for Fontan patients after ambulatory surgery [12]

Oxygen saturations in air maintained at preoperative values
No bleeding
Excellent pain control
No nausea or vomiting
Patient drinking normally
Adequate home support
Patient lives within 30-minute drive from hospital

Acknowledgment The author would like to acknowledge Dr. Isabelle Vonder Muhll, Associate Professor, University of Alberta, for her contribution to this chapter.

References

1. Rychik J, Atz AM, Celermajer DS, Deal BJ, Gatzoulis MA, Gewillig MH, et al. American heart association council on cardiovascular disease in the young and council on cardiovascular and stroke nursing. Evaluation and management of the child and adult with Fontan circulation: a scientific statement from the American heart association. Circulation. 2019;140(6):e234–84.
2. Eagle SS, Daves SM. The adult with Fontan physiology: systematic approach to perioperative management for noncardiac surgery. J Cardiothorac Vasc Anesth. 2011;25(2):320–34.
3. Mori M, Aguirre AJ, Elder RW, Kashkouli A, Farris AB, Ford RM, Book WM. Beyond a broken heart: circulatory dysfunction in the failing Fontan. Pediatr Cardiol. 2014;35(4):569–79.
4. Cannesson M, Earing MG, Collange V, Kersten JR. Anesthesia for noncardiac surgery in adults with congenital heart disease. Anesthesiology. 2009;111(2):432–40.
5. Houska NM, Schwartz LI. The year in review: anesthesia for congenital heart disease 2019. Semin Cardiothorac Vasc Anesth. 2020;24(2):175–86.
6. Warnes CA, Williams RG, Bashore TM, Child JS, Connolly HM, Dearani JA, et al. ACC/AHA 2008 guidelines for the management of adults with congenital heart disease: executive summary: a report of the American college of cardiology/American heart association task force on practice guidelines (writing committee to develop guidelines for the management of adults with congenital heart disease). J Am Coll Cardiol. 2008;52(23):e143–263.
7. Rabbitts JA, Groenewald CB, Mauermann WJ, Barbara DW, Burkhart HM, Warnes CA, et al. Outcomes of general anesthesia for noncardiac surgery in a series of patients with Fontan palliation. Paediatr Anaesth. 2013;23(2):180–7.
8. Stout KK, Daniels CJ, Aboulhosn JA, Bozkurt B, Broberg CS, Colman JM, et al. 2018 AHA/ACC guideline for the management of adults with congenital heart disease: executive summary: a report of the American college of cardiology/American heart association task force on clinical practice guidelines. J Am Coll Cardiol. 2019;73(12):1494–563. Erratum in: J Am Coll Cardiol. 2019;73(18):2361.
9. Kothandan H, Leanne LM, Sharad Shah SK. Fontan physiology: anaesthetic implications for non-cardiac surgery: a case report. Int J Anesthetic Anesthesiol. 2015;2:020.
10. Pans SJ, van Kimmenade RR, Ruurda JP, Meijboom FJ, Sieswerda GT, van Zaane B. Haemodynamics in a patient with Fontan physiology undergoing laparoscopic cholecystectomy. Neth Heart J. 2015;23(7–8):383–5.
11. Pursnani KG, Bazza Y, Calleja M, Mughal MM. Laparoscopic cholecystectomy under epidural anesthesia in patients with chronic respiratory disease. Surg Endosc. 1998;12(8):1082–4.
12. Nayak S, Booker PD. The Fontan circulation. Continuing education in anaesthesia. Crit Care Pain. 2008;8(1):26–30.

4 Hypertension

Derek Dillane

A 48-year-old female presented for optimization to the anesthesia preassessment clinic 1 month prior to ankle arthrodesis. She was diagnosed as being hypertensive 3 months before this consultation. In addition, she had a 7-year history of rheumatoid arthritis, which involved her hands, wrists, and ankles. She denied rheumatoid involvement of the cervical spine.

Medications: Perindopril 4 mg daily, aspirin, hydroxychloroquine, and methotrexate. She had previously been taking leflunomide, but this had been stopped at the time she was found to be hypertensive.

Physical Examination: Blood pressure (BP) was 158/102. Radial artery pulse examination revealed a heart rate of 80 bpm with a regular rhythm. Mallampati I mouth opening was documented on examination of the airway, along with a full range of cervical spine movement.

Investigations: Laboratory tests were normal. Electrocardiogram (ECG) showed a sinus rhythm with a rate of 79 and was otherwise normal. An echocardiogram and myocardial perfusion imaging (MIBI) were performed at the time of diagnosis of hypertension. Both were normal and demonstrated an ejection fraction of 60%. Myocardial perfusion imaging showed normal regional wall motion and a normal-sized left ventricle.

What Is Considered Abnormally High Blood Pressure (Hypertension)?

The American College of Cardiology and American Heart Association (ACC/AHA) categorize hypertension into four levels; normal, elevated, stage 1, and stage 2 hypertension (Table 4.1) [1]. This is based on average BP measurements in a healthcare (as opposed to a home or ambulatory) setting with ≥2 careful readings obtained on ≥2 occasions. These recommendations are based on interpretation of clinical trials and meta-analyses of observational studies on the increased risk of cardiovascular disease, end-stage renal disease, subclinical atherosclerosis and mortality associated with hypertension, as well as the benefit associated with BP reduction [1].

Table 4.1 Classification of high blood pressure according to American College of Cardiology/American Heart Association [1]

Blood pressure (BP) Category	Systolic BP (mmHg)	Diastolic BP (mm Hg)
Normal	<120	<80
Elevated	120–129	<80
Stage 1 hypertension	130–139	80–89
Stage 2 hypertension	≥140	≥90

What Are the Current Pharmacological Treatment Strategies for Control of Hypertension?

Hypertension is treated with one or more of the following:

- Diuretics (thiazide-type diuretics e.g. hydrochlorthiazide; thiazide-like diuretics, e.g., chlorthalidone, indapamide; potassium-sparing spironolactone; loop diuretics)
- ACE inhibitors (ACEi) or angiotensin-2 receptor blockers (ARBs)
- Beta-blockers
- Calcium channel blockers

Initial treatment is with monotherapy, and additional antihypertensive agents are added if target BP is not achieved. Choice of initial agent or combinations is dependent upon several factors, e.g., age, race, comorbidities (heart failure,

D. Dillane (✉)
Department of Anesthesiology & Pain Medicine, University of Alberta, Edmonton, AB, Canada

D. Dillane, B. A. Finegan (eds.), *Preoperative Assessment*, https://doi.org/10.1007/978-3-030-58842-7_4

chronic kidney disease, stroke, peripheral artery disease, diabetes mellitus, atrial fibrillation, valvular heart disease) [2].

The amount of BP reduction provided by any of the above antihypertensive agents is what determines cardiovascular risk reduction, rather than any independent benefit conferred by the agent outside of its antihypertensive properties. This is based on findings from a number of large randomized controlled trials [3, 4]. The only caveat to this is when a comorbidity predicates treatment with one antihypertensive agent over another.

In the absence of a specific clinical indication for a particular agent, thiazide-type diuretics, e.g., low-dose hydrochlorothiazide, or thiazide-like diuretics are commonly used as first-line therapy. The Antihypertensive and Lipid-Lowering Treatment to Prevent Heart Attack Trial (ALLHAT) of 33,357 participants randomized to receive chlorthalidone, amlodipine, lisinopril, or doxazocin over 5 years [5]. The doxazocin arm was terminated early due to an increased risk of heart failure – as a result, alpha-blockade is not recommended for monotherapy in the initial treatment of hypertension. Otherwise, the primary outcome (a composite of fatal coronary heart disease and nonfatal MI) was the same for all study groups. The thiazide-type diuretic was superior at preventing heart failure compared with amlodipine and lisinopril, and was less expensive [5]. Chlorthalidone has a greater potency and longer duration of action than chlorothiazide at a similar dose. Patients on either agent must be monitored for hypokalemia and hyponatremia [1]. A lack of evidence regarding long-term cardiovascular benefit prevents the use of loop diuretics as first-line treatment for hypertension, though they may be seen in hypertensive patients with heart failure and end-stage renal disease.

ACE inhibitors are first-line treatment in patients with heart failure, stable ischemic heart disease (previous MI or stable angina), and chronic kidney disease. There is no compelling evidence in favor of one antihypertensive monotherapy agent over another for secondary stroke prevention.

All first-line agents are effective in the treatment of the diabetic patient with hypertension [6]. ACE inhibitors are the preferred agent in the presence of albuminuria.

Nondihydropyridine calcium channel blockers, i.e., verapamil and diltiazem, are not recommended in heart failure patients due to their myocardial depressant properties. The dihydropyridines, amlodipine and felodipine, appear to be safe in patients with heart failure with reduced ejection fraction and can be used in addition to ACE inhibitors and beta-blockers for treatment-resistant hypertension and angina.

Beta-blockers are not recommended as first-line antihypertensive agents unless the patient has ischemic heart disease or heart failure. Beta-blockade is associated with less protection against stroke when compared with other antihypertensive agents [7, 8].

What Is the Goal for Long-Term Pharmacological Treatment of Hypertension?

The goal varies according to society guidelines. Results from The Systolic Blood Pressure Intervention Trial (SPRINT) have been somewhat influential [9]. This was a randomized controlled trial of 9361 patients showing that a more aggressive lowering of systolic BP to <120 mm Hg compared with the standard goal of 140 mm Hg resulted in lower rates of major cardiovascular events and death from any cause. Though providing a single BP target is somewhat reductive when treatment is individualized for multiple factors, e.g., severity of hypertension, patient age, presence of end-organ damage, established cardiovascular disease, diabetes, or renal disease, the following is an indication of current goals of treatment:

- ACC/AHA recommend a treatment goal of <130/80 [1].
- The British and Irish Hypertension Society and the National Institute for Health and Care Excellence (NICE) advocate for a target clinic BP <140/90 mm Hg in patients under 80 years and below 150/90 mm Hg in those over 80 years [2].
- The European Society of Cardiology (ESC) and the European Society of Hypertension (ESH) recommend that the first objective of treatment should be to lower BP to <140/90 mm Hg in all patients and subsequently to 130/80 mm Hg if treatment is tolerated. In patients over 65 years, it is recommended that systolic BP target range is 130–139 mm Hg [10].

Is There Any Evidence That Aggressive Therapeutic Lowering of BP Is Harmful?

Analysis of data from the Clinical Practice Research Datalink database in the UK reveals a significant association between low preoperative arterial BP and increased postoperative mortality. The threshold for increased risk was a preoperative systolic BP of 119 mm Hg and a diastolic BP of 63 mm Hg [11]. Outside the perioperative arena, in the SPRINT trial, adverse events such as syncope, electrolyte abnormalities, and renal failure occurred more frequently in the intensive (BP <120 mm Hg) treatment group [9].

What Are the Perioperative Risks for the Hypertensive Patient?

Untreated or undertreated hypertension at the time of surgery has been shown to increase the risk of intraoperative BP lability and possibly presage subsequent myocardial injury, heart failure, cerebrovascular events, renal impairment, bleeding, and mortality. However, the question of perioperative risk for the hypertensive patient is not as straightforward as it might first appear as a number of landmark studies delineating an association between hypertension and specific complications are several decades old. Subsequent studies have failed to show that hypertension on the day of surgery significantly increases the risk of adverse outcomes [12–14].

Which Long-Term Consequences of Hypertension Are Associated with an Adverse Perioperative Outcome?

- Occult coronary artery disease (Q waves on the ECG) – ischemic heart disease is the most common form of end-organ damage associated with hypertension [15].
- Left ventricular hypertrophy [16, 17].
- Congestive heart failure [15].
- Cerebrovascular events [18, 19].
- Renal impairment (serum creatinine >176.8 μmol/L or 2.0 mg/dL) [18].

How Successful Is Treatment of Hypertension in Prevention of These Long-Term Consequences?

Appropriate medical treatment can reduce the risk of stroke by up to 40%, MI by up to 25%, and heart failure by as much as 64% [20].

How Should the Hypertensive Patient Be Optimized Preoperatively?

Assessment of target end-organ damage is an important part of preoperative evaluation of the patient with hypertension. Ischemic heart disease is the most common form of end-organ damage. Other consequences of long-term hypertension include heart failure, renal impairment, and cerebrovascular disease.

Antihypertensive medications should be continued up to and including the morning of surgery. This is especially relevant for beta-blockade and centrally acting adrenergic blockers, e.g., clonidine and methyldopa, whose abrupt withdrawal can lead to rebound hypertension.

Should Perindopril Be Continued Throughout the Operative Period?

Continuation of ACE inhibitors and ARBs up to the morning of surgery can lead to significant intraoperative hypotension, which may be refractory to the usual means of treatment with vasopressor medication [21, 22]. There is limited evidence to suggest that perioperative continuation may be beneficial due to a renoprotective effect [23]. The decision to continue or discontinue should be individualized to the patient's BP variability and severity as well as estimated blood loss and hemodynamic variability associated with the surgery. If ACE inhibitors or ARBs are stopped preoperatively, immediate postoperative resumption is recommended [22].

Is There a Cutoff for Systolic or Diastolic BP Above Which Elective Surgery Should Be Cancelled?

Recommended cutoffs are overarchingly based on expert opinion and a handful of studies over 20 years old. The ACC/AHA guidelines recommend giving consideration to deferral of elective major surgery in patients with a systolic BP ≥180 mm Hg or a diastolic BP ≥110 mm Hg [1]. The Joint Guidelines from the Association of Anaesthetists of Great Britain and Ireland (AAGBI) and the British Hypertension Society recommend that patients should proceed to surgery if preoperative assessment clinic BP is <180/110 mm Hg or mean BP measured in primary care is <160/100 mm Hg [24]. The AAGBI further states that BP does not have to be measured in the preoperative assessment clinic if it is documented at below 160/100 mm Hg in the referral letter from the primary carer nor should secondary care attempt to diagnose hypertension in patients who are normotensive in primary care.

What Do We Know About Perioperative Complications and Degree of Hypertension?

An increase in perioperative complications, e.g., myocardial ischemia, dysrhythmias, renal failure and neurological complications, has been found when the immediate preoperative diastolic blood pressure is ≥110 mm Hg [25]. There is a more opaque relationship between severe systolic hypertension and postoperative outcome. Among patients undergoing carotid endarterectomy, there was an increased risk of severe postoperative hypertension leading to neurologic deficit and death in the presence of preoperative systolic BP ≥200 mm Hg [26].

How Do You Manage a Patient Who Has Not Previously Been Diagnosed with Hypertension Whose BP Is Significantly Elevated at the Anesthesia Preassessment Clinic?

This depends on the severity of hypertension and the urgency of surgery. A patient who has not been diagnosed with hypertension in primary care who is discovered in the preoperative assessment clinic to have a systolic BP ≥180 mm Hg or a diastolic BP ≥110 mm Hg should be referred to primary care for diagnosis and possible treatment if surgery is not of a pressing nature. Treatment of hypertension in primary care is based on the evidence that cardiovascular morbidity is reduced over many years. There is no substantial evidence that short-term BP reduction in the immediate preoperative period affects postoperative cardiovascular morbidity [24].

Should This Patient Continue on Aspirin Therapy?

The POISE-2 study concluded that in patients with increased perioperative cardiovascular risk, aspirin does not reduce all-cause mortality or the incidence of non-fatal MI when compared with placebo. It does increase the risk of major bleeding [27]. Therefore, aspirin should be stopped perioperatively in this patient.

Why Did This Patient Have Echocardiography and Nuclear Stress Myocardial Perfusion Imaging at the Time of Diagnosis of Hypertension? Are Any Other Investigations Indicated?

The newly diagnosed hypertensive patient is evaluated to determine the presence or extent of end-organ damage, to assess general cardiovascular disease risk, and to look for possible causes of secondary hypertension if the clinical picture points toward this. Indicated basic and optional investigations are outlined in Table 4.2 [1]. TSH is performed to look for hypo- or hyperthyroidism, two correctable causes of secondary hypertension. Urinalysis is used to detect hematuria and the urinary albumin-to-creatinine ratio to determine albumin secretion. Cardiac magnetic resonance imaging (MRI) can be used to look for left ventricular hypertrophy. The anesthesiologist performing the preoperative assessment will usually not be ordering or interpreting these investigations, but it is helpful to know what has been performed in the newly diagnosed hypertensive and whether or not there is any indication of end-organ injury.

The patient was asked to stop taking aspirin 7 days before surgery and to not take her perindopril on the morning of surgery. We did note that leflunomide was stopped upon diagnosis of hypertension. Leflunomide is an immunosuppressive agent where associated hypertension has been recorded in up to 10% of patients; this can either be aggravation of preexisting hypertension or onset of de novo hypertension [28]. *Methotrexate, conversely, has been associated with a blood pressure lowering effect* [29]. *As there were no indicators of hypertension-induced end-organ damage, this patient proceeded to an uneventful surgery without further investigation.*

Table 4.2 Preliminary basic and optional tests performed in a new diagnosis of hypertension [1]

Basic testing	Complete blood count Serum electrolytes Serum creatinine and GFR Fasting blood glucose Lipid profile Thyroid-stimulating hormone Urinalysis ECG
Optional testing	Echocardiogram Urinary albumin-to-creatinine ratio Cardiac MRI Carotid ultrasound

True/False Questions

1. Regarding the diagnosis of hypertension
   (a) The American College of Cardiology and American Heart Association (ACC/AHA) categorize hypertension into 5 levels: normal, elevated, stage 1, stage 2, and stage 3 hypertension.
   (b) Hypertension can be diagnosed in the preoperative assessment clinic.
   (c) Stage 2 hypertension is diagnosed when the systolic BP ≥140.
   (d) Nonpharmacological interventions, e.g., weight loss, diet, exercise, and sodium restriction, may be the only treatment recommendation for patients with stage 2 hypertension.
   (e) Thyroid-stimulating hormone is a first-line investigation after hypertension has been diagnosed.
2. Regarding the treatment of hypertension
   (a) The ACC/AHA recommend a treatment goal of <130/80.
   (b) More aggressive lowering of BP to <120 mm Hg compared with the standard goal of 140 mm Hg may result in lower rates of major cardiovascular events and death from any cause.
   (c) Beta-blockers are recommended as first-line therapy in the absence of cardiovascular comorbidities.
   (d) ACE inhibitors are first-line treatment in hypertensive patients with heart failure.
   (e) Nondihydropyridine calcium channel blockers are not recommended in heart failure patients.

References

1. Whelton PK, Carey RM, Aronow WS, Casey DE Jr, Collins KJ, Dennison Himmelfarb C, et al. 2017 ACC/AHA/AAPA/ABC/ACPM/AGS/APhA/ASH/ASPC/NMA/PCNA Guideline for the Prevention, Detection, Evaluation, and Management of High Blood Pressure in Adults: A Report of the American College of

Cardiology/American Heart Association Task Force on Clinical Practice Guidelines. Hypertension. 2018;71(6):e13–e115.
2. Excellence NIfHaC. Hypertension in adults: diagnosis and management 2011. Available from: https://www.nice.org.uk/guidance/cg127.
3. Dahlof B, Sever PS, Poulter NR, Wedel H, Beevers DG, Caulfield M, et al. Prevention of cardiovascular events with an antihypertensive regimen of amlodipine adding perindopril as required versus atenolol adding bendroflumethiazide as required, in the Anglo-Scandinavian Cardiac Outcomes Trial-Blood Pressure Lowering Arm (ASCOT-BPLA): a multicentre randomised controlled trial. Lancet. 2005;366(9489):895–906.
4. Nissen SE, Tuzcu EM, Libby P, Thompson PD, Ghali M, Garza D, et al. Effect of antihypertensive agents on cardiovascular events in patients with coronary disease and normal blood pressure: the CAMELOT study: a randomized controlled trial. JAMA. 2004;292(18):2217–25.
5. ALLHAT Officers and Coordinators for the ALLHAT Collaborative Research Group. The Antihypertensive and Lipid-Lowering Treatment to Prevent Heart Attack Trial. Major outcomes in high-risk hypertensive patients randomized to angiotensin-converting enzyme inhibitor or calcium channel blocker vs diuretic: The Antihypertensive and Lipid-Lowering Treatment to Prevent Heart Attack Trial (ALLHAT). JAMA. 2002;288(23):2981–97. Erratum in: JAMA 2003;289(2):178. Erratum in: JAMA. 2004;291(18):2196. 763.
6. Emdin CA, Rahimi K, Neal B, Callender T, Perkovic V, Patel A. Blood pressure lowering in type 2 diabetes: a systematic review and meta-analysis. JAMA. 2015;313(6):603–15.
7. Wiysonge CS, Bradley HA, Volmink J, Mayosi BM, Mbewu A, Opie LH. Beta-blockers for hypertension. Cochrane Database Syst Rev. 2012;(11):CD002003.
8. Gupta A, Mackay J, Whitehouse A, Godec T, Collier T, Pocock S, et al. Long-term mortality after blood pressure-lowering and lipid-lowering treatment in patients with hypertension in the Anglo-Scandinavian Cardiac Outcomes Trial (ASCOT) Legacy study: 16-year follow-up results of a randomised factorial trial. Lancet. 2018;392(10153):1127–37.
9. Group SR, Wright JT, JR., Williamson JD, Whelton PK, Snyder JK, Sink KM, et al. A randomized trial of intensive versus standard blood-pressure control. N Engl J Med. 2015;373(22):2103–16.
10. Williams B, Mancia G, Spiering W, Agabiti Rosei E, Azizi M, Burnier M, et al. 2018 ESC/ESH guidelines for the management of arterial hypertension. Eur Heart J. 2018;39(33):3021–104.
11. Venkatesan S, Myles PR, Manning HJ, Mozid AM, Andersson C, Jorgensen ME, et al. Cohort study of preoperative blood pressure and risk of 30-day mortality after elective non-cardiac surgery. Br J Anaesth. 2017;119(1):65–77.
12. Prys-Roberts C, Greene LT, Meloche R, Foex P. Studies of anaesthesia in relation to hypertension. II. Haemodynamic consequences of induction and endotracheal intubation. Br J Anaesth. 1971;43(6):531–47.
13. Howell SJ, Sear YM, Yeates D, Goldacre M, Sear JW, Foex P. Hypertension, admission blood pressure and perioperative cardiovascular risk. Anaesthesia. 1996;51(11):1000–4.
14. Wax DB, Porter SB, Lin HM, Hossain S, Reich DL. Association of preanesthesia hypertension with adverse outcomes. J Cardiothorac Vasc Anesth. 2010;24(6):927–30.
15. Fleisher LA. Preoperative evaluation of the patient with hypertension. JAMA. 2002;287(16):2043–6.
16. Landesberg G, Einav S, Christopherson R, Beattie C, Berlatzky Y, Rosenfeld B, et al. Perioperative ischemia and cardiac complications in major vascular surgery: importance of the preoperative twelve-lead electrocardiogram. J Vasc Surg. 1997;26(4):570–8.
17. Hollenberg M, Mangano DT, Browner WS, London MJ, Tubau JF, Tateo IM. Predictors of postoperative myocardial ischemia in patients undergoing noncardiac surgery. The Study of Perioperative Ischemia Research Group. JAMA. 1992;268(2):205–9.
18. Lee TH, Marcantonio ER, Mangione CM, Thomas EJ, Polanczyk CA, Cook EF, et al. Derivation and prospective validation of a simple index for prediction of cardiac risk of major noncardiac surgery. Circulation. 1999;100(10):1043–9.
19. Boersma E, Poldermans D, Bax JJ, Steyerberg EW, Thomson IR, Banga JD, et al. Predictors of cardiac events after major vascular surgery: role of clinical characteristics, dobutamine echocardiography, and beta-blocker therapy. JAMA. 2001;285(14):1865–73.
20. Neal B, MacMahon S, Chapman N. Effects of ACE inhibitors, calcium antagonists, and other blood-pressure-lowering drugs: results of prospectively designed overviews of randomised trials. Blood Pressure Lowering Treatment Trialists' Collaboration. Lancet. 2000;356(9246):1955–64.
21. Bertrand M, Godet G, Meersschaert K, Brun L, Salcedo E, Coriat P. Should the angiotensin II antagonists be discontinued before surgery? Anesth Analg. 2001;92(1):26–30.
22. Bradic N, Povsic-Cevra Z. Surgery and discontinuation of angiotensin converting enzyme inhibitors: current perspectives. Curr Opin Anaesthesiol. 2018;31(1):50–4.
23. Shah M, Jain AK, Brunelli SM, Coca SG, Devereaux PJ, James MT, et al. Association between angiotensin converting enzyme inhibitor or angiotensin receptor blocker use prior to major elective surgery and the risk of acute dialysis. BMC Nephrol. 2014;15:53.
24. Hartle A, McCormack T, Carlisle J, Anderson S, Pichel A, Beckett N, et al. The measurement of adult blood pressure and management of hypertension before elective surgery: Joint Guidelines from the Association of Anaesthetists of Great Britain and Ireland and the British Hypertension Society. Anaesthesia. 2016;71(3):326–37.
25. Wolfsthal SD. Is blood pressure control necessary before surgery? Med Clin North Am. 1993;77(2):349–63.
26. Towne JB, Bernhard VM. The relationship of postoperative hypertension to complications following carotid endarterectomy. Surgery. 1980;88(4):575–80.
27. Devereaux PJ, Mrkobrada M, Sessler DI, Leslie K, Alonso-Coello P, Kurz A, et al. Aspirin in patients undergoing noncardiac surgery. N Engl J Med. 2014;370(16):1494–503.
28. Karras G. Leflunomide induced hypertension. J Hypertens. 2015;33:e244.
29. Mangoni AA, Baghdadi LR, Shanahan EM, Wiese MD, Tommasi S, Elliot D, et al. Methotrexate, blood pressure and markers of arterial function in patients with rheumatoid arthritis: a repeated cross-sectional study. Ther Adv Musculoskelet Dis. 2017;9(9):213–29.

Cardiac Failure

5

Derek Dillane

A 68-year-old man was seen at the preoperative evaluation clinic 1 month prior to transurethral resection of bladder tumor. He had a past history of anterior myocardial infarct, hypertension, and diabetes mellitus (type 2). Six weeks prior to this anesthesia consultation, the patient had a 2-week admission for treatment of an acute exacerbation of congestive cardiac failure. He was noted to belong to New York Heart Association (NYHA) Functional Classification III during this hospitalization period. This had not changed in the intervening 6-week period. He has been compliant with prescribed medications since discharge.
Medications: Ramipril, aspirin, atorvastatin, furosemide, metformin, gliclazide, and metoprolol.
Physical Examination: BP was 131/70, heart rate 92, sinus rhythm, and respiratory rate 14, and the patient appeared comfortable at rest.
Investigations: Laboratory values revealed a hemoglobin of 108 g/L, creatinine 139 μmol/L, potassium 5.0 mmol/L, estimated GFR 45 mL/min/1.73 m^2, HbA1C 6.7%, and BNP 736 pg/mL.
Electrocardiogram (ECG) (Fig. 5.1) showed sinus rhythm with a rate of 93, probable left atrial enlargement, old inferior infarct, and no conduction delay.
During the course of his recent admission for stabilization of congestive cardiac failure, the patient had an echocardiogram and coronary angiography. Echocardiogram showed moderate left ventricular (LV) enlargement, severely impaired systolic function with regional wall motion abnormality, LV ejection fraction (EF) of 15–20%, and moderate pulmonary hypertension with a right ventricular systolic pressure (RVSP) estimate of 64 mmHg. Coronary angiogram (Fig. 5.2) showed a 100% left anterior descending artery stenosis and a large dilated left ventricle with anteroapical akinesia. A cardiovascular magnetic resonance image with and without enhancement demonstrated akinesis/dyskinesis of the anterior and anteroseptal mid-ventricular and apical segments in addition to the apex and inferior apex. This was associated with transmural delayed enhancement of these segments. No myocardial edema was detected in keeping with an established infarct.

D. Dillane (✉)
Department of Anesthesiology & Pain Medicine, University of Alberta, Edmonton, AB, Canada

What Complications Is the Patient with Cardiac Failure Subject to in the Perioperative Period?

Postoperatively, patients with heart failure are subject to myocardial ischemia and infarction, atrial fibrillation and ventricular arrhythmias, pulmonary congestion leading to hypoxemia, thromboembolic stroke, and hepatic congestion and dysfunction.

A large retrospective multicenter cohort study from 2019 found that patients with heart failure undergoing elective noncardiac surgery had a significantly higher 90-day mortality compared to those without heart failure (crude mortality rate 5.49% compared with 1.22%) [1]. The risk increased progressively with decreasing systolic function.

How Is Cardiac Failure Classified?

There is no universally accepted method for classification of heart failure. The NYHA Functional Classification of the stages of heart failure according to symptomology is often utilized [2]:

- Class I: No symptoms and no limitation of ordinary physical activity
- Class II: Mild symptoms, e.g., mild dyspnea or angina and slight limitation of ordinary activity
- Class III: Marked limitation of physical activity due to symptoms even during less than ordinary activity and comfortable at rest
- Class IV: Severe limitation and marked symptoms of heart failure at rest

D. Dillane, B. A. Finegan (eds.), *Preoperative Assessment*, https://doi.org/10.1007/978-3-030-58842-7_5

HR	93	. Sinus rhythm
RR	644	. Ventricular premature complex
PR	167	. Probable left atrial enlargement
QRSD	107	. Probable inferior infarct, old
QT	379	. Probable anteroseptal infarct, recent
QTcB	472	
QTcF	439	
-- AXIS --		
P	77	
QRS	14	
T	97	

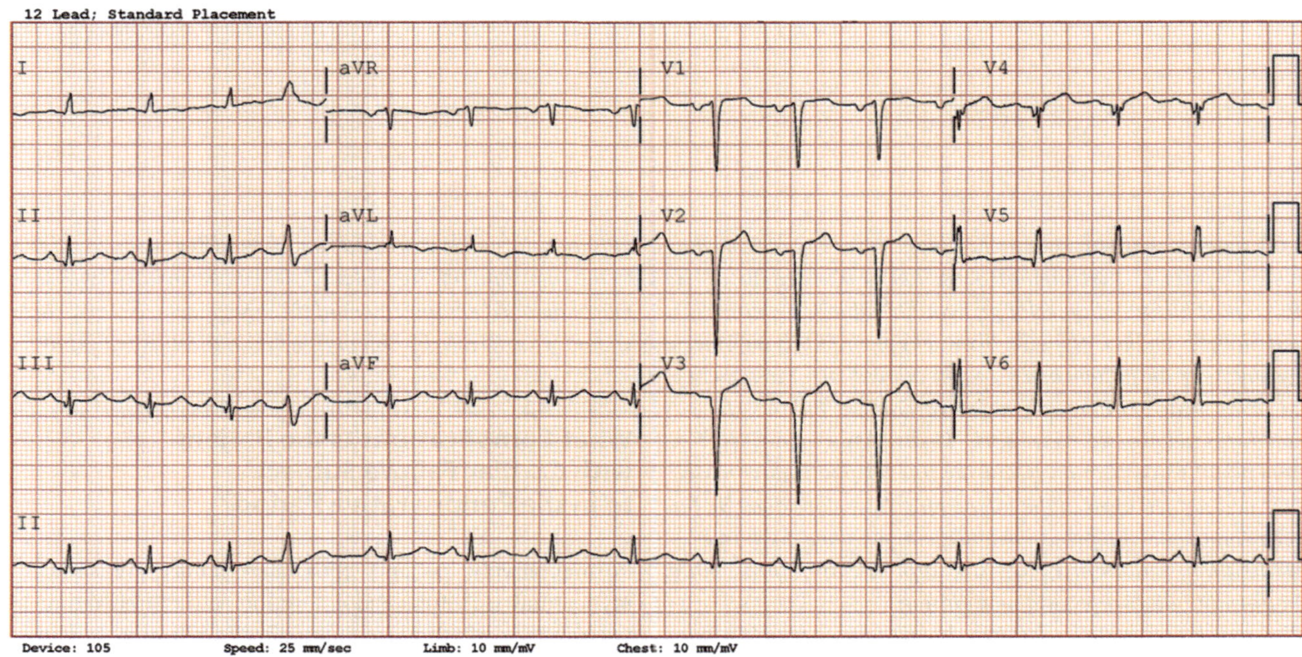

Fig. 5.1 Electrocardiogram (ECG) showed sinus rhythm with a rate of 93, probable left atrial enlargement, old inferior infarct, and no conduction delay

The American College of Cardiology (ACC) and the American Heart Association (AHA) classify heart failure according to disease progression [3]:

- Stage A: Patients at risk of developing heart failure but without structural changes or symptoms of heart failure
- Stage B: Structural heart disease but no symptoms or signs of heart failure
- Stage C: Structural heart disease with current or prior symptomatic heart failure
- Stage D: Advanced heart failure and marked symptoms despite maximal medical therapy

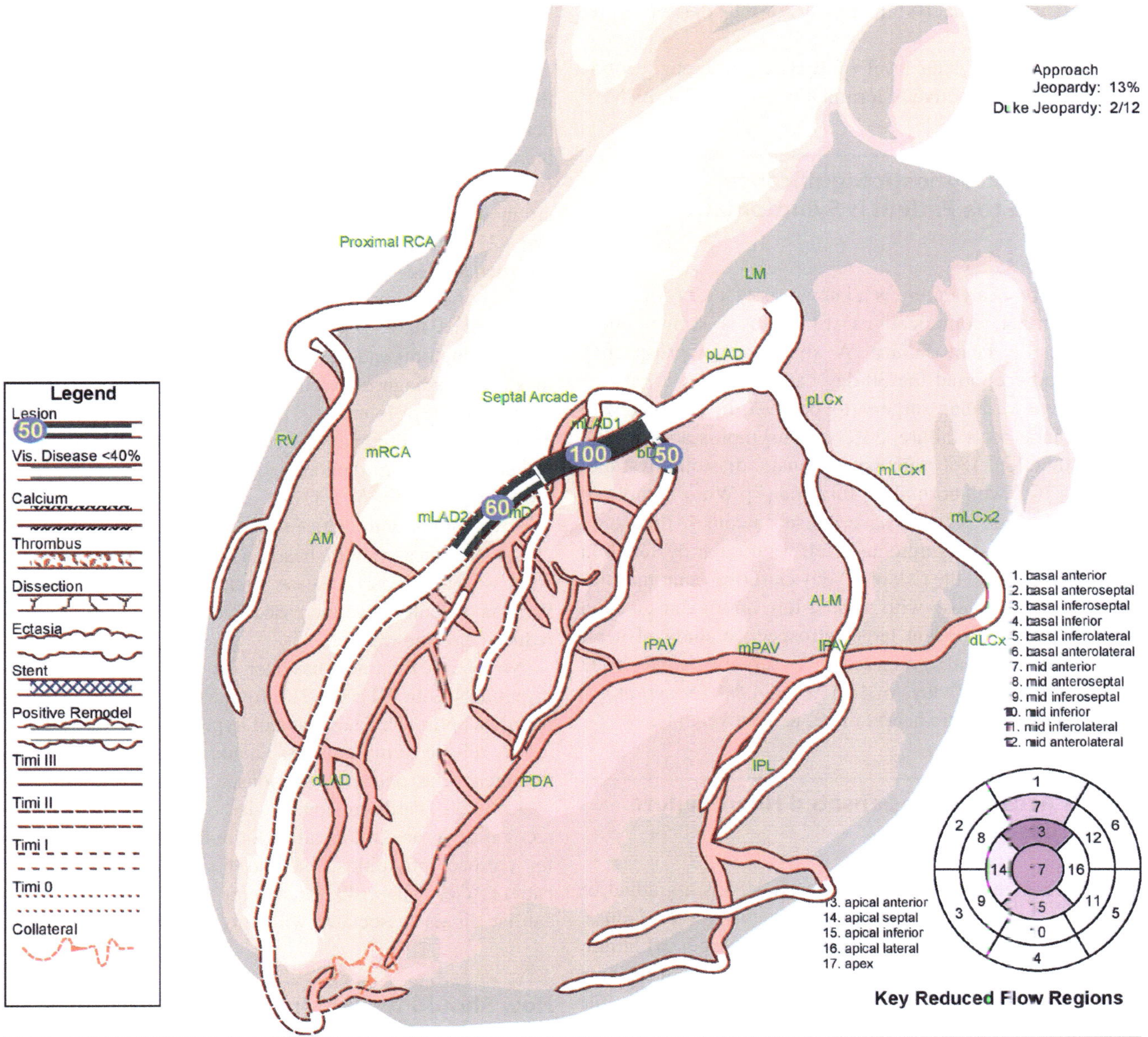

Fig. 5.2 Coronary angiogram showed a 100% left anterior descending artery stenosis and a large dilated left ventricle with anteroapical akinesia. The diagram was created with CARAT® (Coronary Artery Reporting and Archiving Tool, Alberta Provincial Project for Outcome Assessment in Coronary Heart Disease [APPROACH], Cohesic Inc., Calgary, Alberta, Canada)

In Which Patient Populations Should We Maintain a High Index of Suspicion for the Presence of Cardiac Failure?

The commonest underlying causes of cardiac failure include hypertension; coronary artery disease; valvular disease, e.g., aortic stenosis and mitral regurgitation; atrial fibrillation; and dilated cardiomyopathy [4].

What Are Prognostic Indicators in the Heart Failure Patient Presenting for Elective Surgery?

We will address the following prognostic indicators in the next several questions:

- Is the patient symptomatic?
- Is cardiac failure compensated or decompensated? [5]

- Is left ventricular dysfunction systolic or diastolic (preserved EF)?
- What is the plasma level of B-type natriuretic peptide (BNP) or the inactive N-terminal fragment NT-proBNP?

What Is the Prognostic Significance of Whether the Patient Is Symptomatic or Not?

Symptomatic heart failure is a known risk factor for postoperative cardiac complications [6]. Less is known about asymptomatic heart failure. A single-center prospective cohort study reported the 30-day cardiovascular event rate for elective vascular surgery to be 49% in patients with symptomatic heart failure, 23% with asymptomatic systolic LV dysfunction, 18% with asymptomatic diastolic dysfunction, and 10% with normal LV function [7]. While symptomatic heart failure patients have worse outcomes, this study demonstrated that asymptomatic left ventricular dysfunction more than doubled the risk of 30-day cardiovascular morbidity compared to those with normal left ventricular ejection fractions. A more recent large retrospective study of heart failure patients undergoing elective surgery found crude mortality rates at 90 days of 10.1% and 4.8% for symptomatic and asymptomatic heart failure, respectively [1].

How Is Acute Decompensated Heart Failure Recognized?

Acute decompensated heart failure (ADHF) is a gradual or sudden worsening of the symptoms and signs of heart failure. It is most often due to a deterioration in chronic heart failure (70% ADHF presentations). However, up to 20% of patients hospitalized with ADHF are presenting with heart failure for the first time [8]. Clinical findings are related to pulmonary and systemic congestion. Clinical manifestations of ADHF range from mild, e.g., progressive dyspnea, ankle swelling, abdominal distension, or tenderness (secondary to hepatic congestion), to severe pulmonary edema and cardiogenic shock. ADHF may be precipitated by myocardial infarction or ischemia, arrhythmias, uncontrolled hypertension, noncompliance with medications, and infective exacerbations of COPD. No known precipitating factor has been identified in up to 50% of ADHF episodes [9]. There is a high prevalence of atrial fibrillation, valvular disease, and dilated cardiomyopathy in patients presenting with ADHF, which is commensurate with the chronic nature of their underlying heart failure. Patients presenting for surgery with ADHF should have the procedure postponed in all cases except when lifesaving surgery is necessary.

What Is Heart Failure with Preserved Ejection Fraction?

Previously termed diastolic dysfunction, the prevalence of heart failure with preserved ejection fraction (HFpEF) is increasing such that approximately half of hospital admissions for heart failure have preserved LVEF [10]. HFpEF patients are more likely to be female, hypertensive, and of advanced age [11]. Other associated conditions include obesity, obstructive sleep apnea, and lung disease. Not all patients with echocardiographic evidence of diastolic dysfunction and preserved EF have HFpEF. The clinical constellation of heart failure symptoms and signs must accompany these findings to make such a diagnosis. Echocardiographic findings typically seen with HFpEF include LV hypertrophy and left atrial enlargement. Definitive diagnosis is made during cardiac catheterization on demonstration of elevated LV filling pressures with EF ≥50% [12].

Heart failure with reduced ejection fraction (HFrEF), previously known as systolic heart failure, is typically associated with ischemic heart disease and valvular heart disease. Patients typically have increased left ventricular volume and reduced ejection fraction.

No specific treatment has been shown to improve survival in patients with HFpEF. The foundations of treatment are based on optimal management of hypertension, use of diuretics to relieve symptoms associated with congestion, and treatment of associated conditions, e.g., atrial fibrillation.

Amyloid cardiomyopathy is becoming increasingly recognized as an etiological factor in HFpEF [13]. Screening for cardiac amyloidosis should be considered in at-risk patients (see Chap. 49 for a more detailed discussion on cardiac disease associated with amyloidosis).

How Should the Patient with Cardiac Failure Be Evaluated Preoperatively?

Clinical evaluation of severity of symptoms and stability of disease can be performed in the office. Functional capacity can be determined using the metabolic equivalent score or Duke Activity Status Index (see Chap. 2). Symptoms and signs of heart failure which can be used to ascertain severity are outlined in Table 5.1. As we have seen above, lack of symptoms does not mean that risk is negligible. As outlined in Chap. 2, the Revised Cardiac Risk Index and NSQIP Surgical Risk Calculator are useful tools for evaluating perioperative risk [14, 15].

ECG may provide important information relating to the etiology of heart failure, e.g., prior myocardial infarction, atrial fibrillation, and LV hypertrophy associated with hypertension. A diagnosis of chronic heart failure due to LV

Table 5.1 Symptoms and signs of heart failure

Symptoms	Signs
Dyspnea	Elevated jugular venous pressure
Orthopnea	Displaced apex beat
Paroxysmal nocturnal dyspnea	Third heart sound or gallop rhythm
Fatigue	Pulmonary crackles
Palpitations	Hepatomegaly
Ankle swelling	Ascites
Cachexia, anorexia	Peripheral edema

systolic dysfunction is unlikely in the presence of a normal ECG or one that shows only minor abnormalities [16].

CXR findings that help to differentiate heart failure from pulmonary causes of dyspnea include the presence of cardiomegaly, alveolar pulmonary edema (initially seen as perihilar batwing opacities but becoming more generalized over time), Kerley B lines of interstitial edema, prominence of the upper zone vessels, and pleural effusions. However, in the setting of optimization for elective surgery, a change or new findings on CXR would likely correlate with a clinical picture indicating acute decompensation, in which case surgery will almost certainly become deprioritized.

Brain natriuretic peptide (BNP) and N-terminal fragment of proBNP (NT-proBNP) are cardiac biomarkers released from the myocardium in response to stimuli such as ischemia or cardiomyocyte stretch. BNP is synthesized as a prehormone, proBNP, which upon release into the circulation is cleaved into the biologically active BNP and an inactive N-terminal fragment NT-proBNP [17]. These biomarkers have excellent sensitivity but limited specificity for diagnosing heart failure. Moreover, BNP level may be proportionate to the risk. This is especially relevant for the perioperative physician. Much of the literature pertaining to BNP and cardiac failure concerns the acute phase of the condition. With this in mind, a systematic review of 19 studies where plasma BNP from patients at all stages of the disease was used to determine the relative risk of cardiac events or death reported that every 100 pg/ml increase was associated with a 35% increase in the relative risk of death [18]. There is ample evidence that persistently elevated plasma BNP, despite optimal medical treatment, is a poor prognosticator [19, 20].

Echocardiography can provide useful information regarding cardiac function and structure. A reduced EF is an independent predictor of mortality in heart failure patients [21]. However, a normal ejection does not rule out heart failure, considering that approximately half of hospital admissions for heart failure have preserved EF. Echocardiographic demonstration of preserved EF with concomitant structural abnormalities, e.g., LV hypertrophy or left atrial enlargement, is required, along with clinical findings, to confirm the presence of HFpEF. Echocardiography is also useful for

Table 5.2 Revised Cardiac Risk Index (RCRI) score calculation (From Duceppe et al. [24], with permission from Elsevier)

Variable	Points
History of ischemic heart disease[a]	1
History of congestive heart failure[b]	1
History of cerebrovascular disease[c]	1
Use of insulin therapy for diabetes	1
Preoperative serum creatinine >177 μmol/[>2.0 mg/dL]	1
High-risk surgery[d]	1

[a]History of myocardial infarction, positive exercise test, current complaint of ischemic chest pain or nitrate use, electrocardiogram with pathological Q waves; patients with previous revascularization procedure meet criteria if they have such findings after coronary artery bypass or percutaneous coronary intervention (PCI)
[b]History of heart failure, pulmonary edema, or paroxysmal nocturnal dyspnea; an S3 gallop or bilateral rales on physical examination; chest radiograph showing pulmonary vascular redistribution
[c]Previous stroke or transient ischemic attack (TIA)
[d]Intraperitoneal, intrathoracic, or suprainguinal vascular surgery)

evaluation of valvular dysfunction, right ventricular function, and pulmonary artery pressure – all prognostic indicators in heart failure [22].

Though LVEF is an established prognostic indicator in cardiac failure, BNP measurement may be more accessible. Preoperative NT-proBNP has been shown to be more predictive of major perioperative cardiac complications compared to echocardiography [23]. The Canadian Cardiovascular Society (CCS) recommends measuring NT-proBNP or BNP before noncardiac surgery in patients over 65 years or those between 45 and 64 years who have a Revised Cardiac Risk Index (RCRI) score of ≥1 (Table 5.2) [24]. CCS also recommends against obtaining a resting echocardiogram preoperatively to enhance cardiac risk estimation unless clinical examination suggests an undiagnosed, severe obstructive abnormality, e.g., aortic stenosis.

What Are the Goals of Optimization?

- Identify patients with asymptomatic heart failure.
- Identify and minimize symptoms, especially those related to pulmonary congestion and low output failure.
- Identify and treat precipitating factors, e.g., ischemia, hypertension, arrhythmia, and valvular disease.
- Enhance end-organ perfusion and oxygenation.

What Medical Therapy Is Used to Optimize the Heart Failure Patient?

Angiotensin-converting enzyme inhibitors (ACEi) or angiotensin receptor blockers (ARBs) are first-line therapies for the patient with heart failure with reduced EF. ARBs are used in patients intolerant to ACEi. These medications should be withheld on the day of surgery to minimize excessive intraoperative hypotension. Based on more recent data, a combination of a neprilysin inhibitor and ARB, angiotensin receptor blocker-neprilysin inhibitor (ARNI), sacubitril/valsartan, may be substituted for ACEi or ARB single therapy when the following conditions are met: LVEF <40%, BNP or NT-proBNP has been elevated or the patient has been hospitalized for the treatment of heart failure in the past year, and serum potassium <5.2 mmol/L [25]. Neprilysin inhibition decreases the degradation of atrial and brain natriuretic peptide and bradykinin – peptides that evoke vasodilation, natriuresis, and diuresis.

Specific beta-blockers for heart failure management are bisoprolol, extended-release metoprolol, and carvedilol. These specific beta-blockers have been shown to reduce mortality, hospitalization rate, and symptoms in patients with reduced LVEF [26]. Beta-blockers should be continued in patients already taking them but should not be started for the first time in the preoperative period.

Aldosterone receptor antagonists, e.g., spironolactone, reduce mortality in patients with LVEF <35% and NYHA Class II–IV heart failure [3]. Careful monitoring of serum potassium and renal function is required as there is a risk of life-threatening hyperkalemia and renal insufficiency.

Diuretics are used for symptomatic relief of fluid retention. Patients taking diuretic therapy are at increased risk for perioperative hypovolemia and hypokalemia. This warrants a preoperative electrolyte screen.

Digoxin can be beneficial in patients with heart failure with reduced EF who are on optimal evidence-based medical therapy (ACEi or ARB or ARNI and beta-blocker and aldosterone receptor antagonist) but remain symptomatic.

What Is the Role of Implantable Cardioverter-Defibrillators and Permanent Pacemakers in the Heart Failure Patient?

Patients with LV dysfunction are at risk of sudden cardiac death secondary to ventricular arrhythmias. This risk increases as LVEF decreases [27]. Implantable cardioverter-defibrillator (ICD) devices reduce mortality through prevention of sudden cardiac death in certain patients: those with LVEF of ≤35%, at least 40 days post myocardial infarction, NYHA Class II or III symptoms, on long-term guideline-directed medical therapy, and expected to live for 1 year or longer [3]. ICD devices can also act as pacemakers.

Cardiac resynchronization therapy (CRT) may be useful in certain heart failure patients, e.g., those with reduced EF (≤35%), who are in sinus rhythm with a QRS duration of ≥150 ms [3]. Specific indications and contraindications for CRT in heart failure are detailed in the 2013 ACCF/AHA Heart Failure Guidelines [3].

How Should the Decision-Making Process Be Approached Regarding the Appropriateness of the Proposed Surgery for This Patient?

Both surgical and patient factors need to be assessed. The proposed surgery is elective and low risk. It is not particularly time-sensitive and subsequently could be delayed for a period of time if optimization was deemed possible. Is optimization necessary or possible? The patient does not have symptoms and signs to suggest that he is in acute decompensated heart failure. Dyspnea at rest and non-compliance with cardiac failure medications are usually highly suggestive of this. Atrial fibrillation is seen in greater than 30% of patients with acute heart failure. This patient was in sinus rhythm. He is compliant with guideline-directed medical therapy. His hypertension and diabetes are controlled. Therefore, even though he is a high-risk patient with a plasma BNP of 736 pg/mL and LVEF of 15–20%, he is stable and may proceed for this procedure as booked without further evaluation or intervention, once a thorough discussion has taken place with the patient outlining the risks and benefits of proceeding.

True/False Questions

1. Heart failure with preserved ejection fraction (HFpEF)
   (a) Was previously known as diastolic dysfunction.
   (b) All patients with diastolic dysfunction and preserved EF have HFpEF.
   (c) Is commonly associated with hypertension.
   (d) Is a clinical diagnosis.
   (e) Has a better prognostic outcome when compared with heart failure with reduced ejection fraction.
2. Plasma brain natriuretic peptide (BNP)
   (a) Is a neurotransmitter released by the cardioaccelerator center in the cerebral medulla in response to myocyte stretch.
   (b) Is only of prognostic value in patients with acute heart failure.
   (c) Is more predictive of perioperative cardiac complications compared to echocardiography.
   (d) Is not of prognostic value in preoperative patients between 45 and 64 years with an RCRI <2.
   (e) Renal failure causes elevated BNP and NT-proBNP.

References

1. Lerman BJ, Popat RA, Assimes TL, Heidenreich PA, Wren SM. Association of left ventricular ejection fraction and symptoms with mortality after elective noncardiac surgery among patients with heart failure. JAMA. 2019;321(6):572–9.
2. American Heart Association. Classes of heart failure. Last reviewed 31 May 2017. https://www.heart.org/en/health-topics/heart-failure/what-is-heart-failure/classes-of-heart-failure
3. Yancy CW, Jessup M, Bozkurt B, Butler J, Casey DE Jr, Drazner MH, et al. 2013 ACCF/AHA guideline for the management of heart failure: executive summary: a report of the American College of Cardiology Foundation/American Heart Association Task Force on practice guidelines. Circulation. 2013;128(16):1810–52.
4. Baldasseroni S, Opasich C, Gorini M, Lucci D, Marchionni N, Marini M, et al. Left bundle-branch block is associated with increased 1-year sudden and total mortality rate in 5517 outpatients with congestive heart failure: a report from the Italian network on congestive heart failure. Am Heart J. 2002;143(3):398–405.
5. Patel AY, Eagle KA, Vaishnava P. Cardiac risk of noncardiac surgery. J Am Coll Cardiol. 2015;66(19):2140–8.
6. Fleisher LA, Fleischmann KE, Auerbach AD, Barnason SA, Beckman JA, Bozkurt B, et al. 2014 ACC/AHA guideline on perioperative cardiovascular evaluation and management of patients undergoing noncardiac surgery: a report of the American College of Cardiology/American Heart Association Task Force on practice guidelines. J Am Coll Cardiol. 2014;64(22):e77–137.
7. Flu WJ, van Kuijk JP, Hoeks SE, Kuiper R, Schouten O, Goei D, et al. Prognostic implications of asymptomatic left ventricular dysfunction in patients undergoing vascular surgery. Anesthesiology. 2010;112(6):1316–24.
8. Joseph SM, Cedars AM, Ewald GA, Geltman EM, Mann DL. Acute decompensated heart failure: contemporary medical management. Tex Heart Inst J. 2009;36(6):510–20.
9. Opasich C, Rapezzi C, Lucci D, Gorini M, Pozzar F, Zanelli E, et al. Precipitating factors and decision-making processes of short-term worsening heart failure despite “optimal” treatment (from the IN-CHF Registry). Am J Cardiol. 2001;88(4):382–7.
10. Metra M, Teerlink JR. Heart failure. Lancet. 2017;390(10106):1981–95.
11. Yancy CW, Lopatin M, Stevenson LW, De Marco T, Fonarow GC, Committee ASA, et al. Clinical presentation, management, and in-hospital outcomes of patients admitted with acute decompensated heart failure with preserved systolic function: a report from the Acute Decompensated Heart Failure National Registry (ADHERE) Database. J Am Coll Cardiol. 2006;47(1):76–84.
12. Zakeri R, Cowie MR. Heart failure with preserved ejection fraction: controversies, challenges and future directions. Heart. 2018;104(5):377–84.
13. van den Berg MP, Mulder BA, Klaassen SHC, Maass AH, van Veldhuisen DJ, van der Meer P, et al. Heart failure with preserved ejection fraction, atrial fibrillation, and the role of senile amyloidosis. Eur Heart J. 2019;40(16):1287–93.
14. Lee TH, Marcantonio ER, Mangione CM, Thomas EJ, Polanczyk CA, Cook EF, et al. Derivation and prospective validation of a simple index for prediction of cardiac risk of major noncardiac surgery. Circulation. 1999;100(10):1043–9.
15. American College of Surgeons National Surgical Quality Improvement Program. ACS NSQIP surgical risk calculator 2020. https://riskcalculator.facs.org/RiskCalculator/index.jsp. Accessed 16 May 2020.
16. Davie AP, Francis CM, Love MP, Caruana L, Starkey IR, Shaw TR, et al. Value of the electrocardiogram in identifying heart failure due to left ventricular systolic dysfunction. BMJ. 1996;312(7025):222.
17. Weber M, Hamm C. Role of B-type natriuretic peptide (BNP) and NT-proBNP in clinical routine. Heart. 2006;92(6):843–9.
18. Doust JA, Pietrzak E, Dobson A, Glasziou P. How well does B-type natriuretic peptide predict death and cardiac events in patients with heart failure: systematic review. BMJ. 2005;330(7492):625.
19. Berger R, Huelsman M, Strecker K, Bojic A, Moser P, Stanek B, et al. B-type natriuretic peptide predicts sudden death in patients with chronic heart failure. Circulation. 2002;105(20):2392–7.
20. Logeart D, Thabut G, Jourdain P, Chavelas C, Beyne P, Beauvais F, et al. Predischarge B-type natriuretic peptide assay for identifying patients at high risk of re-admission after decompensated heart failure. J Am Coll Cardiol. 2004;43(4):635–41
21. Pocock SJ, Ariti CA, McMurray JJ, Maggioni A, Kober L, Squire IB, et al. Predicting survival in heart failure: a risk score based on 39 372 patients from 30 studies. Eur Heart J. 2013;34(19):1404–13.
22. Cikes M, Solomon SD. Beyond ejection fraction: an integrative approach for assessment of cardiac structure and function in heart failure. Eur Heart J. 2016;37(21):1642–50.
23. Park SJ, Choi JH, Cho SJ, Chang SA, Choi JO, Lee SC, et al. Comparison of transthoracic echocardiography with N-terminal pro-brain natriuretic Peptide as a tool for risk stratification of patients undergoing major noncardiac surgery. Korean Circ J. 2011;41(9):505–11.
24. Duceppe E, Parlow J, MacDonald P, Lyons K, McMullen M, Srinathan S, et al. Canadian cardiovascular society guidelines on perioperative cardiac risk assessment and management for patients who undergo noncardiac surgery. Can J Cardiol. 2017;33(1):17–32.
25. Moe GW, Ezekowitz JA, O'Meara E, Lepage S, Howlett JG, Fremes S, et al. The 2014 Canadian cardiovascular society heart failure management guidelines focus update: anemia, biomarkers, and recent therapeutic trial implications. Can J Cardiol. 2015;31(1):3–16.
26. Fonarow GC, Yancy CW, Hernandez AF, Peterson ED, Spertus JA, Heidenreich PA. Potential impact of optimal implementation of evidence-based heart failure therapies on mortality. Am Heart J. 2011;161(6):1024–30, e3.
27. Doval HC, Nul DR, Grancelli HO, Varini SD, Soifer S, Corrado G, et al. Nonsustained ventricular tachycardia in severe heart failure. Independent marker of increased mortality due to sudden death. GESICA-GEMA Investigators. Circulation. 1996;94(12):3198–203.

6 Atrial Arrhythmias

Derek Dillane

A 72-year-old man presented to the preoperative assessment clinic 4 weeks prior to laparoscopic colectomy. Atrial fibrillation (AF) had been diagnosed 6 years previously. In addition, he had a history of hypertension, hyperlipidemia, and diabetes mellitus (type 2), well controlled on oral hypoglycemic medication. He had a remote history of occupation-related asbestosis. He was an active individual with an estimated metabolic equivalent of task (MET) score of 6.

Medications: Rivaroxaban, metformin, pioglitazone, bisoprolol, perindopril, rosuvastatin, and tamsulosin.

Physical Examination: Blood pressure was 146/92. He had a soft ejection systolic murmur radiating bilaterally to the carotids. There was no evidence of cardiac failure.

Investigations: Electrocardiogram (ECG) and chest radiograph can be seen in Figs. 6.1 and 6.2.

Laboratory values revealed a hemoglobin of 108 g/L, platelet count 138 × 10^9/L, creatinine 152 μmol/L, estimated glomerular filtration rate 39 mL/min/1.73 m^2, and INR 2.8.

An echocardiogram performed at the time of the original diagnosis of AF showed left atrial dilatation with no evidence of mitral valve disease, mild tricuspid regurgitation, and an ejection fraction of 70% with no evidence of regional wall motion abnormalities or left ventricular hypertrophy.

D. Dillane (✉)
Department of Anesthesiology & Pain Medicine, University of Alberta, Edmonton, AB, Canada

What Complications Is the Patient with Atrial Fibrillation Subject to in the Perioperative Period?

- Increased risk of thromboembolic stroke secondary to atrial thrombus formation
- Bleeding due to prophylactic anticoagulation
- Intra- and postoperative hemodynamic instability due to fast AF and rapid ventricular response
- Intra- and postoperative cardiac ischemia due to fast AF and rapid ventricular response
- Congestive cardiac failure and reduction in cardiac output
- Diastolic heart failure (heart failure with preserved ejection fraction)

What Potentially Modifiable Conditions Associated with AF Should Be Optimized in This Patient Prior to Surgery?

Coronary heart disease, hypertension, diabetes mellitus, obstructive sleep apnea, alcohol consumption, and hyperthyroidism may be seen in the patient with atrial fibrillation and each condition is potentially modifiable.

Are There Any Other Factors Which May Contribute to the Development of AF?

- Valvular disease especially mitral stenosis/rheumatic heart disease
- Previous cardiac or thoracic surgery
- Age > 65 years
- Caucasian ethnicity
- Male sex (despite a lower incidence of atrial fibrillation, women have a significantly higher risk of stroke and cardiovascular death secondary to atrial fibrillation).

D. Dillane, B. A. Finegan (eds.), *Preoperative Assessment*, https://doi.org/10.1007/978-3-030-58842-7_6

HR 75 . ATRIAL FIBRILLATION, V-RATE 55-90
RR 800 . BORDERLINE R WAVE PROGRESSION, ANTERIOR LEADS

QRSD 88
QT 364
QTc 407

-- AXIS --

QRS 50 - ABNORMAL ECG -
T 15 Previous ECG:08-Sep-2010 08:01:00 - Borderline Confirmed

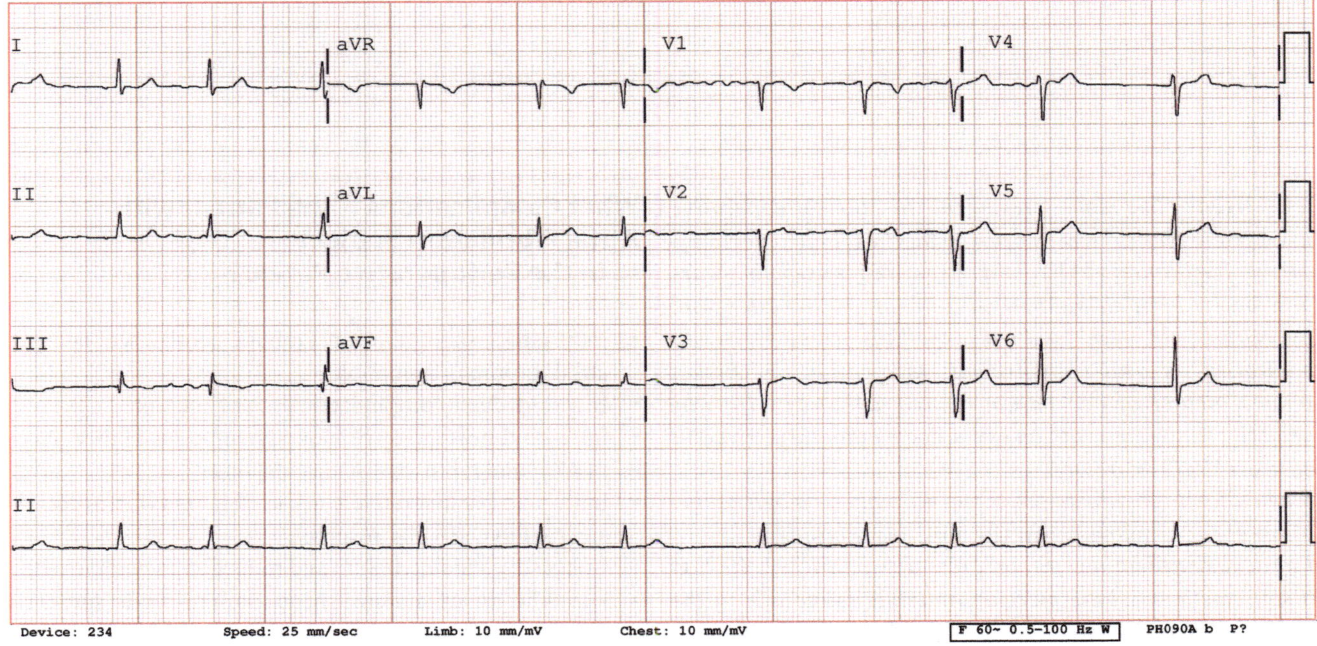

Fig. 6.1 Electrocardiogram showing rate controlled atrial fibrillation without left ventricular hypertrophy

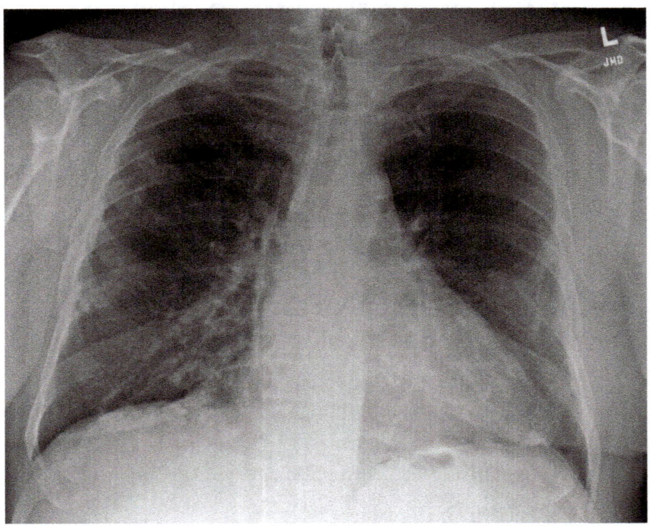

Fig. 6.2 Mild cardiomegaly is seen on the preoperative chest radiograph. Calcified pleural plaque, most likely associated with asbestosis, can be seen in both bases, and within the right hemithorax, especially along the mediastinal pleura

Age >65 years, Caucasian ethnicity, and male sex (despite their lower incidence of atrial fibrillation, women have a significantly higher risk of stroke and cardiovascular death secondary to atrial fibrillation)

How Should the Patient with AF Atrial Be Evaluated Preoperatively?

History

The following should be noted:

- Onset, duration, and severity of AF.
- AF may be classified as paroxysmal, persistent, or permanent. Paroxysmal AF terminates spontaneously or with intervention within 7 days of onset. Persistent AF does not terminate spontaneously within 7 days of onset and lasts from months to years. It may be stopped with treatment. Permanent AF is unresponsive to treatment.
- Precipitating factors: alcohol, exercise, and emotion.

- Medications: rate control/antiarrhythmic/anticoagulation/anti-platelet.
- Coexisting cardiovascular disease, i.e., heart failure, hypertension, valvular heart disease, history of transient ischemic attack (TIA), or cerebrovascular accident (CVA).

Not all patients are symptomatic. Typical symptoms include palpitations, tachycardia, fatigue, lightheadedness, or mild dyspnea. More severe symptoms include dyspnea at rest, angina, or syncopal attacks.

Physical Exam

A complete cardiovascular examination should be performed focusing in particular on pulse rate and rhythm, heart sounds, and murmurs (e.g., mitral stenosis). Signs of heart failure should also be sought. AF and heart failure share common mechanisms and treatment strategies and often occur together. The causative relationship between the two conditions has not been elucidated, i.e., is atrial fibrillation a cause or a consequence of heart failure [1].

Investigations

A baseline ECG is a prerequisite. In addition to elucidating information pertaining to rate control and rhythm, other electrocardiographic markers of cardiac disease, e.g., ischemic or hypertensive changes, must be sought. A chest radiograph should be performed looking at heart size and signs of heart failure. A transthoracic echocardiogram (TTE) may be considered in new or recent onset atrial fibrillation looking at right and left atrial size, right and left ventricular size and function, valvular disease, and left ventricular hypertrophy. The value of echocardiography in persistent AF is less well defined and decided on a case by case basis.

Table 6.1 CHA_2DS_2-VASc scoring system for determination of embolic stroke risk [4]

Risk factor	CHA_2DS_2-VASc (Maximum score, 9) Points
Congestive cardiac failure	1
Hypertension	1
Vascular disease	1
Diabetes	1
Ages 65–74	1
Age ≥75	2
Female sex	1
Previous stroke/TIA	2

TIA Transient ischemic attack

How Is the Stroke Risk in Patients with AF Calculated?

Estimation of embolic risk determines whether long-term oral anticoagulation is indicated in the patient with AF [2]. Reduction in risk of embolization should exceed the risk of bleeding associated with anticoagulation, in particular, intracranial bleeding. CHA_2DS_2-VASc (Table 6.1) is a scoring system used to identify which patients should and should not be placed on thromboprophylaxis [3, 4].

ACC/AHA guidelines recommend use of the CHA_2DS_2-VASc score for assessment of stroke risk in nonvalvular AF patients [5]. Patients with AF and an elevated CHA_2DS_2-VASc score of 2 or greater in men and 3 or greater in women should be anticoagulated. DOACs are recommended over warfarin except in patients with moderate to severe mitral stenosis or a mechanical heart valve. In patients with severe end-stage chronic renal disease or are on dialysis, warfarin and apixaban are reasonable choices for anticoagulation [6]. For moderate-risk patients, the recommendations are more ambivalent with a risk/benefit assessment performed on an individual basis to determine whether the patient is anticoagulated or not. However, expert opinion leans toward full anticoagulation for this intermediate category [7].

How Would the Presence of Valvular Heart Disease with AF Impact Preoperative Optimization?

Patients with moderate to severe mitral stenosis and AF should be anticoagulated with warfarin. There is insufficient evidence at this time to treat these patients with non-vitamin K oral anticoagulants, i.e., the direct thrombin inhibitor dabigatran, and the factor Xa inhibitors rivaroxaban, apixaban and edoxaban [6].

DOACs are contraindicated in patients with mechanical heart valves. This recommendation is based on the observed increase in ischemic stroke rate and bleeding complications in patients receiving dabigatran compared with warfarin in the RE-ALIGN trial [8]. The American College of Cardiology/American Heart Association (ACC/AHA) guidelines recommend warfarin anticoagulation for patients with AF who have mechanical heart valves [5, 6].

What Specific Medications for Rate and Rhythm Control Should We Expect to See in the Preoperative Patient with AF?

The principal goals of long-term management of AF are symptom control and the prevention of thromboembolism. Pharmacological therapy is based on rate or rhythm control and anticoagulation. Rhythm- and rate-control strategies are

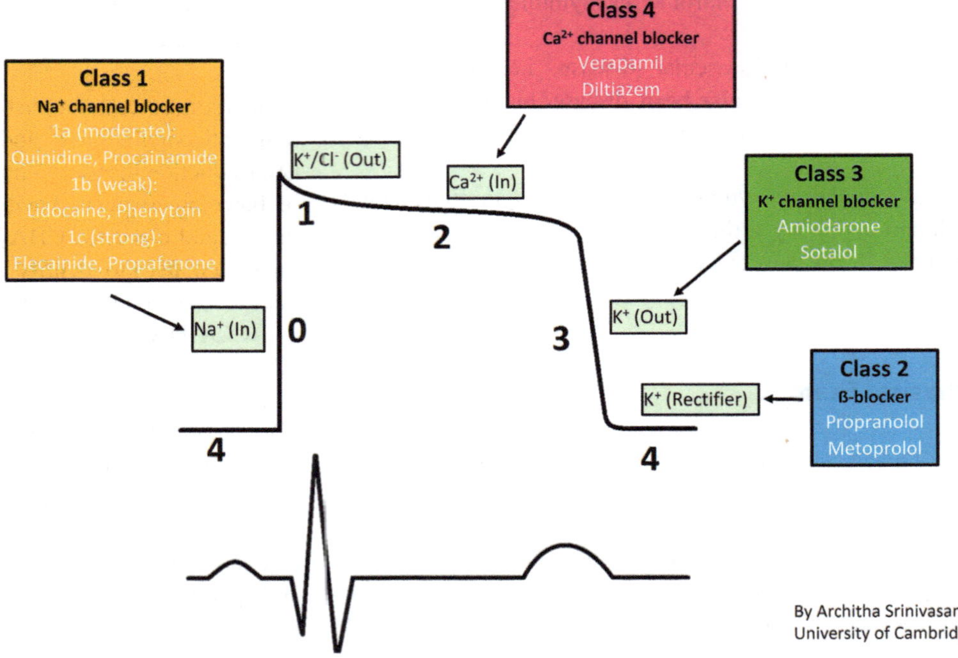

Fig. 6.3 Antiarrhythmic agents. Drugs affecting the cardiac action potential (Courtesy of Architha Srinivasan, University of Cambridge (CC BY-SA 4.0))

associated with similar rates of mortality and serious morbidity, such as embolic risk. As we have seen above, each patient is risk stratified on an individual basis and assessed for suitability for anticoagulation prophylaxis.

Patients over 65 years are normally managed using a rate-control strategy. This is due to concerns about the side effects of antiarrhythmic drug therapy or radiofrequency catheter ablation. A rate-control strategy generally uses drugs that block the atrioventricular node, e.g., beta-blockers, rate-slowing calcium channel blockers, and digoxin. A rhythm-control strategy may be reasonable for older patients who continue to experience clinically significant symptoms on a rate-control strategy.

For most patients with AF younger than age 65, particularly those who are symptomatic, a rhythm-control strategy is frequently used, primarily for symptom relief as AF is not well tolerated in this population. A rhythm-control strategy uses either antiarrhythmic drug therapy (Fig. 6.3) or percutaneous catheter ablation. Electrical cardioversion may be necessary to maintain sinus rhythm. Antiarrhythmic medications are generally started before cardioversion and continued to maintain sinus rhythm. Typical antiarrhythmic medications include amiodarone, propafenone, sotalol, and flecainide.

Does This Patient Need to Be Bridged?

Temporary disruption of anticoagulation increases risk of perioperative thromboembolism, while continuation of anticoagulation increases the risk of bleeding. The decision to discontinue anticoagulation and whether to bridge with a short-acting parenteral agent is made on a case-by-case basis after estimates of thromboembolic and bleeding risk are taken into account.

For patients taking warfarin, bridging is typically reserved for those at very high risk of thromboembolism, e.g., recent stroke or patients with a mechanical heart valve. Bridging with a low-molecular-weight (LMW) heparin is started 3 days before surgery (Figs. 6.4 and 6.5) [9]. Warfarin may be restarted the evening of surgery or the first postoperative day at the same dose as the patient was taking preoperatively. Bridging may need to be continued until INR reaches therapeutic values. Our patient did not need to be bridged; the much more rapid offset and onset times for DOACs eliminate the need for bridging in most cases (Fig. 6.6) [9].

Surgery and DOACs: An Approach

Decide if interruption of DOAC therapy is required by determining the risk of bleeding during the proposed procedure. Surgery with a low risk of bleeding (e.g., cataract/dental extraction) usually does not require any change in DOAC management. Whereas, other procedures (e.g., prostate/vascular/major orthopedic) carry a high risk of hemorrhage in the anticoagulated patient, and temporary cessation of DOAC treatment is warranted.

Determine the half-life of the DOAC that is being discontinued, the impact of renal function on elimination of that DOAC, and the renal function of the patient. The

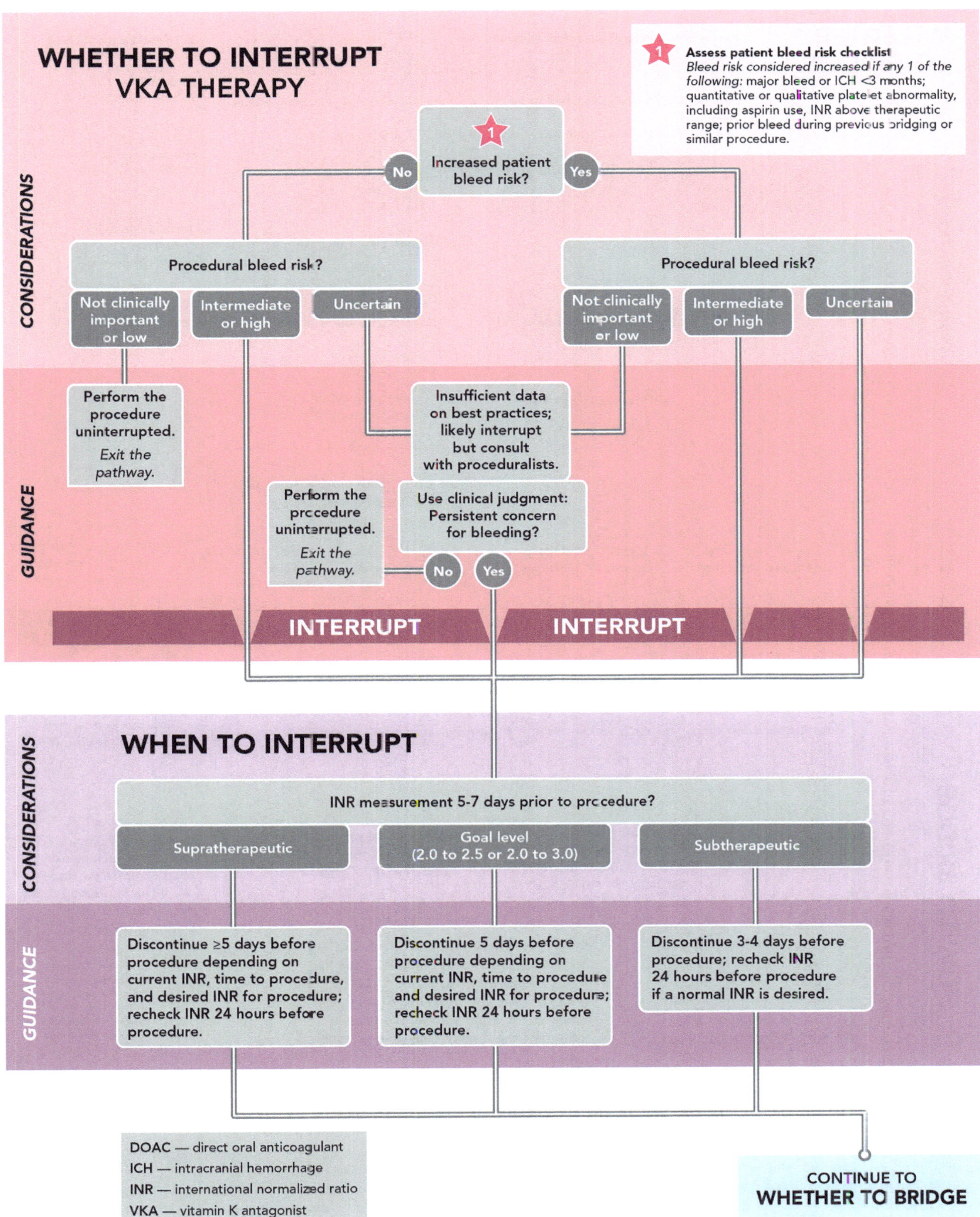

Fig. 6.4 2017 American College of Cardiology Expert Consensus Decision Pathway. Whether and how to interrupt warfarin therapy (From Doherty et al. [9] with permission Elsevier)

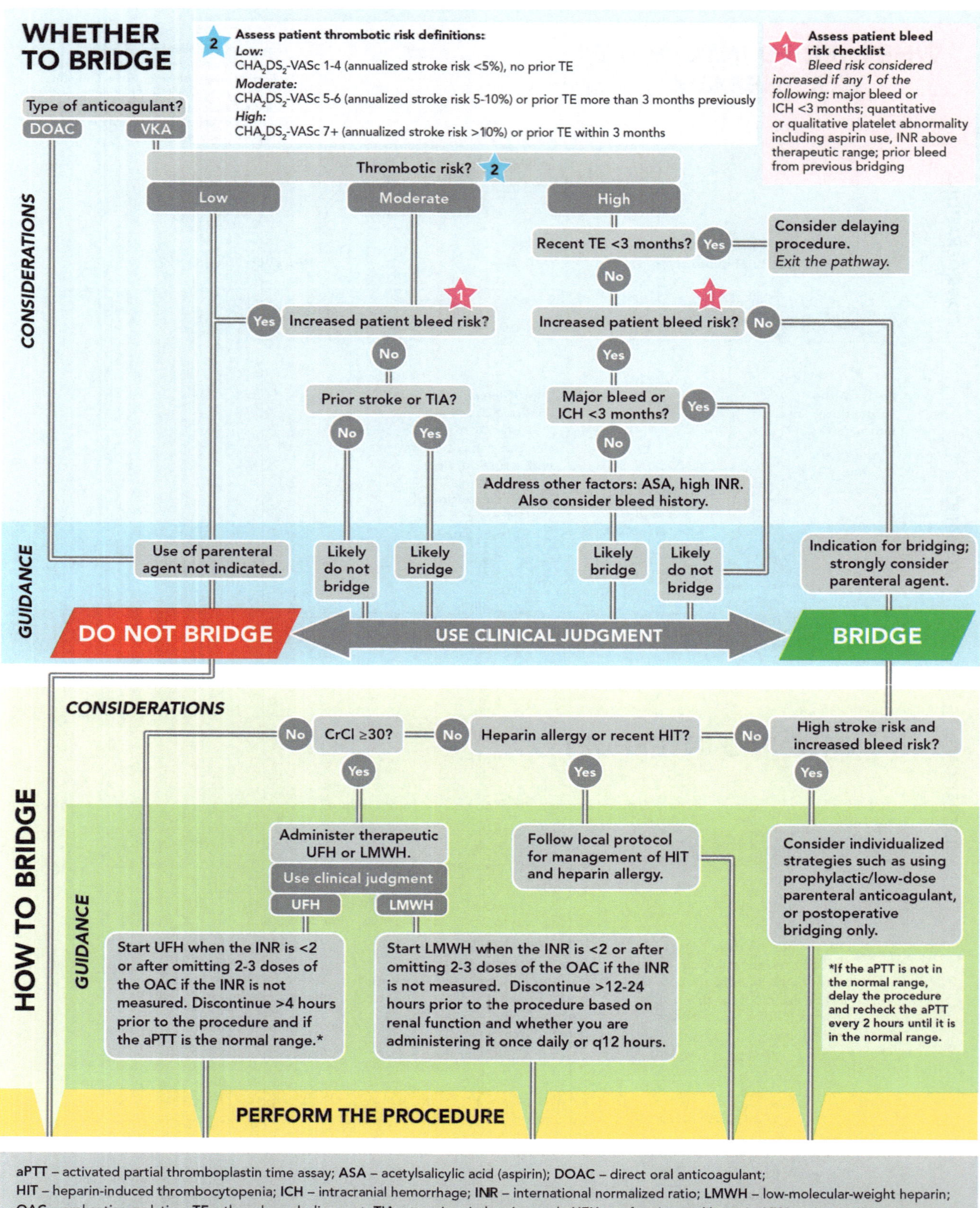

Fig. 6.5 2017 American College of Cardiology Expert Consensus Decision Pathway. Whether and how to bridge (From Doherty et al. [9] with permission Elsevier)

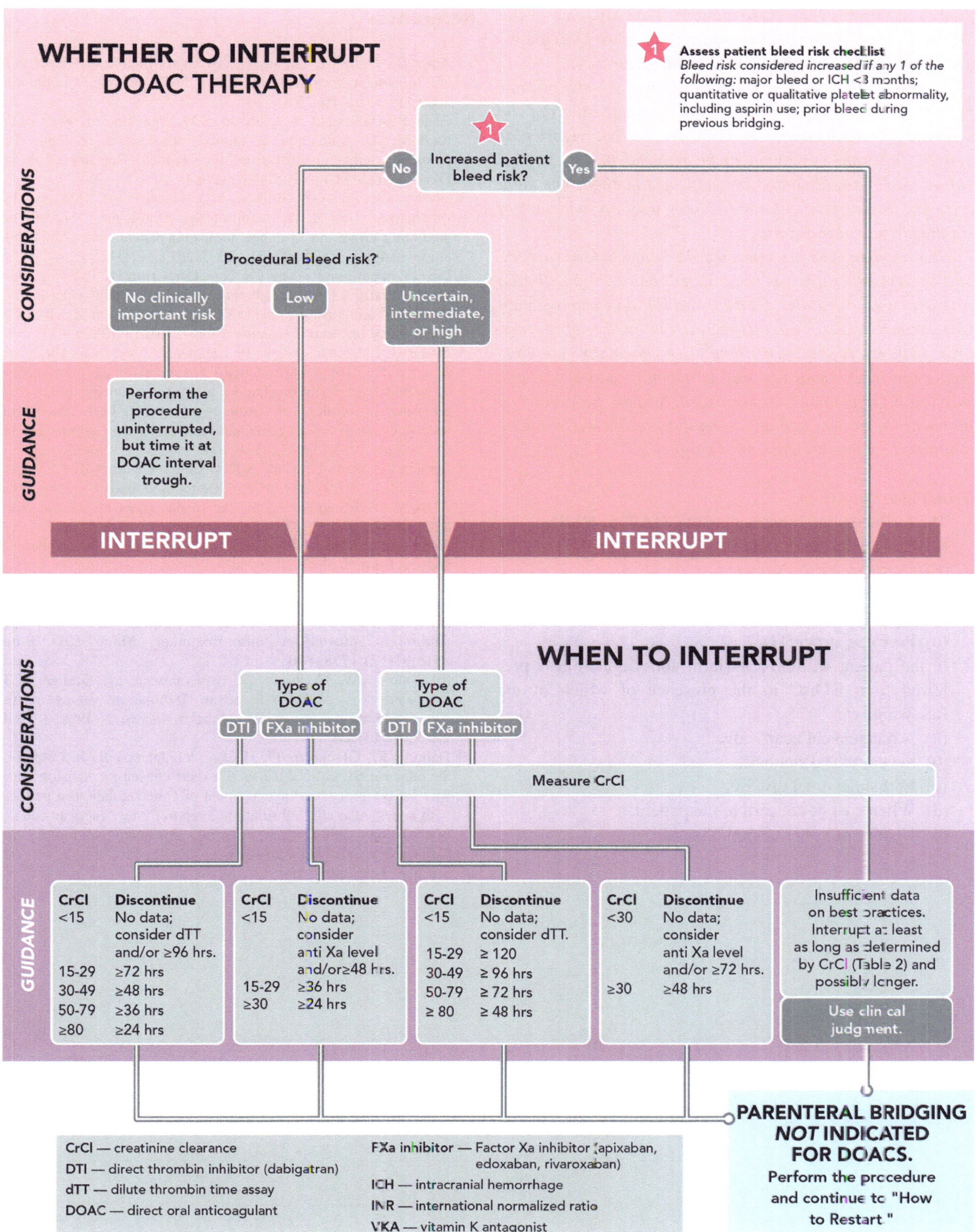

Fig. 6.6 2017 ACC Expert Consensus Decision Pathway. Whether and when to interrupt DOAC therapy (From Doherty et al. [9] with permission Elsevier)

goal is to allow a time equivalent to five half-lives of the DOAC (adjusted for renal function if necessary) to elapse after the last dose of the DOAC prior to surgery.

A repeat TTE was performed preoperatively on our patient to assess left ventricular function and rule out the presence of significant valvular disease. Left ventricular systolic function was found to be reduced to low normal values (50%) as calculated by Simpson's method. The right atrium was severely enlarged. There was no evidence of significant valvular disease.

Rivaroxaban was discontinued 48 hours before surgery, and bridging therapy was not utilized. As atrial fibrillation rate was well controlled with bisoprolol, no further action was deemed necessary in this regard. On the day of surgery, oral hypoglycemics were held (we normally continue metformin when renal function is normal), and a variable rate insulin infusion was commenced. Surgery proceeded as planned; the patient had an uneventful postoperative course and was discharged 4 days after surgery.

True/False Questions

1. The following are components of CHA_2DS_2-VASc
   (a) Congestive heart failure.
   (b) Coronary heart disease.
   (c) Hypertension.
   (d) Age ≥60.
   (e) Previous stroke/TIA.
2. In the patient with AF, warfarin anticoagulation is preferred to a DOAC in the presence of which of the following?
   (a) A mechanical heart valve.
   (b) Severe mitral stenosis.
   (c) End-stage renal disease.
   (d) When cost of concern to the patient.
   (e) History of systemic embolization.

References

1. Anter E, Jessup M, Callans DJ. Atrial fibrillation and heart failure: treatment considerations for a dual epidemic. Circulation. 2009;119(18):2516–25.
2. Gage BF, Waterman AD, Shannon W, Boechler M, Rich MW, Radford MJ. Validation of clinical classification schemes for predicting stroke: results from the National Registry of Atrial Fibrillation. JAMA. 2001;285(22):2864–70.
3. Olesen JB, Lip GY, Hansen ML, Hansen PR, Tolstrup JS, Lindhardsen J, et al. Validation of risk stratification schemes for predicting stroke and thromboembolism in patients with atrial fibrillation: nationwide cohort study. BMJ. 2011;342:d124.
4. Lip GY, Nieuwlaat R, Pisters R, Lane DA, Crijns HJ. Refining clinical risk stratification for predicting stroke and thromboembolism in atrial fibrillation using a novel risk factor-based approach: the euro heart survey on atrial fibrillation. Chest. 2010;137(2):263–72.
5. January CT, Wann LS, Alpert JS, Calkins H, Cigarroa JE, Cleveland JC Jr, et al. 2014 AHA/ACC/HRS guideline for the management of patients with atrial fibrillation: executive summary: a report of the American college of cardiology/American heart association task force on practice guidelines and the heart rhythm society. Circulation. 2014;130(23):2071–104.
6. January CT, Wann LS, Calkins H, Chen LY, Cigarroa JE, Cleveland JC Jr, et al. 2019 AHA/ACC/HRS focused update of the 2014 AHA/ACC/HRS guideline for the management of patients with atrial fibrillation: a report of the American college of cardiology/American heart association task force on clinical practice guidelines and the heart rhythm society in collaboration with the society of thoracic surgeons. Circulation. 2019;140(2):e125–e51.
7. Morin DP, Bernard ML, Madias C, Rogers PA, Thihalolipavan S, Estes NA. The state of the art: atrial fibrillation epidemiology, prevention, and treatment. Mayo Clin Proc. 2016;91(12):1778–810.
8. Eikelboom JW, Connolly SJ, Brueckmann M, Granger CB, Kappetein AP, Mack MJ, et al. Dabigatran versus warfarin in patients with mechanical heart valves. N Engl J Med. 2013;369(13):1206–14.
9. Doherty JU, Gluckman TJ, Hucker WJ, Januzzi JL Jr, Ortel TL, Saxonhouse SJ, et al. 2017 ACC expert consensus decision pathway for periprocedural management of anticoagulation in patients with nonvalvular atrial fibrillation: a report of the American college of cardiology clinical expert consensus document task force. J Am Coll Cardiol. 2017;69(7):871–98.

Aortic Stenosis

7

Derek Dillane

A 77-year-old female scheduled to have a right ankle fusion presented to the anesthesia preadmission clinic 2 weeks prior to surgery. She had previously been diagnosed with aortic stenosis. The most recent echocardiogram had been done 4 years preceding this visit and showed a valve area of 0.9 cm^2, peak gradient across the aortic valve of 45 mm Hg, and a mean gradient of 23 mm Hg. Ejection fraction (EF) was 60%, and left ventricular hypertrophy was identified. Thereafter she had been lost to follow up as she had left the country for an extended period. She was obese with a body weight of 109 kg and BMI 45, hypertensive, and prediabetic. She was noted to have a history of chronic renal insufficiency. She denied any history of presyncope, syncope, or chest pain. She did complain of shortness of breath on exertion and had previously been designated New York Heart Association (NYHA) II.

Medications: Metoprolol, amlodipine, furosemide, dipyridamole/aspirin, levothyroxine, and colchicine.

Physical Examination: A blood pressure of 145/90 was recorded with a resting heart rate of 68 beats per minute. Heart sounds S1 and S2 were decreased in intensity. A grade 3/6 ejection systolic murmur was heard along the right upper sternal border which radiated to the carotid arteries. Jugular venous pressure (JVP) was 5–6 cm, and significant peripheral edema was seen.

Investigations: Laboratory values showed hemoglobin of 108 g/L, platelet count 138 × 10^9/L, sodium 129, creatinine 98, estimated GFR 48, albumin 31, and HbA1C 6.2.

Electrocardiography (ECG) showed sinus bradycardia with 1st degree AV block, left axis deviation, and incomplete left bundle branch block (Fig. 7.1). *Chest radiograph demonstrated mild cardiomegaly.*

What Complications Is the Patient with AS Subject to in the Perioperative Period?

- Myocardial ischemia: The left ventricle responds to chronic outflow obstruction in a gradual, compensatory manner by becoming concentrically hypertrophic [1]. Associated diastolic dysfunction and subsequent decreased coronary perfusion pressure eventually result in myocardial ischemia, i.e., there is inadequate oxygen supply to an enlarged muscle. This is a slow process, and patients can remain asymptomatic for many years. Unmasking of the disease process and sudden decompensation may occur in states of increased cardiac output, e.g., perioperative hemodynamic stress response. A study of over 5000 patients with AS undergoing noncardiac surgery reported a significantly higher incidence of acute myocardial infarction when compared with controls (3.86% vs. 2.03%) [2].
- Heart failure
- Stroke
- Mortality: Due to the large number of heterogeneous patient and surgery factors, there is considerable debate regarding the association – or at any rate the degree of association – between aortic stenosis and increased perioperative mortality. In a large meta-analysis of 29,327 subjects, patients with AS, regardless of severity, were not shown to be at increased risk of mortality when undergoing noncardiac surgery [3]. However, they did have significantly higher rates of adverse cardiovascular events.
- Bleeding: von Willebrand factor abnormalities are common in patients with severe aortic stenosis and are improved by valve replacement [4].

D. Dillane (✉)
Department of Anesthesiology & Pain Medicine, University of Alberta, Edmonton, AB, Canada

D. Dillane, B. A. Finegan (eds.), *Preoperative Assessment*, https://doi.org/10.1007/978-3-030-58842-7_7

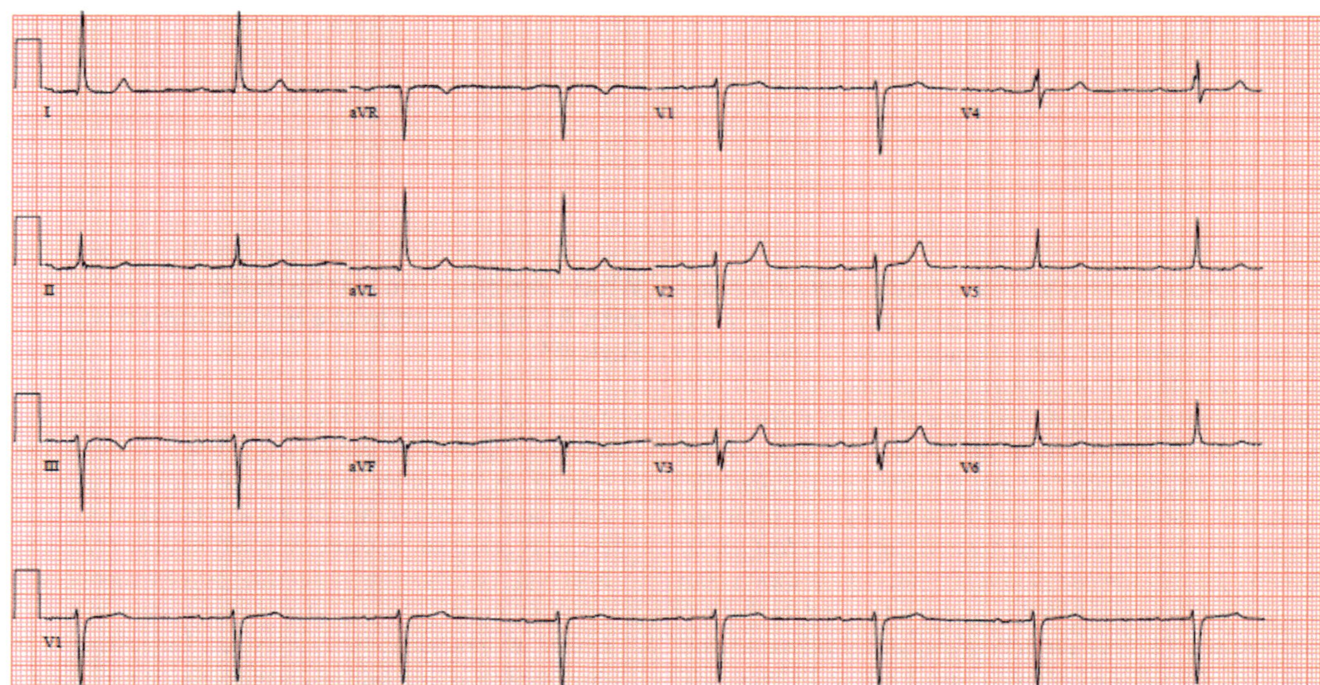

Fig. 7.1 Preoperative ECG showing sinus bradycardia, 1st degree AV block, left axis deviation, and incomplete left bundle branch block

How Should the Patient with AS Be Evaluated Preoperatively?

History and physical examination provide important indicators of disease severity, but echocardiography will be most useful for categorizing the extent of AS and its hemodynamic effects. The complexity of the surgical procedure and associated risks are additional factors to consider.

History

The classic symptoms of AS are those associated with angina, presyncope or syncope, and congestive cardiac failure, i.e., exertional chest pain, dizziness, and dyspnea on exertion. Angina is the first to appear in 50–75% of AS patients, but only 25–50% of these patients have coronary artery disease [5]. Life expectancy, in the untreated patient, is typically 5 years after onset of angina, 3 years after onset of syncope, and 2 years after development of cardiac failure.

Physical Exam

When undiagnosed, findings suggestive of AS include ejection systolic murmur, reduced intensity of the second heart sound, and a carotid pulse with a slow rate of rise and reduced peak [1].

Findings associated with cardiac failure should be recorded at the preoperative visit.

Investigations

Transthoracic echocardiography Recommended in patients with clinical evidence of moderate to severe AS who have not had an echocardiogram within 1 year or if there has been a significant clinical change since the last echocardiographic examination [6].

Coronary angiography Time-permitting, recommended in patients with symptomatic chest pain to distinguish between obstructive coronary artery disease and supply/demand imbalance secondary to compensatory myocardial hypertrophy.

ECG Useful for diagnosis of left ventricular hypertrophy, ischemia, conduction abnormalities, and arrhythmias.

What Is the Etiology of AS?

AS is either congenital or acquired. A congenital bicuspid (rather than the normal tricuspid) valve may become calcified in adults. A normal tricuspid aortic valve can become degeneratively calcified with age. Rheumatic aortic valve disease is usually associated with mitral valve disease.

How Is the Severity of AS Categorized?

AS is classified as mild, moderate, or severe. Aortic valve area, mean and peak pressure gradient across the aortic valve, as well as jet velocity can be used to assess severity (Table 7.1) [7]. Patients with a low ejection fraction and severe AS will have a small transvalvular pressure gradient and subsequently are at risk for underestimation of disease severity

Which Patients with AS Are Considered Candidates for Surgical Repair/Replacement?

The need for aortic valve replacement (AVR) is determined by taking account of (1) whether the patient is symptomatic, (2) severity of disease, and (3) left ventricular ejection fraction (LVEF).

Surgery should be offered to patients with symptomatic severe AS (mean pressure gradient >40 mm Hg). Patients with asymptomatic severe AS with LVEF <50% or having other cardiac surgery should also be offered AVR surgery. Patients with asymptomatic severe AS and an abnormal exercise tolerance test are reasonable candidates for surgery (Fig. 7.2) [7].

Patients with moderate AS (mean pressure gradient 20–39 mm Hg) who are asymptomatic are considered surgical candidates only if having other cardiac surgery. Patients with moderate AS who are symptomatic are considered for surgery if LVEF <50% and/or valve area is <1 cm^2.

Patients may proceed to transcatheter aortic valve implantation if suitable, rather than open surgery requiring cardiopulmonary bypass.

Table 7.1 Stages of the severity of aortic stenosis [7]

Stage	Disease severity	Hemodynamics	Cardiac function	Symptoms
A	At risk of AS, e.g., bicuspid aortic valve or aortic sclerosis	Normal	Normal	None
B	Progressive AS	Mild AS: mean ΔP <20 mmHg Moderate AS: mean ΔP 20–39 mmHg	Possible early LV diastolic dysfunction Normal LVEF	None
C1	Asymptomatic severe	Mean ΔP ≥40 mmHg AVA ≤1.0 cm^2	LV diastolic dysfunction Mild LV hypertrophy Normal LVEF	None: exercise testing can confirm
C2	Asymptomatic severe with LV dysfunction	Mean ΔP ≥40 mmHg AVA ≤1.0 cm^2	LVEF <50%	None
D1	Symptomatic severe high gradient	Mean ΔP ≥40 mmHg AVA ≤1.0 cm^2 Aortic Vmax ≥4 m/s	LV diastolic dysfunction LV hypertrophy	Exertional dyspnea or decreased exercise tolerance Exertional angina Exertional syncope or presyncope
D2	Symptomatic severe low gradient with reduced LVEF	AVA ≤1.0 cm^2 Aortic Vmax <4 m/s	LV diastolic dysfunction LV hypertrophy LVEF <50%	HF Angina Syncope or presyncope
D3	Symptomatic severe low gradient with normal LVEF or paradoxical low-flow severe	AVA ≤1.0 cm^2 with aortic Vmax <4 m/s or mean ΔP <40 mmHg	Increased LV relative wall thickness Restrictive diastolic filling LVEF ≥50%	HF Angina Syncope or presyncope

AS aortic stenosis, *AVA* aortic valve area, *HF* heart failure, *LV* left ventricular, *LVEF* left ventricular ejection fraction, *ΔP* pressure gradient, *Vmax* maximum aortic velocity

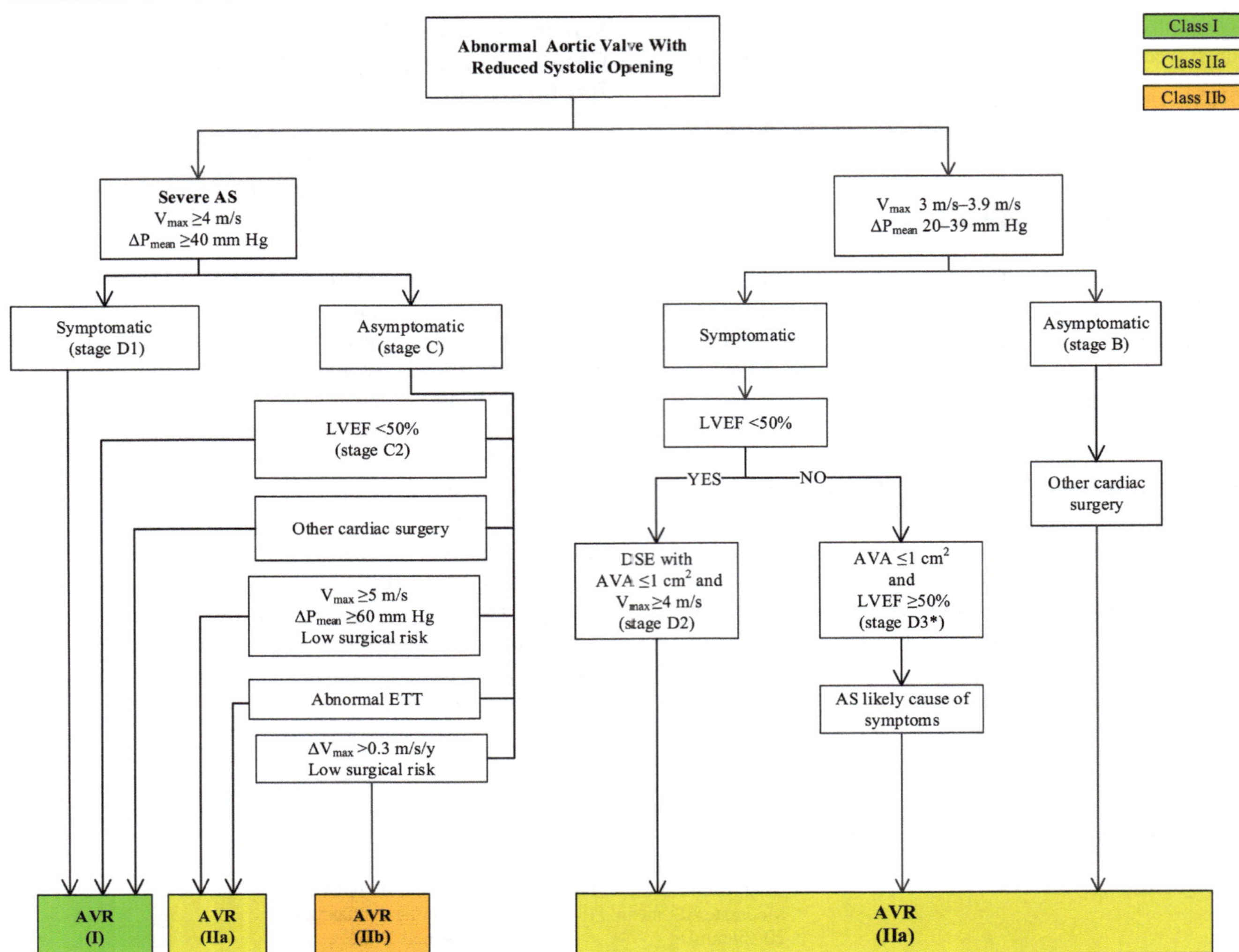

Fig. 7.2 Indications for aortic valve replacement in patients with aortic stenosis. AS aortic stenosis, AVA aortic valve area, AVR aortic valve replacement by either surgical or transcatheter approach, BP blood pressure, DSE dobutamine stress echocardiography, ETT exercise treadmill test, LVEF left ventricular ejection fraction, ΔPmean mean pressure gradient, and Vmax maximum velocity. Class of recommendation I: procedure should be performed. Class of recommendation IIa: it is reasonable to perform the procedure. Class IIb: procedure may be considered (From Nishimura et al. [7], with permission from Elsevier)

What Are the Reasons for Not Replacing a Severely Stenotic Valve Prior to Noncardiac Surgery?

- Very short life expectancy
- Lack of symptoms related to AS and patient aware and willing to accept the increased perioperative risk
- Emergency noncardiac surgery or cancer surgery
- Patient refusal of AVR procedure

What Potentially Modifiable Conditions Associated with AS Should Be Considered/Optimized in This Patient Prior to Surgery?

Coexisting *coronary artery disease* (CAD) has been reported as being significantly greater in patients with AS compared with controls (54.7% vs 34.4%) [8]. Patients with concomitant CAD and AS may represent a particularly high-risk group who are at increased risk for perioperative adverse outcomes including acute myocardial infarction [3].

Arrhythmias can be associated with hemodynamic decompensation in patients with AS. Atrial contraction normally contributes approximately 15–20% to stroke volume. This increases to 40–50% in AS patients where reduced left ventricular compliance secondary to hypertrophy leads to reduced passive diastolic filling. A heart rate of 70–80 beats per minute is targeted, slow enough for diastolic filling and fast enough to maintain cardiac output even with a fixed reduced stroke volume.

Is Spinal Anesthesia an Option for This Patient?

The sympatholysis associated with spinal anesthesia may cause decreased systemic vascular resistance with subsequent reduced coronary perfusion pressure, myocardial ischemia, and systemic hypotension. While single shot spinal anesthesia is not absolutely contraindicated, the successful and safe use of more gradual techniques, e.g., continuous spinal or epidural blockade, has been previously described [9, 10] and may be more prudent in this case.

What Is the Significance of Prediabetes in This Patient?

Prediabetes is an intermediate state between normoglycemia and diabetes. It includes patients with impaired glucose tolerance, impaired fasting glucose, and mildly raised hemoglobin A1C. It is associated with an increased risk of all-cause mortality and cardiovascular disease [11]. The mainstay of treatment is lifestyle modification.

As this patient's most recent echocardiogram was 4 years old, transthoracic echocardiography was repeated shortly after this preadmission clinic visit. This showed severe aortic stenosis (AS) with peak and mean pressure gradients across the aortic valve of 74 mm Hg and 45 mm Hg, respectively, and an aortic valve area by continuity equation of 0.8 cm^2. Moderate diastolic dysfunction was noted. Left ventricle size and wall thickness were within normal limits. Left ventricular systolic function was judged to be normal with an EF greater than 55%. Putting this altogether, our patient had asymptomatic severe AS with normal left ventricular function. She was advised of the risks of proceeding but was adamant she wanted to have the surgery. She underwent general anesthesia for her ankle surgery. Her perioperative course was uneventful, and she was discharged home 5 days after surgery. As recommended in the 2014 AHA/ACC Guideline for the Management of Patients with Valvular Heart Disease, periodic monitoring of her AS continued in this patient postoperatively. She became symptomatic 6 months after her ankle surgery and proceeded to have an AVR at this time [7].

True/False Questions

1. The following are clinical elements associated with AS
   (a) Normal S2.
   (b) Dyspnea on exertion.
   (c) Pansystolic murmur.
   (d) Fainting episodes.
   (e) Atrial fibrillation.
2. Regarding severity of AS
   (a) Disease severity is best assessed using dobutamine stress test.
   (b) Severe disease is frequently present in the absence of symptoms.
   (c) Patients with a low EF and severe AS are at risk of overestimation of disease severity.
   (d) A mean pressure gradient across the aortic valve of greater than 20 mm Hg is considered severe AS.
   (e) Patients with asymptomatic severe AS and LVEF <50% are candidates for surgery.

References

1. Vaishnava P, Eagle K. Noncardiac surgery in patients with aortic stenosis. In: Post TW, editor. UpToDate. Waltham: UpToDate; 2020.
2. Zahid M, Sonel AF, Saba S, Good CB. Perioperative risk of noncardiac surgery associated with aortic stenosis. Am J Cardiol. 2005;96(3):436–8.
3. Kwok CS, Bagur R, Rashid M, Lavi R, Cibelli M, de Belder MA, et al. Aortic stenosis and non-cardiac surgery: a systematic review and meta-analysis. Int J Cardiol. 2017;240:145–53.
4. Vincentelli A, Susen S, Le Tourneau T, Six I, Fabre O, Juthier F, et al. Acquired von Willebrand syndrome in aortic stenosis. N Engl J Med. 2003;349(4):343–9.
5. Reed AP. Clinical cases in anesthesia. 2nd ed. New York: Churchill Livingstone; 1995.
6. Fleisher LA, Fleischmann KE, Auerbach AD, Barnason SA, Beckman JA, Bozkurt B, et al. 2014 ACC/AHA guideline on perioperative cardiovascular evaluation and management of patients undergoing noncardiac surgery: a report of the American College of Cardiology/American Heart Association Task Force on Practice Guidelines. Circulation. 2014;130(24):e278–333.
7. Nishimura RA, Otto CM, Bonow RO, Carabello BA, Erwin JP 3rd, Guyton RA, et al. 2014 AHA/ACC guideline for the management of patients with valvular heart disease: executive summary: a report of the American College of Cardiology/American Heart Association Task Force on Practice Guidelines. J Am Coll Cardiol. 2014;63(22):2438–88. Erratum in: J Am Coll Cardiol. 2014;63(22):2489.
8. Tashiro T, Pislaru SV, Blustin JM, Nkomo VT, Abel MD, Scott CG, et al. Perioperative risk of major non-cardiac surgery in patients with severe aortic stenosis: a reappraisal in contemporary practice. Eur Heart J. 2014;35(35):2372–81.
9. Collard CD, Eappen S, Lynch EP, Concepcion M. Continuous spinal anesthesia with invasive hemodynamic monitoring for surgical repair of the hip in two patients with severe aortic stenosis. Anesth Analg. 1995;81(1):195–8.
10. Ho MC, Beathe JC, Sharrock NE. Hypotensive epidural anesthesia in patients with aortic stenosis undergoing total hip replacement. Reg Anesth Pain Med. 2008;33(2):129–33.
11. Huang Y, Cai X, Mai W, Li M, Hu Y. Association between prediabetes and risk of cardiovascular disease and all cause mortality: systematic review and meta-analysis. BMJ. 2016;355:i5953.

Pulmonary Hypertension

8

Barry A. Finegan

A 55-year-old female presented for elective cholecystectomy. Apart from three episodes of abdominal pain over the last year, she indicated that she had never been in hospital or seen a physician since she was a child. On standard questioning about her exercise tolerance, she indicated that she had a relatively sedentary lifestyle, working as a mid-level executive for a logistics provider. She had, however, noticed that she was somewhat more tired than usual. Ascending the two flights of stairs to her office downtown had become more difficult over the last year, leaving her quite breathless (NYHA Class II). She attributed these changes to her gallbladder disease, because before these events, she had been "totally fine." She denied any syncopal episodes but had experienced bouts of chest pain unrelated to exercise in the last year. She was a nonsmoker. Systems review was otherwise noncontributory. She had no previous operative procedures and was on no medications. She had no allergies. She denied ingestion of street drugs or any herbal compounds.

Physical Examination: There was no evidence of central cyanosis, but the patient had obvious signs of Raynaud's phenomenon peripherally in both upper limbs. Inspection of her jugular venous pressure (JVP) revealed a prominent v wave. Her pulse was regular and of normal volume. Her pulse rate was 76/min, respiratory rate 14/min, and BP 155/80. Oxygen saturation on room air was 95%.

Auscultation of the heart revealed normal S_1 and a loud S_2, the latter being particularly noticeable on auscultation over the left sternal border at the second intercostal space. A soft holosystolic (III/VI) and brief early diastolic murmur was heard over the left lower sternal border augmented during inspiration. Otherwise, her examination was unremarkable.

Investigations: The ECG showed evidence of sinus tachycardia, right axis deviation, and right ventricular hypertrophy (Fig. 8.1). CXR demonstrated cardiomegaly, prominent central pulmonary arteries, and mild peripheral hypovascularity (Fig. 8.2).

A BNP was ordered and revealed a raised level of 420 pg/ml. These data in tandem with the symptoms and signs, confirmed a diagnosis of heart failure.

A subsequent urgent echocardiogram was requested which demonstrated severe right ventricular (RV) enlargement and a shift of the intraventricular septum toward the D-shaped left ventricle (LV). The measured tricuspid regurgitant velocity (TRV) was 4 m/sec (normal TRV ≤2.5 m/sec). Estimated PA systolic (PAPs) and mean (PAPm) pressures were 100 and 63 mmHg, respectively. A dilated inferior vena cava was seen in the subcostal view.

What Are the Symptoms/Signs That Might Suggest the Presence of Severe PAH?

Presentation is nonspecific, but symptoms of right heart failure are usually predominant – dyspnea, fatigue, angina-like chest pain, and syncope.

Physical signs include left parasternal lift, loud S_2, a tricuspid regurgitant murmur, elevated JVP, hepatomegaly, and ankle edema [1].

What Is the Definition of PAH?

PAH is said to be present when PAPm is ≥25 mmHg at rest when *measured directly* via *right heart catheterization* [2]. The upper resting value for normal PAPm is 20 mmHg (usual range 9–18 mmHg). PAPm is calculated by using the following equation:

$$(\text{PA systolic pressure} + [2 \times \text{PA diastolic pressure}])/3$$

B. A. Finegan (✉)
Department of Anesthesiology & Pain Medicine, University of Alberta, Edmonton, AB, Canada
e-mail: bfinegan@ualberta.ca

D. Dillane, B. A. Finegan (eds.), *Preoperative Assessment*, https://doi.org/10.1007/978-3-030-58842-7_8

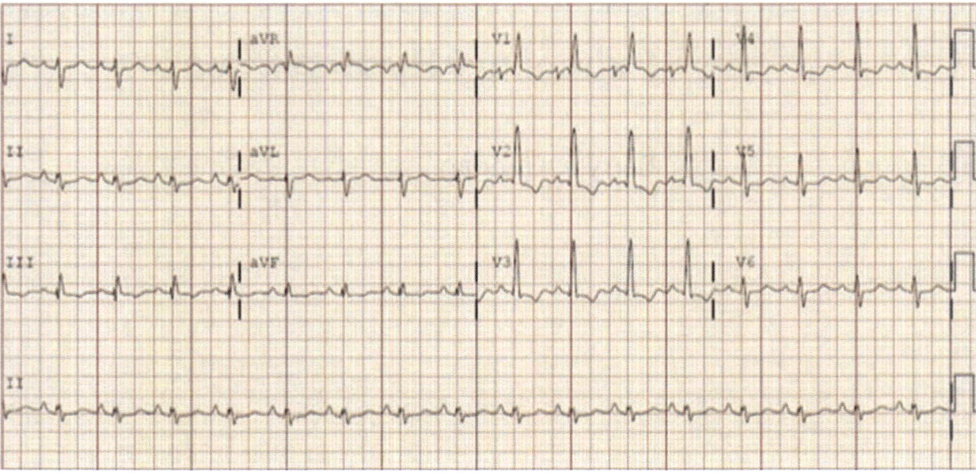

Fig. 8.1 Electrocardiogram showing evidence sinus tachycardia, right axis deviation, and right ventricular hypertrophy

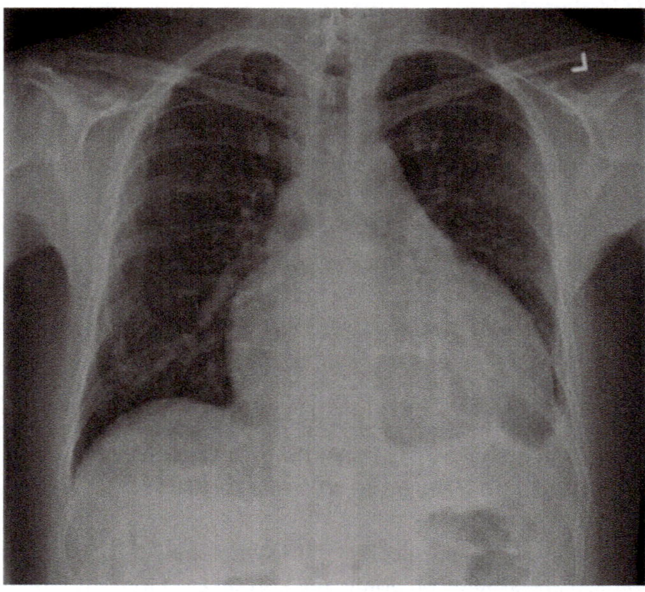

Fig. 8.2 Chest radiograph showing cardiomegaly, prominent central pulmonary arteries, and mild peripheral hypovascularity

How Should "Elevated" PAP Reported in a Routine Echocardiogram Be Interpreted?

Echocardiography is a vital noninvasive screening and diagnostic tool in the assessment of cardiac function and hemodynamics. As part of a complete echocardiographic examination, estimated PAP values (using validated formulas) are reported if the quality of the study and appropriate Doppler-/2D-derived data can be obtained. While the sensitivity of Doppler echocardiography in estimating PAP is adequate, specificity/accuracy is relatively low when compared to direct measurement during right heart catheterization [3]. This is particularly true in the presence of severe tricuspid regurgitation where there is a very high likelihood (>50%) of overestimating PAPm [4]. In interpreting Doppler-derived elevated values of PAP, clinical correlates and other 2D echocardiographic findings suggestive of RV chronic pressure overload (dilated/rounded right atrium (RA), PA enlargement, RV dilatation/dysfunction, and D-shaped LV) should be sought to support a potential diagnosis of PAH. It is generally agreed that echocardiographic-derived estimated PAPs values of <40 mmHg, in the absence of any other clinical or echocardiographic findings suggestive of PAH, are reassuring and in most cases obviate the need for invasive right heart catheterization [5].

What Are the Causes of PH?

Multiple pathophysiological processes can lead to the development of PH (Fig. 8.3) [6]. A clinical classification of PH into groups that share characteristics and management has been developed by the World Symposium on Pulmonary Hypertension Group [7]. The groups are outlined as follows:

- *Group 1. Pulmonary arterial hypertension (PAH)*
  - Can be idiopathic, heritable, drug-/toxin-induced, or associated with connective tissue disease and multiple other disorders.
  - PAH patients have precapillary PH. This is characterized by PAPm ≥25 mmHg at rest, an end-expiratory pulmonary wedge pressure (PAWP) ≤15 mmHg, and pulmonary vascular resistance (PVR) >3 Woods units (WU). WU is calculated using the equation: PAPs – PAWP/cardiac output (CO) expressed in l/min. A PVR >3 WU is considered abnormal [3].
- *Group 2. Pulmonary hypertension due to left heart disease*
  - These patients have postcapillary PH.
  - Postcapillary PH is characterized hemodynamically by PAPm ≥25 and PAWP >15 mmHg

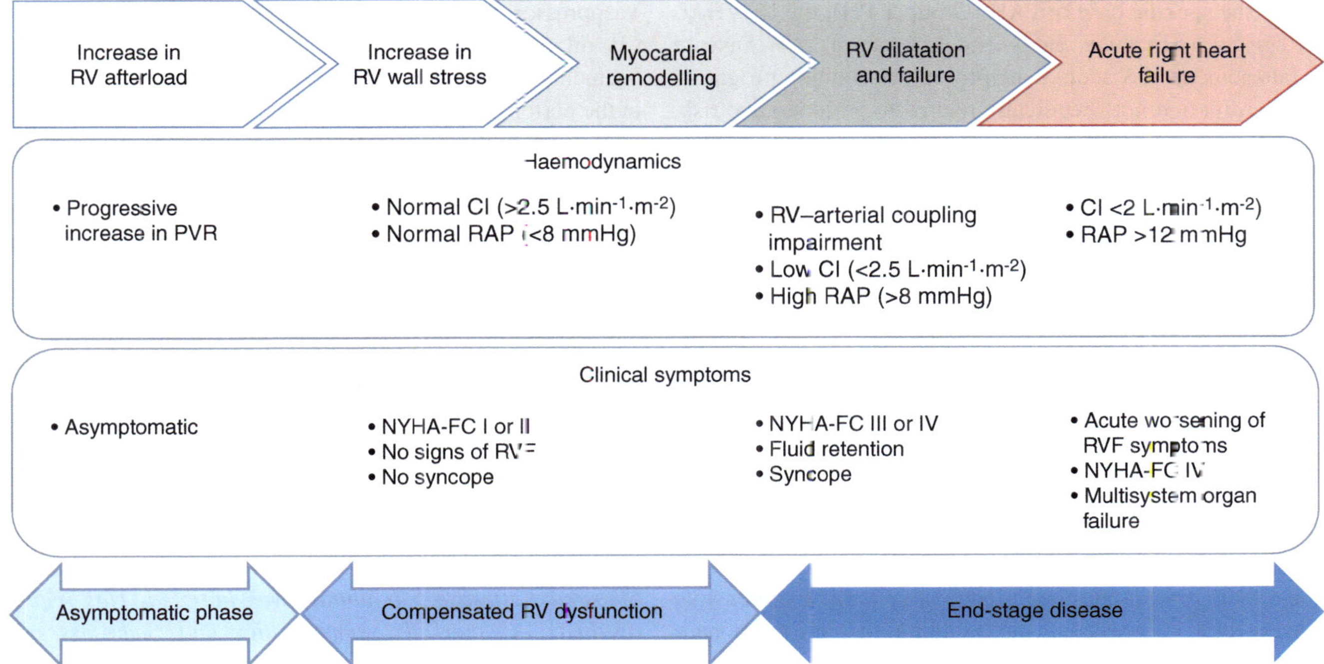

Fig. 8.3 Gradual evolution toward end-stage pulmonary hypertension (*RV* right ventricle, *PVR* pulmonary vascular resistance, *CI* cardiac index, *RAP* right atrial pressure, *NYHA-FC* New York Heart Association functional class, *RV* right ventricular failure) (From Savale et al. [6], Reproduced with permission of the © ERS 2020: European Respiratory Review 26 (146) 170092; DOI: https://doi.org/10.1183/16000617.0092-2017 Published 15 November 2017)

- *Group 3. Pulmonary hypertension due to lung disease/hypoxia*
  - These patients have precapillary PH.
- *Group 4. Chronic thromboembolic pulmonary hypertension*
  - These patients have precapillary PH.
- *Group 5. Pulmonary hypertension with unclear multifactorial mechanisms*
  - These patients have mixed pre-/postcapillary PH.

What Are the Treatment Options for Patients with PH?

There are specific medications directed at patients who fall into Groups 1 and 4. There are no specific therapies other than management of the underlying disease state responsible for the development of PH for Groups 2, 3, and 5.

In Group 1 patients, as in this case, the goal is to achieve improved exercise capacity, quality of life, and good RV function [2]. Pharmacological therapy aimed at the three signaling pathways currently known to be involved in the development of PAH is the mainstay of management. Drugs are available to target the prostacyclin pathway (proteinoids), the endothelin pathway (endothelin receptor antagonists), and the nitric oxide (NO) pathway (phosphodiesterase 5 inhibitors and soluble guanylate cyclase stimulators). Combination therapy directed at these pathways is becoming standard [8].

In Group 4, patients' lifelong anticoagulant therapy is recommended, and, if technically operable and has a suitable risk/benefit outcome, pulmonary endarterectomy is an appropriate option. Balloon pulmonary angioplasty is a less invasive option for nonsurgical candidates. The ultimate surgical intervention is lung transplantation. Medical care includes anticoagulants, diuretics, and O_2.

Is This Patient at "Normal" Risk for Elective Surgery?

PAH is associated with an increased risk of death or adverse outcome during the perioperative period. A recent single-center retrospective review detailed a morbidity of 27% and a 30-day mortality of 5.4% associated with noncardiac surgery in patients with PAH [9].

Reassuringly, in the context of this patient, an adverse outcome is usually associated with emergency surgery, advanced NYHA functional classification, and the presence of coexisting cardiac and renal disease [9]. With current multidisciplinary management of PAH, patients with advanced disease, if functionally stable, can undergo elective surgery reasonably safely.

In the specific case of PAH (Group 1 PH), the REVEAL (Registry to Evaluate Early and Long-term PAH Disease Management) risk score is helpful in determining prognosis [10]. Although not specifically related to perioperative risk, it is clear that overall prognosis is diminished in the presence of deteriorating functional status, abnormally high resting heart rate, systolic hypotension, and elevated BNP levels. The presence of any of these should prompt pause and reconsideration of proceeding with elective surgery.

Should Regional Anesthesia Be Discussed as an Option for Patients with PH?

It is generally agreed that, if the choice is available, peripheral regional anesthesia (PRA)/monitored anesthetic care (MAC) should be the preferred route of anesthetic management for patients with PH. The unique benefits of PRA/MAC (avoiding general anesthetic-induced systemic hypotension, myocardial depression, and alteration in pulmonary ventilation-perfusion [V/Q] status) should be emphasized. However, in the case of PH associated with lung disease, impaired pulmonary function could preclude the use of a supraclavicular block, given the known risk of temporary phrenic nerve paralysis with this approach.

Central neuraxial blockade can be accompanied by preload and afterload reduction of the right ventricle and, in the case of thoracic epidural or high spinal anesthesia, inhibition of the enhanced cardiac sympathetic tone that forms part of the adaptive response to PH. Nevertheless, appropriately performed and monitored, this mode of anesthesia is recommended over general anesthesia if this is a feasible option [1].

How Should This Patient's Medications Be Managed Preoperatively?

Pulmonary vasodilator therapy should be continued up to and after the day of the procedure.

What Is the Preferred Location to Perform Elective Invasive Surgery in Patients with Severe PH?

Patients with PH who fall into World Health Organization (WHO) Functional Assessment for Pulmonary Hypertension Class III (marked limitation of physical activity, less than ordinary activity causing undue dyspnea or fatigue) or IV (inability to carry out any physical activity without symptoms; dyspnea and fatigue may even be present at rest) are particularly challenging to manage intraoperatively. Vasopressor (vasopressin/norepinephrine), pulmonary artery vasodilator therapy (NO/epoprostenol), and inotropic management of right heart failure are not infrequently employed in the perioperative period.

Surgery in these patients should be performed in a center where expertise and resources are immediately available to manage an acute deterioration in functional status, up to and including the use of right ventricular assist devices and extracorporeal membrane oxygenation (ECMO).

The patient's echocardiographic findings were compatible with a diagnosis of severe pulmonary hypertension (PAH). The patient was urgently referred to cardiology for further assessment and treatment. Surgery was deferred.

She underwent a full work up, including right heart catherization and assessment of vasoreactivity. Pulmonary arterial hypertension (Group 1) secondary to systemic sclerosis was the final diagnosis. Treatment with ambrisentan (an endothelin type A receptor inhibitor) and tadalafil (phosphodiesterase 5 inhibitor) was initiated. This regime resulted in marked symptomatic and echo-assessed hemodynamic improvement. The patient was rebooked for surgery and returned for reevaluation.

She reported remarkable improvement in exercise function (NYHA Class I) and was no longer in heart failure. A repeat BNP value was 45 pg/ml and an echocardiogram performed 2 weeks before the assessment visit revealed a tricuspid regurgitant velocity (TRV) of 2.1 m/sec, a calculated PAPs value of 58 mmHg, and a PAPm of 37 mmHg. The patient indicated that she could carry out normal activities without limitation and had no recent episodes of chest pain or syncope.

The patient was transferred to a center with expertise in PAH management and underwent cholecystectomy under general anesthesia without incident. She was monitored for 24 hours postoperatively in an intermediate care unit. She was discharged at 72 hours postoperatively, having been able to tolerate oral medication for 36 hours.

True/False Questions

1. In a patient with suspected PAH
   (a) Symptoms may include gradual onset of dyspnea.
   (b) A tricuspid regurgitant murmur is frequently heard.
   (c) An estimated PAPm obtained by Doppler echocardiography of 35 mmHg is diagnostic.
   (d) The diagnosis is ruled out if the PAPm by heart catherization is <25 mmHg.
   (e) Thromboembolic disease may coexist.
2. A patient with PAH presenting for surgery
   (a) A normal resting heart rate is reassuring.
   (b) BNP determination is helpful in assessment.
   (c) Pulmonary vasodilator therapy should be held on the day of surgery to avoid hypotension.

(d) Regional anesthesia is usually preferable to general anesthesia.
(e) A supraclavicular block is always preferred for upper limb procedures.

References

1. Galiè N, Humbert M, Vachiery JL, Gibbs S, Lang I, Torbicki A, ESC Scientific Document Group, et al. 2015 ESC/ERS guidelines for the diagnosis and treatment of pulmonary hypertension: The Joint Task Force for the Diagnosis and Treatment of Pulmonary Hypertension of the European Society of Cardiology (ESC) and the European Respiratory Society (ERS): Endorsed by: Association for European Paediatric and Congenital Cardiology (AEPC), International Society for Heart and Lung Transplantation (ISHLT). Eur Heart J. 2016;37(1):67–119.
2. Hoeper MM, Bogaard HJ, Condliffe R, Frantz R, Khanna D, Kurzyna M, et al. Definitions and diagnosis of pulmonary hypertension. J Am Coll Cardiol. 2013;62(25 Suppl):D42–50.
3. Taleb M, Khuder S, Tinkel J, Khouri SJ. The diagnostic accuracy of doppler echocardiography in assessment of pulmonary artery systolic pressure: a meta-analysis. Echocardiography. 2013;30(3):258–65.
4. Özpelit E, Akdeniz B, Özpelit EM, Tas S, Alpaslan E, Bozkurt S, et al. Impact of severe tricuspid regurgitation on accuracy of echocardiographic pulmonary artery systolic pressure estimation. Echocardiography. 2015;32(10):1483–90.
5. Ahmed M, Dweik RA, Tonelli AR. What is the best approach to a high systolic pulmonary artery pressure on echocardiography? Cleve Clin J Med. 2016;83(4):256–60.
6. Savale L, Weatherald J, Jaïs X, Vuillard C, Boucly A, Jevnikar M, et al. Acute decompensated pulmonary hypertension. Eur Respir Rev. 2017;26(146):170092.
7. Simonneau G, Gatzoulis MA, Adatia I, Celermajer D, Denton C, Ghofrani A, et al. Updated clinical classification of pulmonary hypertension. J Am Coll Cardiol. 2013;62(25 Suppl):D34–41.
8. Sundaram SM, Chung L. An update on systemic sclerosis-associated pulmonary arterial hypertension: a review of the current literature. Curr Rheumatol Rep. 2018;20(2):10.
9. Díaz-Gómez JL, Ripoll JG, Mira-Avendano I, Moss JE, Divertie GD, Frank RD, Burger CD. Multidisciplinary perioperative management of pulmonary arterial hypertension in patients undergoing noncardiac surgery. South Med J. 2018;111(1):64–73.
10. Raina A, Humbert M. Risk assessment in pulmonary arterial hypertension. Eur Respir Rev. 2016;25(142):390–8.

Cardiac Implantable Electronic Devices

9

Derek Dillane

A 93-year-old man with a history of complete heart block presented to the anesthesia preoperative assessment clinic 1 day prior to a transurethral resection of the prostate (TURP) for benign prostatic hyperplasia. He had a dual-chamber pacemaker for an unknown period of time. He was unaware of when the device was last interrogated. The medical notes indicated that the generator had been replaced 7 years prior to this visit. He had longstanding hypertension, glaucoma, and back pain. As expected, he led a very sedentary lifestyle, and mobility was limited. Metabolic equivalent capability was estimated at no greater than 2.5, i.e., not capable of anything greater than the activities of daily living.

Medications: Irbesartan, tamsulosin, hydrochlorothiazide, and timolol maleate/travoprost ophthalmic drops.

Physical Examination: Blood pressure was 118/62 mmHg. Radial artery pulse examination revealed a heart rate of 68 bpm with a regular rhythm. Oxygen saturation was 95% on room air. Ele.ctrocardiogram and chest radiograph can be seen in Figs. 9.1 and 9.2.

Investigations: Laboratory values revealed a hemoglobin of 136 g/L, platelet count 196 × 10^9/L, white blood cell count (WBC) 15.5 × 10^9/L, sodium (Na) 138 mmol/L, potassium (K) 3.9 mmol/L, creatinine 102 umol/L, and estimated glomerular filtration rate (eGFR) 54 ml/min/1.73 m^2. Prothrombin time (INR) was 1.0 and partial thromboplastin time (PTT) 32.

An echocardiogram was not available.

What Is a Cardiac Implantable Electronic Device (CIED)?

There are two main categories of CIED that we are concerned about in the perioperative period: pacemaker devices and implantable defibrillators.

What Are the Indications for Permanent Cardiac Pacing?

The American College of Cardiology Foundation/American Heart Association and the European Society of Cardiology/European Heart Rhythm Association have developed guidelines for pacemaker implantation that discuss indications for permanent pacing in considerable detail [1, 2]. The most common indication is *persistent symptomatic* bradycardia secondary to sinus node disease or symptomatic atrioventricular (AV) block, e.g., complete or third-degree heart block and symptomatic Mobitz I or II second-degree heart block. Patients with *intermittent* bradycardia secondary to sinus node disease, paroxysmal AV block, reflex asystolic syncope, and asymptomatic pauses (>6 s) are usually considered for pacemaker therapy.

What Do the Letters of the Pacemaker Code Signify?

The North American Society of Pacing and Electrophysiology (NASPE)/British Pacing and Electrophysiology Group (BPEG) device coding system is universally accepted. There are five letters to the pacemaker code. Only the first three are commonly used (Table 9.1) [3]. The first letter describes the chamber being paced (*A = atrium, V = ventricle, D = dual*).

D. Dillane (✉)
Department of Anesthesiology & Pain Medicine, University of Alberta, Edmonton, AB, Canada

D. Dillane, B. A. Finegan (eds.), *Preoperative Assessment*, https://doi.org/10.1007/978-3-030-58842-7_9

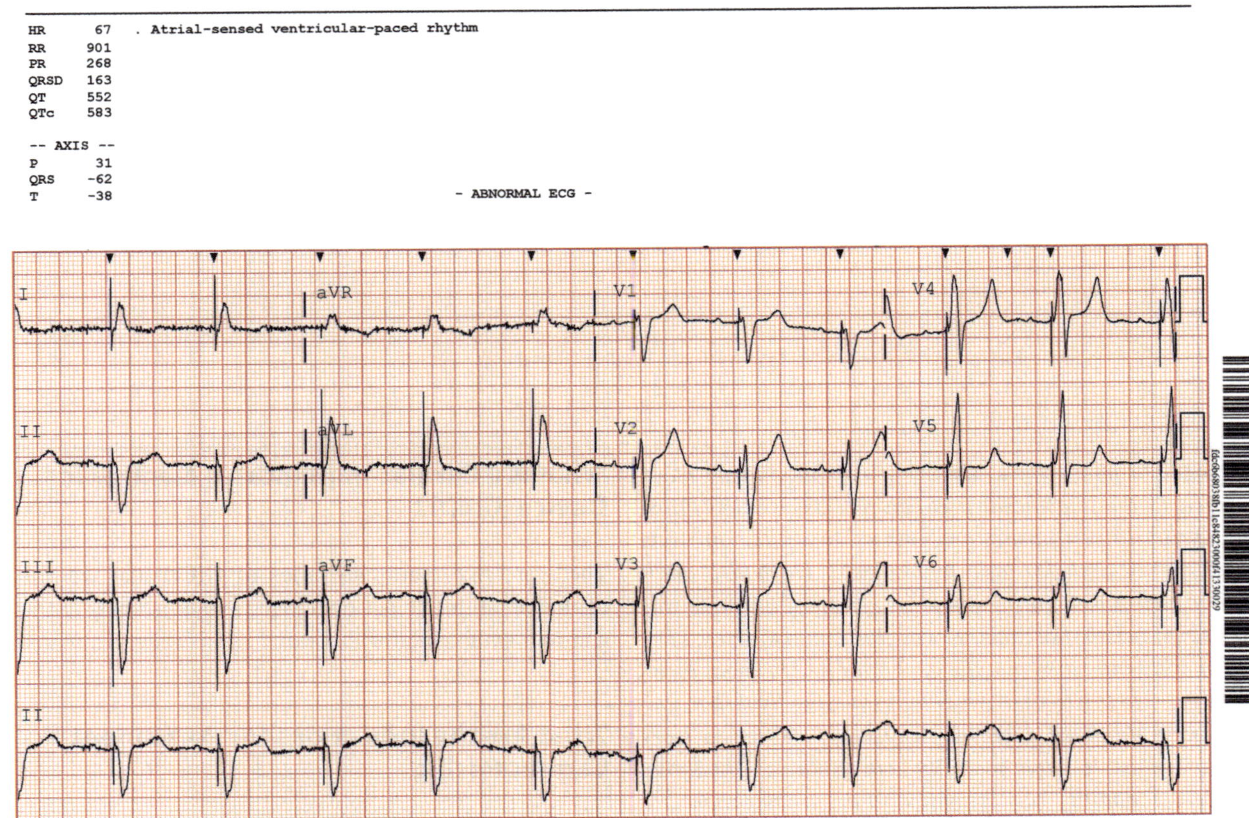

Fig. 9.1 Electrocardiogram showing atrial sensed ventricular rhythm

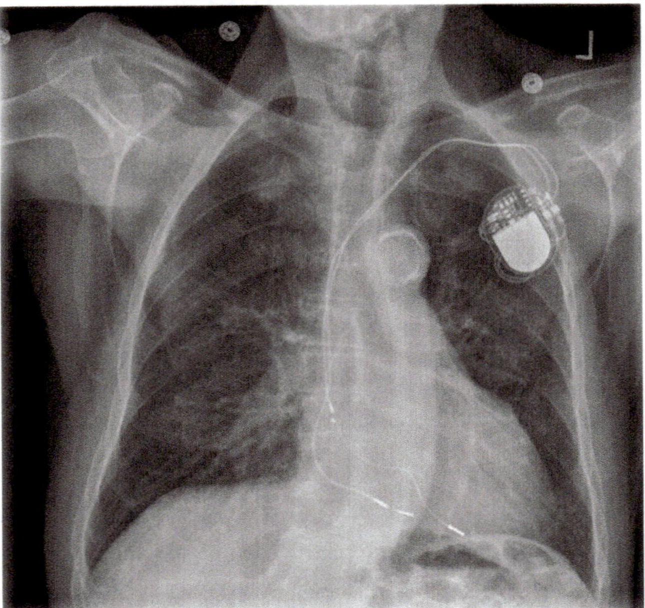

Fig. 9.2 Chest radiograph with a dual-chamber transvenous pacemaker entering from the left in an acceptable position. An abandoned tip of a former atrial lead can be seen within the atrial appendage as well as an abandoned ventricular lead extending from the ventricular apex into the lower superior vena cava. Lungs are well inflated and clear of active disease. The cardiomediastinal silhouette, hilar contours, pulmonary vasculature, and pleural spaces are normal

The second letter describes the sensing chamber, and the third letter represents the pacemaker response to sensed events (*I = inhibition, T = triggered, D = dual, O = no response*). The fourth letter describes programmability, i.e., can the pacemaker adapt its rate in response to patient exercise (*O = none, R = rate modulation*), and the fifth letter signifies multisite pacing, typically used in cardiac resynchronization therapy for patients with intraventricular conduction delay (*V = ventricle, A = atrium, D = dual, O = none*).

Our Patient Has a VDD Pacemaker. What Does This Mean?

The ventricle is the chamber being paced. Sensing occurs in both the atrium and ventricle. The response may be to inhibit or trigger pacing. Ventricular activity is triggered in response to sensed atrial activity, thus preserving AV synchrony. This mode is useful in patients with a slow ventricular rate or AV nodal block. Conversely, asynchronous modes, e.g., *AOO*, *VOO*, and *DOO*, pace at a predetermined rate regardless of underlying activity. These are the modes of choice in an emergency or perioperatively when the pacemaker is subject to electromagnetic interference.

Table 9.1 North American Society of Pacing and Electrophysiology (NASPE)/British Pacing and Electrophysiology Group (BPEG) Generic Pacemaker Code (NBG Code) [3]

Pacing chamber	Sensing chamber	Response to sensing	Programmability	Multisite pacing
O = None	O = None	O = None	O = None	O = None
A = Atrium	A = Atrium	I = Inhibition	R = Rate modulation	A = Atrium
V = Ventricle	V = Ventricle	T = Triggered	C = Communicating	V = Ventricle
D = Dual (A + V)	D = Dual (A + V)	D = Dual (T and I)		D = Dual (A + V)

What Complications Is a Patient with a CIED Subject to in the Perioperative Period?

Pacemaker devices and implantable defibrillators are subject to malfunction or failure secondary to electromagnetic interference. This is manifest as pacemaker inhibition due to oversensing (pacemaker fails to deliver pacing), inadvertent software or electrical reset to backup pacing modes (*VVI* or *VOO*), or sudden asynchronous pacing. Inappropriate delivery of a shock is the principle risk for patients with an implantable cardioverter-defibrillator (ICD).

What Are Potential Sources of Electromagnetic Interference in the Perioperative Setting?

- Electrocautery
- Radiofrequency ablation
- Magnetic resonance imaging
- Nerve stimulators
- Extracorporeal shock wave lithotripsy

Is Electroconvulsive Therapy (ECT) a Source of Electromagnetic Interference?

This field is not very well studied. The American Society of Anesthesiologists (ASA) Task Force notes that no clinical studies were found that report electromagnetic interference or permanent CIED malfunction associated with ECT [4]. However, the recommendation is that the CIED be comprehensively interrogated by the ordering CIED physician or team before the procedure. Pacemakers may have to be programmed to an asynchronous mode to avoid inhibition in pacemaker-dependent patients. ICD functions should be disabled for shock therapy. Ventricular arrhythmias may occur secondary to ECT, and a high degree of preparedness is advised.

Are There Any Guidelines to Aid in Decision-Making with Regard to the Safety of Patients with CIEDs in the Perioperative Period?

A practice advisory has been published by the ASA, and an expert consensus statement has been jointly issued by the Heart Rhythm Society (HRS), the ASA, and the Society of Thoracic Surgeons [4, 5]. The Canadian Cardiovascular Society and the Canadian Anesthesiologists' Society have published a society position statement as a perioperative reference for physicians and surgeons [6]. The British Heart Rhythm Society has provided guidelines for the management of CIEDs around the time of surgery [7].

Who Is Responsible for Ensuring that the Patient's CIED Functions Appropriately Throughout the Perioperative Period?

A multidisciplinary team-based approach is advocated [8]. Recommendations should be sought well in advance, if possible, from the physician who usually manages the patient's CIED. An individualized approach is taken based on patient- and surgery-specific information communicated to the CIED team by the anesthesiologist or surgeon. The resultant plan can be subsequently implemented on the day of surgery by the CIED technician or nurse. However, in case of emergency and out-of-hours surgery that precludes preoperative consultation with the CIED team, it is incumbent on the anesthesiologist to manage the device.

What Information Should Be Communicated to the CIED Team in Advance of Surgery?

- Surgical procedure
- Type of electrocautery to be used
- Other possible sources of electromagnetic interference
- Patient position for the surgery
- Location of the pulse generator

What Factors Must Be Established Preoperatively in the Patient with a CIED?

1. Establish the presence of a CIED from patient history, physical examination, health record, chest radiograph, or ECG.
2. Determine device type from the manufacturer's identification card (usually available from the patient), chest radiograph, or from the patient's cardiologist. The chest radiograph can provide information on lead configuration and subsequently whether the device is single or dual chamber, biventricular, or an ICD [8].
3. Determine the degree of pacemaker dependence [4]:
   - Has the patient experienced symptomatic bradycardia requiring pacemaker insertion?
   - Is there absence of spontaneous ventricular activity when the pacemaker is reprogrammed to *VVI* mode at the lowest programmable rate?
   - Has the patient undergone successful AV nodal ablation with pacemaker placement?
   - A pacemaker spike before every P-wave and/or QRS complex on the ECG indicates pacemaker dependence.
4. Date of last device interrogation.
5. Indication for device, e.g., third-degree heart block, sick sinus syndrome, or second-degree AV block after acute myocardial infarct
6. Estimated battery life must be documented as 3 months or greater.
7. Pacing mode and programmed lower rate.
8. Underlying rhythm and heart rate.
9. Response of device to magnet placement – asynchronous pacing in most cases unless the magnet response parameter has been reprogrammed.
10. Last pacing threshold, i.e., the minimum amount of electrical energy that consistently produces cardiac depolarization. To ensure an adequate pacing safety margin, the pacemaker output should be two to three times the pacing threshold.
11. Presence of any new leads less than 3 months old – these are at risk of dislodgement during cardiac surgery and central line placement.

What Is the Significance of Unipolar Versus Bipolar Pacemaker Leads?

Unipolar leads have a negative electrode in the heart, and the casing of the generator serves as the positive electrode. With bipolar leads, the negative electrode is located at the tip of the lead in the heart and the positive electrode is approximately 1 cm proximal to the tip. Bipolar pacemaker leads are less prone to electromagnetic interference because a large enough voltage change is unlikely to be generated in the small space between the two electrodes. Most modern pacemaker devices have bipolar leads.

Do CIEDs Have Any Other Inbuilt Protective Mechanisms to Prevent Electromagnetic Interference?

Modern devices have noise protection algorithms and use electrical filters and circuit shields that protect against electrical noise outside of the expected physiologic cardiac frequency range.

Does This Patient's Device Need to Be Interrogated Prior to Surgery?

According to the HRS/ASA expert consensus statement, all patients with pacemakers undergoing elective surgery should have had a device check in the past 12 months [5]. This is reduced to 6 months for patients with ICDs. In this instance, the patient does not know when the device was last interrogated.

The CIED Programmer Was Previously Concerned About a "Failure to Capture." What Is "Failure to Capture"?

Pacemaker capture is defined as depolarization and resultant contraction of the atria and/or ventricles in response to a pacemaker stimulus.

Is There a Requirement for the Pacemaker Device to Be Reprogrammed Prior to Surgery?

Reprogramming of a pacemaker to an asynchronous mode is only required for pacemaker-dependent patients who are expected to be subject to significant electromagnetic interference. In contrast, regardless of the expected degree of electromagnetic interference, patients with an ICD must have the anti-tachyarrhythmia functions suspended for surgery. This can be done with a magnet.

The CIED Team Tells You to Apply a Magnet to the Pacemaker Intraoperatively. How Do You Respond?

Application of a magnet over a CIED induces an asynchronous mode in a pacemaker, and an ICD will have its tachycardia detection disabled, thus preventing discharge. Magnet application *will not* reprogram the ICD to an asynchronous mode, i.e., defibrillation will be deactivated but pacing behavior will not change. If an asynchronous pacing mode is deemed prudent for surgery in a patient with an ICD, this will need to be programmed in advance.

Magnet application is convenient as the perioperative team is not dependent on the availability of a technician from the electrophysiology laboratory. In addition, the magnet can be easily removed if, for instance, a patient with a CIED develops a competing rhythm or a patient with an ICD develops a malignant tachycardia. The main disadvantages of magnet use relate to dependence on patient positioning and body habitus. For instance, magnet application is less than reassuring in an obese patient undergoing spinal instrumentation in a prone position. Conversely, CIED reprogramming preoperatively has the disadvantage that changes cannot be made expeditiously in the absence of a programmer.

Reports of magnet placement having unexpected results, i.e., inadequate pacemaker capture or failure of expected disabling of tachyarrhythmia therapy in an ICD [9, 10], demonstrate how this is not a panacea for the perioperative management of these devices. There are reasons why magnet use may be inappropriate or not work as intended, e.g., magnet responsiveness can be disabled in CIED programming. Asynchronous pacing rates vary. Some can be in the range of 90–100, which is ill advised for patients with coronary artery disease or valvular heart disease. Once these shortcomings are appreciated and the anesthesiologist has the knowledge to perform basic device assessment, magnet application can be appropriate and may be necessary in emergency situations, and a magnet should be available for all cases involving CIEDs even when reprogramming has been deemed unnecessary.

Should an Echocardiogram Be Performed Preoperatively in This Patient?

Current evidence is not strongly supportive of routine preoperative resting echocardiography for noncardiac surgery unless clinical examination is suggestive of an undiagnosed, severe obstructive intracardiac abnormality (e.g., aortic stenosis, mitral stenosis, hypertrophic obstructive cardiomyopathy), or severe pulmonary hypertension [11].

What Valvular Abnormality Is Not Uncommonly Associated with Transvalvular ICD/Pacemaker Lead Presence?

The vast majority of CIED leads are placed transvenously into the right side of the heart. It is now recognized that tricuspid valve dysfunction/damage can occur in the CIED population [12]. Tricuspid valve leaflets can be perforated by a lead, entanglement of a lead in one of the three cusps that make up the valve can occur, or a lead can become adherent to a cusp by fibrous attachment. The hemodynamic consequences of the aforementioned are the development of tricuspid regurgitation (TR) and volume overload. While the TR may be mild initially, TR induces volume retention, tricuspid annular, and atrial dilatation, events that are a harbinger of right-sided heart failure. This may be of particular concern in the patient with poor left-sided heart function, a frequent indication for ICD placement. A history suggestive of right-sided failure should always be sought and the tricuspid area examined by auscultation. Evidence of significant TR is an indication for screening echocardiography.

Is Spinal Anesthesia Contraindicated for This Patient?

The sympathectomy induced by neuraxial blockade results in a decrease in stroke volume and, subsequently, in cardiac output. A reduction in preload, secondary to venodilatation, is a greater contributory factor in comparison to the reduction in afterload resulting from decreased arterial resistance. The resultant hypotension may be more pronounced in older patients with greater sympathetic tone. This hypotension is normally treated with a sympathomimetic agent, e.g., ephedrine. However, this chronotropic response is unpredictable in patient with a pacemaker, e.g., it will depend on how pacemaker-dependent the patient is.

We communicated with the cardiology/electrophysiology care team and discovered that the most recent pacemaker assessment took place 8 months prior to the proposed TURP procedure. As a result, formal interrogation was not required in this instance.

According to the most recent interrogation, the patient was intermittently pacemaker-dependent. The device was noted to be pacing and sensing appropriately with satisfactory thresholds. No programming changes were deemed necessary after this evaluation. Monopolar cautery is commonly utilized for TURP procedures. This combination of intermittent dependence and significant potential for electromagnetic interference led to the decision that this particular patient's CIED should be reprogrammed to an asynchronous mode prior to surgery.

Spinal anesthesia was not contraindicated – he was intermittently pacemaker-dependent. Low-dose spinal anesthesia with arterial pressure monitoring was an option available to the intraoperative anesthesiologist. However, this was decided against in view of the

patient's WBC count of 15.5 × 10^9/L, taken to be an indication of systemic infection.

True/False Questions

1(a) Magnet application will reprogram an ICD to an asynchronous mode.
1(b) A pacemaker with the code DDD is considered to have an asynchronous mode.
1(c) Sick sinus node syndrome is a common indication for permanent cardiac pacing.
1(d) Signs of pacemaker dependence are often visible on examination of the ECG.
1(e) The first letter of the generic NAPSE / BPEG pacemaker code describes the chamber being sensed.

2. In the preoperative setting, cardiac implantable electronic devices should be formally reprogrammed to asynchronous modes in the following scenarios:
(a) The patient is not pacemaker dependent.
(b) Monopolar cautery will be utilized by the surgical team.
(c) Distance from CIED to source of electromagnetic interference < 15 cm.
(d) Patient is undergoing electroconvulsive therapy and is not pacemaker dependent.
(e) The patient is undergoing an emergency laparotomy at 3 am.

References

1. European Society of Cardiology (ESC); European Heart Rhythm Association (EHRA), Brignole M, Auricchio A, Baron-Esquivias G, Bordachar P, Boriani G, et al. 2013 ESC guidelines on cardiac pacing and cardiac resynchronization therapy: the task force on cardiac pacing and resynchronization therapy of the European Society of Cardiology (ESC). Developed in collaboration with the European Heart Rhythm Association (EHRA). Europace. 2013;15(8):1070–118.
2. Epstein AE, DiMarco JP, Ellenbogen KA, Estes NA 3rd, Freedman RA, Gettes LS, et al. 2012 ACCF/AHA/HRS focused update incorporated into the ACCF/AHA/HRS 2008 guidelines for device-based therapy of cardiac rhythm abnormalities: a report of the American College of Cardiology Foundation/American Heart Association Task Force on Practice Guidelines and the Heart Rhythm Society. J Am Coll Cardiol. 2013;61(3):e6–75.
3. Bernstein AD, Daubert JC, Fletcher RD, Hayes DL, Luderitz B, Reynolds DW, et al. The revised NASPE/BPEG generic code for antibradycardia, adaptive-rate, and multisite pacing. North American Society of Pacing and Electrophysiology/British Pacing and Electrophysiology Group. Pacing Clin Electrophysiol. 2002;25(2):260–4.
4. American Society of Anesthesiology. Practice advisory for the perioperative management of patients with cardiac implantable electronic devices: pacemakers and implantable cardioverter-defibrillators: an updated report by the American Society Of Anesthesiologists Task Force on Perioperative Management of Patients With Cardiac Implantable Electronic Devices. Anesthesiology. 2011;114(2):247–61.
5. Crossley GH, Poole JE, Rozner MA, Asirvatham SJ, Cheng A, Chung MK, et al. The Heart Rhythm Society (HRS)/American Society of Anesthesiologists (ASA) Expert Consensus Statement on the perioperative management of patients with implantable defibrillators, pacemakers and arrhythmia monitors: facilities and patient management this document was developed as a joint project with the American Society of Anesthesiologists (ASA), and in collaboration with the American Heart Association (AHA), and the Society of Thoracic Surgeons (STS). Heart Rhythm. 2011;8(7):1114–54.
6. Healey JS, Merchant R, Simpson C, Tang T, Beardsall M, Tung S, et al. Society position statement: Canadian Cardiovascular Society/Canadian Anesthesiologists' Society/Canadian Heart Rhythm Society joint position statement on the perioperative management of patients with implanted pacemakers, defibrillators, and neurostimulating devices. Can J Anaesth. 2012;59(4):394–407.
7. Thomas H, Turley A, Plummer C on behalf of BHRS Council. British heart rhythm society guidelines for the management of patients with cardiac implantable electronic devices (CIEDS) Around the time of surgery. 2016. http://www.bhrs.com/files/files/Guidelines/160216-Guideline%2CPeri-operative management of CIEDs.pdf. Accessed 11 Sept 2018.
8. Stone ME, Salter B, Fischer A. Perioperative management of patients with cardiac implantable electronic devices. Br J Anaesth. 2011;107(Suppl 1):i16–26.
9. Schulman PM, Rozner MA. Case report: use caution when applying magnets to pacemakers or defibrillators for surgery. Anesth Analg. 2013;117(2):422–7.
10. Rooke GA, Bowdle TA. Perioperative management of pacemakers and implantable cardioverter defibrillators: it's not just about the magnet. Anesth Analg. 2013;117(2):292–4.
11. Duceppe E, Parlow J, MacDonald P, Lyons K, McMullen M, Srinathan S, et al. Canadian cardiovascular society guidelines on perioperative cardiac risk assessment and management for patients who undergo noncardiac surgery. Can J Cardiol. 2017;33(1):17–32.
12. Chang JD, Manning WJ, Ebrille E, Zimetbaum PJ. Tricuspid valve dysfunction following pacemaker or cardioverter-defibrillator implantation. JACC. 2017;69(18):2331–41.

Part II

Vascular

Carotid Endarterectomy

10

Susan Halliday

A 77-year-old male scheduled for a left carotid endarterectomy (CEA) for an ulcerated, moderately stenotic internal carotid artery plaque presented for preoperative optimization. He had experienced two previous transient ischemic attacks (TIA) affecting the left and right cerebral hemispheres, 10 and 4 months, respectively, prior to his visit to the clinic. A right CEA was performed after the second TIA from which he had made a positive recovery. Follow-up ultrasound at 6 weeks showed no residual stenosis. His past medical history included paroxysmal atrial fibrillation, dyslipidemia, early chronic obstructive airway disease, well-controlled ulcerative colitis, and gastroesophageal disease. He was an ex-smoker for 12 years with a 40-pack-year history. Other past procedures included a right total knee replacement, left total hip replacement, and right rotator cuff repair. There were no problems with previous anesthetics. He had an active lifestyle with greater than four metabolic equivalents of activity without any cardiovascular or respiratory symptoms.

Medications: Rosuvastatin, tiotropium bromide, mesalamine, and apixaban.

Physical Examination: On examination, oxygen saturation on room air was 97%, blood pressure was 128/80, and heart rate was 62.

Investigations: The ECG was as seen in Fig. 10.1. The chest radiograph was unremarkable. A recent echocardiogram showed normal left and right ventricular sizes and function with a left ventricular ejection fraction greater than 55%. No valvular disease was identified, and estimated pulmonary pressures were within normal limits.

Hematological and biochemistry laboratory results are shown in Table 10.1.

What Is the Primary Objective of CEA Surgery?

Carotid artery stenosis from atheromatous plaque is responsible for 10–20% of ischemic strokes [1]. Rupture of the atheromatous plaque initiates thrombus formation that can lead to embolization and ischemic infarction. Carotid endarterectomy (CEA) is performed to remove atheromatous plaque from within the carotid artery to reduce the incidence of further embolic strokes in symptomatic patients.

What Are the Indications for Carotid Endarterectomy?

The Canadian Stroke Best Practice Guidelines for secondary prevention recommend that all patients with a recent TIA or non-disabling stroke and ipsilateral 50–90% carotid stenosis should be evaluated by an experienced physician and that selected patients be offered CEA as soon as feasible [2]. They also recommend consideration of CEA for carefully selected patients with 60–99% stenosis who are asymptomatic or remotely symptomatic for events occurring more than 6 months prior. The patient presented above came under the latter category, having a remotely symptomatic, moderate plaque.

Guidelines from the American Heart Association and American Stroke Association recommend CEA in two situations [3].

- For patients experiencing a TIA or ischemic stroke within the past 6 months with ipsilateral severe (70–99%) carotid artery stenosis identified on noninvasive imaging, i.e., carotid duplex ultrasound, computed tomography angiography (CTA), or magnetic resonance angiography (MRA), CEA is recommended if the perioperative morbidity and mortality rate is estimated to be less than 6%.
- Secondly, CEA is recommended for patients with a recent TIA or ischemic stroke in the presence of ipsilateral moderate (50–69%) carotid stenosis identified on conventional catheter-based angiography or noninvasive imaging

S. Halliday (✉)
Department of Anesthesiology & Pain Medicine, University of Alberta Hospital, Edmonton, AB, Canada
e-mail: halliday@ualberta.ca

D. Dillane, B. A. Finegan (eds.), *Preoperative Assessment*, https://doi.org/10.1007/978-3-030-58842-7_10

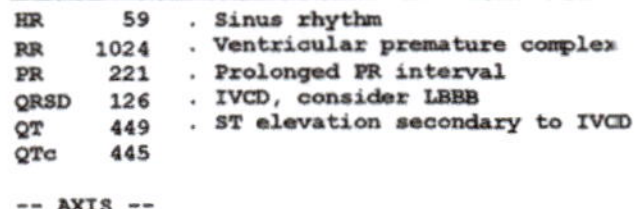

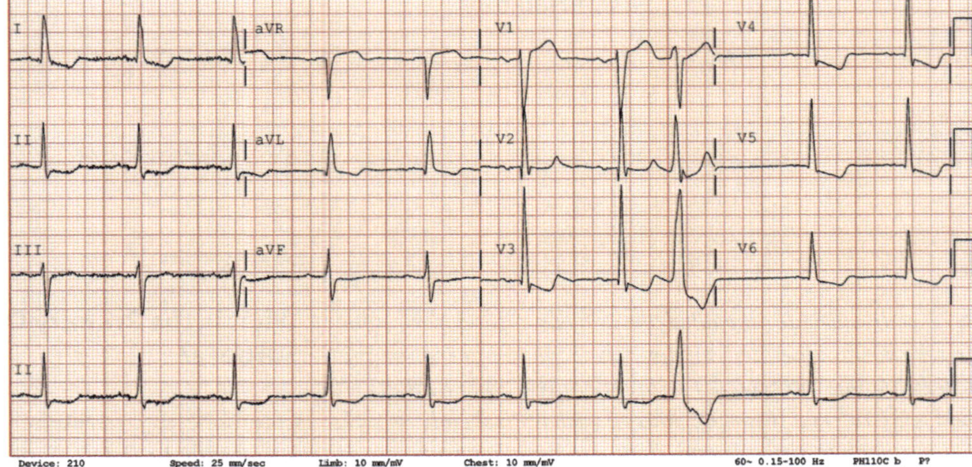

Fig. 10.1 Electrocardiogram showing sinus rhythm with premature ventricular complexes, PR prolongation, and intraventricular conduction delay. ST changes secondary to intraventricular conduction delay

Table 10.1 Hematology and biochemistry laboratory results

Laboratory parameter	Result
Hemoglobin	136 g/L
Platelet count	122 × 10^9/L
White blood cell count	7.4 × 10^9/L
Sodium	136 mmol/L
Potassium	4.0 mmol/L
Creatinine	62 μmol/L
INR	1.0
PTT	29
Cholesterol	2.38
Triglycerides	1.3
HDL	0.86
LDL	0.93
Hemoglobin A1C	5.6%

INR International normalized ratio, *PTT* partial thromboplastin time, *LDL* low-density lipoprotein, *HDL* high-density lipoprotein

with corroboration (e.g., on MR or CT angiogram) in the presence of certain patient-specific factors, e.g., age, sex, and comorbidities. Again, CEA is recommended for this class of patient when the perioperative morbidity and mortality rate is estimated to be less than 6%.

- CEA is not recommended when degree of stenosis is less than 50%.

Should the Patient with Acute Ischemic Stroke Have Invasive or Noninvasive Neurovascular Imaging?

Brain imaging and noninvasive vascular imaging from the aorta to the vertex should be undertaken for patients presenting with an acute or recent stroke or TIA. As CT angiography is now widely available, vascular imaging can be performed at the same time as the initial head CT. MR with angiography or carotid ultrasound are suitable alternatives.

Due to the risk of stroke with conventional catheter-based angiography, it is rarely performed in the acute setting despite providing superior images. Moreover, noninvasive imaging, i.e., carotid duplex ultrasound, CTA, and MRA, provides immediate images that are adequate for visualization of intra- and extracranial vascular disease.

When Is the Optimum Time for Surgery Relative to the Onset of Neurological Symptoms?

Analysis of data pooled from the European Carotid Surgery Trial and North American Symptomatic Carotid Endarterectomy Trial showed improved neurological outcomes in patients undergoing CEA within 2 weeks of the onset of neurological deficits [4]. Subsequently, the American Heart Association and American Stroke Association guidelines recommend revascularization within 2 weeks of the TIA or non-disabling stroke. The Canadian Stroke Best Practice guidelines reiterate this and recommend that those with a 70–99% symptomatic stenosis have an endarterectomy performed within the first days following the initial event and within the first 14 days if the patient's clinical condition precludes it occurring within first few days. A recent meta-analysis, however, showed that CEA within 48 hours was associated with a significantly increased risk of stroke compared to CEA undertaken after 48 hours (OR 2.35; 95% CI 1.61e3.45, $p < .001$) [5].

Patient optimization before surgery may be limited by time constraints. By understanding the benefits of expedited surgery, anesthesiologists have to be pragmatic in their approach to patient optimization preoperatively.

When Is Carotid Angioplasty and Stenting Favored Over CEA?

Carotid stenting should be considered for patients who are not suitable for CEA due to medical, technical, or anatomical reasons. The peri-procedural morbidity and mortality rates (for stenting) for the interventionist and/or center should be less than 5% for symptomatic stenosis and 3% for asymptomatic stenosis [2]. Carotid stenting is associated with an increased risk of peri-procedural stroke and death in older patients when compared to endarterectomy [6]. Endarterectomy is, therefore, more appropriate for patients over 70 years.

What Complications Is the CEA Patient Subject to in the Perioperative Period?

The North American Symptomatic Carotid Endarterectomy Trial (NASCET) Surgical Results of 1415 patients found an overall rate of 6.5% for perioperative events including death, disabling stroke, and non-disabling stroke. At 30 days, the rates were 1.8% for disabling stroke, 3.7% for non-disabling stroke, and 1.1% for death. Following neurological recovery of patients deemed to be disabled at 30 days, by 90 days, the rates of disabling and non-disabling stroke had changed to 0.9% and 4.5%, respectively. Death rate at 90 days remained the same at 1.1%. Thromboembolism was the cause of most strokes. One-third of events occurred intraoperatively. Increased surgical risk was predicted by the following variables: symptomatic hemispheric versus retinal TIA, contralateral carotid occlusion, ipsilateral ischemic lesion on CT scan, and irregular or ulcerated ipsilateral plaque [7].

Cranial nerve injuries occurred in 8.6%. The majority (7.9%) were mild, resulting in no delay in discharge and had resolved on follow-up. The incidence of vagus nerve injury was 2.5%.

Airway edema requiring reintubation was a rare event, occurring in only 0.4%. Wound hematomas occurred in 7.1% of patients. Wound hematoma was demonstrated to be a statistically significant risk factor for perioperative stroke and death (14.9% risk versus 5.9% without a wound hematoma).

How Should This Patient Be Evaluated Preoperatively?

Most stroke patients will have been thoroughly evaluated by the stroke team by the time they come to the attention of the anesthesiologist. The timing of initial evaluation by stroke expert will depend on the duration between symptom onset and presentation to a healthcare facility. As the time elapsed between the initial TIA or non-disabling stroke and presentation to a healthcare facility increases, the risk of recurrent stroke decreases. The highest risk of recurrent TIA or stroke is within 48 hours of the initial symptoms [8]. Ultimately, investigations undertaken as part of the assessment include brain imaging and noninvasive vascular imaging, the latter to identify any thrombus or carotid stenosis amenable to thrombectomy or surgery. Head CT and CTA from aortic arch to vertex are most commonly performed. If CTA is not available, carotid ultrasound or MRA with angiography can be performed. MRA has an increased diagnostic sensitivity when compared to CT for detecting small strokes. Invaluable information for the anesthesiologist can be gleaned from angiography or ultrasound regarding patency of the non-operative internal carotid artery and vertebral arteries. Of particular interest is the degree of blood flow through the contralateral internal carotid artery and both vertebral arteries. Global cerebral perfusion intraoperatively is dependent on this contralateral flow, while the operative internal carotid artery is clamped. This will impact the surgeon's decision to use intraoperative carotid shunting.

Standard laboratory investigations include complete blood count, electrolyte, creatinine, coagulation screen, troponin, and random glucose. Lipid profiles and hemoglobin A1C level are routine to identify modifiable stroke risk factors.

A 12-lead ECG is essential in all patients to detect cardiac arrhythmias and/or ECG changes indicative of structural heart disease that may be present following acute stroke. ECG changes have been reported following ischemic strokes as well as those from a hemorrhagic origin. The incidence of arrhythmias following acute ischemic stroke has been reported to be up to 25% in the first 72 hours [9]. Atrial fibrillation is the most common arrhythmia and is identified more frequently following cardioembolic stroke.

The stroke assessment may also have included an echocardiogram. This is generally considered in cases where the mechanism of stroke has not been identified.

How Should Hypertension Be Managed Perioperatively in This Patient Population?

Poorly controlled hypertension is an indicator for labile intraoperative blood pressure. Significant postoperative hypertension is a risk factor for cerebral hyperperfusion syndrome. Hypertension in the setting of acute ischemic stroke (in those not eligible for thrombolytic therapy) or TIA is not routinely treated. Extreme blood pressures with a systolic pressure greater than 220 mmHg or diastolic greater than 120 mmHg are treated carefully to ensure a gradual reduction of 15% but no more than 25% within the first 24 hours. In addition to being the most important risk factor for stroke, hypertension is also a significant risk factor for further stroke. Secondary prevention guidelines therefore recommend a blood pressure target below 140/90 mm Hg [2]. In the presence of small subcortical strokes, the target systolic pressure is 130 mm Hg. Frequently, due to the short time period between occurrence of the stroke and surgery, it is difficult to achieve optimal blood pressure control preoperatively in patients with previously undiagnosed or poorly controlled hypertension. For those on antihypertensive medications, the current practice in our center is to hold angiotensin-converting enzyme inhibitors and angiotensin II receptor antagonists on the day of surgery because of their potential to cause intraoperative hypotension.

How Are Arrhythmias Managed?

Patients with an identified arrhythmia, most commonly atrial fibrillation, should have the ventricular response rate controlled to a preoperative target of 100 beats per minute. Any rate-controlling medications such as beta-blockers and rate-limiting calcium channel blockers should be taken on the day of surgery.

Describe an Approach to Anticoagulant Medications in the Perioperative Period

Antiplatelet therapy with aspirin is recommended for all patients with acute ischemic strokes and TIAs. Those not already on an antiplatelet are usually commenced with a loading dose of 160–320 mg. This is commenced as soon as any intracranial hemorrhage has been excluded on imaging. The daily dose thereafter ranges from 80 to 325 mg. If alteplase is given, then an antiplatelet agent is not given until 24 hours after this has been administered.

Dual-antiplatelet therapy with aspirin and clopidogrel may be considered for patients with a minor stroke (National Institute of Health Stroke Score (NIHSS) of 3 or less), or a high-risk TIA (ABCD2 (age, blood pressure, clinical features, diabetes)) score of 4 or greater [10]. This is not continued for longer than 21–30 days due to the increased risk of bleeding. In very high-risk TIA or minor ischemic stroke patients caused by a high-grade carotid stenosis in whom endarterectomy may be indicated, consultation with the surgical team should be sought to determine the time of commencement of dual-antiplatelet therapy. In a large retrospective review, dual-antiplatelet therapy was associated with a significant increased risk of major bleeding requiring reoperation, although there was a significant reduction in neurological events [11]. The risk of bleeding has subsequently been contested in a smaller prospective study [12]. The surgical team may opt to continue single therapy with aspirin until following surgery or continue dual therapy, depending on the individual patient case.

Anticoagulation for patients with atrial fibrillation or paroxysmal atrial fibrillation is recommended. Direct oral anticoagulants (DOACs) such as apixaban and rivaroxaban are now used in preference over warfarin. As was the case with our patient who was on apixaban for paroxysmal atrial fibrillation, DOACs should be discontinued 2 days prior to surgery. Warfarin should be held for 5 days. In the face of acute ischemic stroke and atrial fibrillation alone, there is no requirement to bridge with heparin; therefore our patient did not receive any bridging therapy.

Should This Patient Continue Statin Therapy in the Perioperative Period?

Dyslipidemia is a well-known cause of atherosclerosis and a risk factor for ischemic stroke. The use of statins in primary and secondary prevention of stroke is irrefutable. Statin therapy is recommended following an ischemic stroke or TIA. Lifestyle modifications should also be made. A reasonable target to strive for is a low-density lipoprotein (LDL) cholesterol level less than 2.0 mmol/L or a greater than 50% reduction from baseline [2]. Observational studies have shown benefits of statin therapy in the perioperative period in patients undergoing CEA. Benefits include reduced in-hospital mortality and stroke [13] and long-term protection against myocardial infarction (MI) and stroke [14]. These beneficial effects have been contested in a smaller prospective study [15]. On balance, given that discontinuation of statin therapy increases risk of MI following major vascular surgery, it seems prudent to continue statin therapy throughout the perioperative period [16].

Is Glucose Control in the Perioperative Period in This Cohort of Patients Important?

Diabetes mellitus is a risk factor for stroke and an independent risk factor for stroke recurrence [17]. Hyperglycemia at the time of CEA is associated with significant morbidity and mortality. With blood glucose levels greater than 11.1 mmol/l, patients are 2.8-fold, 4.3-fold, and 3.3-fold more likely to experience a stroke or TIA, MI, or death, respectively [18]. The exception to this may be with lacunar infarcts where moderate hyperglycemia (8–12 mmol/l) has been associated with better outcomes. However, outcomes were worse in the cohort with more severe hyperglycemia (>12 mmol/l) [19]. Given the importance of glucose control in the perioperative period, consultation with a diabetologist may be beneficial for those with previously undiagnosed diabetes or poorly controlled diabetes. At our institution, we use a variable rate insulin infusion with a concurrent low volume infusion of 10% dextrose.

The Patient Has Read on the Internet That He Can Be Awake for His Carotid Endarterectomy. How Do You Advise Him?

The type of anesthetic, general anesthesia versus regional anesthesia, for CEA, has long been debated. There are many perceived benefits to both techniques. Local anesthesia allows the patient to act as their own neurological monitor, reduces the rate of arterial shunt intervention, avoids the need for intubation and stress response associated with it (unless there is need to convert to general anesthesia), and may result in less hemodynamic instability. General anesthesia provides immobility not requiring patient cooperation, potential neurological protection from general anesthetic agents, and control of ventilation and arterial carbon dioxide. Despite these perceived benefits, a large randomized controlled trial published in 2008 demonstrated no difference in 30-day outcomes for stroke, including retinal infarction, MI, or death [20]. The primary outcome, stroke, occurred in 4.8% of patients who had undergone general anesthesia and 4.5% who had their procedure under regional anesthesia. Note though that his study was not powered for mortality. As the debate continued, an updated Cochrane review published in 2013 that included 14 randomized controlled trials (although 3526 of the 4596 surgeries were from the GALA trial) found no difference in 30-day stroke rates between the two anesthetic groups [21]. There was also no statistically significant difference between the two groups for the following: MI or death within 30 days of surgery, local hemorrhage, and cranial nerve injury. The length of hospital stay and patient satisfaction were also not different between the groups. More recently a non-randomized comparison of general and regional anesthesia from the Carotid Revascularization Endarterectomy versus Stenting Trial (CREST) showed that general anesthesia presented twice the risk of MI compared to regional anesthesia. The sample size, however, was small and at risk of confounding [22]. Careful patient selection for each type of anesthesia and the manner in which the anesthetic of choice are conducted may well be more important than the actual choice of anesthetic.

What Approaches Are Available for a Regional Anesthetic Technique?

Awake CEA may be undertaken using local anesthetic infiltration, superficial cervical plexus block, and/or deep cervical plexus block. The author's regional anesthesia experience for this procedure is with superficial cervical plexus blocks performed under ultrasound guidance. No matter which regional approach is used, it is important that the patient be fully briefed on what to expect and has an established rapport with the operating room team. Communication with the patient needs to be maintained throughout the procedure, not only to monitor cerebral function but to help alleviate any anxiety the patient may be experiencing.

Is Assessment of Neurocognitive Function During Cross-Clamping Important During Awake Carotid Endarterectomy?

Neurocognitive function assessment determines the adequacy of collateral circulation from the circle of Willis. Adequate collateral circulation mitigates the need for shunting. Although the purpose of placing a shunt is to maintain cerebral blood flow, therefore protecting against ischemia, it has associated complications, including arterial dissection, acute occlusion, and distal embolization. It can also make surgical exposure difficult at the distal ends of the incision. Shunt rates during CEA are substantially reduced in regional techniques compared to during general anesthesia (14% versus 43%) [20]. Neurocognitive monitoring in awake patients undergoing CEA has been shown to be more sensitive and specific for identifying the need for shunt placement compared to electroencephalography and stump pressure in this cohort [23]. Prior to, immediately after, and throughout cross-clamping of the carotid artery, neurocognitive assessment should be made by assessing level of consciousness, presence of confusion, alterations in speech, and contralateral motor function. A new deficit indicates the need for shunt placement. In the event of new deficits that do not revert quickly with shunt placement and manipulation of cerebral perfusion, general anesthesia will be required.

The patient requested that he be given a general anesthetic. An arterial line was placed prior to induction. He was hemodynamically stable during the subsequent procedure and was discharged 48 hours later without incident.

True/False Questions

1(a) Carotid endarterectomy is recommended for patients who have experienced a TIA within the past 6 months in the presence of severe ipsilateral carotid artery stenosis when perioperative morbidity and mortality is estimated to be less than 6%.

1(b) Carotid endarterectomy is not recommended when carotid artery stenosis is less than 50%.

1(c) Catheter-based angiography is the imaging modality of choice in the patient with acute ischemic stroke.

1(d) The American Heart Association and American Stroke Association guidelines recommend revascularization 2 weeks after a TIA or non-disabling stroke.

1(e) Carotid stenting is preferred to endarterectomy surgery in patients over 70 years old.
2(a) Magnetic resonance angiography has an increased diagnostic sensitivity when compared to CT for detecting small strokes.
2(b) Antiplatelet therapy with aspirin is contraindicated for patients with acute ischemic strokes and TIAs.
2(c) Dual-antiplatelet therapy with aspirin and clopidogrel for up to 30 days can be considered for patients with a minor stroke or a high-risk TIA.
2(d) Warfarin is the preferred method of anticoagulation for the stroke patient with atrial fibrillation.
2(e) Superficial cervical plexus blockade offers clear benefits over general anesthesia for 30-day outcomes after carotid endarterectomy.

References

1. Flaherty ML, Kissela B, Khoury JC, Alwell K, Moomaw CJ, Woo D, et al. Carotid artery stenosis as a cause of stroke. Neuroepidemiology. 2013;40(1):36–41.
2. Wein T, Lindsay MP, Côté R, Foley N, Berlingieri J, Bhogal S, et al. Heart and Stroke Foundation Canadian Stroke Best Practice Committees. Canadian stroke best practice recommendations: secondary prevention of stroke, sixth edition practice guidelines, update 2017. Int J Stroke. 2018;13(4):420–43.
3. Kernan WN, Ovbiagele B, Black HR, Bravata DM, Chimowitz MI, Ezekowitz MD, et al. American Heart Association Stroke Council, Council on Cardiovascular and Stroke Nursing, Council on Clinical Cardiology, and Council on Peripheral Vascular Disease. Guidelines for the prevention of stroke in patients with stroke and transient ischemic attack: a guideline for healthcare professionals from the American Heart Association/American Stroke Association. Stroke. 2014;45(7):2160–236.
4. Rothwell PM, Eliasziw M, Gutnikov SA, Warlow CP, Barnett HJ. Carotid Endarterectomy Trialists Collaboration. Endarterectomy for symptomatic carotid stenosis in relation to clinical subgroups and timing of surgery. Lancet. 2004;363(9413):915–24.
5. Milgrom D, Hajibandeh S, Hajibandeh S, Antoniou SA, Torella F, Antoniou GA. Editor's choice—systematic review and meta-analysis of very urgent carotid intervention for symptomatic carotid disease. Eur J Vasc Endovasc Surg. 2018;56(5):622–31.
6. Hobson RW 2nd, Howard VJ, Roubin GS, Brott TG, Ferguson RD, Popma JJ, et al. CREST Investigators. Carotid artery stenting is associated with increased complications in octogenarians: 30-day stroke and death rates in the CREST lead-in phase. J Vasc Surg. 2004;40(6):1106–11.
7. Ferguson GG, Eliasziw M, Barr HW, Clagett GP, Barnes RW, Wallace MC, et al. for the North American Symptomatic Carotid Endarterectomy Trial (NASCET) Collaborators. The North American symptomatic carotid endarterectomy trial: surgical results in 1415 patients. Stroke. 1999;30(9):1751–8.
8. Boulanger JM, Lindsay MP, Gubitz G, Smith EE, Stotts G, Foley N, et al. Canadian stroke best practice recommendations for acute stroke management: prehospital, emergency department, and acute inpatient stroke care, 6th edition, update 2018. Int J Stroke. 2018;13(9):949–84.
9. Kallmünzer B, Breuer L, Kahl N, Bobinger T, Raaz-Schrauder D, Huttner HB, et al. Serious cardiac arrhythmias after stroke: incidence, time course, and predictors—a systematic, prospective analysis. Stroke. 2012;43(11):2892–7.
10. Galvin R, Geraghty C, Motterlini N, Dimitrov BD, Fahey T. Prognostic value of the ABCD(2) clinical prediction rule: a systematic review and meta-analysis. Fam Pract. 2011;28(4):366–76.
11. Jones DW, Goodney PP, Conrad MF, Nolan BW, Rzucidlo EM, Powell RJ, et al. Dual antiplatelet therapy reduces stroke but increases bleeding at the time of carotid endarterectomy. J Vasc Surg. 2016;63(5):1262–70.
12. Illuminati G, Schneider F, Pizzardi G, Masci F, Calio' FG, Ricco JB. Dual antiplatelet therapy does not increase the risk of bleeding after carotid endarterectomy: results of a prospective study. Ann Vasc Surg. 2017;40:29–43.
13. Kennedy J, Quan H, Buchan AM, Ghali WA, Feasby TE. Statins are associated with better outcomes after carotid endarterectomy in symptomatic patients. Stroke. 2005;36(10):2072–6.
14. Arinze N, Farber A, Sachs T, Patts G, Kalish J, Kuhnen A, Kasotakis G, Siracuse JJ. The effect of statin use and intensity on stroke and myocardial infarction after carotid endarterectomy. J Vasc Surg. 2018;68(5):1398–405.
15. Ballotta E, Toniato A, Farina F, Baracchini C. Effects of preoperative statin use on perioperative outcomes of carotid endarterectomy. Brain Behav. 2017;7:e00597.
16. Schouten O, Hoeks SE, Welten GM, Davignon J, Kastelein JJ, Vidakovic R, et al. Effect of statin withdrawal on frequency of cardiac events after vascular surgery. Am J Cardiol. 2007;100(2):316–20.
17. Shou J, Zhou L, Zhu S, Zhang X. Diabetes is an independent risk factor for stroke recurrence in stroke patients: a meta-analysis. J Stroke Cerebrovasc Dis. 2015;24(9):1961–8.
18. McGirt MJ, Woodworth GF, Brooke BS, Coon AL, Jain S, Buck D, Huang J, et al. Hyperglycemia independently increases the risk of perioperative stroke, myocardial infarction, and death after carotid endarterectomy. Neurosurgery. 2006;58(6):1066–73.
19. Uyttenboogaart M, Koch MW, Stewart RE, Vroomen PC, Luijckx GJ, De Keyser J. Moderate hyperglycaemia is associated with favourable outcome in acute lacunar stroke. Brain. 2007;130(Pt 6):1626–30.
20. GALA Trial Collaborative Group, Lewis SC, Warlow CP, Bodenham AR, Colam B, Rothwell PM, Torgerson D, et al. General anesthesia versus local anesthesia for carotid surgery (GALA): a multicentred, randomised controlled trial. Lancet. 2008;72(9656):2132–42.
21. Vaniyapong T, Chongruksut W, Rerkasem K. Local versus general anesthesia for carotid endarterectomy. Cochrane Database Syst Rev. 2013;12:CD000126.
22. Hye RJ, Voeks JH, Malas MB, Tom M, Longson S, Blackshear JL, Brott TG. Anesthetic type and risk of myocardial infarction after carotid endarterectomy in the Carotid Revascularization Endarterectomy versus Stenting Trial (CREST). J Vasc Surg. 2016;64(1):3–8.e1.
23. Hans SS, Jareunpoon O. Prospective evaluation of electroencephalography, carotid artery stump pressure, and neurologic changes during 314 consecutive carotid endarterectomies performed in awake patients. J Vasc Surg. 2007;45(3):511–5.

Abdominal Aortic Aneurysm

11

Barry A. Finegan

An 86-year-old male was assessed on the day before scheduled urgent endovascular abdominal aortic aneurysm repair (EVAR). An infra-renal abdominal aortic aneurysm (AAA) with a transverse diameter of 6.2 cm was observed by abdominal ultrasound 1 week previously as part of surveillance screening. When assessed 6 months previously, the AAA was measured at 5.6 cm. The patient was offered but declined surgical intervention at that time and elected to continue screening at 6- rather than 12-month intervals. He had a history of known cardiac disease, having had drug-eluting stents placed in his mid-left anterior descending (LAD), the obtuse marginal branch of the circumflex artery, and the mid-right coronary artery 3 years prior to presentation. Other comorbidities included paroxysmal atrial fibrillation (last episode 2 years prior to presentation), long-standing hypertension, moderate chronic obstructive pulmonary disease, and mild renal insufficiency (GFR 25 ml/min/1.7m^3*). He was a 40-pack-year smoker, having quit 5 years prior to this event.*

He indicated on questioning that over the last 2 months he had experienced back and flank pain that was dull and constant. He denied any sudden increase in the pain, groin discomfort (a sign of retroperitoneal expansion and femoral nerve compression), bladder issues, or syncope.

Review of systems revealed reasonable exercise tolerance (he was able to golf and pull a cart without chest pain or dyspnea), no admissions to hospital for management of his COPD, or use of oral steroids in the past 24 months. His blood pressure was well controlled on home monitoring, and he had only mild reflux disease. His STOP/BANG score was three.

Medications: Losartan/hydrochlorothiazide (100 mg/12.5 mg OD), atorvastatin 80 mg OD, metoprolol 25 mg BID, ASA 81 mg OD, tiotropium bromide 2.5 mg OD, and fluticasone propionate/salmeterol 100 µg/50 µg BID.

Physical Examination: Vital signs and oxygen saturation were normal, including erect and supine BP. BP measured on the left and right arm did not vary. An obvious pulsatile abdominal mass was observed, but this was non-tender on gentle palpation. Auscultation of the chest revealed distant breath sounds but no localized wheeze. Heart sounds were normal apart from an S4 audible at the apex on expiration. Carotids were easily palpable with no bruits detected. Radial pulses were strong and of normal character bilaterally.

Investigations: Apart from the abnormal renal function data (vide supra), other laboratory tests were within normal limits.

When Is an Enlargement of the Aorta Considered Aneurysmal?

The size of the normal aorta decreases in a tapering manner from the aortic valve to its termination. The normal diameter of the ascending and descending aorta is defined as <2.1 cm/m^2 and 1.6 cm/m^2, respectively [1]. However, aorta dimensions enlarge in tandem with increasing body surface area and with advancing age. Descending aorta dimensions >3 cm/m^2 are abnormal.

What Are the Risk Factors, Screening Recommendations, Time Course of Enlargement, and Point of Consideration of Surgical Intervention for AAA?

The main risk factors for AAA are male sex, age >65 years, smoking, a coronary artery disease and/or peripheral vascular disease history, first-degree relative with AAA, or presence of aneurysms elsewhere. The US Preventive Services Taskforce recommends one-time ultrasonographic screening for AAA in all males between the ages of 65–75 years with

B. A. Finegan (✉)
Department of Anesthesiology & Pain Medicine, University of Alberta, Edmonton, AB, Canada
e-mail: bfinegan@ualberta.ca

D. Dillane, B. A. Finegan (eds.), *Preoperative Assessment*, https://doi.org/10.1007/978-3-030-58842-7_11

an ever-smoking history. The prevalence of AAA in this population is 1.2–3.3% in men over 60 years of age [2].

The average annual expansion rate for aneurysms between 3.0 to 3.9 cm, 4.0 cm to 6.0 cm, and >6.0 cm is 1 to 4 mm, 3 to 5 mm, and 7 to 8 mm, respectively. The greater the dimension of the aneurysm, the higher the risk of rupture. Referral for a surgical opinion should be considered when an AAA reaches 5 cm in diameter, particularly in females, and definitive repair is indicated when AAA is > 5.4 cm in diameter if the patient is a suitable surgical candidate [3].

Are There Validated AAA Perioperative Risk Assessment Tools?

The Vascular Quality Initiative (VQI) perioperative risk score suite, which is freely available for use at https://www.vqi.org/resources/vqi-risk-calculators-2/ [4], provides an opportunity to estimate mortality and perioperative myocardial infarction risk for individuals undergoing either open AAA repair (OAR) or EVAR [5, 6]. Individuals with high VQI risk scores should be considered for high dependency unit admission following surgery.

Is There a Mortality Difference in Outcome Between OAR and EVAR?

There is a clear short-term survival benefit with EVAR compared to OAR, but this appears to be gradually lost over periods ranging from 2 to 10 years due to EVAR catch-up morbidity and mortality [7, 8]. This finding may change given the evolving nature of EVAR technology, the development of specialized vascular surgery referral centers, and enhanced operator expertise. Given current survival data, there is some support, particularly in Europe, in offering OAR to patients with a reasonable chance of long-term survival and directing those with a shorter life expectancy to EVAR management [9]. However, in North America, EVAR has replaced OAR as the method of choice for AAA surgical management. Not all patients are suitable for EVAR due to anatomic requirements, excessive thrombus, multiple accessory renal arteries, or other issues.

What Specific Preoperative Assessment/Investigations/Interventions Are Recommended Prior to AAA?

The Society for Vascular Surgery has recently (2018) published updated guidelines on the preoperative care and assessment of patients with AAA [3]. These include a "strong" recommendation that the following apply to patients being considered for either elective OAR or EVAR:

1. Cardiology consultation in patients with active cardiac conditions (unstable angina, decompensated heart failure, severe valvular heart disease, and significant dysrhythmias).
2. A 12-lead electrocardiogram (ECG) within 30 days of planned surgery.
3. Echocardiography for those with dyspnea of unknown origin or increasing dyspnea.

   In the absence of a clear indication, cardiac stress testing of patients prior to vascular surgical intervention is not indicated and of doubtful value in improving outcome [10]. There is no role for "elective" coronary revascularization prior to AAA repair in patients who otherwise would not have been considered for it [11].
4. Discontinuation of smoking 2 weeks prior to surgery. Smoking-related pulmonary disease is common in patients with AAA. Smoking is a key risk factor for the development of AAA, infection following surgery, impaired wound healing, and OAR/EVAR early and late complications. Assessment and optimal preoperative management of COPD is addressed in Chap. 14.
5. Preoperative hydration of patients with renal insufficiency and those at risk of contrast-induced nephropathy undergoing EVAR.

Acute kidney injury (AKI) is a frequent complication of AAA repair, especially OAR, and is one of the key complications of both OAR and EVAR that leads to morbidity and death. Multiple risk calculators have been developed that address the propensity for AKI to develop postoperatively in AAA patients [12, 13]. Key factors that increase the risk of AKI are advanced age, supra-/juxta-renal aneurysm location, OAR vs. EVAR, and a history of preexisting hypertension/respiratory/renal disease. There are few validated interventions that effectively prevent AKI from developing following surgery, but the recommendations of the Kidney Disease Improving Global Outcomes (KDIGO) group deserve consideration [14]. These recommendations include preoperative discontinuation of nephrotoxic drugs (if feasible), adequate perioperative hydration, functional hemodynamic monitoring to aid in avoiding hypotension, intraoperative euglycemia, following creatinine and urine output levels perioperatively, and minimizing use of contrast dye. In the preoperative setting, pausing ACE inhibitors/ACE receptor blockers, diuretics, and NSAIDs would seem to be prudent. Susceptible patients should be informed of the risk of postoperative AKI and the probable need for invasive intraoperative BP monitoring.

What Forms of Anesthetic Management Should Be Discussed with the Patient Scheduled for Elective EVAR?

Local infiltration, regional block, and general anesthesia have all been used successfully in patients undergoing EVAR. Selection of the form of anesthesia usually depends on the experience of the anesthesiologist, institutional practice, and the preferences of the anesthesiologist and operating surgeon. However, there is emerging evidence that the use of local/regional anesthesia techniques rather than general anesthesia in EVAR decreases pulmonary morbidity, operating time, and length of stay [15, 16]. These data echo the demonstrated advantage of locoregional techniques on mortality in the endovascular management of ruptured AAA [17]. A general discussion with the patient regarding available anesthetic options at the time of the preoperative visit is appropriate.

What Anesthetic Management Strategy Should Be Discussed with the Patient Scheduled for an Elective OAR?

General anesthesia is almost universally used to facilitate OAR. There is compelling evidence from retrospective analysis of prospectively collected data that general anesthesia should be combined with thoracic epidural anesthesia to provide intraoperative and postoperative pain management [18]. This approach appears to be associated with reduced postoperative renal and pulmonary morbidity and improved 5-year survival in OAR [18].

Invasive monitoring including arterial line placement and central venous access in selected cases are appropriate. Frequently, transesophageal echocardiography is used intraoperatively to assess cardiac function and volume status.

The calculated VQI postoperative mortality risk score after elective EVAR was 2.6% for this patient, and his VQI cardiac risk index score was 1.7%. These were reassuring data suggesting that the patient would undergo an uneventful procedure, which indeed transpired.

True-False Questions

1. In the case of an AAA:
   (a) Aortic dimensions ≤4.0 cm are reassuring and within normal limits.
   (b) CT angiography is the preferred screening method.
   (c) Annual expansion rate increases in line with enlarging dimensions of the aorta.
   (d) Up to 2 years after surgery, EVAR holds a survival advantage over OAR.
   (e) All patients are suitable for EVAR.
2. In the preoperative assessment and management of AAA patients:
   (a) Cardiac stress testing is warranted and valuable.
   (b) Echocardiography may be helpful.
   (c) Discontinuation of NSAIDs preoperatively is prudent.
   (d) ACE inhibitors should be continued to control intraoperative hypertension.
   (e) Thoracic epidural anesthesia should be considered for those undergoing OAR.

References

1. Erbel R, Eggebrecht H. Aortic dimensions and the risk of dissection. Heart. 2006;92(1):137–42.
2. US Preventive Services Task Force, Owens DK, Davidson KW, Krist AH, Barry MJ, Cabana M, Caughey AB, et al. Screening for abdominal aortic aneurysm: US preventive services task force recommendation statement. JAMA. 2019;322(22):2211–8.
3. Chaikof EL, Dalman RL, Eskandari MK, Jackson BM, Lee WA, Mansour MA, et al. The Society for Vascular Surgery practice guidelines on the care of patients with an abdominal aortic aneurysm. J Vasc Surg. 2018;67(1):2–77.e2.
4. Society for Vascular Surgery. The Vascular Study Group of New England. The Vascular Quality Initiative. VQI Risk Calculators. https://www.vqi.org/resources/vqi-risk-calculators-2/. Accessed 16 Apr 2020.
5. Eslami MH, Rybin DV, Doros G, Siracuse JJ, Farber A. External validation of Vascular Study Group of New England risk predictive model of mortality after elective abdominal aorta aneurysm repair in the Vascular Quality Initiative and comparison against established models. J Vasc Surg. 2018;67(1):143–50.
6. Bertges DJ, Neal D, Schanzer A, Scali ST, Goodney PP, Eldrup-Jorgensen J, Cronenwett JL. Vascular Quality Initiative. The Vascular Quality Initiative Cardiac Risk Index for prediction of myocardial infarction after vascular surgery. J Vasc Surg. 2016;64(5):1411–1421.e4.
7. Patel R, Sweeting MJ, Powell JT, Greenhalgh RM, EVAR trial investigators. Endovascular versus open repair of abdominal aortic aneurysm in 15-years' follow-up of the UK endovascular aneurysm repair trial 1 (EVAR trial 1): a randomised controlled trial. Lancet. 2016;388(10058):2366–74.
8. Lederle FA, Kyriakides TC, Stroupe KT, Freischlag JA, Padberg FT Jr, Matsumura JS, Huo Z, Johnson GR, Veterans Affairs OVER. Cooperative Study Group. Open versus endovascular repair of abdominal aortic aneurysm. N Engl J Med. 2019;380(22):2126–35.
9. Antoniou GA, Antoniou SA, Torella F. Editor's choice - endovascular vs. open repair for abdominal aortic aneurysm: systematic review and meta-analysis of updated peri-operative and long term data of randomised controlled trials. Eur J Vasc Endovasc Surg. 2020;59(3):385–97.
10. Chan K, Abou-Zamzam AM, Woo K. Preoperative cardiac stress testing in the Southern California Vascular Outcomes Improvement Collaborative. Ann Vasc Surg. 2018;49:234–40.
11. Fleisher LA. Preoperative assessment of the patient with cardiac disease undergoing noncardiac surgery. Anesthesiol Clin. 2016;34(1):59–70.
12. Grant SW, Grayson AD, Grant MJ, Purkayastha D, McCollum CN. What are the risk factors for renal failure following open elec-

tive abdominal aortic aneurysm repair? Eur J Vasc Endovasc Surg. 2012;43(2):182–7.
13. Dang T, Dakour-Aridi H, Rizwan M, Nejim B, Malas MB. Predictors of acute kidney injury after infrarenal abdominal aortic aneurysm repair in octogenarians. J Vasc Surg. 2019;69(3):752–762.e1.
14. Romagnoli S, Ricci Z, Ronco C. Perioperative acute kidney injury: prevention, early recognition, and supportive measures. Nephron. 2018;140(2):105–10.
15. Van Orden K, Farber A, Schermerhorn ML, Goodney PP, Kalish JA, Jones DW, et al. Vascular Quality Initiative. Local anesthesia for percutaneous endovascular abdominal aortic aneurysm repair is associated with fewer pulmonary complications. J Vasc Surg. 2018;68(4):1023–9.e2.
16. Harky A, Ahmad MU, Santoro G, Eriksen P, Chaplin G, Theologou T. Local versus general anesthesia in nonemergency endovascular abdominal aortic aneurysm repair: a systematic review and meta-analysis. J Cardiothorac Vasc Anesth. 2020;34(4):1051–9.
17. Mouton R, Rogers CA, Harris RA, Hinchliffe RJ. Local anaesthesia for endovascular repair of ruptured abdominal aortic aneurysm. Br J Surg. 2019;106(1):74–81.
18. Bardia A, Sood A, Mahmood F, Orhurhu V, Mueller A, Montealegre-Gallegos M, et al. Combined epidural-general anesthesia vs general anesthesia alone for elective abdominal aortic aneurysm repair. JAMA Surg. 2016;151(12):1116–23.

Marfan Syndrome

12

Derek Dillane

A 33-year-old male patient with Marfan syndrome (MFS) presented for preoperative assessment before elective total thyroidectomy. One month prior to this presentation, he had undergone an uneventful aortic valve replacement (AVR) for severe aortic valve insufficiency and removal of Nuss bars. He had previously undergone an aortic valve-sparing root replacement and mitral valve repair, 15 and 8 years prior, respectively. He had a background of polymorphic ventricular tachycardia that required insertion of an implantable cardioverter-defibrillator (ICD). Day 1 post AVR, he developed rapid atrial fibrillation and decompensated heart failure requiring inotropic support. He was cardioverted successfully and started on amiodarone. One month later, he re-presented with amiodarone-induced hyperthyroidism.

Medications: Prednisone 40 mg daily, ramipril, aspirin, bisoprolol, methimazole 20 mg twice daily, warfarin, spironolactone, pregabalin, and hydromorphone 1 mg twice daily.

Physical Examination: The patient was noted to be 195 cm tall with disproportionately long arms and long, thin fingers. He weighed 59 kg. He had a partially repaired pectus excavatum. He was in atrial fibrillation with a rate between 116 and 145 bpm. There were no other obvious clinical signs of hyperthyroidism.

Investigations: Laboratory findings on first anesthesia encounter, i.e., the day prior to thyroidectomy, can be found in Table 12.1.

ECG on admission and on the day prior to surgery can be seen in Figs. 12.1 and 12.2, *respectively. Preoperative chest radiograph is shown in* Fig. 12.3.

Table 12.1 Laboratory findings the day prior to thyroidectomy

Test	Results	Reference range (units)
Hgb	90	140–175 (g/L)
WBC	16	4.0–10.0 (×10⁹/L)
PLT	232	145–450 (×10⁹/L)
INR	2.4	0.8–1.2
TSH	< 0.01	0.2–4 (mIU/L)
Free T3	8.1	3.5–6.5 (pmol/L)
Free T4	49.5	9–23 (pmol/L)
Total Calcium	2.26	2.1–2.6 (mmol/L)

Hgb hemoglobin, *WBC* white blood cell count, *PLT* platelet count, *INR* international normalized ratio, *TSH* thyroid-stimulating hormone, *Free T3* thyroxine, *Free T4* thyroxine

Transthoracic echocardiography showed severe left ventricular hypertrophy with severely reduced left ventricular function. Left ventricular ejection was estimated at 20–25%, and severe global hypokinesis was noted. The left atrium was severely dilated. A mitral annuloplasty ring was noted in good position. There was mild to moderate mitral regurgitation. The recently replaced aortic valve appeared well seated, and there was no evidence of aortic regurgitation. The right ventricular cavity was noted to be small and hypokinetic. The pulmonic valve appeared grossly normal. Due to technical difficulties associated with the patient's scoliosis and pectus deformity, it was difficult to comment on right-sided pressures, but right ventricular systolic pressure was estimated to be at least 30–40 mmHg.

Computed tomography (CT) of the chest confirmed the presence of a bioprosthetic valve and ascending aortic graft. The remainder of the aorta was noted to be dilated measuring up to 5.5 cm at the suprarenal abdominal location. A type B aortic dissection, of long-standing presence, was again noted, with a dissection flap to the aortic bifurcation.

Technetium 99m-MIBI thyroid scan findings were in keeping with Type II amiodarone-induced thyrotoxicosis.

D. Dillane (✉)
Department of Anesthesiology & Pain Medicine, University of Alberta, Edmonton, AB, Canada

D. Dillane, B. A. Finegan (eds.), *Preoperative Assessment*, https://doi.org/10.1007/978-3-030-58842-7_12

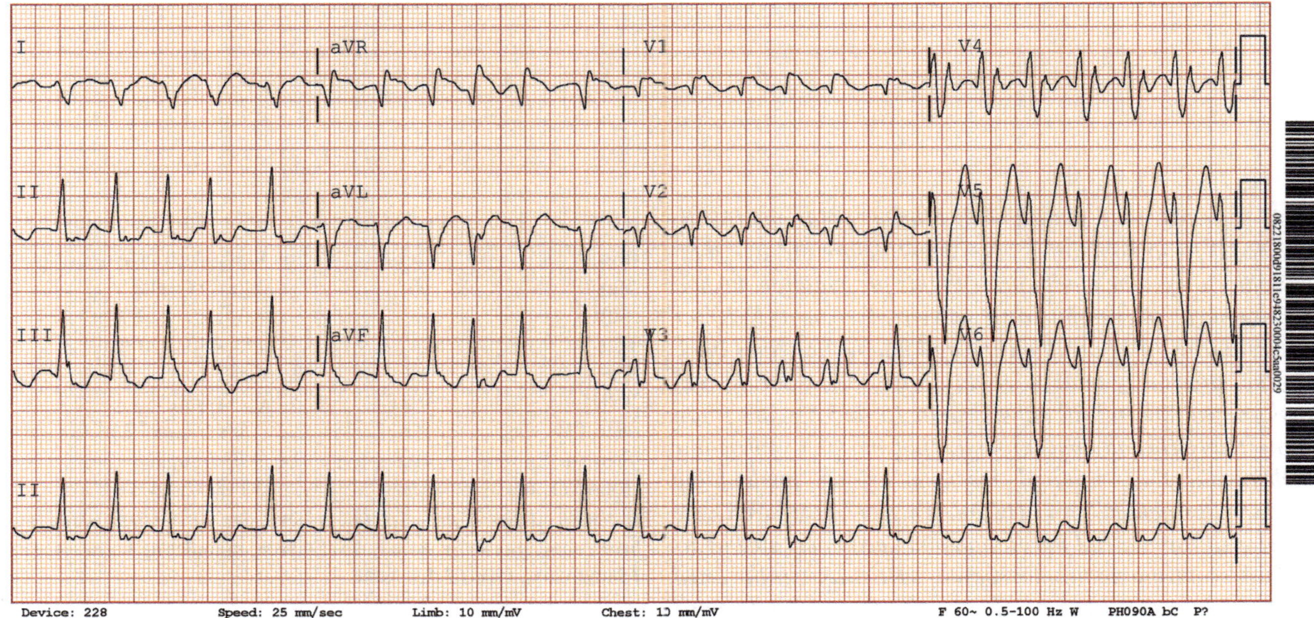

Fig. 12.1 Atrial fibrillation on electrocardiogram on readmission with amidarone-induced thyrotoxicosis

What Is Marfan Syndrome?

MFS is a disorder of connective tissue. It is usually associated with mutations in the fibrillin-1 gene (*FBN-1*). MFS is inherited in an autosomal dominant fashion, although about 25% of cases are due to sporadic new mutations; a family history is not always present [1]. The incidence of MFS is reported as 2–3/10,000 individuals [1]. Fibrillin is a large glycoprotein that is an important component of connective tissue in arteries, lung, skin, the ocular lens, and dura mater [2]. The diagnosis of MFS is primarily a clinical one. Genetic testing for mutations in the fibrillin-1 gene is available and may be used to confirm diagnosis. However, genetic testing is neither sensitive nor specific enough to make a reliable diagnosis. To put this in context, more than 1800 different mutations of the fibrillin-1 gene have been identified. Some of these mutations do not result in a typical Marfan phenotype but are associated with a milder disease.

What Are the Clinical Manifestations of MFS?

MFS is a multisystem disorder with abnormalities mainly involving the skeletal, cardiovascular, ocular, and pulmonary systems in addition to the skin and dura. A set of defined diagnostic criteria, known as the Ghent nosology, comprising major and minor manifestations, has been developed to aid recognition and diagnosis [3]. Aortic root dilatation/dissection and ocular lens dislocation (ectopia lentis) are the cardinal clinical features. The revised Ghent criteria are summarized in Tables 12.2 and 12.3.

What Is the Aortic Root?

The aortic root is defined as that part of the left ventricular outflow tract that supports the leaflets of the aortic valve.

```
HR      66   . Sinus rhythm
RR     912   . Repol abnrm, global ischemia, diffuse leads
PR     160
QRSD   134
QT     453
QTc    475

-- AXIS --
P       76
QRS    103
```

- ABNORMAL ECG -

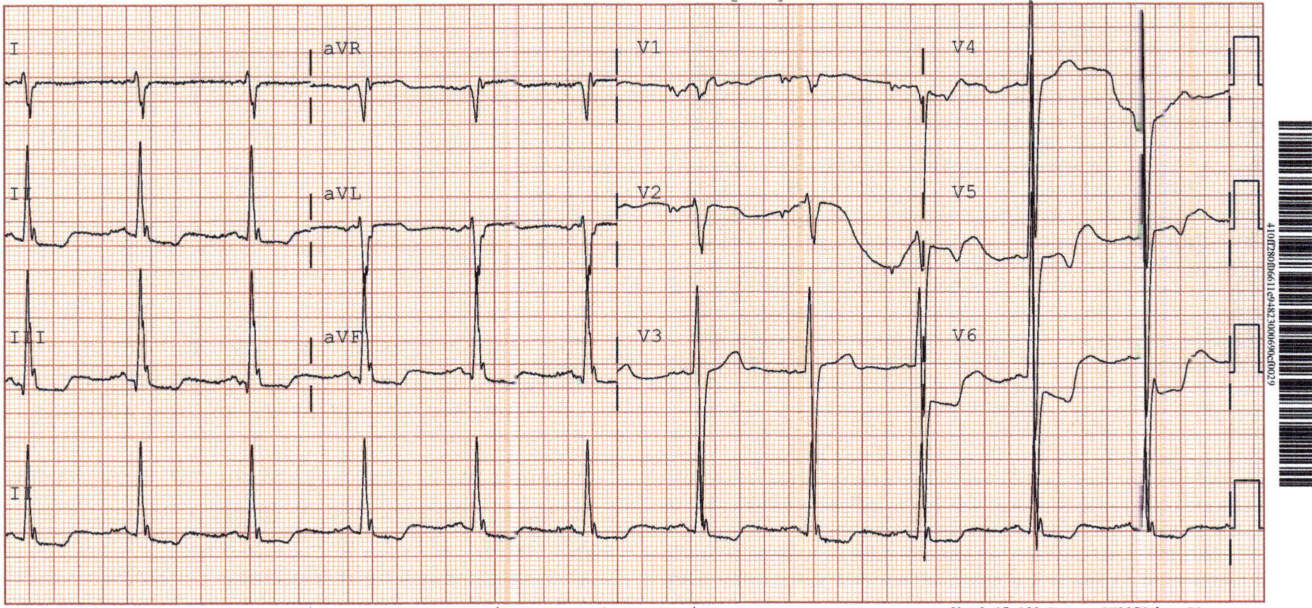

Device: 235 Speed: 25 mm/sec Limb: 10 mm/mV Chest: 10 mm/mV 60~ 0.15-100 Hz PH110C

Fig. 12.2 Electrocardiogram reverted to sinus rhythm after 3 weeks of treatment with methimazole and prednisone for thyrotoxicosis

What Are Nuss Bars?

The Nuss procedure is a surgical procedure performed to correct pectus excavatum. It is considered a minimally invasive procedure where one to three curved metal bars are inserted behind the sternum. They are usually removed after approximately 3 years [4].

What Pulmonary Manifestations May Be Relevant Perioperatively?

Early onset of emphysema is common. These emphysematous changes may exacerbate the restrictive changes associated with kyphoscoliosis. Associated upper lobe bullae can predispose to pneumothorax. A history of recurrent pneumothorax can be found in up to 10% of MFS patients [5].

What Cardiac Findings Are Associated with MFS?

Cardiac disease is the major cause of morbidity and mortality in MFS.

(a) The atrioventricular (AV) valves are most commonly affected. Thickening of either the mitral, tricuspid, or both AV valves is common and associated with variable degrees of prolapse and regurgitation (MVR) [1]. Mitral valve prolapse has a high prevalence in the general population (2–3%) [6]. In a population-based cohort study of 204 patients with MFS, mitral valve prolapse was identified in 40% and severe MVR in 12% of study subjects. Severe MVR was associated with concomitant tricuspid valve prolapse and the sporadic form of MFS. The incidence of mitral valve prolapse was found to increase with advancing age [7]. In children with early-onset severe MFS, MVR can lead to congestive cardiac failure, pulmonary hypertension, and death. It is

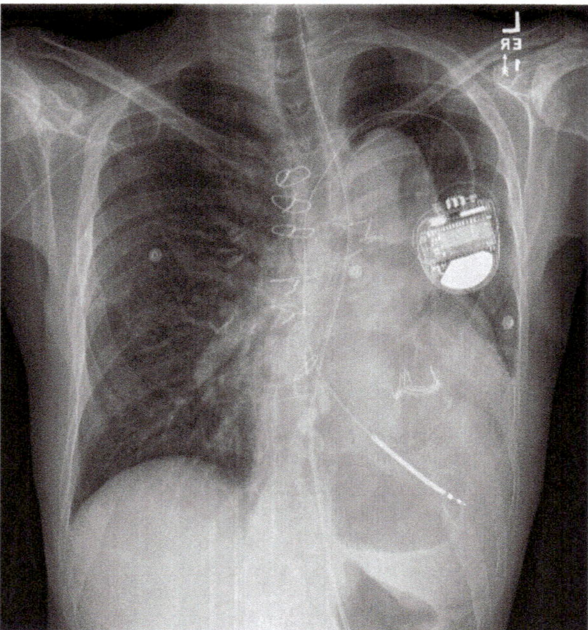

Fig. 12.3 Chest radiograph. The heart is displaced into the left hemithorax. The anteroposterior diameter of the thorax was noted to be very narrow secondary to moderate thoracic lordosis and the pectus excavatum deformity. A minor scoliosis of the upper thoracic spine, convex left, can also be seen. The aortic arch and descending thoracic aorta are tortuous and moderately ectatic. A Keofeed catheter terminates in the distal gastric body. A single-lead implantable cardioverter-defibrillator is visible in the upper left chest wall. A peripherally inserted central catheter (PICC) is seen entering the right hemithorax. Sequelae of recent surgery are evident – midline sternotomy wires and multiple mediastinal surgical clips

Table 12.2 Revised Ghent criteria outlining the distinct features for diagnosis of Marfan syndrome. The presence of any of the following criteria is diagnostic. Z-score describes the number of standard deviations by which a given measurement lies above or below a size- or age-specific population mean [3]

No family history of Marfan syndrome	Family history of Marfan syndrome
Aortic diameter $Z \geq 2$ and ectopia lentis	Ectopia lentis
Aortic diameter $Z \geq 2$ and fibrillin-1 mutation	System score ≥7 (see Table 12.3)
Aortic diameter $Z \geq 2$ and systemic score ≥7 (see Table 12.3)	Aortic diameter $Z \geq 2$ above 20 years old, ≥3 below 20 years
Ectopia lentis and fibrillin-1 mutation with known aortic root dilatation or dissection	

the leading cause of mortality in early childhood MFS [1, 8].

(b) Aneurysmal dilatation of the aortic root results in aortic regurgitation, dissection, or rupture. Aortic aneurysm and dissection are the most life-threatening complications of MFS. In contrast to atherosclerotic aortic aneurysm, dilatation is greatest at – and may even be restricted to – the aortic root. The most important considerations when calculating risk of rupture are maximal diameter and family history of dissection. Monitoring is performed annually with echocardiography or cross-sectional imaging with magnetic resonance imaging (MRI) or CT. Surgery is recommended when the diameter of the ascending aorta at the level of the aortic sinuses is ≥5 cm [9]. Surgery may be performed earlier in the presence of a family history of dissection, increased rate of dilatation, or severe aortic regurgitation with left ventricular dilatation. The standard surgical approach is the Bentall procedure, which involves composite graft replacement of the aortic valve, aortic root, and ascending aorta with reimplantation of the coronary arteries into the graft [9]. A valve-sparing root and ascending aortic replacement can be performed in the presence of a normal aortic valve. Undiagnosed MFS frequently leads to aortic dissection. Dissection in MFS usually begins proximally, just above the origin of the coronary arteries, and can extend throughout the entire aorta (type A dissection). According to the Stanford classification, type A dissections affect the ascending aorta and the arch. Type B dissections do not involve the ascending aorta. Type A dissection is a surgical emergency. Type B dissection (descending aorta) can often be managed conservatively. Surgery may be required in the event of development of complications of the dissection or failure of medical management.

(c) Dilatation may also involve the distal thoracic aorta, the abdominal aorta, the pulmonary artery, and the carotid arteries [10].

(d) Dilated cardiomyopathy unrelated to valvular disease has been described but is an unusual finding in MFS [1, 11].

Table 12.3 Scoring of systemic features of Marfan syndrome for use in Ghent criteria for diagnosis. Maximum total is 20 points. A score ≥7 indicates systemic involvement [3]

Systemic feature	Score
Wrist ***and*** thumb sign	3
Wrist ***or*** thumb sign	1
Pectus carinatum deformity	2
Hindfoot deformity	1
Pneumothorax	2
Dural ectasia	2
Reduced upper segment/lower segment ratio ***and*** increased arm/height	2
Scoliosis or thoracolumbar kyphosis	1
Reduced elbow extension	1
Facial features	1
Skin striae	1
Myopia	1
Mitral valve prolapse	1

What Is the Medical Management for MFS?

- Annual monitoring of aortic growth, including absolute size and rate of growth by echocardiography or CT/MRI, if echocardiography is technically difficult due to the presence of a pectus deformity or kyphoscoliosis
- Beta-adrenergic blockade is the standard of care to delay or prevent aortic aneurysm and dissection. Treatment with beta-blockers is thought to reduce aortic wall stress and the rate of aortic dilatation. Treatment should be started early in the disease process regardless of the diameter of the aorta.
- Angiotensin-converting enzyme (ACE) inhibitors or angiotensin receptor blocker (ARBs) can be used for blood pressure control in patients who are intolerant of beta-blockade. The 2010 American College of Cardiology/ American Heart Association/ American Association for Thoracic Surgery Guidelines for the Diagnosis and Management of Patients with Thoracic Aortic Disease recommend a combination of beta-blockade and ACE inhibitor/ARB therapy titrated to the lowest blood pressure tolerable without adverse effects [12].
- Calcium channel blockade may increase the risk of aortic dissection compared to other antihypertensive agents, and its use for the medical management of MFS is not widely agreed upon [13].

What Is the Life Expectancy for Individuals with MFS?

Improvements in early diagnosis and effective medical and surgical management have resulted in a near normal life expectancy for patients with MFS. This is a dramatic improvement from that seen in the early 1970s when the average age of death was in the fourth and fifth decades [14].

How Should the Patient with MFS Be Evaluated Preoperatively?

Preoperative history, physical examination, and investigations will, to a large extent, be directed by the presence and extent of cardiopulmonary disease. This includes assessment for atrioventricular and aortic valve regurgitation and associated congestive cardiac failure and aortic dilatation and dissection. MFS patients have an annual assessment of aortic diameter by echocardiography or CT/MRI. This usually includes echocardiographic evaluation of ventricular function. This should be performed preoperatively if an appropriately recent study is not available for review. Optimization of arrhythmia management, whether medically or by implantable device, needs to occur at the preoperative evaluation stage (see below for implantable cardioverter-defibrillator [ICD] discussion). The degree to which the lungs have been altered by emphysematous changes and restrictive kyphoscoliosis can be assessed by chest radiograph and pulmonary function testing. Airway evaluation may reveal abnormalities that predispose to difficult intubation, e.g., high palate, overcrowding of the teeth, prognathism, and ligamentous hyperlaxity of the temporomandibular joints and cervical spine. All joints should be assessed for laxity in order to avoid dislocation during intraoperative patient positioning.

How Should This Patient's ICD Be Managed Perioperatively?

This topic is addressed in detail in Chap. 9. Ensure that the ICD has undergone a device check in the previous 6 months. The anti-tachyarrhythmia function must be suspended for surgery and resumed in the post-anesthesia care unit postoperatively. This can be performed with a magnet in an emergency.

Why Was This Patient on Warfarin?

He had undergone bioprosthetic aortic valve replacement 1 month prior to this episode of thyrotoxicosis. Anticoagulation is maintained in this population for 3–6 months in patients with risk factors for thromboembolic events [15] This patient had a history of atrial fibrillation and, in addition, was known to have a severely dilated left atrium and was thus deemed to be at high enough risk to warrant anticoagulation.

This patient had his anticoagulation reversed with prothrombin complex concentrate 80 ml on the morning of surgery. Warfarin was restarted 24 hours postoperatively. He proceeded to total thyroidectomy after the anti-tachyarrhythmia function of his ICD was disabled by the pacemaker technician. He was given a stress steroid dose of methylprednisolone 125 mg on induction (see Chap. 19 *for detailed discussion on surgical stress dosing of steroids). He had an arterial line placed prior to induction, and it was noted that he was easy to intubate with a video laryngoscope. He returned to the cardiac intensive care unit after uneventful surgery.*

True/False Questions

1. (a) Autosomal dominant inheritance is a pattern of inheritance where a parent with the condition has a 50% chance of having a child with the condition.
   (b) MFS is definitively diagnosed by genetic testing for a mutation on the fibrillin-1 gene.
   (c) A history of ocular lens dislocation is a major diagnostic criterion for MFS.

   (d) Pneumothorax is a rare finding in Marfan syndrome.
   (e) Aortic aneurysm and dissection are the major cause of morbidity and mortality in MFS.
2. (a) Beta-adrenergic blockade is the standard of care to delay aortic dilatation.
   (b) ACE inhibitors and ARBs are contraindicated in patients with aortic dilatation.
   (c) Type A aortic dissection does not affect the ascending aorta.
   (d) Type A aortic dissection is a surgical emergency.
   (e) Dilated cardiomyopathy unrelated to valvular disease is an unusual finding in MFS.

References

1. Judge DP, Dietz HC. Marfan's syndrome. Lancet. 2005;366(9501):1965–76.
2. Grecu L, Chawla N, Disease V. In: Hines R, Marschall K, editors. Stoelting's anesthesia and co-existing disease. Philadelphia: Elsevier; 2018. p. 239–40.
3. Loeys BL, Dietz HC, Braverman AC, Callewaert BL, De Backer J, Devereux RB, et al. The revised Ghent nosology for the Marfan syndrome. J Med Genet. 2010;47(7):476–85.
4. Pilegaard HK. Short Nuss bar procedure. Ann Cardiothorac Surg. 2016;5(5):513–8.
5. Wood JR, Bellamy D, Child AH, Citron KM. Pulmonary disease in patients with Marfan syndrome. Thorax. 1984;39(10):780–4.
6. Delling FN, Vasan RS. Epidemiology and pathophysiology of mitral valve prolapse: new insights into disease progression, genetics, and molecular basis. Circulation. 2014;129(21):2158–70.
7. Rybczynski M, Mir TS, Sheikhzadeh S, Bernhardt AM, Schad C, Treede H, et al. Frequency and age-related course of mitral valve dysfunction in the Marfan syndrome. Am J Cardiol. 2010;106(7):1048–53.
8. Sisk HE, Zahka KG, Pyeritz RE. The Marfan syndrome in early childhood: analysis of 15 patients diagnosed at less than 4 years of age. Am J Cardiol. 1983;52(3):353–8.
9. Castellano JM, Silvay G, Castillo JG. Marfan syndrome: clinical, surgical, and anesthetic considerations. Semin Cardiothorac Vasc Anesth. 2014;18(3):260–71.
10. Wright MJ, Connolly HM. Genetics, clinical features, and diagnosis of Marfan syndrome and related disorders. In: Post TW, editor. UpToDate. Waltham MA: UpToDate; 2020.
11. Alpendurada F, Wong J, Kiotsekoglou A, Banya W, Child A, Prasad SK, et al. Evidence for Marfan cardiomyopathy. Eur J Heart Fail. 2010;12(10):1085–91.
12. Hiratzka LF, Bakris GL, Beckman JA, Bersin RM, Carr VF, Casey DE Jr, et al. 2010 ACCF/AHA/AATS/ACR/ASA/SCA/SCAI/SIR/STS/SVM guidelines for the diagnosis and management of patients with thoracic aortic disease: a report of the American College of Cardiology Foundation/American Heart Association Task Force on Practice Guidelines, American Association for Thoracic Surgery, American College of Radiology, American Stroke Association, Society of Cardiovascular Anesthesiologists, Society for Cardiovascular Angiography and Interventions, Society of Interventional Radiology, Society of Thoracic Surgeons, and Society for Vascular Medicine. Circulation. 2010;121(13):e266–369.
13. Doyle JJ, Doyle AJ, Wilson NK, Habashi JP, Bedja D, Whitworth RE, et al. A deleterious gene-by-environment interaction imposed by calcium channel blockers in Marfan syndrome. elife. 2015;4:e08648.
14. Pyeritz RE. Marfan syndrome: 30 years of research equals 30 years of additional life expectancy. Heart. 2009;95(3):173–5.
15. Cremer P, Barzilai B. Anticoagulation strategies after bioprosthetic valve replacement: what should we do? American College of Cardiology. Latest in cardiology. Expert analysis. 19 Dec 2016. Available from: https://www.acc.org/latest-in-cardiology/articles/2016/12/19/08/44/anticoagulation-strategies-after-bioprosthetic-valve-replacement. Accessed 27 Oct 2019.

Part III

Pulmonary

Obstructive Sleep Apnea

13

Derek Dillane

A 52-year-old male patient was seen at the preadmission clinic 2 weeks in advance of a scheduled ambulatory arthroscopic repair of a rotator cuff tear. He had a history of hypertension for which he had been prescribed losartan. He was not taking any other prescribed medication. He denied any history or symptoms related to coronary artery disease, congestive cardiac failure, or carotid artery disease. He was a lifelong smoker. His STOP-Bang score was 7/8 (Fig. 13.1) [1].

Physical Examination: Body mass index (BMI) was 38.5 and blood pressure was 154/108. Physical examination was otherwise normal. Airway examination revealed Mallampati II mouth opening, reduced neck extension, thyromental distance greater than 6 cm, and neck circumference of 46 cm.

Investigations: Normal CBC, electrolytes, creatinine, and random glucose. Triglyceride level was elevated at 1.89 mmol/L. Urinalysis and electrocardiogram (ECG) were normal.

How Is Obstructive Sleep Apnea (OSA) Defined?

According to the American Academy of Sleep Medicine, OSA is a breathing disorder characterized by narrowing of the upper airway that impairs normal ventilation during sleep [2]. Recurrent episodes of complete upper airway obstruction (apnea) or partial upper airway obstruction (hypopnea) may occur [3]. The number of these episodes occurring per hour, the apnea-hypopnea index (AHI), determines the severity of the condition.

Is There Any Difference Between OSA and OSA Syndrome?

OSA resulting in excessive daytime sleepiness (hypersomnolence) is known as OSA syndrome. It is associated with systemic hypertension, pulmonary hypertension, coronary artery disease, atrial fibrillation, cerebrovascular disease, and diabetes mellitus type 2 [3].

How Is Severity of OSA Classified?

OSA is classified according to the number of apneas and/or hypopneas per hour of sleep observed during a sleep study. This frequency is called the apnea-hypopnea index (AHI). Scoring is outlined in Table 13.1 [4]. Apnea is defined as cessation of air flow for 10 seconds. Hypopnea is a reduction of air flow (≥30%) for 10 seconds.

What Is the Prevalence of OSA in the General Population? How Does the Prevalence Change in the Presence of Obesity?

The prevalence of OSA in the general population is approximately 10–20% [5]. In the obese population, the prevalence of OSA is increased markedly especially in those undergoing bariatric surgery where the prevalence of OSA approaches 70% [3, 6]. OSA is undiagnosed, and subsequently untreated, in many patients, including those who are scheduled for surgery [7, 8].

D. Dillane (✉)
Department of Anesthesiology & Pain Medicine, University of Alberta, Edmonton, AB, Canada

D. Dillane, B. A. Finegan (eds.), *Preoperative Assessment*, https://doi.org/10.1007/978-3-030-58842-7_13

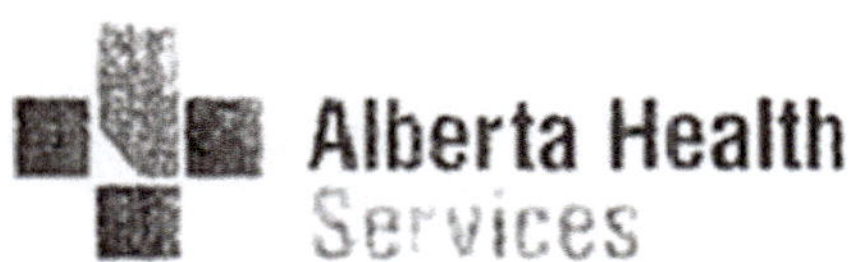

STOP-BANG Sleep Apnea Questionnaire
Chung F et al Anesthesiology 2008 and BJA 2012

STOP		
Do you SNORE loudly (louder than talking or loud enough to be heard through closed doors)?	Yes	No
Do you often feel TIRED, fatigued, or sleepy during daytime?	Yes	No
Has anyone OBSERVED you stop breathing during your sleep?	Yes	No
Do you have or are you being treated for high blood PRESSURE?	Yes	No
BANG		
BMI more than 35kg/m2?	Yes	No
AGE over 50 years old?	Yes	No
NECK circumference > 16 inches (40cm)?	Yes	No
GENDER: Male?	Yes	No
TOTAL SCORE	7	

High risk of OSA: Yes 5 - 8 Intermediate risk of OSA: Yes 3 - 4 Low risk of OSA: Yes 0 – 2

Fig. 13.1 A STOP-Bang questionnaire demonstrated that the patient was at high risk for OSA with an overall score of 7/8 [1]

Table 13.1 Apnea-hypopnea index (AHI)/obstructive sleep apnea (OSA) scale [4]

AHI	Degree of OSA
0–5	None
6–20	Mild
21–40	Moderate
> 40	Severe

What Are the Risk Factors for the Development of OSA?

1. Obesity.
2. Advancing age – risk for development of OSA increases from the third decade and peaks in 60–80-year-olds.
3. Males are more prone than females [9].
4. Medical conditions – congestive heart disease, renal failure, COPD, hypothyroidism, and polycystic ovarian disease are some medical disorders that are associated with an increased incidence of OSA.
5. Smoking – this is controversial. While the association is plausible, the evidence is less than conclusive [10].
6. Craniofacial abnormalities – more of a concern with children, e.g., adenotonsillar hypertrophy, cleft lip/palate, and abnormalities of the mandible or maxilla.

How Is OSA Diagnosed?

For a diagnosis of OSA, the American Academy of Sleep Medicine's *International Classification of Sleep Disorders* (3rd edition) [11] requires either:

1. *Signs and symptoms* (e.g., associated sleepiness, insomnia, fatigue, snoring, observed apnea) or an associated medical or psychiatric disorder (e.g., hypertension, atrial fibrillation, coronary artery disease, congestive heart failure, stroke, diabetes, mood disorder) *coupled with an AHI of 5*

   or
2. *AHI ≥ 15*

The gold standard for measurement of AHI is a Level 1 sleep study (full-night polysomnography). This requires considerable resources including the attendance of a trained technician overnight in a sleep laboratory. Level 1 studies capture multiple points of data: EEG (minimum of three channels), air flow, chin muscle tone, leg movement, eye movement, heart rate and rhythm, oxygen saturation, and chest and abdominal movement. The technician observes live video feed of the subject and comments contemporaneously on the data being recorded. Level 1 sleep studies provide a comprehensive assessment of changes occurring during sleep.

Level 2 studies capture similar data to Level 1 studies but without the presence of a technician. Level 3 studies use portable monitors which the patient can take home; they usually record at least three channels of data: oxygen saturation, air flow, and respiratory effort. There are no EEG data to determine sleep or arousal. According to the American Academy of Sleep Medicine Clinical Practice Guidelines, a Level 3 study (termed in the guideline "home sleep apnea testing") is appropriate for the diagnosis of uncomplicated adult patients thought to be at risk of moderate to severe sleep apnea [2]. Level 1 studies are recommended for those with "significant cardiorespiratory disease, potential respiratory muscle weakness due to a neuromuscular condition, awake hypoventilation or suspicion of sleep-related hypoventilation, chronic opioid medication use, history of stroke, or severe insomnia." Level 3 studies provide reasonable diagnostic accuracy compared to Level 1 studies in adult patients with a high probability of OSA and no unstable comorbidities [12].

What Is Central Sleep Apnea (CSA)?

As distinct from OSA, an obstructive issue, CSA occurs as a consequence of lack of ventilatory drive. It accounts for <10% of patients referred for Level 1 sleep studies. Examples include Cheyne-Stokes respiration (seen in patients with heart failure, dementia, and neuromuscular disorders) and the use of CNS depressants such as opioids, alcohol, and benzodiazepines. OSA and CSA can be present in the same patient. Level 1 studies are required to assess patients suspected to have CSA or combined OSA/CSA.

How Is OSA Screened for Preoperatively?

A number of questionnaires and screening tools have been developed to identify patients at high risk of OSA. These screening tools tend to have higher sensitivity than specificity, i.e., a low score indicates that the patient is unlikely to have OSA, but a high score warrants further consideration for a sleep study.

1. STOP-Bang is a validated screening tool for pre-surgery patients [1, 3] (see Fig. 13.1). STOP is an acronym for **S**noring, **T**iredness, **O**bserved apnea during sleep, and high blood **P**ressure. Bang is an acronym for **B**MI > 35 kg m^{-2}, **A**ge > 50 years, **N**eck circumference >16 inches/40 cm, and male **G**ender. Patients with five or more positive responses are deemed to be high risk for OSA. It has a sensitivity of 93% and 100% for AHI > 15 and AHI > 30, respectively.
2. The Berlin questionnaire is comprised of questions on snoring, excessive daytime sleepiness, sleepiness while driving, hypertension, age, sex, and BMI. The questionnaire is meant to be self-administered and is not as straightforward as the STOP-Bang questionnaire, with a slightly reduced sensitivity of 87% for AHI > 30 [13].
3. The Perioperative Sleep Apnea Prediction Score (P-SAP) was derived from an observational study of over 43,000 adult anesthesia cases [14]. Three demographic variables (age > 43 years, male sex, and obesity), three history variables (snoring, diabetes mellitus type 2, and hypertension), and three airway measures (large neck circumference, Mallampati score 3 or 4, and reduced thyromental distance) were identified as independent predictors for a diagnosis of OSA.

What Percentage of Patients Who Screen Positive for OSA with STOP-Bang Test Positive with Sleep Studies?

A retrospective study by Guralnick et al. reported that, of 211 patients who screened high risk for OSA with STOP-Bang (≥5) over a 2-year period, 2.5% did not have OSA, 16.1% had mild OSA, 26.3% had moderate OSA, and 55.1% had severe OSA on completion of a diagnostic polysomnogram [15].

What Comorbidities Are Associated with OSA?

- Cardiovascular complications, including hypertension, coronary artery disease, arrhythmia, and stroke, are more common in OSA [16, 17].
- Type 2 diabetes has been shown in a number of studies to be independently associated with OSA [18, 19]. Several possible explanations for this link have been posited, including sympathetic activation, oxidative stress, inflammation, and hypothalamic-pituitary-adrenal axis dysfunction [19].
- Pulmonary hypertension has been shown to occur to varying degrees in 20–40% of OSA patients in the absence of other known cardiopulmonary disorders. Pulmonary artery pressure (PAP) responds well to CPAP treatment in these patients [20]. However, the elevation in PAP appears to be mild (mean PAP of 20–30 mm Hg), similar to that seen in COPD patients with pulmonary hypertension.
- Gastroesophageal reflux disease (GERD) is frequently seen in OSA patients [21].

How Can the OSA Patient Be Optimized Preoperatively?

- Associated comorbidities should be assessed and optimized.
- Compliance with preoperative use of CPAP, as prescribed, should be emphasized.
- Consideration should be given to commencement of CPAP therapy preoperatively in the newly diagnosed OSA patient, particularly when OSA is severe.
- There is insufficient evidence to recommend weight loss as a means of preoperative optimization [4].

What Are the Perioperative Complications of OSA?

- Cardiovascular complications
  - OSA increases the risk of myocardial ischemia and infarction, arrhythmias, pulmonary embolism, and cardiac arrest. A large meta-analysis of 13 studies with almost 4000 patients demonstrated that the risk of a postoperative cardiac event was over twice as high in OSA patients [22].
- Respiratory complications
  - OSA has been associated with difficult mask ventilation and intubation [23, 24]. This may be independent of BMI [25].
  - Postoperative oxygen desaturation, respiratory failure requiring noninvasive or invasive ventilation, reintubation, acute respiratory distress syndrome (ARDS), and aspiration and bacterial pneumonia are seen with increased frequency postoperatively in patients with OSA [3, 26].
- Longer duration of stay [27]
- Unanticipated ICU transfer [22]
- Acute renal failure [27]
- Delirium [28]

What Circumstances May Exacerbate the Risk of Perioperative Complications Occurring in the OSA Patient?

Patients undergoing major surgery, general anesthesia, surgery requiring postoperative opioids, and those with higher grades of OSA may be at increased risk. A scoring system developed by the American Society of Anesthesiologists (Table 13.2) can be useful in determining the overall risk of postoperative OSA-related complications, but it is not evidence-based or clinically validated [3, 4].

Table 13.2 Scoring system for perioperative risk from OSA: Example* (From ASA Task Force on Perioperative Management of Patients With Obstructive Sleep Apnea [4], with permission of Wolters Kluwer and the American Society of Anesthesiologists)[a]

A. Severity of sleep apnea based on sleep study (or clinical indicators if sleep study is not available) Point score: (0–3)[b, c]	Points
Severity of OSA (see Table 13.1)	
None	0
Mild	1
Moderate	2
Severe	3
B. Invasiveness of surgery and anesthesia	Points
Point score: (0–3)	
Type of surgery and anesthesia	
Superficial surgery under local or peripheral nerve block anesthesia without sedation	0
Superficial surgery with moderate sedation or general anesthesia	1
Peripheral surgery with spinal or epidural anesthesia (with no more than moderate sedation)	1
Peripheral surgery with general anesthesia	2
Airway surgery with moderate sedation	2
Major surgery, general anesthesia	3
Airway surgery, general anesthesia	3
C. Requirement for postoperative opioids	Points
Point score: (0–3)	
Opioid requirement	
None	0
Low-dose oral opioids	1
High-dose oral opioids, parenteral or neuraxial opioids	3
D. Estimation of perioperative risk:	
Overall point score: The score for A plus the greater of the score for either B or C: (0–6)[d]	

CPAP Continuous positive airway pressure, *NIPPV* noninvasive positive pressure ventilation, *OSA* obstructive sleep apnea

[a]A scoring system similar to the above may be used to estimate whether a patient is at increased perioperative risk of complications from OSA. This example, which has not been clinically validated, is meant only as a guide, and clinical judgment should be used to assess the risk of an individual patient

[b]One point may be subtracted if a patient has been on CPAP or NIPPV before surgery and will be using his or her appliance consistently during the postoperative period

[c]One point should be added if a patient with mild or moderate OSA also has a resting >PaCO2 50 mmHg

[d]Patients with score of 4 may be at increased perioperative risk from OSA; patients with a score of 5 or 6 may be at significantly increased perioperative risk from OSA

Is There Any Reason Why This Patient Should Not Have an Interscalene Brachial Plexus (ISBP) Block to Reduce Perioperative Opioid Use?

ISBP blockade, as a result of a concomitant phrenic nerve block, is associated with diaphragmatic hemiparesis, the incidence of which approaches 100%. This is usually subclinical but may become problematic in the presence of chronic respiratory disease. OSA patients with a predisposition toward postoperative hypoxia might be considered at greater risk after ISBP block. However, the benefit of avoidance or reduction of postoperative opioid analgesia must also be taken into account. A large retrospective review of over 15,000 shoulder surgery patients who received ISBP blockade showed that the incidence of respiratory complications was similar in OSA and non-OSA populations [29, 30]. When particularly concerned about postoperative respiratory compromise, a low-volume block with a short-/medium-acting local anesthetic, e.g., lidocaine, can be injected as a bolus via an ISBP catheter followed by a continuous low-dose infusion. This can be calibrated to the patient's pain needs as tolerated.

What Factors Determine Whether Surgery Should Be Performed on an Inpatient or Outpatient Basis?

This decision must be individualized to each patient. Factors taken into consideration include OSA severity, invasiveness and nature of the surgery, presence of coexisting diseases, general versus regional anesthesia, postoperative opioid use, and patient age.

The patient was high risk for OSA based on his STOP-Bang score. A Level 3 study was requested, and the surgery was postponed. The Level 3 home sleep apnea test was inconclusive. Because of the persisting strong clinical suspicion for OSA, Level 1 studies/split-night polysomnography protocol was requested. The patient was found to have severe OSA requiring CPAP 10 cm H2O to establish a stable breathing pattern with elimination of snoring and obstructive hypopneas (Fig. 13.2). *Surgery was rescheduled for 4 weeks after the patient commenced CPAP therapy and proceeded without incident.*

True/False Questions

1. (a) The apnea-hypopnea index (AHI) is the number of episodes of complete or partial upper airway obstruction occurring per day.
   (b) An AHI of 15–25 signifies severe sleep apnea.
   (c) Males are more prone to OSA than females.
   (d) OSA can be diagnosed with an AHI ≥ 15.
   (e) Full-night polysomnography is never used in the diagnosis of OSA.
2. (a) The STOP-Bang screening tool is a highly sensitive questionnaire for the diagnosis of OSA
   (b) The STOP component of STOP-Bang is an acronym for Snoring, Tiredness, Obesity, and high blood Pressure
   (c) CPAP therapy should not be commenced in newly diagnosed OSA patients preoperatively.
   (d) Pulmonary hypertension is seen in up to 40% of OSA patients.
   (e) Interscalene brachial plexus block is contraindicated in OSA patients undergoing arthroscopic shoulder surgery.

a

Split Night Diagnostic PSG

RESPIRATORY EVENTS	Cen. Apneas	Obs. Apneas	Mxd. Apneas	Hypopneas	Total Apneas	Apnea+ Hypopnea	RERA	All Resp. Events*
Count:	0	0	0	157	0	157	0	157
Index (events/hr.):	0.0	0.0	0.0	90.9	0.0	90.9	0.0	90.9
Mean Duration (sec.):	N/A	N/A	N/A	21.5	N/A	21.5	N/A	21.5
Longest Event (sec.):	N/A	N/A	N/A	41.4	N/A	41.4	N/A	41.4
REM Count:	N/A	N/A	N/A	N/A	N/A	N/A	N/A	N/A
Non-REM Count:	0	0	0	157	0	157	0	157
REM Index:	N/A	N/A	N/A	N/A	N/A	N/A	N/A	N/A
Non-REM Index:	0.0	0.0	0.0	90.9	0.0	90.9	0.0	90.9

* Note: Does not contain Cheyne Stokes Breathing, Hypoventilation, or Periodic Breathing.

Fig. 13.2 (**a**) Diagnostic polysomnography revealed severe obstructive sleep apnea (OSA) with an apnea-hypopnea index (AHI) of 90.9. (**b**) Oxygen saturation was recorded between 60 and 69% for 5.3% of total sleep time (TST), 70 and 79% for 52% of TST, 80 and 89% for 38.3% 0f TST, and 90 and 100% for 4.4% of TST. The maximum transcutaneous partial pressure of carbon dioxide (TcpCO2) was 53.6 mmHg, signifying mild sleep hypoventilation

b

OXYGEN SATURATION	Wake	Non-REM	REM	TST	TIB
Max. SpO2%:	97.0	95.0	N/A	95.0	97.0
Mean SpO2%:	86.6	79.6	N/A	79.6	80.0
Min. SpO2%:	71.0	61.0	N/A	61.0	61.0
SpO2% <= 89% (min)	0.1	97.2	0.0	97.2	102.4
		% Time in range			
90 – 100%:	19.8%	4.4%	0.0%	4.4%	5.4%
80 – 89%:	60.5%	38.3%	0.0%	38.3%	39.8%
70 – 79%:	17.0%	52.0%	0.0%	52.0%	49.7%
60 – 69%:	0.0%	5.3%	0.0%	5.3%	4.9%
50 – 59%:	0.0%	0.0%	0.0%	0.0%	0.0%
< 50%:	0.0%	0.0%	0.0%	0.0%	0.0%
% Artifact / Bad Data:	2.7%	0.0%	N/A	0.0%	0.2%

TCPCO2 RESULTS	Wake	Non-REM	REM	TST	TIB
Max. TcpCO2 (mmHg):	51.5	53.6	N/A	53.6	53.6
Mean TcpCO2 (mmHg):	43.9	50.3	N/A	50.3	49.9
Min. TcpCO2 (mmHg):	33.0	41.2	N/A	41.2	33.0
		% Duration of TcpCO2 in Range			
Above 60 (mmHg):	0.0%	0.0%	0.0%	0.0%	0.0%
55 - 60 (mmHg):	0.0%	0.0%	0.0%	0.0%	0.0%
50 - 55 (mmHg):	17.5%	63.1%	0.0%	63.1%	60.1%
45 - 50 (mmHg):	31.3%	33.1%	0.0%	33.1%	33.0%
40 - 45 (mmHg):	18.4%	3.8%	0.0%	3.8%	4.8%
Bad Data Time:	0.0%	0.0%	N/A	0.0%	0.0%

Fig. 13.2 (continued)

References

1. Chung F, Yegneswaran B, Liao P, Chung SA, Vairavanathan S, Islam S, et al. STOP questionnaire: a tool to screen patients for obstructive sleep apnea. Anesthesiology. 2008;108(5):812–21.
2. Kapur VK, Auckley DH, Chowdhuri S, Kuhlmann DC, Mehra R, Ramar K, et al. Clinical practice guideline for diagnostic testing for adult obstructive sleep apnea: an American Academy of Sleep Medicine Clinical Practice Guideline. J Clin Sleep Med. 2017;13(3):479–504.
3. Roesslein M, Chung F. Obstructive sleep apnoea in adults: peri-operative considerations: a narrative review. Eur J Anaesthesiol. 2018;35(4):245–55.
4. American Society of Anesthesiologists Task Force on Perioperative Management of patients with obstructive sleep a. Practice guidelines for the perioperative management of patients with obstructive sleep apnea: an updated report by the American Society of Anesthesiologists Task Force on Perioperative Management of patients with obstructive sleep apnea. Anesthesiology. 2014;120(2):268–86.
5. Lang LH, Parekh K, Tsui BYK, Maze M. Perioperative management of the obese surgical patient. Br Med Bull. 2017;124(1):135–55.
6. Ravesloot MJ, van Maanen JP, Hilgevoord AA, van Wagensveld BA, de Vries N. Obstructive sleep apnea is underrecognized and underdiagnosed in patients undergoing bariatric surgery. Eur Arch Otorhinolaryngol. 2012;269(7):1865–71.
7. Romero-Corral A, Caples SM, Lopez-Jimenez F, Somers VK. Interactions between obesity and obstructive sleep apnea: implications for treatment. Chest. 2010;137(3):711–9.
8. Singh M, Liao P, Kobah S, Wijeysundera DN, Shapiro C, Chung F. Proportion of surgical patients with undiagnosed obstructive sleep apnoea. Br J Anaesth. 2013;110(4):629–36.
9. Tufik S, Santos-Silva R, Taddei JA, Bittencourt LR. Obstructive sleep apnea syndrome in the Sao Paulo Epidemiologic Sleep Study. Sleep Med. 2010;11(5):441–6.
10. Krishnan V, Dixon-Williams S, Thornton JD. Where there is smoke...there is sleep apnea: exploring the relationship between smoking and sleep apnea. Chest. 2014;146(6):1673–80.
11. Sateia MJ. International classification of sleep disorders-third edition: highlights and modifications. Chest. 2014;146(5):1387–94.
12. El Shayeb M, Topfer LA, Stafinski T, Pawluk L, Menon D. Diagnostic accuracy of level 3 portable sleep tests versus level 1 polysomnography for sleep-disordered breathing: a systematic review and meta-analysis. CMAJ. 2014;186(1):E25–51.
13. Netzer NC, Stoohs RA, Netzer CM, Clark K, Strohl KP. Using the Berlin Questionnaire to identify patients at risk for the sleep apnea syndrome. Ann Intern Med. 1999;131(7):485–91.
14. Ramachandran SK, Kheterpal S, Consens F, Shanks A, Doherty TM, Morris M, et al. Derivation and validation of a simple

perioperative sleep apnea prediction score. Anesth Analg. 2010;110(4):1007–15.
15. Guralnick AS, Pant M, Minhaj M, Sweitzer BJ, Mokhlesi B. CPAP adherence in patients with newly diagnosed obstructive sleep apnea prior to elective surgery. J Clin Sleep Med. 2012;8(5):501–6.
16. Konecny T, Kara T, Somers VK. Obstructive sleep apnea and hypertension: an update. Hypertension. 2014;63(2):203–9.
17. Drager LF, Togeiro SM, Polotsky VY, Lorenzi-Filho G. Obstructive sleep apnea: a cardiometabolic risk in obesity and the metabolic syndrome. J Am Coll Cardiol. 2013;62(7):569–76.
18. Kent BD, Grote L, Ryan S, Pepin JL, Bonsignore MR, Tkacova R, et al. Diabetes mellitus prevalence and control in sleep-disordered breathing: the European Sleep Apnea Cohort (ESADA) study. Chest. 2014;146(4):982–90.
19. Bakker JP, Weng J, Wang R, Redline S, Punjabi NM, Patel SR. Associations between obstructive sleep apnea, sleep duration, and abnormal fasting glucose. he multi-ethnic study of atherosclerosis. Am J Respir Crit Care Med. 2015;192(6):745–53.
20. Sajkov D, McEvoy RD. Obstructive sleep apnea and pulmonary hypertension. Prog Cardiovasc Dis. 2009;51(5):363–70.
21. Olson E, Chung F, Ping E. Surgical risk and the preoperative evaluation and management of adults with obstructive sleep apnea. In: Post TW, editor. UpToDate. Waltham: UpToDate; 2020.
22. Kaw R, Chung F, Pasupuleti V, Mehta J, Gay PC, Hernandez AV. Meta-analysis of the association between obstructive sleep apnoea and postoperative outcome. Br J Anaesth. 2012;109(6):897–906.
23. Hiremath AS, Hillman DR, James AL, Noffsinger WJ, Platt PR, Singer SL. Relationship between difficult tracheal intubation and obstructive sleep apnoea. Br J Anaesth. 1998;80(5):606–11.
24. Brousseau CA, Dobson GR, Milne AD. A retrospective analysis of airway management in patients with obstructive sleep apnea and its effects on postanesthesia care unit length of stay. Can J Respir Ther. 2014;50(1):23–6.
25. Kheterpal S, Healy D, Aziz MF, Shanks AM, Freundlich RE, Linton F, et al. Incidence, predictors, and outcome of difficult mask ventilation combined with difficult laryngoscopy: a report from the multicenter perioperative outcomes group. Anesthesiology. 2013;119(6):1360–9.
26. Memtsoudis S, Liu SS, Ma Y, Chiu YL, Walz JM, Gaber-Baylis LK, et al. Perioperative pulmonary outcomes in patients with sleep apnea after noncardiac surgery. Anesth Analg. 2011;112(1):113–21.
27. Memtsoudis SG, Stundner O, Rasul R, Chiu YL, Sun X, Ramachandran SK, et al. The impact of sleep apnea on postoperative utilization of resources and adverse outcomes. Anesth Analg. 2014;118(2):407–18.
28. Flink BJ, Rivelli SK, Cox EA, White WD, Falcone G, Vail TP, et al. Obstructive sleep apnea and incidence of postoperative delirium after elective knee replacement in the nondemented elderly. Anesthesiology. 2012;116(4):788–96.
29. Wallisch W, Jackson D, Orebaugh S, Luke S, ML K, Taormina D. Outcomes for ambulatory shoulder surgery patients with sleep apnoea. Ambul Surg. 2018;24:1.
30. Rohrbaugh M, Kentor ML, Orebaugh SL, Williams B. Outcomes of shoulder surgery in the sitting position with interscalene nerve block: a single-center series. Reg Anesth Pain Med. 2013;38(1):28–33.

Chronic Obstructive Pulmonary Disease (COPD)

14

Barry A. Finegan

A 59-year-old female, having suffered from osteoarthritis of her left hip for many years, presented for assessment prior to an elective total hip replacement. She had a 40-pack-year smoking history and an established diagnosis of COPD, made 4 years previously when she was admitted to hospital following an episode of severe dyspnea. She had successfully quit smoking 1 year prior to this visit. Her only other comorbidity was hypertension.

On closer questioning, the patient indicated that she had two admissions to hospital due to exacerbation of her predominant COPD symptom—dyspnea. The most recent episode, 3 months previously, necessitated a 2-day ICU admission.

The patient indicated that she experienced breathlessness when hurrying but could walk on the level at a reasonable pace without difficulty. She denied any history of hemoptysis, weight loss, excessive fatigue, or symptoms suggestive of angina or gastric reflux.

Medications: Tiotropium bromide 2.5 mg OD, fluticasone propionate/salmeterol 100 μg/50 μg BID, albuterol 100 μg PRN Q6H, and amlodipine 5 mg OD.

The patient was concerned about developing an exacerbation of COPD following surgery and inquired if there was any way of reducing the risk of this occurring other than taking her medications as prescribed.

Physical Examination: The patient had a respiratory rate of 14/minute. Vital signs were otherwise stable. Oxygen saturation on room air was 93%. There was no evidence of cyanosis. The chest was barrel-shaped and hyper-resonant to percussion. Breath sounds were distant. There were scattered rales in both lung fields but no wheezing. There were no distended neck veins or hepatomegaly. There was mild bilateral ankle edema.

The ankle edema began shortly after she initiated amlodipine therapy some years ago and was unchanged in degree since that time.

Investigations: Laboratory values were within normal limits.

Spirometry data obtained on the day of her clinic visit are shown in Table 14.1.

A chest radiograph taken 1 month prior to the clinic visit was available for evaluation (Fig. 14.1).

Table 14.1 Spirometry data of patient presenting for assessment prior to an elective total hip replacement

FEV_1	FVC	PEF	FEV_1/FVC	Quality
0.84	2.44	1.51	34%	Good blow

FEV_1 forced expiratory volume in the first second (of expiration), *FVC* forced vital capacity, *PEF* peak expiratory flow

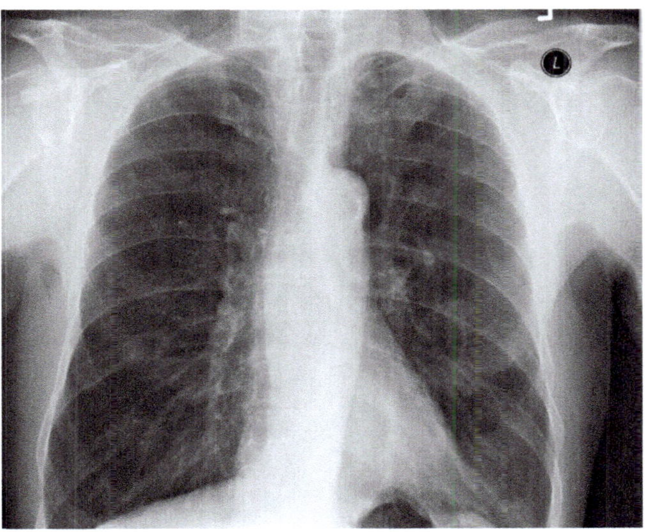

Fig. 14.1 Chest radiograph taken 1 month before presentation to clinic

B. A. Finegan (✉)
Department of Anesthesiology & Pain Medicine, University of Alberta, Edmonton, AB, Canada
e-mail: bfinegan@ualberta.ca

D. Dillane, B. A. Finegan (eds.), *Preoperative Assessment*, https://doi.org/10.1007/978-3-030-58842-7_14

What Is COPD?

COPD is a progressive inflammatory disease of the airways and/or alveoli. It is characterized by expired airflow limitation that arises because of chronic long-term exposure to smoke or occupational/environmental air pollution. Inhalation of smoke produced by combustible tobacco products is the key risk factor in over 75% of cases.

Patients suffer from persistent respiratory symptoms, chronic and progressive dyspnea, which may be accompanied by cough and sputum production. The diagnosis of COPD is confirmed by spirometry (post-bronchodilator $FEV_1/FVC < 0.7$). A normal and a COPD spirometry trace is shown in Fig. 14.2 [1].

Due to the insidious nature of the disease, COPD-related symptoms, particularly dyspnea, are frequently underreported.

Susceptibility to develop COPD is influenced by genetic factors, reduced intrauterine and childhood lung growth (low birth weight, prematurity, and exposure to smoke), and a history of airway hyperresponsiveness, particularly asthma.

What Are the Pathophysiological Consequences of COPD?

The chronic inflammatory process induces (1) obstructive bronchiolitis, a narrowing and obstruction of small airways with gas trapping during expiration leading to hyperinflation; (2) emphysematous change, destruction of lung parenchyma with minimal fibrosis, breakdown of elastin (loss of elastic recoil), and remodeled enlarged acinar units with a reduced blood/gas exchange interface; (3) mucus hypersecretion in some but not all individuals; and (4) pulmonary vascular bed destruction and hypoxic vasoconstriction leading over time to pulmonary hypertension and right ventricular dysfunction.

How Is the Severity of COPD Assessed?

The Global Initiative for Chronic Obstructive Lung Disease (GOLD) (https://goldcopd.org/) provides a structured process for quantification of disease status incorporating the

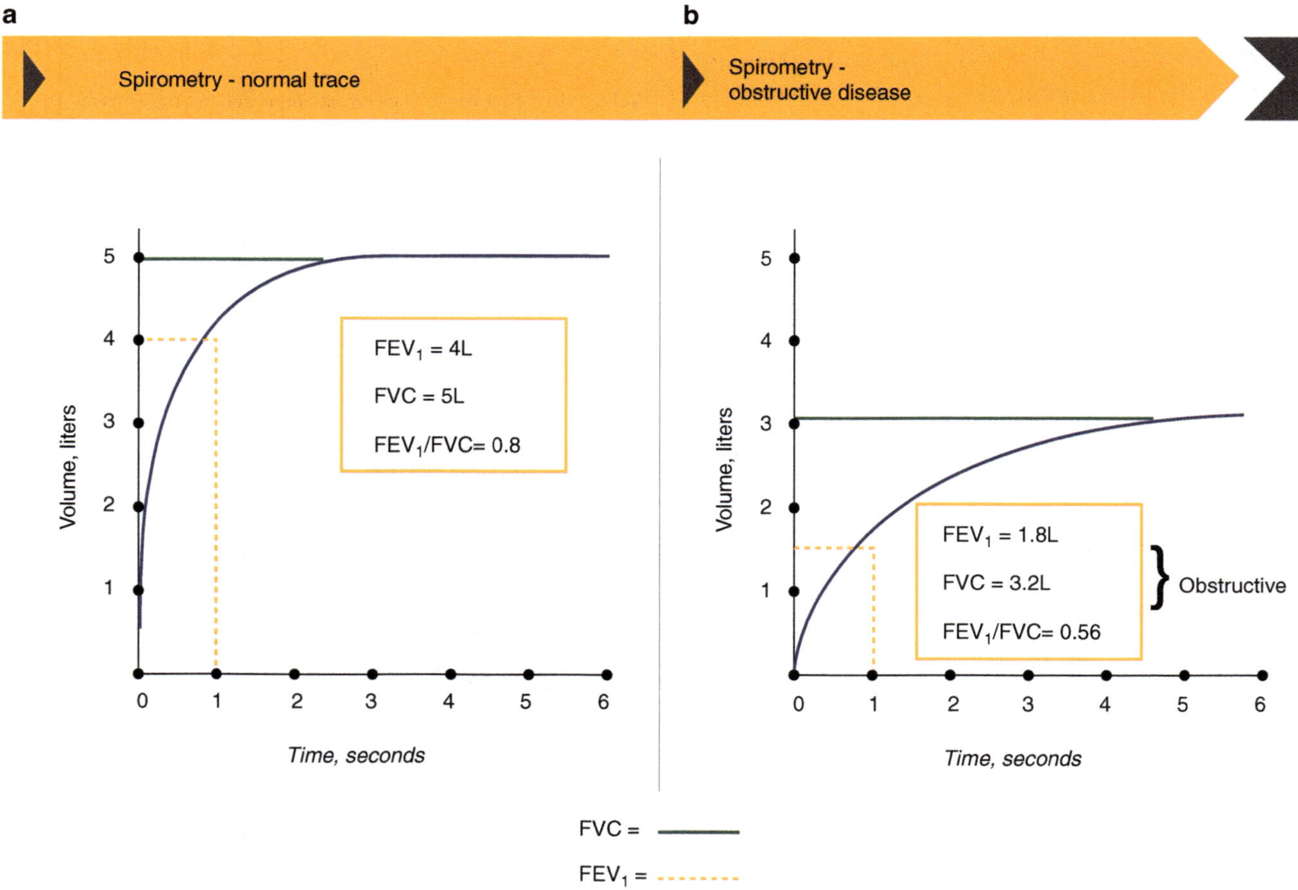

Fig. 14.2 Spirometry, normal trace, (**a**) and spirometry, obstructive disease (**b**). (From Global Strategy for the Diagnosis, Management and Prevention of COPD, Global Initiative for Chronic Obstructive Lung Disease (GOLD) 2017 [1], with permission)

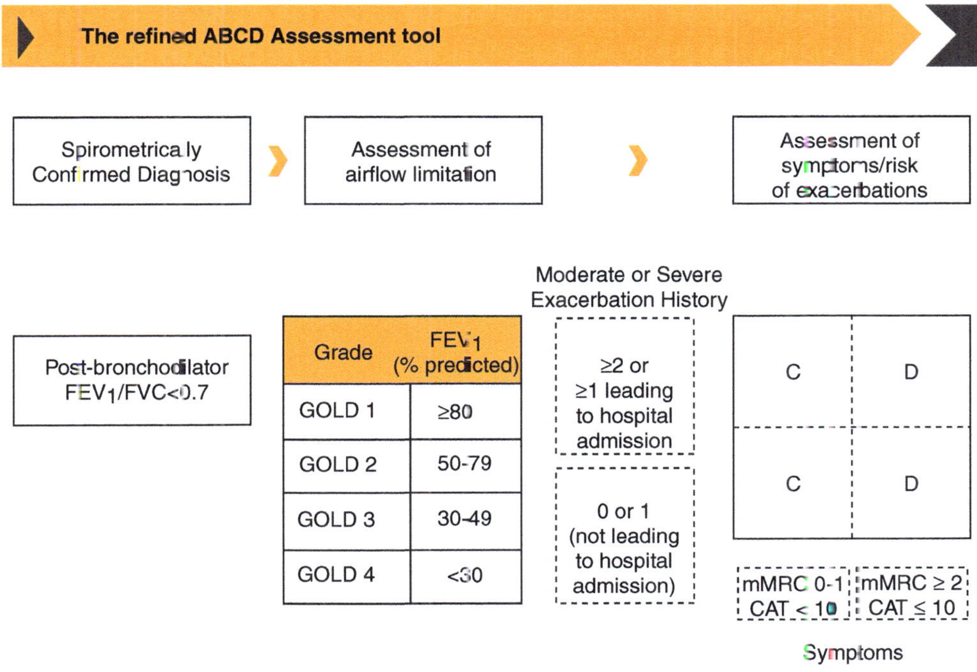

Fig. 14.3 The refined ABCD assessment tool. (From Global Strategy for the Diagnosis, Management and Prevention of COPD, Global Initiative for Chronic Obstructive Lung Disease (GOLD) 2017 [1], with permission)

Refined ABCD assessment tool (Fig. 14.3) [1]. This involves the following:

1. Determining the FEV_1, the key ongoing metric for severity of airflow limitation.

   Grades of airflow limitation range in severity from 1 to 4:
   (a) GOLD 1 (mild) individuals have an $FEV_1 \geq 80\%$ of predicted values.
   (b) GOLD 2 (moderate) $50\% \leq FEV_1 < 80\%$ predicted.
   (c) GOLD 3 (severe) $30\% \leq FEV_1 < 50\%$ predicted.
   (d) GOLD 4 (very severe) $FEV_1 < 30\%$ of predicted.
2. Eliciting a history of exacerbation episodes in the previous 12 months.

   An exacerbation of COPD is defined as an *"acute worsening of respiratory symptoms that results in additional therapy"* [1]. Exacerbations can be considered:
   (a) Mild/moderate (treated medically out of hospital)
   (b) Severe (hospital emergency room treatment or admission)

   A history of two mild/moderate exacerbations or one severe exacerbation in the last 12 months places the patient in the severe, as opposed to the moderate, exacerbation category in the GOLD assessment schema.
3. Assessing symptom severity.

   Dyspnea is the most common presenting symptom of COPD. A simple well-validated measure of COPD-related dyspnea is the Modified Medical Research Council (mMRC) Dyspnea Scale [1]. This scale involves self-assessment of breathlessness severity experienced during physical activities ranging from strenuous exercise to dressing and undressing. Details of symptom equivalence are shown in Table 14.2 [2].

   A score of ≥2 in the mMRC places the patient in the higher-risk groupings according to the GOLD assessment schema. A weakness of mMRC is the focus on dyspnea solely, exclusive of cough and sputum production.

Table 14.2 mMRC Dyspnea Scale [2]

Symptom	Grade
Breathless on strenuous exertion	0
Breathless when hurrying or walking up a slight hill	1
Walks slower than contemporaries on the level or must stop for breath when walking at own pace	2
Stops for breath after walking 100 yards or after a few minutes on the level	3
Breathless when dressing/undressing or too breathless to leave home	4

What Is the Utility of GOLD Grading and Grouping in the Perioperative Period?

COPD is underdiagnosed and undertreated in the community. Appropriate pharmacological interventions decrease symptoms and the risk and severity of exacerbations, also reducing perioperative morbidity and mortality. The GOLD assessment structure allows the application of appropriate treatment algorithms tailored to the stage of the disease in the individual patient.

Furthermore, there is emerging evidence that GOLD grouping can be helpful in predicting perioperative complications. Patients in high-risk GOLD groups (C and D) have been shown to be a higher risk of postoperative complications, especially infection and wound issues, than those in low-risk GOLD groups (A and B) [2].

What Coexisting Conditions Should One Consider in a Patient with COPD?

Lung cancer, cardiovascular diseases (especially right-sided heart failure and coronary artery disease), obstructive sleep apnea, gastroesophageal reflux disease (GERD), and depression are all associated with COPD and are important causes of morbidity and mortality in this population.

What Are the Two Classes of Bronchodilators Commonly Used in the Treatment of COPD?

Bronchodilators are either short-acting bronchodilator (SAB) or long-acting bronchodilator (LAB). The former is used for immediate relief of symptoms and the latter for long-term management. SABs and LABs in current use are muscarinic antagonists or beta-agonists. In more severe cases, combination therapy involving administration of both classes is employed. The prototypical long-acting muscarinic antagonist (LAMA) is tiotropium and is frequently co-prescribed with long-acting beta-agonist (LABA), salmeterol. Both these drugs have been extensively studied, and, although concern has been raised about possible adverse cardiovascular effects involving both classes of drugs, they are considered very safe for long-term administration.

What Are the Current Recommendations for Maintenance Bronchodilator and Steroid Therapy in COPD?

The GOLD groupings are very helpful in guiding pharmacological therapy in COPD. For group A (few symptoms and mild exacerbation history), a SAB, taken as needed, is indicated. For group B (more symptoms but mild exacerbation history), a LAB is suggested. For group C (few symptoms and severe exacerbation history), single or dual LAB is recommended ± inhaled steroid (IS). For group D (more symptoms and severe exacerbation history), dual LAB with IS ± roflumilast (a PDE-4 inhibitor) ± macrolide antibiotic therapy is recommended.

If My Patient Is *not* on Current Recommended Therapy, Should I Initiate Treatment in the Preoperative Period?

Appropriate bronchodilator therapy decreases the risk of perioperative respiratory failure and postoperative exacerbations in patients with COPD [3]. Postoperative pulmonary complications in patients with COPD, in particular pneumonia and respiratory failure, are associated with very significant morbidity and mortality [4]. Patients with mild COPD do not require any special management perioperatively apart from advice to quit smoking and continue on usual medications. However, it is essential in patients with GOLD group C and D diseases presenting for major elective procedures, to optimize medical management of COPD before proceeding to surgery. If the patient is not under the care of a respiratory physician or internist, referral to same is indicated. In general, dual LAB ± IS has proven to be safe and effective in reducing both symptoms and exacerbations of COPD in these patient populations [5].

How Useful Is a Chest Radiograph in the Diagnosis and Assessment of COPD?

The classic chest radiograph findings associated with COPD are hyperinflation, hyperlucency of the lungs, and rapid tapering of the vascular markings. A chest radiograph is not considered useful in making the diagnosis of COPD [1]. If coexisting conditions are suspected, for example, lung cancer, a chest radiograph may be helpful in management.

Does the Type of Anesthetic Influence Postoperative Outcome in Patients with COPD?

It is clear from analysis of the American College of Surgeons National Surgical Quality Improvement Program (ACS NSQIP) database that patients undergoing hip arthroplasty who have COPD are more likely to have a postoperative complication, including mortality, myocardial infarction, pneumonia, and readmission, than those patients without COPD [6]. Hausman et al. [7], using the same database and propensity score matching, have convincingly demonstrated a reduction in complications, but not mortality, if regional rather than general anesthesia is used in patients with COPD undergoing an array of surgical procedures.

The patient's airflow limitation was GOLD Grade 3 (severe), her exacerbation history was severe and her mMRC grade was 1. This placed her in the GOLD Grade 3, Group C category, indicating that she was at moderately high risk for perioperative exacerbation of COPD. A respiratory physician was consulted who agreed that her current therapy consisting of dual LAB (tiotropium bromide and salmeterol) and inhaled steroid (fluticasone) was adequate in view of the fact that she was currently stable.

She agreed to spinal anesthesia for the procedure. She was advised to take her COPD medications as per her usual practice on the morning of the procedure. The procedure was completed without incident and the patient discharged on postoperative day 4.

True/False Questions

1. The following should be considered in assessing a stable COPD patient preoperatively:
   (a) A FEV_1 determination
   (b) A chest radiograph
   (c) The mMRC dyspnea score
   (d) A pulmonary CT
   (e) An ECHO to rule out pulmonary hypertension
2. Appropriate management of a COPD patient with GOLD Grade 4 and Group D diseases presenting for elective major surgery should include:
   (a) Smoking cessation
   (b) Tiotropium bromide 2.5 mg OD
   (c) Fluticasone propionate/salmeterol 100 μg/50 μg BID
   (d) Preferential choice of regional/local anesthesia
   (e) An ICU consultation

References

1. Global Strategy for the Diagnosis, Management and Prevention of COPD, Global Initiative for Chronic Obstructive Lung Disease (GOLD) 2020. https://goldcopd.org. Accessed 20 May 2020.
2. Kim HJ, Lee J, Park YS, Lee CH, Lee SM, Yim JJ, et al. Impact of GOLD groups of chronic pulmonary obstructive disease on surgical complications. Int J Chron Obstruct Pulmon Dis. 2016;11:281–7.
3. Shin B, Lee H, Kang D, Jeong BH, Kang HK, Chon HR, et al. Airflow limitation severity and post-operative pulmonary complications following extra-pulmonary surgery in COPD patients. Respirology. 2017;22(5):935–41.
4. Fernandez-Bustamante A, Frendl G, Sprung J, Kor DJ, Subramaniam B, Martinez Ruiz R, et al. Postoperative pulmonary complications, early mortality, and hospital stay following noncardiothoracic surgery: a multicenter study by the perioperative Research Network Investigators. JAMA Surg. 2017;152(2):157–66.
5. Papi A, Vestbo J, Fabbri L, Corradi M, Prunier H, Cohuet G, et al. Extrafine inhaled triple therapy versus dual bronchodilator therapy in chronic obstructive pulmonary disease (TRIBUTE): a double-blind, parallel group, randomised controlled trial. Lancet. 2018;391(10125):1076–84.
6. Yakubek GA, Curtis GL, Sodhi N, Faour M, Klika AK, Mont MA, et al. Chronic obstructive pulmonary disease is associated with short-term complications following total hip arthroplasty. J Arthroplast. 2018;33(6):1926–9.
7. Hausman MS Jr, Jewell ES, Engoren M. Regional versus general anesthesia in surgical patients with chronic obstructive pulmonary disease: does avoiding general anesthesia reduce the risk of postoperative complications? Anesth Analg. 2015;120(6):1405–12.

Asthma

15

Barry A. Finegan

The patient was a 62-year-old male scheduled to undergo endoscopic sinus surgery and septoplasty. He indicated that he had anosmia and obstructive nasal issues for the last 3 years and had undergone a trial of nasal steroid therapy without resolution of his symptoms. Review of patient history revealed a remote history of pulmonary tuberculosis as a child, hypertension well controlled on medication for 20 years, and recent-onset asthma (within the last 2 years).

His asthma was diagnosed after he developed wheezing, dyspnea, and cough when visiting a major urban city when the air pollution was intense. His symptoms responded to outpatient nebulized salbutamol, a 5-day course of oral steroids, and 10 days of inhaled short-acting β-agonist (SABA) therapy. He was advised to use the SABA as required if the wheeze recurred. Since his initial episode, he had three episodes of prolonged wheezing associated with a nighttime cough, the last occurring 6 months previously; these episodes responded to inhaled corticosteroids (ICS) and SABA use for 2 weeks. After these events, he was advised to use his ICS daily and take his SABA as required to control symptoms. In addition, he was started on montelukast, a leukotriene receptor antagonist (LTRA).

The patient denied any exacerbation of symptoms with nonsteroidal anti-inflammatory drug (NSAID) exposure. He confirmed he had never been admitted to hospital for asthma. He admitted to discontinuing his ICS and LTRA mediations after his symptoms resolved.

He indicated that he had been using his SABA 3–4 times a week over the last month as he noticed he was wheezing/coughing when walking to and from work, especially on climbing stairs. This was the only medication he was taking. The cough was minimally productive of clear sputum. He had stopped working out in the gym because of his breathing.

Physical Examination: His respiratory rate was 14 breaths/min, his temperature was normal, O_2 saturation was 96% on room air, and his pulse rate 80 beats/min. Physical examination was normal apart from bilateral expiratory wheeze audible in both lung fields. There was no evidence of use of accessory muscles of respiration or of a pulmonary infection.

Investigations: A peak expiratory flow (PEF) rate was determined on the day of his clinic visit. His reading was 420 liters/min. He indicated his "usual" value was 550 liters/min. His laboratory data were normal, including his white cell count and ESR.

What Is Asthma?

The Global Initiative for Asthma has termed asthma as "a heterogeneous disease, usually characterized by airway inflammation. It is defined by the history of respiratory symptoms such as wheeze, shortness of breath, chest tightness and cough that vary over time and in intensity, together with variable expiratory airflow limitation" [1]. There has been an evolution in our understanding of asthma with the recognition that different phenotypes exist that can, to a degree, be characterized by biomarkers and responsiveness to particular therapies. Overlap between phenotypes frequently occurs [2]. Commonly described phenotypes include asthma where allergic mechanisms predominate (childhood and seasonal asthma), asthma where allergy does not appear to be the dominant mechanism (obesity- and exercise-induced asthma), drug-induced asthma (aspirin and NSAIDs), adult-onset asthma (includes the eosinophilic cohort and that associated with upper airway allergic pathology), and asthma-COPD overlap syndrome [3].

B. A. Finegan (✉)
Department of Anesthesiology & Pain Medicine, University of Alberta, Edmonton, AB, Canada
e-mail: bfinegan@ualberta.ca

D. Dillane, B. A. Finegan (eds.), *Preoperative Assessment*, https://doi.org/10.1007/978-3-030-58842-7_15

How Is Asthma Diagnosed?

Asthma is a probability-based diagnosis, made after consideration of the presenting symptoms and the presence of variable airflow limitation [4]. In routine practice, airflow characteristics are determined by measuring the forced expiratory volume in 1 second (FEV_1), the forced vital capacity (FVC), and peak expiratory flow (PEF). A significant decrease in the FEV_1/FVC (compared to standardized data for equivalent age, sex, and ethnicity), evidence of reversibility of the decrease in FEV_1 in response to bronchodilator therapy, a positive provocation test, and evidence of week-to-week FEV_1/FVC and PEF variability all support the diagnosis of asthma.

How Is Asthma Managed?

While there are differences in asthma management depending on the phenotype at presentation, the standard approach is to reduce exposure to environmental triggers, modify lifestyle (e.g., obesity management), and, if appropriate, initiate pharmacological therapy.

A stepwise pharmacological approach to asthma symptom control is recommended involving the use of "controller" and "reliever" medications [1].

The cornerstone of "controller" therapy is the use of inhaled corticosteroids (ICS) - airway inflammation is a major component of disease pathogenesis in most phenotypes.

The key "reliever" medications are short-acting β-agonists and long-acting β-agonists (SABA/LABA).

- *Step 1* (symptoms < twice per month/no waking due to symptoms/no exacerbation risk factors) → no ICS, but this is controversial given the inflammatory nature of the disease [5], use SABA as required.
- *Step 2* (infrequent asthma symptoms but has risk factors for exacerbations) → low-dose ICS with optional use of a leukotriene receptor antagonist (LTRA) is suggested for control and SABA for symptom management.
- *Step 3* (symptoms or need for SABA between twice per month and twice per week or greater or waking with symptoms ≥ once per month) → low-medium dose ICS and LABA with optional LTRA for control and SABA for symptom control.
- *Steps 4 and 5* (symptoms or need for SABA more than twice per week/symptoms most day and escalating) → medium-high dose ICS and LABA with add-on therapy which may include oral steroids and specific inflammatory mediator management.

What Are Leukotriene Receptor Antagonists?

LTRAs such as montelukast are selective antagonists at the cysteinyl leukotriene-1 receptor (cysLT1R) [6]. Cysteinyl leukotrienes are eicosanoids released via the 5-lipoxygenase pathway within inflammatory cells including mast cells, eosinophils, and basophils. CysLT1R agonists mediate edema formation, airway smooth muscle proliferation/bronchoconstriction, and mucus production. CysLT1R are found in abundance in the upper airway in patients with allergic rhinitis and in the large and small airways in patients with asthma. LTRAs are not as effective as ICS in the management of asthma but are a useful adjunctive therapy, particularly in the subset of patients who present with asthma and concomitant allergic rhinitis.

What Other Pathogenesis-Modifying Agents Are Available to Treat Asthma Phenotypes?

There are several agents in development targeted at specific pathways responsible for asthma symptoms [7]. One drug, omalizumab, an anti-immunoglobulin E monoclonal antibody, is approved for treating severe allergic asthma not well controlled with standard agents. Interleukin 5 monoclonal antibodies mepolizumab and reslizumab are available for the treatment of severe asthma in patients where eosinophilia is a predominant feature.

How Is Asthma Control Assessed?

Optimal asthma control involves reducing or eliminating the symptoms of asthma and decreasing the risk of future exacerbations.

The occurrence and frequency of asthma symptoms in the 4 weeks prior to the clinic visit provide a good indication of symptom control status. The Global Initiative for Asthma (GINA) symptom control questionnaire provides a simple and valuable tool in this regard [1]. Ask the following questions:

1. Any daytime symptoms?
2. Any night waking due to asthma?
3. Have you needed to use your SABA more than twice/week?
4. Any activity limitation due to asthma?

An individual who is *well* controlled will have none of the above, *partly* controlled patients will answer yes to one to two questions, while those in a *poorly* controlled state will have positive responses to three to four of the above.

Determine the PEF – it is helpful if the patient is aware of his baseline value when asymptomatic. A nomogram of height-, age-, and sex-adjusted values is widely available. A reduction to 50–79% of baseline "usual" values is concerning, and consideration should be given to adjusting medication dosing or adding another agent. A >50% reduction is indicative of severe bronchoconstriction, and medical assistance should be sought immediately.

What Are the Risk Factors for a Future Exacerbation of Asthma?

The major risk factors for exacerbation of asthma are as follows:

1. Uncontrolled current status as determined by GINA symptom assessment score (vide supra)
2. Low lung volumes
3. Previous history of intubation or admission to an ICU for asthma management
4. Requirement for oral corticosteroid therapy in the past 12 months
5. Recent or ongoing upper airway infection
6. Severe asthma uncontrolled with standard therapy (patient on monoclonal antibody therapy)

Is Medication Compliance a Problem in Asthma Management?

Poor compliance with ICS, incorrect technique of administration of ICS, and erroneous use of a SABA rather than an ICS are ongoing issues in asthma management [5].

Patients should be advised to use all their prescribed asthma medications (except SABA) for at least 5 days before an elective surgical procedure even if that is not their usual practice.

What Is Samter's Triad?

Nasal polyps, asthma, and sensitivity to aspirin (or other NSAIDs) constitute Samter's triad, otherwise known as aspirin-exacerbated respiratory disease (AERD). This diagnosis should be considered in patients who have asthma and sinus disease, as many may be sensitive to NSAIDs. NSAID or aspirin use precipitating respiratory symptoms is suggestive in this setting, and further investigation is indicated, as NSAID use perioperatively would be contraindicated and the long-term outcome of surgery could be compromised [8].

What Is a Suggested Approach to the Asthmatic Patient Presenting for Surgery?

1. Determine factors that trigger asthmatic attack.
2. Determine symptom control status using the GINA questionnaire.
3. Determine the risk of exacerbation.
4. Postpone elective surgery if symptom control is not optimal:
   (a) Determine compliance with the current treatment.
   (b) If clinically indicated, obtain simple spirometry to assess FEV_1 and FVC:
      (i) Compare with previously obtained values and assess reversibility.
      (ii) If marked deterioration, refer for further assessment.
5. Strongly encourage smoking cessation as this is a risk factor for perioperative bronchospasm.
6. Advise daily use of prescribed asthma medications (except SABA) for 5 days before the day of surgery in all patients even if they are asymptomatic at the time of assessment.
7. Supplement with oral methylprednisolone 20–40 mg 5 days preoperatively if patient has risks factors for exacerbation.
8. Initiate preoperative intravenous steroid therapy if patient has uncontrolled asthma and requires urgent surgery and cannot take oral medication.

The patient's account of the past month combined with his responses to the GINA questionnaire (answering in the affirmative three out of four questions) indicated poor current symptom control. He was judged to be not having a severe exacerbation as his normal respiratory rate, O_2 saturation, and heart rate combined no evidence of use of accessory muscles of respiration and relatively moderate reduction in PFR was reassuring. Surgery was deferred for 2 weeks. He was instructed to take his ICS (budesonide 360 mcg) twice daily to get control of his asthma and use his SABA daily to achieve symptom relief. On telephone review 7 days after his initial assessment, he indicated that he was much improved. The need to continue ICS until the day of surgery was emphasized. Three days prior to surgery, the patient confirmed that he was asymptomatic and had been able to resume his exercise workouts. On the day of admission, both lung fields were clear. Surgery proceeded uneventfully.

True/False Questions

1. Asthma is well controlled:
   (a) If the patient is no longer taking ICS
   (b) If the patient has had no symptoms in the past year

   (c) If the patient is only using SABA three times a week
   (d) If the only symptom present is cough
   (e) If SABA is effective in managing symptoms
2. The following suggest that the patient is at risk of exacerbation of asthma perioperatively:
   (a) Admission to ICU for asthma management in the past
   (b) Oral corticosteroid use for asthma control in the last 6 months
   (c) Ongoing daily use of ICS
   (d) Ongoing daily use of ICA and leukotriene receptor inhibitors
   (e) Recent upper airway infection

References

1. Global Initiative for Asthma. Global Strategy for Asthma Management and Prevention, 2018. Available from: www.ginasthma.org. Accessed 8 Mar 2019.
2. Wenzel SE. Asthma phenotypes: the evolution from clinical to molecular approaches. Nat Med. 2012;18(5):716–25.
3. Guilleminault L, Ouksel H, Belleguic C, Le Guen Y, Germaud P, Desfleurs E, et al. Personalised medicine in asthma: from curative to preventive medicine. Eur Respir Rev. 2017;26(143):160010. https://doi.org/10.1183/16000617.0010-2016.
4. Papi A, Brightling C, Pedersen SE, Reddel HK. Asthma. Lancet. 2018;391(1022):783–800.
5. O'Byrne PM, Jenkins C, Bateman ED. The paradoxes of asthma management: time for a new approach? Eur Respir J. 2017;50(3):1701103. https://doi.org/10.1183/13993003.01103-2017.
6. Diamant Z, Mantzouranis E, Bjermer L. Montelukast in the treatment of asthma and beyond. Expert Rev Clin Immunol. 2009;5(6):639–58.
7. Chung KF. New treatments for severe treatment-resistant asthma: targeting the right patient. Lancet Respir Med. 2013;1(8):639–52.
8. White AA, Stevenson DD. Aspirin-exacerbated respiratory disease. N Engl J Med. 2018;397(23):2281.

16 Restrictive Lung Disease

Derek Dillane

A 70-year-old man presented 1 week prior to removal of an osteosarcoma of the proximal humerus. He had been diagnosed with idiopathic pulmonary fibrosis (IPF) 8 years previously. He described having dyspnea on moderate exertion, and he had a chronic, mild, nonproductive cough. He did not require home oxygen. In addition, he had a history of hypertension and diabetes mellitus type 2, well controlled on oral hypoglycemic medication. He led a sedentary lifestyle with an estimated MET score ≤3. He was an ex-smoker since the time of the original diagnosis of IPF.
Medications: Metformin, sitagliptin, ramipril, atorvastatin, pirfenidone, pantoprazole, and tamsulosin.
Physical Examination: Weight was 73.5 kg, height 1.81 m, BMI 22.4, SpO2 95% on room air, heart rate 90 bpm and regular, and blood pressure 158/92 mmHg.
A pansystolic murmur, which intensified on inspiration, was heard best over the fourth rib at the left sternal border. Bibasal crackles were detected on auscultation of the lungs.
Investigations: Laboratory values revealed a hemoglobin 138 g/L, platelet count 138 × 10^9/L, creatinine 152 μmol/L, estimated glomerular filtration rate (eGFR) 39 mL/min/1.73m², and HbA1C 6.9%.
His ECG showed typical features of right ventricular hypertrophy, right axis deviation, a dominant R wave in V1, a dominant S wave in V6, and right strain pattern (ST depression) in V1–V4. Chest radiograph showed reticular shadowing bibasally. The cardiac contours were indistinct, a not uncommon finding in pulmonary fibrosis. Key elements of pulmonary function testing, last performed 9 months prior to the current evaluation, are outlined in Table 16.1.

Table 16.1 Pulmonary function tests 9 months prior to preoperative evaluation

	Predicted	Best	% Predicted
FVC (L)	3.68	2.90	79
FEV1 (L)	2.71	2.44	90
FEV_1/FVC (%)	86	84	98
TLC (L)	6.0	5.04	84
DL_{CO} (ml/min/mmHg)	24.50	19.73	80.5

FVC forced vital capacity, *FEV_1* forced expiratory volume in the first second (of expiration), *TLC* total lung capacity, *DL_{CO}* diffusing capacity of the lung for carbon monoxide

How Is Restrictive Lung Disease Classified?

Restrictive lung disease is classified according to whether it is caused by an intrinsic or extrinsic disease process.

Pulmonary restrictive lung disorders include the following:

- Interstitial lung disease (ILD)
- Pulmonary fibrosis
- Lung resection
- Atelectasis
- Pneumonia
- Advanced pneumoconiosis

Extrapulmonary restrictive lung disorders include the following:

- Disorders of the chest wall or body habitus, e.g., ankylosing spondylitis, kyphoscoliosis, pregnancy, and obesity
- Respiratory muscle disorders, e.g., diaphragmatic paralysis, myasthenia gravis, muscular dystrophy, and amyotrophic lateral sclerosis
- Pleural cavity disorders, e.g., pleural effusion, pneumothorax, chronic empyema, and asbestosis

D. Dillane (✉)
Department of Anesthesiology & Pain Medicine, University of Alberta, Edmonton, AB, Canada

D. Dillane, B. A. Finegan (eds.), *Preoperative Assessment*, https://doi.org/10.1007/978-3-030-58842-7_16

What Are the Causes of Interstitial Lung Disease?

Causes of ILD are categorized according to whether the underlying cause is known or unknown. A common approach to classification of ILD is outlined in Fig. 16.1 [1]. IPF is the commonest ILD of unknown cause.

What Are the Characteristics of IPF?

- It is a chronic, progressive, fibrosing, interstitial pneumonia diffusely affecting the lung parenchyma.
- Incidence is estimated at 7–17/100,000 [2].
- It affects males more than females.
- Patients present in sixth and seventh decades.
- It has unknown etiology.
- Diagnosis requires exclusion of identifiable causes of ILD.
- Diagnosis is made using high-resolution computed tomography (CT) +/– biopsy.
- Most cases are spontaneously occurring, but familial disease has been described.
- It is associated with cigarette smoking, exposure to metal and wood dusts, and a particularly high prevalence of gastroesophageal reflux disease.
- The natural history is one of gradual and progressive decline to respiratory failure over a median period of 3–4 years [3]. Approximately 25% of patients with milder disease will survive to 10 years or beyond [3].

What Complications Is the Patient with ILD Subject to in the Perioperative Period?

- Acute exacerbation of ILD
- Pneumonia
- Acute respiratory distress syndrome/acute lung injury

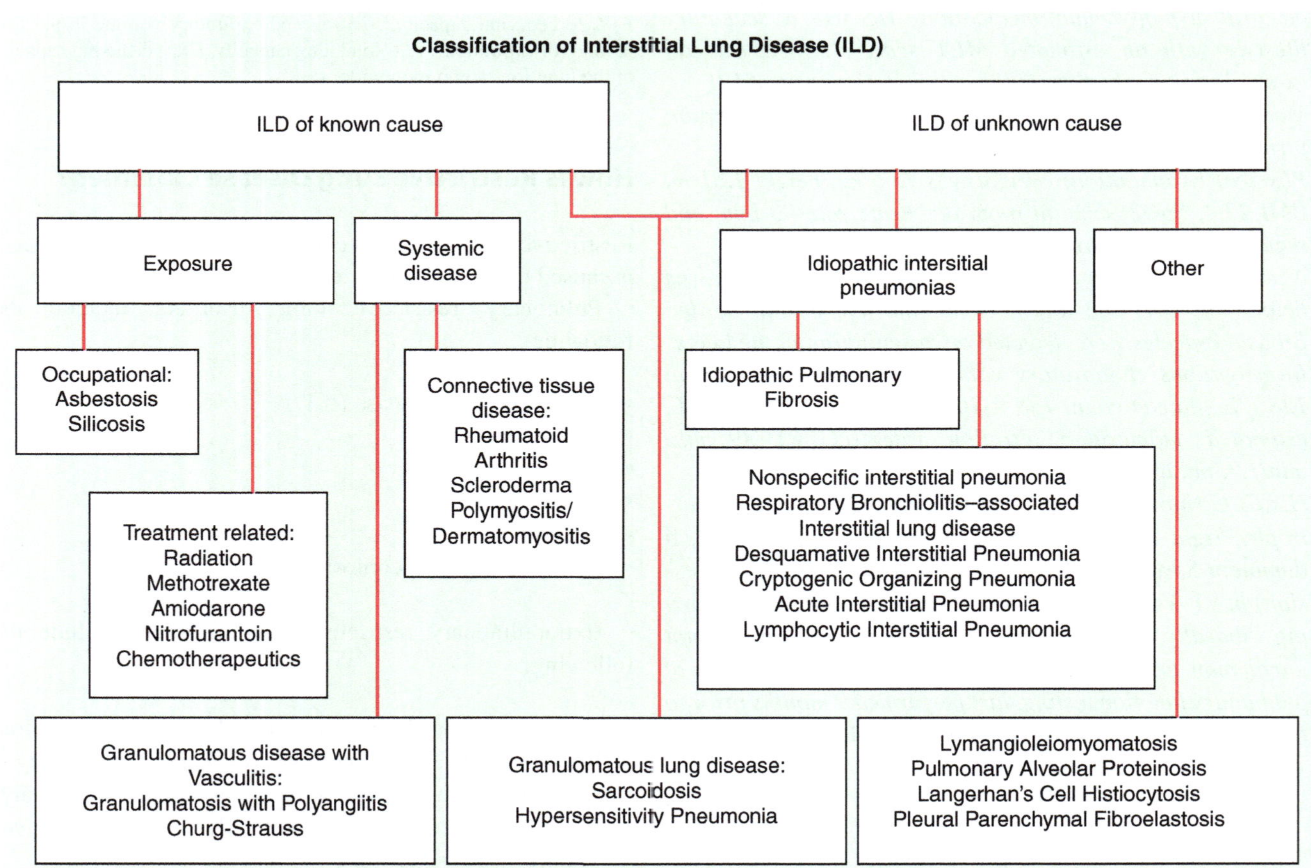

Fig. 16.1 Classification of interstitial lung disease into known and unknown causes. (From Hunninghake GM and Rosas IO [1], with permission McGraw Hill LLC)

- Prolonged mechanical ventilation
- Mortality

What Are the Independent Risk Factors for the Development of Postoperative Pulmonary Complications in Patients with ILD?

Risk factors for postoperative pulmonary complications, regardless of the presence of ILD, can be classified as follows:

Surgical:

- Thoracic and abdominal procedures
- Procedures requiring cardiopulmonary bypass
- Surgery lasting longer than 3 hours

Anesthetic:

- General anesthesia
- Prolonged neuromuscular blockade
- Invasive ventilation

Patient:

- Advanced age (risk significantly increases with each decade after 60 years) [4]
- Smoking
- BMI > 40
- Obstructive sleep apnea
- Pre-existing chronic lung disease

For ILD patients undergoing pulmonary resection for lung cancer, decreased preoperative diffusing capacity of the lung for carbon monoxide (DL_{CO}) and pre-existing comorbidities (e.g., ischemic heart disease, renal failure, and COPD) have been shown to be the most significant risk factors for the development of postoperative pulmonary complications [5]. For all major operative procedures, BMI < 23, emergency surgery, lung surgery, and longer anesthesia time have been associated with an increased risk of postoperative pulmonary complications [6].

What Are the Characteristic Pulmonary Function Test (PFT) Features of Restrictive Lung Disease?

- Reduction in total lung capacity (TLC).
- Forced expiratory volume in the first second (of expiration) (FEV_1) and forced vital capacity (FVC) reduced proportionally.
- FEV_1/FVC normal or increased.
- DL_{CO} is reduced when restrictive lung disease is caused by intrinsic lung disease but is normal when secondary to extrapulmonary causes, e.g., musculoskeletal deformities.

How Should the Patient with Restrictive Lung Disease Be Evaluated Preoperatively?

The purpose of clinical evaluation is to determine the degree of preoperative pulmonary reserve and the severity of pulmonary compromise.

History and Physical Examination

A focused assessment of pulmonary symptoms, including dyspnea, cough, and exercise tolerance, should be performed. Risk factors for postoperative pulmonary complications as discussed above must be ascertained and documented.

Investigations

- Spirometry (especially FEV_1) and DL_{CO} can be predictive of failure to wean from mechanical ventilation.
- Chest radiograph may provide little in the way of new or unexpected information and is unlikely to influence perioperative management.
- Arterial blood gas analysis is frequently performed to obtain a preoperative baseline. However, arterial hypoxia and hypercapnia are not significant independent predictors for postoperative pulmonary complications in respiratory disease [7].
- Echocardiography: Patients with respiratory disease may have comorbid cardiovascular disease. Moderate-to-severe restrictive lung disease may be accompanied by pulmonary hypertension.
- The 6-minute walk test can be used to quantify the clinical significance of restrictive lung disease. It is a submaximal measurement of aerobic capacity that has been shown to be a useful predictor of patient mortality [8].

How Is Disease Severity in IPF Classified?

Disease severity and progression are assessed using a combination of clinical, radiological, and pulmonary function test findings. Clinical parameters used to monitor disease progression are primarily degree of dyspnea, exercise capacity, and severity of cough. Patients with mild IPF may

Table 16.2 GAP staging system for predicting mortality associated with IPF. Patients score 3 points for diffusing capacity of the lung for carbon monoxide (DL_{CO}) if lung function is so poor that it prohibits performance of the test. GAP = gender, age, and physiology. The model predicts 1-, 2-, and 3-year mortality [10]

	Predictor		*Points*
Gender (G)	Female		0
	Male		1
Age (A)	≤60		0
	61–65		1
	>65		2
Physiology (P)	FVC, % predicted		
	>75		0
	50–75		1
	<50		2
	D_{LCO}, % predicted		
	>55		0
	36–55		1
	≤35		2
	Cannot perform		3
Stage	*I*	*II*	*III*
Points	0–3	4–5	6–8
Mortality			
1 year	5.6	16.2	39.2
2 year	10.9	29.9	62.1
3 year	16.3	42.1	76.8

FVC forced vital capacity, D_{LCO} diffusing capacity of the lung for carbon monoxide

Table 16.3 ARISCAT risk index for prediction of postoperative pulmonary complications [11]

Predictor		*Risk score*
Preoperative oxygen saturation		
≥96%		0
91–95%		8
≤90%		24
Respiratory infection in the past month		17
Preoperative hemoglobin ≤10 g/dL		11
Surgical incision		
Upper abdominal		15
Intrathoracic		24
Duration of surgery		
≤2 hours		16
2–3 hours		23
≥3 hours		8
Risk	*Number of points*	*Pulmonary complication rate (%)*
Low	<26	1.6%
Intermediate	26–44	13.3%
High	>45	42.1%

complain of a mild or nonproductive cough and dyspnea on considerable exertion. Patients with severe IPF will have dyspnea on moderate exertion and require oxygen at rest.

Pulmonary function testing is frequently performed every 3–6 months in patients with IPF – varying depending on disease progression. FVC (or more specifically, rate of decline of FVC) and DL_{CO} are especially important, being strong predictors of mortality and need for lung transplantation [9]. The Gender-Age-Physiology (GAP) clinical prediction model uses gender, age, FVC, and DL_{CO} to predict likelihood of mortality at 1-, 2-, and 3-year intervals (Table 16.2) [10].

Chest X-ray may be useful at the time of diagnosis when searching for possible etiologies but is not especially useful for monitoring disease progression. High-resolution CT is useful at the time of diagnosis and can be performed annually to monitor disease progression [9].

What Risk Scores Provide an Estimate of Postoperative Respiratory Failure?

A number of multifactorial risk scores are available that stratify the risk of postoperative pulmonary complications and/or failure to wean from mechanical ventilation. The ARISCAT (Assess Respiratory Risk in Surgical Patients in Catalonia) risk index uses seven independent risk factors that are assigned a weighted score and used to predict the risk of postoperative complications (Table 16.3) [11]. The Gupta validated risk calculator predicts failure to wean from mechanical ventilation within 48 hours of surgery or unplanned reintubation postoperatively [12]. Five preoperative predictors of postoperative respiratory failure were identified: type of surgery, emergency surgery, functional status, preoperative sepsis, and higher American Society of Anesthesiologists (ASA) class.

What Specific Medications Should We Expect to See in the Preoperative Patient with IPF?

Treatment of IPF is largely supportive, consisting of supplemental oxygen, pulmonary rehabilitation programs, education, and vaccination against influenza and pneumococcus. No drug has been found to be curative for IPF. However, two medications, nintedanib and pirfenidone, appear to slow disease progress. These medications are not widely available and are usually restricted to adult patients with mild to moderate IPF confirmed by a respiratory physician and a high-resolution CT scan within the previous 24 months. After an initial approval period, typically around 6 months, PFTs are performed to demonstrate that the disease has not progressed. (For example, in the authors' institution, disease progression is defined as a decline in predicted FVC of ≥10% from initiation of therapy.) The only definitive treatment for IPF is lung transplantation. It is the second most common reason for lung transplant after COPD/emphysema [13]. Among patients awaiting lung transplant, IPF has the highest mortality rate, and, as a result, IPF patients tend to be referred early for transplant [14].

What Complications of IPF Should the Patient Be Evaluated For?

- Emphysema
- Pulmonary hypertension
- Arrhythmias
- Congestive cardiac failure
- Coronary artery disease
- Obstructive sleep apnea
- Lung cancer

A pansystolic murmur was heard at the left sternal border over the fourth rib. At this location a pansystolic murmur that intensifies during inspiration is most likely due to pulmonary hypertension secondary to IPF. An echocardiogram performed on the same day as the preoperative anesthesia visit showed right ventricular hypertrophy, functional tricuspid regurgitation, and pulmonary artery systolic pressure 48 mmHg with a maximum tricuspid regurgitant jet (TRV) of 3.6. We concluded that the patient had moderate pulmonary hypertension.

Using the GAP staging system, it was determined that the patient had stage I IPF. PFTs were repeated and did not differ significantly from those obtained 9 months previously, giving some indication that the disease process was stable. The ARISCAT preoperative pulmonary risk index predicted a 13.3% risk of postoperative pulmonary complications (age 51–80 years, preoperative oxygen saturation 91–95%, no other clinical risk factors, no abdominal or intrathoracic surgery, and duration of surgery 2–3 hours). Due to the risk for prolonged postoperative intubation, the ICU team was consulted.

The patient was asked to take his metformin, pantoprazole, pirfenidone, and atorvastatin on the day of surgery.

At first glance, surgery involving the proximal humerus appears to be ideally suited to interscalene brachial plexus blockade. However, the incidence of concomitant ipsilateral phrenic nerve blockade and associated diaphragmatic hemiparesis approaches 100% with interscalene brachial plexus block. It has been suggested that interscalene block should not performed in patients who cannot tolerate a 25% reduction in pulmonary function [15]. *The incidence of phrenic nerve paralysis may be reduced by using a smaller volume of local anesthetic solution* [16]. *An alternative approach may be to insert an interscalene catheter that can be incrementally blocked and subsequently topped up with a shorter-acting agent such as lidocaine. Therefore, a regional anesthesia technique was not absolutely contraindicated. As we have a number of very experienced practitioners in regional anesthesia at our institution, we decided to proceed with an interscalene catheter through which the interscalene brachial plexus was gradually blocked with 15 ml of a 3:1 mixture of 2% lidocaine and 0.5% bupivacaine. Surgery and postoperative recovery were uneventful.*

True/False Questions

1. Idiopathic pulmonary fibrosis:
   (a) Is a rare cause of interstitial lung disease.
   (b) Affects men more than women.
   (c) Is the commonest reason for patients referred for lung transplant.
   (d) Is usually familial.
   (e) Onset is in the third to fourth decades.
2. Concerning the PFT characteristics of restrictive lung disease:
   (a) FEV_1 is reduced to a greater degree than FVC.
   (b) FVC is normal or increased.
   (c) TLC is reduced.
   (d) DL_{CO} is normal if restrictive lung disease is secondary to extrapulmonary causes.
   (e) DL_{CO} can be used as a predictor of postoperative pulmonary complications.

References

1. Hunninghake GM, Rosas IO. Interstitial lung disease. In: Jameson J, Fauci AS, Kasper DL, Hauser SL, Longo DL, Loscalzo J, editors. Harrison's principles of internal medicine. 20th ed. New York: McGraw Hill Education; 2018. Available at: https://accesspharmacy.mhmedical.com/content.aspx?bookid=2129§ionid=192031469. Accessed 22 May 2020.
2. Ley B, Collard HR. Epidemiology of idiopathic pulmonary fibrosis. Clin Epidemiol. 2013;5:483–92.
3. Nathan SD, Shlobin OA, Weir N, Ahmad S, Kaldjob JM, Battle E, et al. Long-term course and prognosis of idiopathic pulmonary fibrosis in the new millennium. Chest. 2011;140(1):221–9.
4. Smetana GW, Lawrence VA, Cornell JE. American College of P. Preoperative pulmonary risk stratification for noncardiothoracic surgery: systematic review for the American College of Physicians. Ann Intern Med. 2006;144(8):581–95.
5. Park JS, Kim HK, Kim K, Kim J, Shim YM, Choi YS. Prediction of acute pulmonary complications after resection of lung cancer in patients with preexisting interstitial lung disease. Thorac Cardiovasc Surg. 2011;59(3):148–52.
6. Choi SM, Lee J, Park YS, Cho YJ, Lee CH, Lee SM, et al. Postoperative pulmonary complications after surgery in patients with interstitial lung disease. Respiration. 2014;87(4):287–93.
7. Lakshminarasimhachar A, Smetana GW. Preoperative evaluation: estimation of pulmonary risk. Anesthesiol Clin. 2016;34(1):71–88.
8. Lederer DJ, Arcasoy SM, Wilt JS, D'Ovidio F, Sonett JR, Kawut SM. Six-minute-walk distance predicts waiting list survival in idiopathic pulmonary fibrosis. Am J Respir Crit Care Med. 2006;174(6):659–64.
9. Ryerson C, Ley B. Prognosis and monitoring of idiopathic pulmonary fibrosis. In: Post TW, editor. UpToDate. Waltham; 2020.
10. Ley B, Ryerson CJ, Vittinghoff E, Ryu JH, Tomassetti S, Lee JS, et al. A multidimensional index and staging system for idiopathic pulmonary fibrosis. Ann Intern Med. 2012;156(10):684–91.

11. Canet J, Gallart L, Gomar C, Paluzie G, Valles J, Castillo J, et al. Prediction of postoperative pulmonary complications in a population-based surgical cohort. Anesthesiology. 2010;113(6): 1338–50.
12. Gupta H, Gupta PK, Fang X, Miller WJ, Cemaj S, Forse RA, et al. Development and validation of a risk calculator predicting postoperative respiratory failure. Chest. 2011;140(5): 1207–15.
13. Alalawi R, Whelan T, Bajwa RS, Hodges TN. Lung transplantation and interstitial lung disease. Curr Opin Pulm Med. 2005;11(5):461–6.
14. Thabut G, Mal H, Castier Y, Groussard O, Brugiere O, Marrash-Chahla R, et al. Survival benefit of lung transplantation for patients with idiopathic pulmonary fibrosis. J Thorac Cardiovasc Surg. 2003;126(2):469–75.
15. Urmey WF, McDonald M. Hemidiaphragmatic paresis during interscalene brachial plexus block: effects on pulmonary function and chest wall mechanics. Anesth Analg. 1992;74(3):352–7.
16. Riazi S, Carmichael N, Awad I, Holtby RM, McCartney CJ. Effect of local anaesthetic volume (20 vs 5 ml) on the efficacy and respiratory consequences of ultrasound-guided interscalene brachial plexus block. Br J Anaesth. 2008;101(4):549–56.

Part IV

Endocrine

Diabetes Mellitus

17

Derek Dillane

A 69-year-old male with a 6-month history of episodic, transient left-sided monocular amaurosis fugax presented for evaluation 1 week in advance of carotid endarterectomy (CEA). He had type 1 diabetes mellitus (DM), hypertension, and hyperlipidemia. He was a smoker, his weight was 124 kg, and he had a history of obstructive sleep apnea for which he used a continuous positive airway pressure (CPAP) machine.
Medications: Insulin lispro (Humalog) 80 units with meals, insulin glargine (Lantus) 200 units at bedtime, hydrochlorothiazide, losartan, rosuvastatin, and aspirin.
Physical examination: Weight 124 kg, BMI 38.6, heart rate 60 bpm, blood pressure 164/77, and respiratory rate 18/minute.
Investigations: HbA1c was 8.2%. Triglycerides were 1.92 mmol/L, LDL cholesterol was 2.77 mmol/L, and HDL cholesterol was 1.16 mmol/L. Creatinine was 75 umol/L and estimated GFR was 90 ml/min/1.73 m^2.
Chest radiograph was normal, and his ECG can be seen in Fig. 17.1. *Carotid duplex ultrasound reported up to 80% stenosis of the left internal carotid artery and 70% stenosis of the right internal carotid artery. This had been confirmed by a CT angiogram. Echocardiogram showed normal left ventricular size, mild aortic sclerosis without stenosis, and a left ventricular ejection fraction of 56%.*

How Is DM Classified?

DM type 1 (DM1) is an autoimmune process involving pancreatic beta-cell destruction. There is absolute insulin deficiency. Its development is associated with other autoimmune conditions, particularly thyroid disease (15–30% DM1 patients), autoimmune gastritis/pernicious anemia (5–10%), and Addison's disease (0.5%) [1]. DM1 accounts for 5–10% of patients with diabetes.

DM type 2 (DM2) occurs as a consequence of progressive reduction in insulin secretion and the coexisting development of insulin resistance. Risk factors for the development of DM2 include obesity, age > 45 years, positive family history for DM, sedentary lifestyle, and race (indigenous Americans, Hispanic/Latino Americans, and African Americans are at higher risk). DM2 accounts for ≥90% of patients with diabetes.

Gestational DM (GDM) occurs in up to 10% of pregnancies. It is defined as diabetes diagnosed during the second or third trimester of pregnancy that is not clearly overt DM. It almost always resolves after delivery. However, the occurrence of GDM does increase maternal risk for subsequent development of DM2 in later years.

Secondary DM occurs secondary to another medical condition, e.g., cystic fibrosis, hemochromatosis, chronic pancreatitis, Cushing's disease, and drug-/chemical-induced disease.

An important issue for the perioperative physician is the underdiagnosis of DM in the general population. It is estimated that one in five patients with DM is unaware that they have the disease.

What Complications Is the Patient with Diabetes Mellitus (DM) Subject to in the Perioperative Period?

Elevated blood glucose levels are associated with impaired wound healing and increased risk of infection.

Metabolic decompensation secondary to mismanagement of diabetes drugs leads to diabetic ketoacidosis (DKA) or hyperosmolar hyperglycemic state (HHS) [2].

Hypoglycemia may go unrecognized due to its symptoms being masked by general anesthesia.

D. Dillane (✉)
Department of Anesthesiology & Pain Medicine, University of Alberta, Edmonton, AB, Canada

D. Dillane, B. A. Finegan (eds.), *Preoperative Assessment*, https://doi.org/10.1007/978-3-030-58842-7_17

HR 58 . SINUS RHYTHM
RR 1034 . BORDERLINE LEFT AXIS DEVIATION
PR 148 . BORDERLINE R WAVE PROGRESSION, ANTERIOR LEADS
QRSD 86 . NONSPECIFIC T ABNORMALITIES, LATERAL LEADS
QT 388
QTc 382

-- AXIS --
P 68
QRS -27
T 137

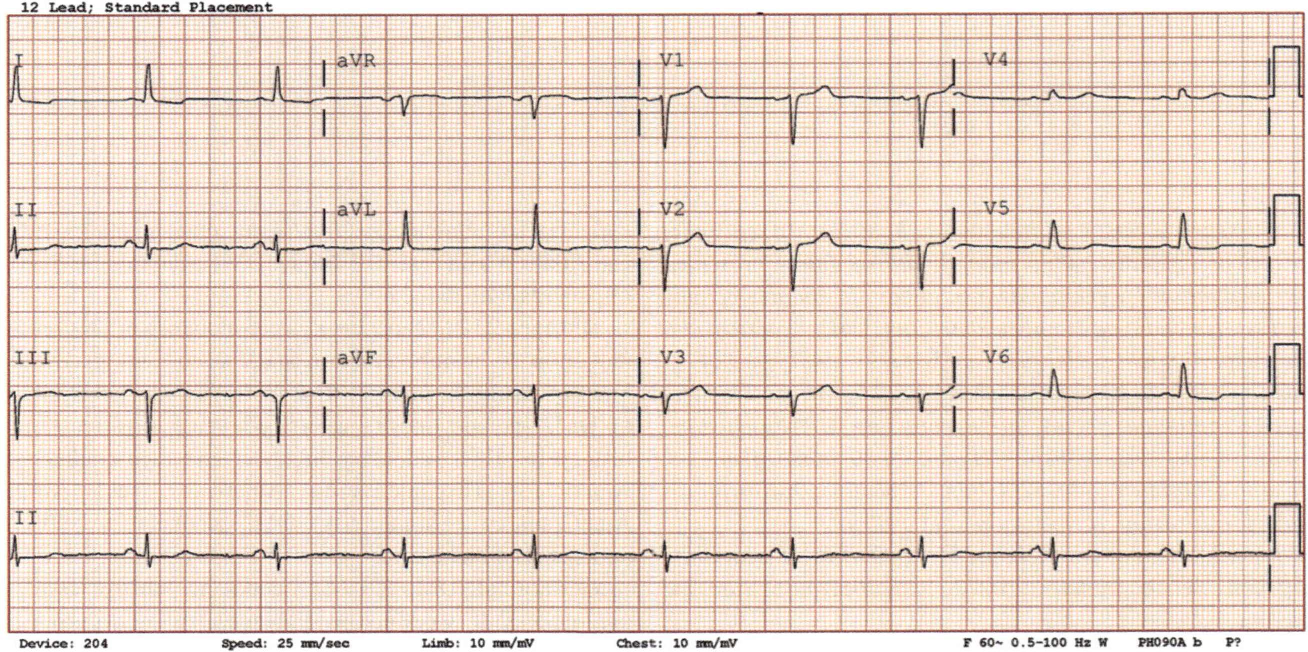

Fig. 17.1 Electrocardiogram of a 69-year-old male with a 6-month history of episodic, transient left-sided monocular amaurosis fugax presented for carotid endarterectomy

Diabetics with autonomic neuropathy are predisposed to intra- and postoperative hemodynamic instability due to impaired mechanisms to compensate for intravascular volume changes.

Patients with diabetic autonomic neuropathy have a high incidence of gastroparesis and silent myocardial ischemia. Autonomic dysfunction and resultant hypercapnia may be responsible for a diminished response to hypoxia and an exaggerated respiratory depressant response to opioids [3].

What Target Blood Glucose Level Should We Aim for Preoperatively?

Optimization of baseline glycemic control is a pivotal concern. The American Diabetes Association guidelines recommend a target glucose range of 80–180 mg/dL (4.4–10.0 mmol/L) for most noncritically ill hospitalized patients [2]. Blood glucose levels that trend persistently or significantly above this should be addressed preoperatively if possible.

What End-Organ Abnormalities Associated with Diabetes Are of Particular Concern Perioperatively?

End-organ abnormalities due to macro- and microangiopathy are responsible for the increased morbidity and mortality associated with DM. Macrovascular complications include coronary artery and cerebrovascular disease. Macrovascular complications are more common if the disease is longstanding, if glucose levels are poorly controlled, or if there is coexisting hypertension, tobacco use, hyperlipidemia, and a sedentary lifestyle [4]. Long-term DM patients should be considered high risk for perioperative myocardial ischemia.

Microvascular complications of particular concern perioperatively include diabetic nephropathy and neuropathy. Autonomic neuropathy with gastroparesis increases the risk of aspiration. If a peripheral or central neuraxial block is planned, a baseline neurological assessment is prudent, to establish the extent (if present) of peripheral neuropathy.

How Should the Patient with DM Be Evaluated Preoperatively?

History

- What type of DM does the patient have?
- Age of onset, long-term control (HbA1c), and fasting/pre-meal glucose values
- History of hyperglycemic emergencies: DKA and HHS
- History of hypoglycemic episodes
- Medications: oral therapy and/or insulin, including basal and corrective doses and time taken
- If available, a diary of the patient's fasting, pre-meal, and nighttime glucose values along with the amount of insulin given
- Long-term noncardiac complications: nephropathy, peripheral neuropathy, autonomic neuropathy (gastro-esophageal reflux disease, reported early satiety, chronic diarrhea, lack of sweating), and retinopathy
- Long-term cardiovascular complications: coronary artery disease, hypertension, cerebrovascular disease, and peripheral vascular disease

Physical Exam

The physical exam should focus on the cardiovascular, pulmonary, renal, and neurologic systems. Assess for signs of diabetic autonomic neuropathy (orthostatic hypotension and resting tachycardia).

Joint mobilization should also be assessed, focusing on mouth opening and cervical spine mobility. DM1 patients may develop stiff joint syndrome with diminished mobility of the cervical spine and resultant difficult intubation [4].

Investigations

Laboratory investigations include HbA1c value, 24-hour urinary albumin, and serum creatinine. Preoperative elevated baseline blood glucose may indicate increased risk for post-operative wound infection [5].

A baseline ECG is a prerequisite. In addition to elucidating information pertaining to rate and rhythm, other markers of cardiac disease, e.g., Q waves indicative of a previous myocardial infarct, or hypertensive changes, may be seen. Many diabetics present with silent ischemia diagnosed on routine ECG. Further cardiac evaluation—e.g., exercise stress test, myocardial perfusion scan, and echocardiography—is performed commensurate with the complexity of the planned surgery and the patient's perioperative risk for a major adverse cardiac event (see Chap. 2 for an overview of preoperative evaluation of the cardiac patient undergoing noncardiac surgery).

Chest radiograph may indicate signs of heart failure, e.g., cardiac enlargement, presence of pleural effusions, or pulmonary vascular congestion.

Should Elective Surgery Be Cancelled Because of a High Preoperative HbA1c Value?

HbA1c is a measure of average blood glucose over a 3-month period (the life of a red blood cell). A high preoperative HbA1c level is associated with poor surgical outcome in cardiac and noncardiac surgery [6]. Several studies have suggested that HbA1c could be used as a risk stratification tool to predict perioperative hyperglycemia and other morbidities postoperatively [8]. Halkos et al. demonstrated that a HbA1c > 7% was associated with a significantly increased risk of renal failure, deep surgical wound infection, and prolonged hospital stay after coronary artery bypass grafting. An HbA1c of 8.6% was associated with a fourfold increase in mortality [7]. The Association of Anaesthetists of Great Britain and Ireland suggests delaying elective surgery for optimization of glycemic control when the HbA1c >8.5% [6] (Table 17.1) [9]. The American Diabetes Association has not provided an optimal HbA1c target for patients undergoing elective surgery but recommends a target of <7% in general [10]. No study has compared the effect of actively reducing HbA1c preoperatively versus not reducing it. However, the observational evidence points toward a target of <7% for elective surgery. Therefore, if the surgery can wait, it seems

Table 17.1 Diagnostic use of glycated hemoglobin (HbA1c)[a]

	HbA1c (%)	HbA1c ($mmol\ mol^{-1}$)
No diabetes	<5.6	<38
Pre-diabetes	5.7–6.4	37–47
Diabetes	>6.5	>48
Well-controlled diabetes	<6	<42
Controlled diabetes	<7	<53
Poorly controlled diabetes	>8.5	>69
Level at which studies show increased risk of complications	>6	>42
Level at which AAGBI and JBDS guidelines suggest optimization before elective surgery	>8.5	69

From Stubbs et al. [9], with permission from Elsevier

AAGBI Association of Anaesthetists of Great Britain and Ireland, *JBDS* Joint British Diabetes Societies

[a]This table highlights the diagnostic interpretation of HbA1c results. Through affecting the red blood cell's lifespan, other comorbidities may affect he usefulness of the test. These disorders include hemolytic anemias, and kidney and liver diseases

reasonable to attain optimal long-term glycemic control as guided by the HbA1c.

What Medications Should We Expect to See in the Preoperative Patient with DM?

Insulin Ultra-short and short-acting, intermediate-acting, and long-acting preparations exist. Most commercial insulin contains beef insulin as the primary component, or a combination of beef and pork. Recombinant DNA techniques have allowed the production of human insulin. Advantages include more rapid absorption, less immunogenicity than beef-pork insulin, and comparable effectiveness to animal insulins. Insulin can be delivered via portable pen injectors, closed-loop systems (e.g., insulin infusion intravenously), or open-loop systems such the insulin pump.

Oral Hypoglycemic Agents Major groups include α-glucosidase inhibitors (e.g., acarbose), meglitinide (e.g., repaglinide or nateglinide), biguanides (e.g., metformin), sulfonylureas (e.g., glibenclamide, glipizide, glimepiride, gliquidone), thiazolidinediones (e.g., pioglitazone), and dipeptidyl peptidase-4 (DPP-IV) inhibitors (e.g., sitagliptin, saxagliptin, vildagliptin) and SGLT-2 inhibitors also known as gliflozins (e.g., dapagliflozin). The FDA released a safety statement in 2015 regarding reports of DKA occurring with SGLT-2 inhibitors. As a result of this statement, the American College of Endocrinology recommends holding the drug 24 hours before elective surgery [12].

Incretin Analogs (Liraglutide) One of the main physiological effects of incretins is to rapidly increase insulin and decrease glucagon secretion in response to an oral glucose load.

Angiotensin-Converting Enzyme (ACE) Inhibitors or Angiotensin Receptor Blockers Either, but not both together, is recommended for the treatment of nonpregnant diabetic patients with modestly elevated urinary albumin excretion (20–299 mg/day) and strongly recommended when urinary albumin excretion ≥300 mg/day or estimated GFR <60 ml/min/1.73 m^2 [11].

What Terminology Is Used to Describe Commonly Used Insulin Regimens Outside of the Operating Room Environment?

Basal Insulin Administered to manage hepatic glucose output. It may be given intravenously or subcutaneously.

Bolus Insulin (Meal Insulin) Administered to cover carbohydrate in a meal. It is short- and fast-acting insulin that is administered subcutaneously.

Correction Insulin Added to or subtracted from meal insulin or given at bedtime to correct for glucose outside of the target range. It is the same insulin as bolus insulin and is administered subcutaneously.

What Is the Significance of Rosuvastatin Use in a Diabetic Patient?

The risk of cardiovascular disease in diabetic patients is increased in the presence of dyslipidemia, in particular that due to elevated LDL cholesterol. The American Diabetes Association, in 2016 guidelines, follows American Heart Association/American College of Cardiology guidelines by setting no LDL cholesterol goal but recommending a 50% reduction from baseline. A moderate to high intensity statin such as rosuvastatin can be used for this purpose [12].

What Factors Contribute to the Development of DKA or HHS Perioperatively?

- Sepsis and infections (urinary tract infections, pneumonia, infected wounds, and upper respiratory tract infections)
- New onset of diabetes
- Treatment noncompliance
- Alcohol and illicit drug use
- Site of injection complications interfering with adequate absorption of insulin, e.g., lipodystrophy

Surgery and Hypoglycemic Agents: An Approach

Perioperative management of the diabetic patient's therapy should be tailored to, among other factors, random glucose values and HbA1c. Intravenous insulin infusion therapy adjusted by sliding scale is not a panacea for the insulin-dependent diabetic.

The goal of treatment is avoidance of hypo- and hyperglycemic episodes from when fasting starts preoperatively until the patient is eating and drinking normally after surgery. Decide if interruption of hypoglycemic therapy is required by determining the fasting time and the projected number of meals that will be missed perioperatively. Patients who are unlikely to miss more than one meal can often be managed by manipulation of their normal medication or even continuation in certain cases [6].

Previously, all oral hypoglycemic drugs were stopped perioperatively. It may be rational—indeed, possibly safer—to continue metformin, a drug that works by preventing glucose levels from rising, in patients undergoing a short starvation period, i.e., scheduled first on the operating slate with one projected missed meal [13].

Metformin *should be* withheld in patients with pre-existing renal impairment or with the use of nephrotoxic agents, e.g., contrast media. Agents that act by lowering glucose concentration, e.g., sulfonylureas and insulin, should be stopped or have their regular dose modified during periods of starvation.

Basal insulin is often inappropriately held in the perioperative setting. The patient described above was on a basal bolus insulin therapy (BBIT) regime with basal long-acting insulin at night in addition to preprandial short-acting insulin. Basal insulin controls hepatic glucose output, which increases with fasting and surgical stress. Continuation of basal insulin in DM1 is imperative to prevent ketoacidosis. Basal insulin improves glycemic control and reduces hospital complications when compared to sliding scale insulin alone in DM1 undergoing general surgery [14].

Time of surgery is important to consider, especially in patients that take 100% of their normal basal insulin dose.

Finally, the Enhanced Recovery After Surgery (ERAS) Society recommends carbohydrate-rich drinks up to 2 hours before surgery [15]. This increases insulin sensitivity and decreases the risk of postoperative hyperglycemia. This is a contentious issue in diabetic patients as there is a risk of aspiration secondary to delayed gastric emptying [16]. Further investigation is required before preoperative carbohydrate loading can be recommended without qualification in diabetic patients.

The patient had symptomatic high-grade internal carotid artery stenosis (80% stenosis on ultrasound carotid Doppler). Indications for CEA are reviewed in Chap. 10—*surgery was indicated in this case. The timing of surgery relative to stroke or TIA is somewhat controversial, but there is evidence that early intervention, i.e., within weeks of stroke or TIA improves outcome* [17]. *Even though his Revised Cardiac Risk Index score was 2 (10.1% risk estimate for MI, cardiac arrest, or death within 30 days of surgery), we decided to proceed to surgery without further intervention or testing, which was felt to have little impact on decision-making. A HbA1c of 8.2% clearly indicates a lot of room for optimization with regard to glycemic control. The patient was referred to a diabetologist in the knowledge that this was a longer-term project than immediate preoperative optimization. He was requested to take 80% of his insulin glargine the evening before surgery, his insulin lispro was held on the morning of surgery, and he was scheduled to be first on the operating list* [13].

True/False Questions

1. (a) Patients with diabetic autonomic neuropathy have a high incidence of silent myocardial ischemia.
   (b) HbA1c is a measure of average blood glucose over a 6-month period.
   (c) A high preoperative HbA1c level is associated with poor surgical outcome in noncardiac surgery.
   (d) The American Diabetes Association suggests delaying elective surgery for optimization of glycemic control when the HbA1c > 8.5%.
   (e) ACE inhibitors are frequently used in diabetic patients with elevated urinary albumin excretion.
2. (a) Basal insulin may only be administered via the intravenous route.
   (b) Bolus insulin is given to cover the carbohydrate ingested in a meal.
   (c) All oral hypoglycemic medications should be discontinued preoperatively on the day of surgery.
   (d) Metformin may be continued preoperatively on the day of surgery if the planned starvation period is of short duration.
   (e) For patients with pre-existing renal impairment, it is safe to administer metformin preoperatively on the day of surgery.

References

1. American Diabetes Association. 2. Classification and diagnosis of diabetes. Diabetes Care. 2015;38(Suppl):S8–S16.
2. American Diabetes Association. 13. Diabetes Care in the Hospital. Diabetes Care. 2016;39(Suppl 1):S99–104.
3. Mustafa HI, Fessel JP, Barwise J, Shannon JR, Raj SR, Diedrich A, et al. Dysautonomia: perioperative implications. Anesthesiology. 2012;116(1):205–15.
4. Nicholson G, GM H. Diabetes and adult surgical inpatients. Continuing education in anaesthesia. Criti Care Pain. 2011;11(6):234–8.
5. Trick WE, Scheckler WE, Tokars JI, Jones KC, Reppen ML, Smith EM, et al. Modifiable risk factors associated with deep sternal site infection after coronary artery bypass grafting. J Thorac Cardiovasc Surg. 2000;119(1):108–14.
6. Barker P, Creasey PE, Dhatariya K, Levy N, Lipp A, Nathanson MH, et al. Peri-operative management of the surgical patient with diabetes 2015: Association of Anaesthetists of Great Britain and Ireland. Anaesthesia. 2015;70(12):1427–40.
7. Halkos ME, Lattouf OM, Puskas JD, Kilgo P, Cooper WA, Morris CD, et al. Elevated preoperative hemoglobin A1c level is associated with reduced long-term survival after coronary artery bypass surgery. Ann Thorac Surg. 2008;86(5):1431–7.
8. O'Sullivan CJ, Hynes N, Mahendran B, Andrews EJ, Avalos G, Tawfik S, et al. Haemoglobin A1c (HbA1C) in non-diabetic and diabetic vascular patients. Is HbA1C an independent risk factor and predictor of adverse outcome? Eur J Vasc Endovasc Surg. 2006;32(2):188–97.
9. Stubbs DJ, Levy N, Dhatariya K. The rationale and strategies to achieve perioperative glycaemic control. BJA Educ. 2017;17(6):185–9.
10. American Diabetes Association. 5. Glycemic targets: standards of medical care in diabetes-2016. Diabetes Care. 2016;39(Supplement 1):S39–46.
11. American Diabetes Association. 9. Microvascular complications and foot care: standards of medical care in diabetes-2016. Diabetes Care. 2016;39:S39–46.
12. American Diabetes Association. 8. Cardiovascular disease and risk management: standards of medical care in diabetes-2016. Diabetes Care. 2016;39:S60–71.
13. Duggan EW, Carlson K, Umpierrez GE. Perioperative hyperglycemia management: an update. Anesthesiology. 2017;126(3):547–60.

14. Umpierrez GE, Smiley D, Jacobs S, Peng L, Temponi A, Mulligan P, et al. Randomized study of basal-bolus insulin therapy in the inpatient management of patients with type 2 diabetes undergoing general surgery (RABBIT 2 surgery). Diabetes Care. 2011;34(2):256–61.
15. Gustafsson UO, Scott MJ, Schwenk W, Demartines N, Roulin D, Francis N, et al. Enhanced Recovery After Surgery (ERAS) Society, for Perioperative Care; European Society for Clinical Nutrition and Metabolism (ESPEN); International Association for Surgical Metabolism and Nutrition (IASMEN). Guidelines for perioperative care in elective colonic surgery: Enhanced Recovery After Surgery (ERAS®) Society recommendations. World J Surg. 2013;37(2):259–84.
16. Albalawi Z, Laffin M, Gramlich L, Senior P, McAlister FA. Enhanced Recovery After Surgery (ERAS®) in individuals with diabetes: a systematic review. World J Surg. 2017;41(8):1927–34.
17. Rothwell PM, Eliasziw M, Gutnikov SA, Warlow CP, Barnett HJ, Carotid Endarterectomy Trialists C. Endarterectomy for symptomatic carotid stenosis in relation to clinical subgroups and timing of surgery. Lancet. 2004;363(9413):915–24.

Hyperthyroidism

18

Derek Dillane

A 34-year-old female patient presented to the anesthesia preoperative assessment clinic 1 week prior to total thyroidectomy for hyperthyroidism secondary to Graves' disease. She reported a history of palpitations, tremor, heat intolerance, and weight gain.
Medications: Propranolol. She had been on methimazole, but it had been discontinued due to a hypersensitivity reaction.
Physical Examination: Sinus tachycardia with a rate of 97 bpm, mild tremor, exophthalmos, and a moderate non-tender goiter.
Investigations: Laboratory findings are shown in Table 18.1.
Her ECG confirmed a sinus tachycardia with a long QT interval (Fig. 18.1). *Chest radiograph showed mild enlargement of the cardiac silhouette. Thyroid ultrasound revealed a prominent hypervascular gland measuring approximately 7 × 2.5 × 3 cm on the right and 5.5 × 2.5 × 3.5 cm on the left. Echocardiography showed normal left ventricular systolic and diastolic function. She was noted to have mild pulmonary hypertension with a pulmonary artery pressure estimated at 50 mm Hg.*

Table 18.1 Laboratory values at pre-admission clinic visit

Thyroid-stimulating hormone (TSH)	*<0.03*	*(0.2–4 mU/L)*
Free T3	*>30*	*(3.5–6.5 pmol/L)*
Free T4	*143.7*	*(9–23 pmol/L)*
Calcium	*2.26*	*(2.1–2.6 mmol/L)*

What Is the Difference Between Thyrotoxicosis and Hyperthyroidism?

Thyrotoxicosis is a condition resulting from the effects of excessive circulating thyroid hormone of any cause or source. Hyperthyroidism is a form of thyrotoxicosis that occurs when the excessive thyroid hormone originates from the thyroid gland. Causes of non-hyperthyroid thyrotoxicosis include excessive levothyroxine use and pharmacologic thyroiditis, e.g., caused by iodine-containing drugs such as amiodarone.

What Is Graves' Disease and What Distinguishes It from Other Causes of Hyperthyroidism?

Graves' disease is the most common cause of hyperthyroidism. It is an autoimmune condition more prevalent in females and in patients between 30 and 60 years old. Thyroid-stimulating hormone (TSH) receptor antibodies stimulate thyroid gland growth and promote thyroid hormone synthesis and secretion (Fig. 18.2). A radioiodine thyroid scan will show normal or high uptake indicating excess new thyroid hormone synthesis. A radioiodine scan that shows near-absent uptake will be seen when hyperthyroidism is due to viral, radiation-, or drug-induced thyroiditis. Laboratory findings seen with Graves' disease include elevated T3 and T4 (T3 is typically higher in Graves' disease and T4 is higher in subacute thyroiditis), decreased TSH, and elevated TSH receptor antibody level (Fig. 18.3) [1].

D. Dillane (✉)
Department of Anesthesiology & Pain Medicine, University of Alberta, Edmonton, AB, Canada

D. Dillane, B. A. Finegan (eds.), *Preoperative Assessment*, https://doi.org/10.1007/978-3-030-58842-7_18

sinus rhythm (rapid)
long QT interval, consider hypocalcaemia or quinidine-like drug
This is especially noticeable in inferior leads
Further assessment strongly advised

Abnormal ECG

P / PQ: 98 ms / 125 ms
QRS: 85 ms
QT / QTc / QTd: 422 ms / 537 ms / 141 ms
P/QRS/T axis: 54° / -2° / 59°
Heartrate: 97 bpm

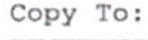

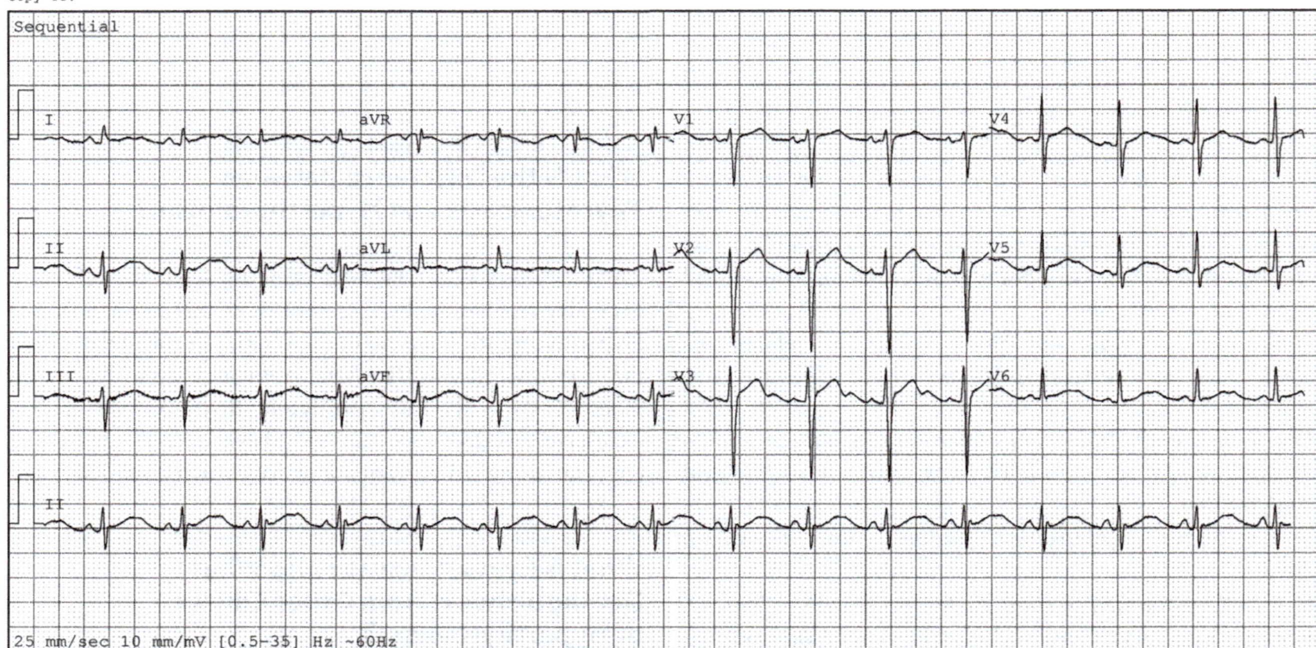

Fig. 18.1 ECG showing sinus tachycardia and prolonged QT interval

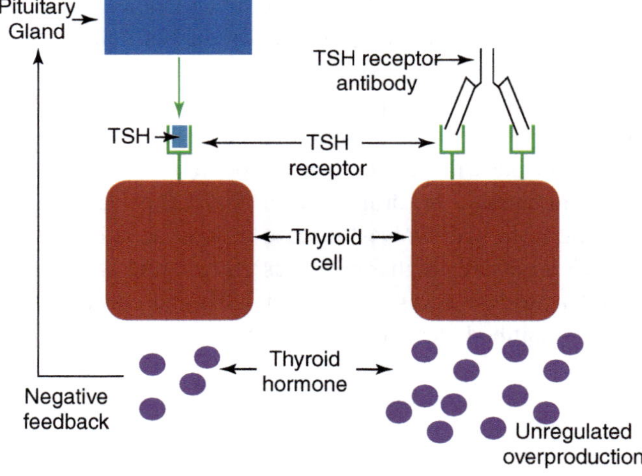

Fig. 18.2 Normal pituitary control of thyroid function via thyroid-stimulating hormone (TSH) on the left. TSH receptor antibodies, on the right of the figure, seen in Graves' disease

How Can a Patient with Hyperthyroidism Gain Weight?

Hyperthyroidism causes weight loss in most patients. Some patients gain weight due to stimulation of the appetite and/or treatment of hyperthyroidism.

What Is the Significance of a Long QT Interval in a Patient with Hyperthyroidism?

Hyperthyroidism is associated with cardiac complications. Atrial fibrillation is the most common cardiac abnormality occurring in approximately 10–25% of hyperthyroid patients [2]. The QT interval represents the time for ventricular depolarization and repolarization. It is dependent on heart rate, i.e., a faster heart rate leads to a shorter QT interval. Therefore, QTc estimates the QT interval corrected for a

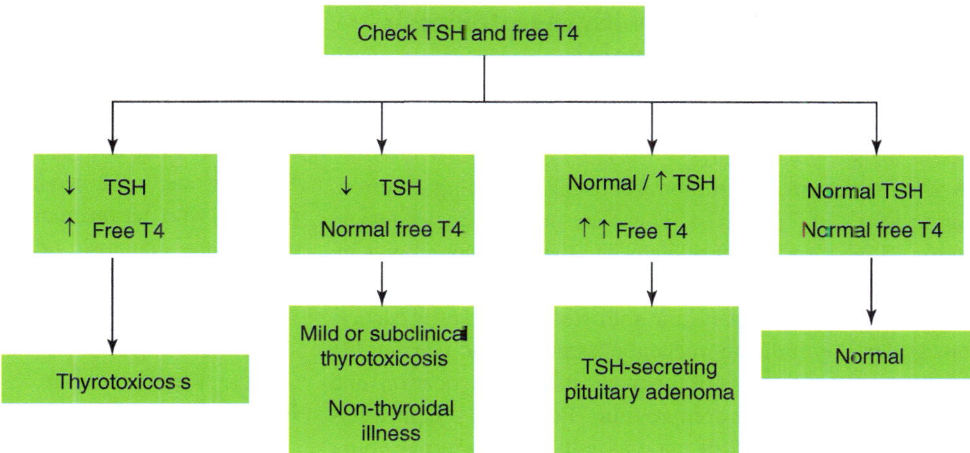

Fig. 18.3 Biochemical abnormalities that aid the diagnosis of thyrotoxicosis. (Adapted from Jonklas and Cooper [1], with permission Elsevier)

heart rate of 60 bpm. A prolonged QT interval places the patient at increased risk for tachyarrhythmias, e.g., *torsades de pointes* and ventricular fibrillation. The correlation between hyperthyroidism and prolonged QT interval has been previously noted [3]. Indeed, there is an association between levels of T4 and QTc [3]. The etiology is not precisely known but may be related to the effect of thyroid hormone on the cardiac myocyte. The QTc frequently reverts to a normal range once the patient becomes biochemically euthyroid [4].

Is There a Link Between Pulmonary Hypertension and Hyperthyroidism?

Hyperthyroidism is associated with changes in cardiac output, blood pressure, and systemic and pulmonary vascular resistance. Most patients with pulmonary hypertension and thyroid disease are older with toxic multinodular goiter. Again, the etiology is not entirely known (see relationship between thyroid and cardiovascular disease in the following question). There may be a direct effect of thyroid hormone on pulmonary vasculature. Patients with hyperthyroidism should be considered at risk for pulmonary hypertension. Patients with newly diagnosed pulmonary hypertension should be investigated for thyroid disease, as it may be a reversible cause of pulmonary hypertension.

What Complications Is the Patient with Thyrotoxicosis Subject to in the Perioperative Period?

1. *Thyroid Storm*

   This is a rare and life-threatening exacerbation of hyperthyroidism brought on by acute illness, trauma, and thyroid or non-thyroid surgery. Discontinuation of, or poor compliance with, antithyroid medication is a risk factor. Thyroid storm can be diagnosed clinically by severe tachycardia, hypotension, cardiac failure, and hyperpyrexia in the patient under anesthesia. Delirium, extreme anxiety, and altered consciousness progressing to coma can be seen in the awake patient.

2. *Cardiovascular Changes*

   Arrhythmias, most frequently sinus tachycardia or atrial fibrillation, systemic and pulmonary hypertension, coronary ischemia, and heart failure can be seen with suboptimal disease control. The extent of involvement of the adrenergic system versus that of direct thyroid hormone stimulation and the interaction between these two systems is unknown. For instance, many of the adrenergic-like effects are mediated via T3 stimulation of cardiac myocytes. In addition, many components of the cardiac beta-adrenergic system are regulated by thyroid hormone. Treatment with beta-blockade improves most of the cardiovascular concerns associated with hyperthyroidism. Of note, treatment of tachyarrhythmia in the thyrotoxic cardiac patient with beta-blockade is the first-line therapy. In the patient with overt cardiac failure, a cautious trial of short-acting beta-blockade (e.g., esmolol) may be used [5].

3. *Airway Complications*

   In addition to concerns regarding intubation at induction of anesthesia as outlined below, the thyroidectomy patient can develop a number of postoperative airway complications. Airway obstruction may occur secondary to hematoma, tracheomalacia, recurrent laryngeal nerve damage, or hypocalcemic laryngeal tetany [6]. Unilateral recurrent laryngeal nerve damage may result in hoarseness or may be asymptomatic. Bilateral recurrent laryngeal nerve damage can result in aspiration pneumonia or complete airway occlusion requiring immediate intubation [7].

How Should the Patient with Thyrotoxicosis Be Evaluated Preoperatively?

History

A wide spectrum of symptoms is seen, depending on circulating levels of T3 and T4. These are outlined by system in Table 18.2. Of particular relevance to the anesthesiologist are symptoms that may indicate a difficult intubation. A goiter causing tracheal compression, retrosternal goiter, or cancerous goiter may indicate tracheal obstruction and warrant CT investigation of the size of the mass, its precise location, and the degree of tracheal compression. Positional dyspnea has been reported by 75% of patients with a retrosternal goiter [8]. Dysphagia has been reported as the second most common symptom (43% patients with retrosternal goiter) [9].

Physical Exam

A thorough airway examination is imperative. Most patients with a large goiter, whether retrosternal or causing tracheal deviation, can be intubated with direct laryngoscopy. An observational study of over 300 patients having thyroid surgery reported that the classic predictive criteria for difficult intubation – small mouth opening, short neck, Mallampati class 3 or 4, reduced neck mobility, and short thyromental distance – were reliable predictors of difficult intubation in patients having thyroid surgery. A large palpable goiter, mediastinal extension, tracheal compression or deviation, and malignancy were not associated with difficult intubation [10]. Regardless, for the authors there are two principal causes for concern that reduce our threshold for awake fiber-optic intubation: (1) malignancy leading to fibrosis and associated immobile larynx and (2) severe tracheal compression.

Retrosternal goiter may be diagnosed clinically by detection of caudal extension of the goiter below the sternal notch. Superior vena cava syndrome has been reported in 5–9% of patients with retrosternal goiter [11]. Pemberton's sign will confirm this diagnosis, i.e., with arms raised for 1–2 minutes, a large goiter will inhibit venous return, causing venous engorgement, facial edema, cyanosis, and respiratory distress.

Table 18.2 Symptoms of hyperthyroidism classified by system

Cardiac
Palpitations secondary to sinus tachycardia or atrial fibrillation
Shortness of breath secondary to cardiac failure
Edema secondary to cardiac failure
Gastrointestinal
Weight loss
Appetite stimulation
Diarrhea
Gynecological
Amenorrhea
Oligomenorrhea
Central nervous system/psychological
Anxiety
Emotional lability
Tremor
Metabolic
Perspiration
Heat intolerance
Hyperpyrexia

Investigations

- Free T3 and T4 (free hormone is the best indicator of thyroid status)
- TSH
- TSH receptor antibody
- Radioactive iodine uptake
- Ultrasound
- CT

What Specific Medications Should We Expect to See in the Preoperative Patient with Thyrotoxicosis?

Two categories of drug are used: (1) those that inhibit thyroid hormone synthesis and (2) those that inhibit the adrenergic-like effects of excess thyroid hormone.

Thyroid hormone synthesis is reviewed in Fig. 18.4. Dietary iodide compounds are trapped in the thyroid epithelial follicular cells and oxidized to iodinium ions (I^+) by thyroid peroxidase. TSH from the anterior pituitary stimulates synthesis of the Na/I transporter, thyroid peroxidase, and thyroglobulin. Thyroglobulin (specifically its tyrosine amino acid) stored in thyroid colloid is iodinated in a process known as organification to monoiodotyrosine (MIT) and diiodotyrosine (DIT). These molecules are then conjugated (again by thyroid peroxidase) to form triiodothyronine (T3) and tetraiodothyronine (T4). The final steps in the process are proteolysis of thyroglobulin and release of T3 and T4. The ratio of T4:T3 release to plasma is approximately 3:1. T4 is subsequently metabolized to T3 by deiodination in the liver and kidney. T3 is 3–5 times more active than T4 and is responsible for most activity attributed to thyroid hormone.

Thionamides *Methimazole and propylthiouracil* inhibit thyroid hormone synthesis at the organification and conjugation steps. As stores of thyroid hormone can last for months, clinical effects of propylthiouracil and methimazole may not be seen for up to 2 months. Methimazole is the

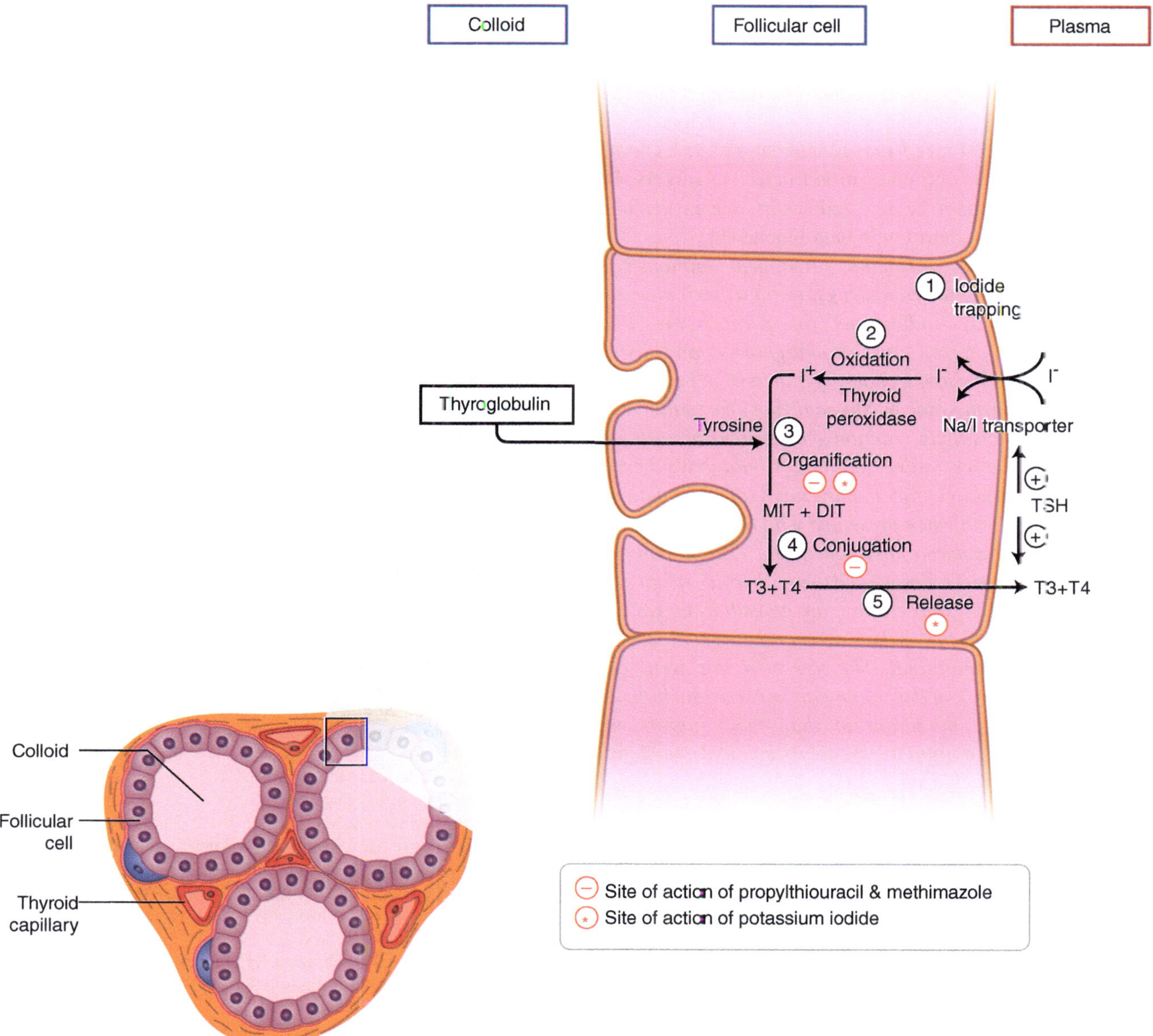

Fig. 18.4 Thyroid follicle (combination of follicular cell and colloid) with molecular mechanism of thyroid hormone synthesis

first line of therapy. It is faster acting (though still expected to take between 3 and 8 weeks to be effective), has less potential for hepatotoxicity, and has a longer half-life that facilitates once-daily dosing [12]. Adverse effects associated with thionamide use include rash, hepatotoxicity, and agranulocytosis [13].

Iodine (e.g., *Lugol's solution/potassium iodide)* inhibits thyroid hormone secretion within hours of administration. It also inhibits thyroid hormone synthesis at the stage of organification/iodination of thyroglobulin tyrosine. Its effect is maximal at 10–20 days but can be short lived. Its use is recommended as an adjunct in the preoperative preparation of the patient with Graves' disease or for the treatment of thyroid storm.

Glucocorticoids inhibit the conversion of T4 to T3 and reduce thyroid hormone secretion.

Beta-blockade is used for control of hyper-adrenergic symptoms. It is frequently started with methimazole to achieve a euthyroid state. The target is a heart rate of 90 bpm.

What Is the Goal of Preoperative Optimization Prior to Surgery?

Whenever possible, the patient should be rendered clinically and biochemically euthyroid prior to surgery. This can take several months. TSH levels may remain suppressed, and this is not considered a contraindication to elective surgery. If a euthyroid state cannot be realized, heart rate is the most important factor to control with beta-blockade.

There are three principal treatment options for hyperthyroidism – antithyroid drugs, radioactive iodine, and thyroidectomy [13]. *Indications for surgery are local compressive symptoms, risk of malignancy, and hyperthyroidism. Our patient had significant clinical and biochemical hyperthyroidism. She could not take methimazole due to a hypersensitivity reaction – an urticarial rash with pruritis. Radioactive iodine ablation would have been a reasonable alternative for management of this patient's hyperthyroidism, but when presented with treatment options, she decided to undergo thyroidectomy. The patient was informed of the risks associated with thyroid storm, and subsequent to this conversation, in consultation with an endocrinologist and the patient's general surgeon, she was started on propylthiouracil. She tolerated this well, even though there is a risk of developing an adverse reaction with one thionamide if intolerant of the other. Surgery was deferred for 2 months until a state of biochemical and clinical euthyroidism was achieved.*

True/False Questions

1. With regard to hyperthyroidism:
   (a) Multinodular goiter is the most common cause.
   (b) Is associated with elevated plasma TSH.
   (c) May be accompanied by weight loss or weight gain.
   (d) When associated with retrosternal goiter is frequently accompanied by dyspnea.
   (e) When caused by Graves' disease will show normal or high uptake on radioiodine thyroid scan.
2. With regard to the management of patients with hyperthyroidism:
   (a) Thyroid storm occurring perioperatively can be mistaken for malignant hyperthermia.
   (b) Beta-blockade is contraindicated in patients with known cardiac disease.
   (c) Thionamides do not affect the release of stored thyroid hormone.
   (d) Propylthiouracil is preferred to methimazole because it is less likely to cause hepatotoxicity.
   (e) Elective surgery should be postponed until TSH levels have returned to normal.

References

1. Jonklaas J, Cooper DS. Thyroid. In: Goldman L, Schafer AI, editors. Goldman-Cecil medicine. 26th ed. Philadelphia: Elsevier; 2020. p. 1462–76.
2. Ertek S, Cicero AF. Hyperthyroidism and cardiovascular complications: a narrative review on the basis of pathophysiology. Arch Med Sci. 2013;9(5):944–52.
3. Kulairi Z, Deol N, Tolly R, Manocha R, Naseer M. QT prolongation due to Graves' disease. Case Rep Cardiol. 2017;2017:7612748.
4. van Noord C, van der Deure WM, Sturkenboom MC, Straus SM, Hofman A, Visser TJ, et al. High free thyroxine levels are associated with QTc prolongation in males. J Endocrinol. 2008;198(1):253–60.
5. Choudhury RP, MacDermot J. Heart failure in thyrotoxicosis, an approach to management. Br J Clin Pharmacol. 1998;46(5):421–4.
6. Buyukcam F, Sonmez FT, Sahinli H. A delayed diagnosis: stridor secondary to hypocalcemia. Int J Emerg Med. 2010;3(4):461–2.
7. Reed AP, Yudkowitz FS. Clinical cases in anesthesia. 2nd ed. London: Churchill Livingstone; 1995.
8. Stang MT, Armstrong MJ, Ogilvie JB, Yip L, McCoy KL, Faber CN, et al. Positional dyspnea and tracheal compression as indications for goiter resection. Arch Surg. 2012;147(7):621–6.
9. Shen WT, Kebebew E, Duh QY, Clark OH. Predictors of airway complications after thyroidectomy for substernal goiter. Arch Surg. 2004;139(6):656–9; discussion 9-60.
10. Amathieu R, Smail N, Catineau J, Poloujadoff MP, Samii K, Adnet F. Difficult intubation in thyroid surgery: myth or reality? Anesth Analg. 2006;103(4):965–8.
11. Chen AY, Bernet VJ, Carty SE, Davies TF, Ganly I, Inabnet WB 3rd, et al. American Thyroid Association statement on optimal surgical management of goiter. Thyroid. 2014;24(2):181–9.
12. Palace MR. Perioperative management of thyroid dysfunction. Health Serv Insights. 2017;10:1178632916689677.
13. Patel KN, Yip L, Lubitz CC, Grubbs EG, Miller BS, et al. The American Association of Endocrine Surgeons Guidelines for the definitive surgical management of thyroid disease in adults. Ann Surg. 2020;271(3):e21–93.

Adrenal Insufficiency

19

Derek Dillane

A 46-year-old female patient scheduled for total thyroidectomy for Graves' hyperthyroidism was seen at the anesthesia preassessment clinic. Eight years previously, she was diagnosed with primary adrenal insufficiency. She had a large multinodular goiter, increasing dysphagia, and mild obstructive airway symptoms. In addition, she had a gastric fundal diverticulum, resulting in severe gastroesophageal reflux disease.

Medications: Methimazole 20 mg daily, atenolol 50 mg/daily, hydrocortisone 10 mg in the morning and 5 mg in the afternoon, fludrocortisone 0.1 mg daily, and esomeprazole 20 mg daily.

Physical examination: Revealed a large goiter but was otherwise unremarkable.

Investigations: Laboratory findings can be seen in Table 19.1. On chest radiograph (Fig. 19.1), a mass effect was seen to the right of the extrathoracic trachea displacing the trachea to the left, which resulted in narrowing of the coronal tracheal diameter. Cardiovascular silhouette, hilar contours, pulmonary vasculature, and lung volumes appeared normal.

Table 19.1 Laboratory values at preadmission clinic visit

Test	Result	Reference range
Thyroid-stimulating hormone	<0.01	0.2–4 (mU/L)
Free T4	12.0	9–23 (pmol/L)
Calcium	2.3	2.1–2.6 (mmol/L)
Sodium	136	133–146 (mmol/L)
Potassium	3.9	3.5–5.0 (mmol/L)
Random glucose	8.2	3.3–11.0 (mmol/L)

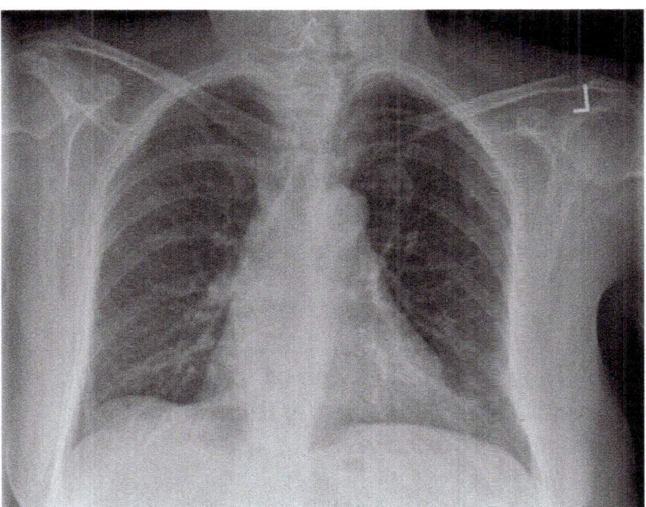

Fig. 19.1 Chest radiograph with displacement of the trachea to the left secondary to the mass effect of a multinodular goiter

What Is Primary Adrenal Insufficiency?

Also known as Addison's disease, primary adrenal insufficiency occurs when the adrenal gland cannot produce sufficient quantities of glucocorticoid and mineralocorticoid hormones. The incidence of Addison's disease in the United States is approximately 1 per 100, 000, and the overall prevalence is thought to be 40–60 per million. Males and females are equally affected, and even though it can occur at any age, it typically presents between the fourth and fifth decades of life. It is most commonly caused by autoimmune destruction of the adrenal cortex. Up to 90% of cases of Addison's disease have been attributed to autoimmune adrenalitis [1]. Tuberculosis, the most common cause when Thomas Addison originally described the condition in 1855, is now an uncommon etiological finding in the western world. Other causes include metastatic malignancy, hemorrhage, heparin-induced thrombocytopenia, trauma,

D. Dillane (✉)
Department of Anesthesiology & Pain Medicine, University of Alberta, Edmonton, AB, Canada

D. Dillane, B. A. Finegan (eds.), *Preoperative Assessment*, https://doi.org/10.1007/978-3-030-58842-7_19

and infection (e.g., HIV) [2]. More than 90% of the adrenal cortex must be damaged bilaterally for symptoms to develop. Subsequently, onset is insidious and presents with nonspecific symptoms, e.g., weakness, fatigue, nausea, and vomiting, as well as more specific signs such as cutaneous and mucosal pigmentation, hypovolemia, and hyponatremia [3].

What Is Secondary Adrenal Insufficiency?

Secondary adrenal insufficiency develops from underproduction of adrenocorticotrophic hormone (ACTH) secondary to pituitary disease or suppression of the hypothalamic-pituitary-adrenal axis (HPAA), rather than damage to the adrenal glands themselves. Insufficient production of corticotropin-releasing hormone (CRH) due to hypothalamic disease is often termed tertiary adrenal insufficiency. Common causes include the use of prolonged steroid therapy (tertiary) and surgery or radiotherapy involving the pituitary (secondary). Due to preserved functional capacity of the adrenal cortex, specifically the ability to function as part of the renin-angiotensin system, secondary adrenal insufficiency produces an isolated glucocorticoid deficiency in contrast to primary disease where mineralocorticoid deficiency is also a feature. Adrenal insufficiency almost exclusively refers to adrenocortical insufficiency. Rare congenital absence of the adrenal cortex may cause a developmental absence of the adrenal medulla. This seldom produces a state of catecholamine deficiency as catecholamines are likely produced elsewhere in the autonomic nervous system, e.g., sympathetic neurons [4].

Provide a Brief Overview of Adrenal Gland Physiology Including Hormone Production

The adrenal gland consists of two distinct components, the outer cortex and the inner medulla. The adrenal cortex is responsible for the production of glucocorticoid, mineralocorticoid, and androgen hormones. CRH produced by the hypothalamus stimulates the anterior pituitary to synthesize ACTH (Fig. 19.2) [5, 6]. ACTH in turn regulates adrenocortical secretion of glucocorticoids. Aldosterone is the main mineralocorticoid secreted by the adrenal cortex in response to regulation by the renin-angiotensin system. The adrenal medulla is a component of the sympathetic nervous system and is responsible for synthesis of catecholamines, e.g., norepinephrine and epinephrine. It is of no significance in the context of adrenal insufficiency, which, as indicated above, may be more appropriately termed adrenocortical insufficiency.

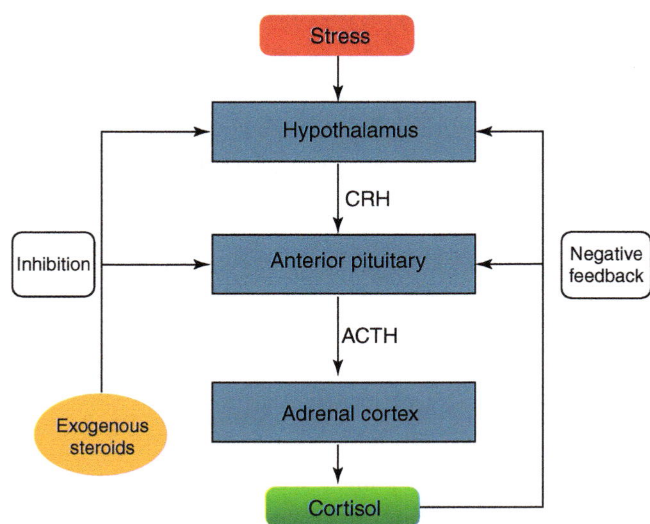

Fig. 19.2 The hypothalamic-pituitary-adrenal axis. Patients using chronic exogenous steroids with resultant low CRH and ACTH levels from negative feedback have atrophy of the adrenal cortex and a decrease in endogenous cortisol production [6]

What Glucocorticoid Hormones Are Produced by the Adrenal Cortex?

Ninety-five percent of the glucocorticoid hormone output of the adrenal gland is comprised of cortisol. Cortisol is administered therapeutically as hydrocortisone. Corticosterone and cortisone account for the remainder [3].

What Is the Physiological Role of Cortisol?

Cortisol is essential for carbohydrate, protein, and fatty acid metabolism, e.g., it is responsible for hepatic gluconeogenesis and antagonizes the actions of insulin, maintaining normal blood glucose concentrations during fasting [6]. Through its actions on glomerular filtration and renal plasma flow, it regulates electrolyte and water homeostasis [7]. It also possesses weak mineralocorticoid activity in this regard. Cortisol modulates the immune system—it is frequently used for the treatment of chronic inflammatory conditions such as rheumatoid arthritis. It facilitates the conversion of norepinephrine to epinephrine in the adrenal medulla and maintains endothelial permeability [7].

What Is the Physiological Role of Aldosterone?

Aldosterone causes sodium and water reabsorption and secretion of potassium ions in the distal renal tubule in response to activation of the renin-angiotensin system and to a lesser extent increased potassium concentration [2]. Aldosterone also plays a significant role in the regulation of vascular tone [8].

What Complications Is the Patient with Adrenal Insufficiency Subject to in the Perioperative Period?

If adequate preoperative preparation has not been performed, an acute adrenal or Addisonian crisis can occur even in the presence of a minor stressor [2]. Surgery is one of the most potent activators of the HPAA. The degree of HPAA activation depends on the nature of the surgical procedure and the type of anesthesia, e.g., regional anesthesia or deep general anesthesia can blunt the stress response. A standard surgical stress response sees ACTH secretion begin to increase at surgical incision and remain elevated for several days postoperatively [3]. In the presence of primary adrenal insufficiency, the adrenal cortex cannot respond to ACTH stimulation, and cortisol secretion does not occur.

Patients may demonstrate the effects of long-term steroid use or overtreatment:

- Cushingoid appearance and weight gain
- Hypertension
- Fluid retention
- Premature atherosclerotic disease with associated risks of myocardial infarction, heart failure, and cerebrovascular disease
- Hyperlipidemia
- Arrhythmias (e.g., atrial fibrillation or flutter) [9]
- Hyperglycemia
- Immunosuppression and increased risk of infection

Other autoimmune conditions are frequently associated with autoimmune primary adrenal insufficiency, including hypothyroidism, hyperthyroidism, hypoparathyroidism, diabetes mellitus type 1, vitiligo, and pernicious anemia [1].

What Are the Features of an Acute Adrenal Crisis?

Acute adrenal crisis is cardiovascular shock due to acute stress (e.g., infection, trauma, surgery, pregnancy), to which the patient with adrenal insufficiency is incapable of mounting an appropriate response as a result of glucocorticoid or mineralocorticoid deficiency. Acute adrenal crisis can occur in the patient receiving adequate glucocorticoid replacement therapy without adequate mineralocorticoid replacement. Adrenal crisis occurs less frequently in the setting of secondary adrenal insufficiency as mineralocorticoid production is preserved, allowing for volume status to be maintained.

Clinical features of adrenal crisis are listed below. Needless to say, some of these features are absent in the anesthetized patient:

- Cardiovascular shock and hypotension that is refractory to vasopressor and fluid therapy
- Hyponatremia
- Hyperkalemia
- Hypoglycemia
- Abdominal, back, or flank pain
- Nausea and/or vomiting
- Confusion

What Are the Options for Steroid Hormone Replacement Therapy in Primary Adrenal Insufficiency?

All patients require glucocorticoid replacement therapy, and most will eventually require mineralocorticoid replacement. There is no commonly accepted approach to glucocorticoid replacement. The short-acting hydrocortisone and longer-acting prednisone are used in different scenarios and patients. Physician preference frequently appears to be of an empirical nature. Features common to all approaches to glucocorticoid replacement are recognition of the importance of mimicking the body's daily fluctuation in cortisol levels and using the lowest possible dose to ameliorate the symptoms of deficiency. Hydrocortisone is typically used in two or three divided daily doses up to a total of 15–25 mg per day. Patients with compliance issues may benefit from once-daily dosing with prednisone 3–5 mg (Table 19.2) [5]. Aldosterone replacement therapy takes the form of fludrocortisone. The usual dose is 0.1 mg daily.

How Can We Ascertain That This Patient Is on the Optimal Dose of Glucocorticoid and Mineralocorticoid Replacement Therapy?

Monitoring should be conducted for both overtreatment and undertreatment with glucocorticoids. Clinical assessment for features of glucocorticoid deficiency (anorexia, weight loss, lethargy, hyperpigmentation) or the Cushingoid features of glucocorticoid excess are the most useful means of monitor-

Table 19.2 Relative potency and dosing of commonly used glucocorticoids

Steroid	Glucocorticoid activity	Mineralocorticoid activity	Equivalent dose (IV/PO)	Half-life (h)
Cortisol (hydrocortisone)	1	1	20	8–12
Cortisone	0.8	0.8	25	8–12
Prednisone	4	0.8	5	18–36
Prednisolone	4	0.8	5	12–36
Methylprednisolone	5	0.5	4	18–36
Dexamethasone	30–40	0	0.5–0.75	36–54

From Liu et al. [5], with permission from Wolters Kluwer

ing treatment. Plasma ACTH can be used as a biochemical index of treatment success; however, its use has been cautioned against, as it often remains elevated in patients treated with glucocorticoids despite adequate therapy, which can lead to overtreatment [10]. Efficacy of mineralocorticoid replacement therapy can be monitored by assessing for salt craving, postural hypotension, edema, and electrolyte balance.

What General Measures Can Be Taken to Ensure That the Patient with Primary Adrenal Insufficiency Is Optimized Prior to Surgery?

General measures that should be undertaken involve monitoring and treatment of hypovolemia, hyponatremia, and hyperkalemia.

How Much Cortisol Is Normally Produced Daily? How Does This Change in the Perioperative Period?

Generally, 8–10 mg/day of cortisol is secreted by the adrenal gland. This will increase during periods of physical and psychological stress. Surgical stress, both the physical and psychological components, increases cortisol output in the healthy individual. The degree of increase varies with the surgical procedure. For minor procedures total cortisol output increases to approximately 50 mg daily. Major procedures are associated with a daily cortisol output of up to 150 mg daily (Table 19.3) [5].

Describe an Appropriate Approach to Surgical Stress Dosing of Glucocorticoid Therapy for the Perioperative Period in the Patient with Primary Adrenal Insufficiency

Patients with primary adrenal insufficiency must receive their baseline steroid therapy and supplemental stress dosing. Several approaches have been described. The protocol advised by the Endocrine Society Clinical Practice Guideline meets our needs in most situations (Table 19.4) [10].

Describe a General Approach to Surgical Stress Dosing of Glucocorticoid Therapy for the Perioperative Period for the Patient with Possible Secondary Adrenal Insufficiency Secondary to Chronic Steroid Use

Chronic steroid use is the most common cause of secondary adrenal insufficiency. Low CRH and ACTH levels lead to atrophy of the adrenal cortex and a decrease in cortisol production (see Fig. 19.2). As the renin-angiotensin-aldosterone pathway is intact, there is no concomitant deficiency of aldosterone. Full recovery of adrenal function after cessation of steroid use, i.e., appropriate endogenous production of glucocorticoids in response to stress, can take several days after a short course of steroids, and between 6 and 12 months after long-term steroid use [3]. Therefore, the perioperative physician must give consideration to the benefits of stress dose steroid administration to prevent the manifestation of adrenal crisis in the perioperative period, versus the risks associated with unnecessary steroid use, e.g., impaired wound healing, immunosuppression, hyperglycemia, and postoperative delirium.

There is no agreed-upon dose or duration of steroid known to cause HPAA suppression, and the precise recovery time from HPAA suppression varies. A recent review on this subject suggests that the patient taking any dose of glucocorticoid for less than 3 weeks, or those taking prednisone 5 mg daily for any period of time, do not need steroid stress dose administration [11]. Conversely, the Endocrine Society, in its Clinical Practice Guideline, takes the view that as no harm has been shown to occur with perioperative stress dose steroid administration, prevention of adrenal crisis is more important than prevention of the potential adverse risks of short-term stress dosing [10].

There are numerous practical approaches to the patient with potential HPAA suppression in the perioperative period. One such approach calls for maintenance of the usual steroid dose throughout the surgical period and treating refractory hypotension with rescue dose steroid [5] [11]. A more nuanced strategy assesses the risk of HPAA suppression

Table 19.3 Recommended dosing by surgery type for patients who may have secondary adrenal insufficiency secondary to steroid use

Surgery type	Endogenous cortisol secretion rate	Examples	Recommended steroid dosing
Superficial	8–10 mg per day (baseline)	Dental surgery Biopsy	Usual daily dose
Minor	50 mg per day	Inguinal hernia repair Colonoscopy Uterine curettage Hand surgery	Usually daily dose *plus* Hydrocortisone 50 mg IV before incision Hydrocortisone 25 mg IV every 8 h × 24 h Then usual daily dose
Moderate	75–150 mg per day	Lower extremity revascularization Total joint replacement Cholecystectomy Colon resection Abdominal hysterectomy	Usual daily dose *plus* Hydrocortisone 50 mg IV before incision Hydrocortisone 25 mg IV every 8 h × 24 h Then usual daily dose
Major	75–150 mg per day	Esophagectomy Total proctocolectomy Major cardiac/vascular Hepaticojejunostomy Delivery Trauma	Usual daily dose *plus* Hydrocortisone 100 mg IV before incision Followed by continuous IV infusion of 200 mg of hycrocortisone more than 24 h *or* Hydrocortisone 50 mg IV every 8 h × 24 h Tape dose by half per day until usual daily dose reached *plus* Continuous IV fluids with 5% dextrose and 0.2–0.45% NaCl (based on degree of hypoglycemia)

From Liu et al. [5], with permission from Wolters Kluwer

Table 19.4 Surgical stress dosing as recommended in the Endocrine Society Clinical Practice Guideline for patients with primary adrenal insufficiency undergoing surgery [10]

Minor to moderate surgery	Major surgery
Hydrocortisone 25–75 mg per 24 h (usually 1–2 d)	Hydrocortisone 100 mg per IV injection followed by continuous IV infusion of hydrocortisone 200 mg per 24 h (alternatively 50 mg every 6 h IV)

Table 19.5 Interpretation of results of the ACTH stimulation test

Serum cortisol	Plasma ACTH	Diagnosis
Low	High	Primary adrenal insufficiency
Low	Low	Secondary adrenal insufficiency

based on the clinical picture and/or the ACTH stimulation test, i.e., patients at high risk of HPAA suppression (e.g., Cushingoid features, prednisone ≥20 mg/day) and those diagnosed with secondary adrenal suppression using the ACTH stimulation test require stress dosing (Table 19.5). Patients at low risk (e.g., prednisone <5 mg/day) do not require stress dosing. An approach to the dosing required according to surgical type is provided in Table 19.3 [5].

True/False Questions

1. (a) Most of the glucocorticoid hormone secreted by the adrenal gland is cortisol.
   (b) Autoimmune destruction of the adrenal cortex is the most frequent cause of primary adrenal insufficiency.
   (c) Aldosterone causes sodium secretion and potassium reabsorption in the renal distal tubule.
   (d) Hyponatremia is a feature of acute adrenal crisis.
   (e) Prednisone should not be used for steroid replacement therapy in primary adrenal insufficiency.
2. (a) Cortisol 50–100 mg/day is the normal output of the adrenal gland in the non-stressed and healthy individual.
   (b) Chronic steroid use is the commonest cause of secondary adrenal insufficiency.
   (c) There is no deficiency of aldosterone in the patient with secondary adrenal insufficiency.
   (d) Patients taking long-term steroids may not need supplementary stress dosing perioperatively.
   (e) Release of aldosterone from the adrenal cortex is primarily regulated by ACTH.

References

1. Zelissen PM, Bast EJ, Croughs RJ. Associated autoimmunity in Addison's disease. J Autoimmun. 1995;8(1):121–30.
2. Fleisher LA, Mythen M. Anesthetic implications of concurrent diseases. In: Miller RD, editor. Miller's anesthesia. 8th ed. Philadelphia: Saunders; 2015. p. 1156–225.
3. Wall R. Endocrine disease. In: Hines RL, Marschall KE, editors. Stoelting's anesthesia and co-existing disease. 7th ed. Philadelphia: Elsevier; 2018. p. 449–75.
4. Fung MM, Viveros OH, O'Connor DT. Diseases of the adrenal medulla. Acta Physiol (Oxf). 2008;192(2):325–35
5. Liu MM, Reidy AB, Saatee S, Collard CD. Perioperative steroid management: approaches based on current evidence.

Anesthesiology. 2017;127(1):166–72. https://doi.org/10.1097/ALN.0000000000001659. PMID: 28452806.
6. Davies M, Hardman J. Anaesthesia and adrenocortical disease. Contin Educ Anaesth Crit Care Pain. 2005;5(4):123–6.
7. Nussey S, Whitehead S. The adrenal gland. Endocrinology: an integrated approach. Oxford: BIOS Scientific Publishers; 2001.
8. Toda N, Nakanishi S, Tanabe S. Aldosterone affects blood flow and vascular tone regulated by endothelium-derived NO: therapeutic implications. Br J Pharmacol. 2013;168(3):519–33.
9. Christiansen CF, Christensen S, Mehnert F, Cummings SR, Chapurlat RD, Sorensen HT. Glucocorticoid use and risk of atrial fibrillation or flutter: a population-based, case-control study. Arch Intern Med. 2009;169(18):1677–83.
10. Bornstein SR, Allolio B, Arlt W, Barthel A, Don-Wauchope A, Hammer GD, et al. Diagnosis and treatment of primary adrenal insufficiency: an Endocrine Society clinical practice guideline. J Clin Endocrinol Metab. 2016;101(2):364–89.
11. Glowniak JV, Loriaux DL. A double-blind study of perioperative steroid requirements in secondary adrenal insufficiency. Surgery. 1997;121(2):123–9.

20 Pituitary Adenoma

Derek Dillane

A 69-year-old man presented to the anesthesia preoperative assessment clinic prior to transsphenoidal excision of a pituitary adenoma. He had undergone partial resection of a pituitary adenoma 15 years previously. He had recently been diagnosed with acromegaly. This followed a series of investigations after he had reported an increase in the size of his hands and jaw in addition to progressive impairment of his peripheral vision. He had a history of type 1 diabetes mellitus, hypertension, hyperlipidemia, and gastroesophageal reflux disease (GERD). He did not have symptoms suggestive of coronary artery disease or heart failure. He had a STOP-Bang score of 6/8, but he did not possess a continuous positive airway pressure (CPAP) machine.

Medications: Thyroxine, rosuvastatin, finasteride, insulin glargine, insulin lispro, metformin, nifedipine, candesartan, and rabeprazole.

Physical Examination: BP was 158/92. Heart rate was 70 bpm with a regular rhythm on examination of the radial pulse. Airway examination revealed obvious mandibular prognathism and Mallampati III mouth opening.

Investigations: Endocrine laboratory values can be seen in Table 20.1 [1, 2]. HBA1c was 10.7%.

ECG and chest radiograph were normal.

Recent magnetic resonance imaging (MRI) reported a large sellar/suprasellar mass consistent with a macroadenoma. This was noted to have expanded into, and destroyed, the sella turcica. There was likely cavernous sinus invasion on the right side. Significant superior displacement of the optic chiasm was observed.

Table 20.1 Biochemical indices available at the preoperative consultation

Biochemical index	Value	Reference range
TSH	5.37	0.20–4.00 (mU/L)
Free T4	11.4	9.0–23.0 (pmol/L)
Free T3	3.8	3.5–6.5 (pmol/L)
Cortisol (AM)	287	120–620 (nmol/L)
ACTH	38	10–46 (ng/L)
Testosterone (AM)	3.1	10.3–29.5 (nmol/L)
Sex hormone binding globulin	37	6–65 (nmol/L)
Testosterone/SHBG ratio	0.08	0.20–1.00
Prolactin	39.8	<21.0 (ug/L)
LH	1.5	<12.0 (U/L)
FSH	3.4	<7.0 (U/L)
IGF-1	402	47–192 (ng/mL)
Growth hormone OGTT 2h 75g	0.4	<1 ng/mL

Random growth hormone measurements are not especially valuable in the diagnosis of acromegaly as its secretion is pulsatile and fluctuates throughout the day. Production of insulin-like growth factor-1 (IGF-1), which usually correlates with mean growth hormone level, is stable and considered the single best biochemical investigation for diagnosis of acromegaly [1]. Some acromegaly patients, such as the patient presented here, have a high IGF-1 level and a normal growth hormone level [2]

TSH thyroid-stimulating hormone, *ACTH* adrenocorticotropic hormone, *SHBG* sex hormone binding globulin, *LH* luteinizing hormone, *FSH* follicle-stimulating hormone, *OGTT* oral glucose tolerance test

What Is Acromegaly?

Acromegaly is a rare chronic endocrine disorder caused by excessive secretion of growth hormone (GH) and secondary elevation of insulin-like growth factor-1 (IGF-1). IGF-1, a protein produced primarily by the liver, mediates the effects of GH. The most common cause of acromegaly is pituitary adenoma (>95% of cases) [3]. Acromegaly has an incidence of up to 11 cases per million per year and a prevalence of 78 cases per million population [4]. Due to the insidious nature of the disease diagnosis may be delayed by up to 10 years [5]. Males and females are affected equally. The usual age of onset is 40–50 years [2].

D. Dillane (✉)
Department of Anesthesiology & Pain Medicine, University of Alberta, Edmonton, AB, Canada

D. Dillane, B. A. Finegan (eds.), *Preoperative Assessment*, https://doi.org/10.1007/978-3-030-58842-7_20

How Are Pituitary Adenomas Classified?

Pituitary adenoma, a benign tumor of the anterior pituitary gland, is the most common pituitary tumor. They are classified according to (1) size, (2) functionality, and (3) endocrine cell of origin.

- Tumors smaller than 1 cm are termed microadenomas, while those 1 cm or larger are termed macroadenomas.
- Microadenomas are more common than macroadenomas (57.4% vs 42.6%) [6].
- Approximately 65–75% of adenomas are functioning, i.e., produce excess hormone [7]. Microadenomas that are non-functioning are likely to be subclinical and may be detected as an incidental finding on radiologic investigation. However, non-functioning tumors are more likely to be macroadenomas and present with headache, visual field defects secondary to compression of the optic chiasm, and/or hypopituitarism due to a compression effect on surrounding pituitary cells.
- Lactotroph adenomas (prolactinomas) secrete prolactin. These are the most common type of pituitary adenoma (25–40% of adenomas) [8] and are the most common pituitary tumor overall.
- Somatotroph adenomas secrete GH (10–20% of adenomas) [9]
- Corticotroph adenomas produce adrenocorticotropic hormone (ACTH) (5–10% of adenomas) and are associated with Cushing disease [8].
- Thyrotroph adenomas secrete thyroid-stimulating hormone (TSH) and are the least common adenoma (<1%) [8].
- Plurihormonal adenomas make more than one hormone. They account for approximately 10–15% of all pituitary adenomas [10].

What Are the Objectives of Preoperative Evaluation?

The anatomical and physiological effects of the tumor must be elucidated, and treatment optimized. These effects are due to the following:

- Hormone overproduction from functional tumours

  or
- Hormone underproduction secondary to a non-functioning compressive tumour

What Complications Is the Patient with Acromegaly Subject to in the Perioperative Period?

- Cardiovascular complications: Hypertension, coronary artery disease, left ventricular hypertrophy, congestive cardiac failure, cardiomyopathy, arrhythmias, and valvular dysfunction due to the effects of excessive GH on the myocardium. Cardiovascular disease is the most frequent comorbidity, accounting for up to 80% of complications and is one of the most common causes of death in acromegaly [11, 12]. The cardiomyopathy seen in these patients mainly affects the left ventricle with ensuing diastolic dysfunction (44% of patients with acromegaly), arrhythmias (48%), and valvular disease (75%) [12]. Cardiac failure is seen in 10% of patients [12]. The etiological mechanisms responsible for hypertension in acromegaly have not been fully clarified. Long-term renal exposure to IGF-1 and GH excess may result in an antidiuretic and antinatriuretic effect [13]. Alternative pathogenic mechanisms attributable to excessive GH and IGF-1 include plasma volume expansion and increasing responsiveness to angiotensin with a subsequent increase in peripheral vascular resistance [14].
- Airway complications: Anatomic changes associated with acromegaly can make direct laryngoscopy and intubation difficult [15]. These changes include mandibular enlargement, macroglossia, hypertrophy of the soft palate, nose, epiglottis, soft tissues of the mouth and aryepiglottic folds, in addition to thickening and/or fixity of the vocal cords [16]. Ali et al. reported that 18/66 (27%) of patients with acromegaly had Mallampati grades III and IV, 11/66 (17%) had Cormack-Lehane grades 3 or 4, and there were two failed intubations [17]. Despite the fact that Mallampati scores have been demonstrated to be of moderate value in predicting difficult laryngoscopy for acromegaly patients, the sensitivity of this test was found to be only 44% in a series of 128 acromegalic patients [18]. Therefore, anatomical changes in airway anatomy visible on CT or MRI scans should be used to supplement clinical airway examination. It may be prudent to perform a diagnostic flexible fiberoptic laryngoscopy during the preoperative consultation.
- There is a high prevalence of obstructive sleep apnea (OSA) in patients with acromegaly. This is due to the changes in airway anatomy described above. The actual prevalence varies, depending on the definition used, but it

appears that over 50% of acromegalic patients have OSA [19]. These patients are frequently candidates for CPAP treatment, but the patient should be warned that there is a risk of pneumocephalus associated with CPAP use after transsphenoidal surgery. Its use is occasionally deferred for several weeks after surgery [20]. OSA is discussed in greater detail in Chap. 13.

- Respiratory insufficiency secondary to altered structure and elasticity of the entire respiratory system can affect 30–80% of patients [12, 21]. Kyphotic changes in the thoracic spine lead to altered respiratory mechanics. This is worsened by respiratory muscle weakness. Many patients have V/Q mismatch due to an increased amount of poorly aerated or non-aerated lung tissue. These patients often report poor exercise tolerance [12].
- Acromegaly is frequently associated with disorders of glucose metabolism. Excess GH leads to increased gluconeogenesis and to both hepatic and peripheral insulin resistance. The preoperative optimization of the diabetic patient is discussed in detail in Chap. 17.
- Disorders of lipid metabolism are commonly seen in acromegaly, possibly related to insulin resistance.
- The compressive effects of non-functioning tumors lead to hypopituitarism. This may lead to adrenocortical insufficiency, hypothyroidism, and diabetes insipidus.
  - Unlike primary adrenocortical insufficiency, adrenocortical insufficiency secondary to pituitary disease (also known as central adrenal insufficiency) is not associated with loss of the renin-angiotensin-aldosterone system, and subsequent fluid and electrolyte disorders are less severe. Glucocorticoid is replaced preoperatively, usually hydrocortisone 15–20 mg total daily dose [22]. Surgical stress dosing of steroid may be given if current recommended criteria are met. Surgical stress dosing of steroids is discussed in greater detail in Chap. 19.
  - Free T4 and TSH should be measured to assess for central hypothyroidism. A low free T4 level together with a low or normal TSH in the presence of pituitary disease is suggestive of central hypothyroidism. Thyroid hormone replacement therapy is usually titrated to a free T4 level in the mid to upper half of the reference range [22].
  - Central diabetes insipidus is due to decreased production of anti-diuretic hormone (ADH /vasopressin) by the posterior pituitary gland. It is treated with desmopressin (DDAVP), a synthetic analog of ADH vasopressin, which lacks its vasoconstricting properties [22].
- The presence of acromegaly increases the risk of extra-pituitary benign and malignant neoplasms [23]. Acromegalic patients may present for surgical management of co-existing tumors. Carcinoma is the third most common cause of death in patients with acromegaly, after cardiovascular and respiratory disease [23]. Most commonly associated with acromegaly are gastrointestinal (especially colorectal), lung, breast, prostate, and female genital tract cancers. Screening for colonic neoplasia at the time of diagnosis of acromegaly is recommended in the Endocrine Society Clinical Practice Guidelines [1]. Multinodular goiter is found in 65% of patients – a thyroid ultrasound is recommended if palpable nodularity is detected [1].
- Osteoarthritis, especially of the knees, hips, shoulders, hands, and back, is very prevalent and has been reported in 77% of patients by Biermasz et al. [24].
- Skin thickening may increase the difficulty of intravenous cannulation.

How Is Acromegaly Treated?

- Transsphenoidal surgery is recommended as the primary mode of therapy in most patients [1].
- Medical therapy is usually reserved for patients with persistent disease after surgery or for patients who have adenomas not amenable to surgical resection.
- Patients with disease extending beyond the sellar region who may not be amenable to complete resection may undergo surgical debulking followed by medical therapy.
- Patients with significant disease after surgery can be treated with somatostatin receptor ligands or the GH receptor antagonist, pegvisomant. Patients with moderate disease after surgery may be treated with a dopamine agonist, e.g., cabergoline.

What Is the Surgical Cure Rate?

As most studies evaluating surgical outcome contain small numbers of patients and are up to 20 years old, it is difficult to say anything more substantial than surgery is not entirely curative for pituitary adenoma resection. Typical rates of success appear to be 50–80%, and surgery appears to be more successful for microadenoma than macroadenoma.

Are the Anatomical and Physiological Changes Associated with Acromegaly Reversible with Treatment?

Many of the anatomical and physiological changes of acromegaly are reversible to a greater or lesser degree with medical and/or surgical therapy. Most of the soft tissue changes subside after surgery; however, the bony changes are irreversible. Surgical treatment of acromegaly can lead to significant improvement in glucose metabolism and insulin sensitivity [25]. Medical and surgical control of acromegaly generally improves cardiac structure and function, hypertension, and vascular damage. In addition, medical and surgical treatment has been shown to improve sleep apnea and respiratory insufficiency in up to 75% of patients [12].

What Investigations Should Be Available Preoperatively in the Patient with Acromegaly Scheduled for Transsphenoidal Excision of Pituitary Adenoma?

- Complete blood count (CBC)
- Electrolyte screen
- Blood glucose
- Blood type and screen +/− crossmatch
  - The potential for bleeding, especially in repeat procedures, is significant considering the proximity of the internal carotid arteries within the cavernous sinus, which forms the lateral walls of the sella turcica.
- Endocrine biochemical indices
  - Often these have been measured prior to the anesthesiologist reviewing the patient. The most important ones are outlined in Table 20.1 [1, 2].
- Electrocardiogram and chest radiograph
- Echocardiography
  - When clinical indicators of cardiomyopathy are present
- Polysomnography / sleep studies
  - For confirmation of presence of OSA
- Spirometry, arterial blood gases (ABG), pulmonary function testing
  - If signs of respiratory insufficiency are present
- Lateral neck radiograph, CT, MRI
  - For evaluation of airway abnormalities

This patient had a prolactin-secreting macroadenoma. There were no clinical indicators of cardiomyopathy; therefore, further cardiac evaluation was deemed unnecessary. He was referred to a diabetologist for optimization of his insulin therapy. Formal polysomnography sleep studies were conducted. OSA was diagnosed and he was commenced on CPAP. He proceeded to surgery 6 weeks later.

True/False Questions

1. (a) Most pituitary adenomas are non-functioning
   (b) Prolactin secreting adenomas are the commonest type of pituitary adenoma
   (c) Pituitary adenomas smaller than 1cm are termed microadenomas
   (d) Non-functioning adenomas are more likely to be microadenomas
   (e) Thyrotroph adenomas are the least common pituitary adenoma
2. (a) Acromegaly most commonly presents in the age range of 20–30 years
   (b) The most common cause of acromegaly is pituitary adenoma
   (c) Cardiovascular disease is one of the commonest causes of death in acromegaly
   (d) The prevalence of OSA in acromegaly patients is no higher than in the general population
   (e) Hyposecretion of vasopressin by the anterior pituitary leads to central diabetes insipidus

References

1. Katznelson L, Laws ER Jr, Melmed S, Molitch ME, Murad MH, Utz A, et al. Acromegaly: an endocrine society clinical practice guideline. J Clin Endocrinol Metab. 2014;99(11):3933–51.
2. AlDallal S. Acromegaly: a challenging condition to diagnose. Int J Gen Med. 2018;11:337–43.
3. Vilar L, Vilar CF, Lyra R, Lyra R, Naves LA. Acromegaly: clinical features at diagnosis. Pituitary. 2017;20(1):22–32.
4. Burton T, Le Nestour E, Neary M, Ludlam WH. Incidence and prevalence of acromegaly in a large US health plan database. Pituitary. 2016;19(3):262–7.
5. Colao A, Ferone D, Marzullo P, Lombardi G. Systemic complications of acromegaly: epidemiology, pathogenesis, and management. Endocr Rev. 2004;25(1):102–52.
6. Daly AF, Rixhon M, Adam C, Dempegioti A, Tichomirowa MA, Beckers A. High prevalence of pituitary adenomas: a cross-sectional study in the province of Liege, Belgium. J Clin Endocrinol Metab. 2006;91(12):4769–75.
7. Lake M, Krook L, Crus S. Pituitary adenomas: an overview. Am Fam Physician. 2013;88(5):319–27.
8. Ezzat S, Asa SL, Couldwell WT, Barr CE, Dodge WE, Vance ML, et al. The prevalence of pituitary adenomas: a systematic review. Cancer. 2004;101(3):613–9.
9. Lopes MB. Growth hormone-secreting adenomas: pathology and cell biology. Neurosurg Focus. 2010;29(4):E2.
10. Scheithauer BW, Horvath E, Kovacs K, Laws ER Jr, Randall RV, Ryan N. Plurihormonal pituitary adenomas. Semin Diagn Pathol. 1986;3(1):69–82.
11. Holdaway IM, Rajasoorya RC, Gamble GD. Factors influencing mortality in acromegaly. J Clin Endocrinol Metab. 2004;89(2):667–74.
12. Pivonello R, Auriemma RS, Grasso LF, Pivonello C, Simeoli C, Patalano R, et al. Complications of acromegaly: cardio-

vascular, respiratory and metabolic comorbidities. Pituitary. 2017;20(1):46–62.
13. Feld S, Hirschberg R. Growth hormone, the insulin-like growth factor system, and the kidney. Endocr Rev. 1996;17(5):423–80.
14. Bondanelli M, Ambrosio MR, degli Uberti EC. Pathogenesis and prevalence of hypertension in acromegaly. Pituitary. 2001;4(4):239–49.
15. Dunn LK, Nemergut EC. Anesthesia for transsphenoidal pituitary surgery. Curr Opin Anaesthesiol. 2013;26(5):549–54.
16. Motta S, Ferone D, Colao A, Merola B, Motta G, Lombardi G. Fixity of vocal cords and laryngocele in acromegaly. J Endocrinol Investig. 1997;20(11):672–4.
17. Ali Z, Bithal PK, Prabhakar H, Rath GP, Dash HH. An assessment of the predictors of difficult intubation in patients with acromegaly. J Clin Neurosci. 2009;16(8):1043–5.
18. Schmitt H, Buchfelder M, Radespiel-Troger M, Fahlbusch R. Difficult intubation in acromegalic patients: incidence and predictability. Anesthesiology. 2000;93(1):110–4.
19. Hernandez-Gordillo D, Ortega-Gomez Mdel R, Galicia-Polo L, Castorena-Maldonado A, Vergara-Lopez A, Guillen-Gonzalez MA, et al. Sleep apnea in patients with acromegaly. Frequency, characterization and positive pressure titration. Open Respir Med J. 2012;6:28–33.
20. White-Dzuro GA, Maynard K, Zuckerman SL, Weaver KD, Russell PT, Clavenna MJ, et al. Risk of post-operative pneumocephalus in patients with obstructive sleep apnea undergoing transsphenoidal surgery. J Clin Neurosci. 2016;29:25–8.
21. Luboshitzky R, Barzilai D. Hypoxemia and pulmonary function in acromegaly. Am Rev Respir Dis. 1980;121(3):471–5.
22. Fleseriu M, Hashim IA, Karavitaki N, Melmed S, Murad MH, Salvatori R, et al. Hormonal replacement in hypopituitarism in adults: an endocrine society clinical practice guideline. J Clin Endocrinol Metab. 2016;101(11):3888–921.
23. Ruchala M, Szczepanek-Parulska E, Fularz M, Wolinski K. Risk of neoplasms in acromegaly. Contemp Oncol (Pozn). 2012;16(2):111–7.
24. Biermasz NR, Pereira AM, Smit JW, Romijn JA, Roelfsema F. Morbidity after long-term remission for acromegaly: persisting joint-related complaints cause reduced quality of life. J Clin Endocrinol Metab. 2005;90(5):2731–9.
25. Ferrau F, Albani A, Ciresi A, Giordano C, Cannavo S. Diabetes secondary to acromegaly: physiopathology, clinical features and effects of treatment. Front Endocrinol (Lausanne). 2018;9:358.

Pheochromocytoma

21

Derek Dillane

A 50-year-old man scheduled for laparoscopic resection of a left adrenal pheochromocytoma was admitted for hemodynamic optimization 2 days prior to surgery. He had previously undergone a right-sided adrenalectomy and nephrectomy for a pheochromocytoma 13 years prior to this presentation.

Two drug-eluting stents had been placed 4 months before the proposed surgery for a non-ST segment elevation myocardial infarction (NSTEMI) (Fig. 21.1). *He had a background history of essential hypertension, paroxysmal atrial fibrillation, and hyperlipidemia. He was a lifelong smoker. In addition, he had neurofibromatosis type 1.*

Medications: Valsartan, metoprolol, nitroglycerin, atorvastatin, clopidogrel, aspirin, terazosin. Clopidogrel had been held for 1 week prior to surgery. He had been on terazosin 2 mg twice daily for 2 weeks.

Physical Examination: Initial blood pressure (BP) on admission was 165/94. Heart rate was 80 beats/min. and he was in sinus rhythm. There was no evidence of cardiac failure.

Investigations: Laboratory values revealed a hemoglobin 151 g/L, platelet count 243 × 10^9/L, creatinine 115 μmol/L, estimated GFR 64 mL/min/1.73m^2, and an INR of 1.0.

12-lead ECG showed heart rate 61, sinus rhythm with no evidence of left ventricular hypertrophy, bundle branch block, or ischemia. Chest radiograph was normal with no evidence of cardiomegaly or pulmonary edema.

An echocardiogram performed at the time of NSTEMI 4 months previously showed a left ventricular ejection fraction of 55–60%, a normal right ventricle, mild diastolic dysfunction, and no evidence of valvular disease.

D. Dillane (✉)
Department of Anesthesiology & Pain Medicine, University of Alberta, Edmonton, AB, Canada

What Complications Is the Patient with Pheochromocytoma Subject to in the Perioperative Period?

Due to excess of catecholamine secretion such as epinephrine, norepinephrine and dopamine, patients are subject to significant perioperative hemodynamic and circulatory complications. These include hypertensive and hypotensive crises, arrhythmias—particularly tachycardia— myocardial infarction, cardiomyopathy, cardiac failure, and stroke [1]. The particular pattern of hemodynamic and biochemical effects seen depends on which catecholamines are secreted by the tumor and in what proportion. Secretion from the tumor can either be continuous, episodic, or both and can be precipitated by physical activity (e.g., postural changes) or surgical manipulation (especially until venous drainage from the tumor is interrupted).

What Is the Significance of the Presence of Neurofibromatosis in This Patient?

Pheochromocytomas can be classified as sporadic or familial. Approximately 70% of tumors are sporadic. Familial predisposition is seen in patients with some hereditary conditions, e.g., neurofibromatosis type 1 (NF-1), von Hippel-Lindau disease, multiple endocrine neoplasia type 2, and familial carotid body tumors. Pheochromocytoma occurs in 0.1–5.7% of NF-1 patients and in 50% of patients with multiple endocrine neoplasia type 2 (MEN2) syndrome [2].

Should We Be Surprised That This Patient Previously Had an Adrenalectomy for a Contralateral Pheochromocytoma?

Familial pheochromocytomas are more likely to be bilateral. After unilateral adrenalectomy in MEN2, there is a 30–50% risk of a contralateral tumor developing within 10 years [3].

D. Dillane, B. A. Finegan (eds.), *Preoperative Assessment*, https://doi.org/10.1007/978-3-030-58842-7_21

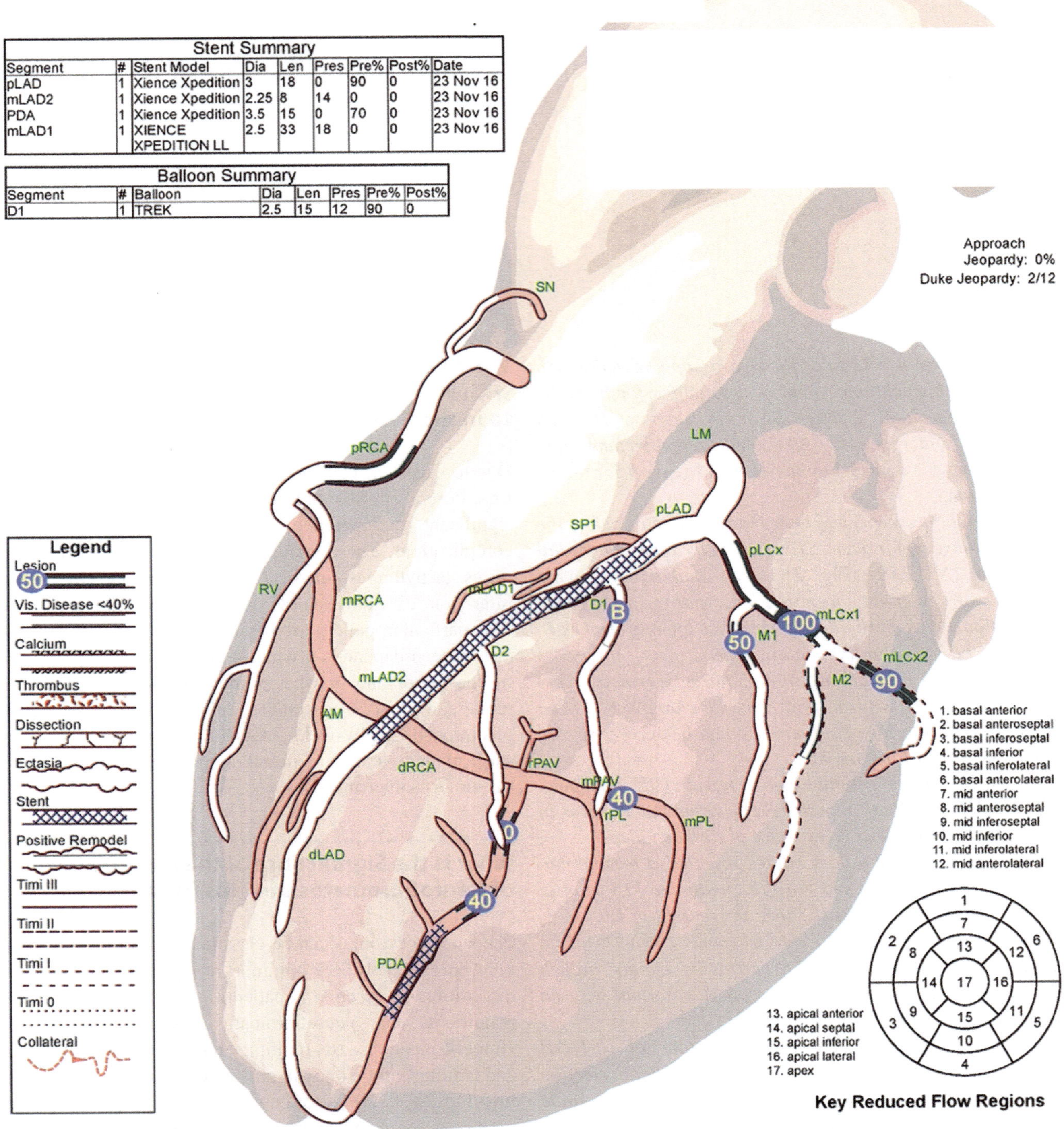

Stent Summary								
Segment	#	Stent Model	Dia	Len	Pres	Pre%	Post%	Date
pLAD	1	Xience Xpedition	3	18	0	90	0	23 Nov 16
mLAD2	1	Xience Xpedition	2.25	8	14	0	0	23 Nov 16
PDA	1	Xience Xpedition	3.5	15	0	70	0	23 Nov 16
mLAD1	1	XIENCE XPEDITION LL	2.5	33	18	0	0	23 Nov 16

Balloon Summary							
Segment	#	Balloon	Dia	Len	Pres	Pre%	Post%
D1	1	TREK	2.5	15	12	90	0

Comments: PCI of LAD with a 2.5X33 and 3.0X18 Xience DES. distal edge of distal stent covered with a 2.25X8 Xience DES. Attmpted CTO of LCx - obviously chronic. PCI of PDA with a 3.5X15 Xience DES in PDA.

Post PCI TIMI-3 flow.

DAPT for at least 3 months - ideallty one year.

Fig. 21.1 Coronary artery angiogram after stenting of left anterior descending and posterior descending arteries with drug-eluting stents. The diagram was created with CARAT®. (Coronary Artery Reporting and Archiving Tool, Alberta Provincial Project for Outcome Assessment in Coronary Heart Disease [APPROACH], Cohesic Inc., Calgary, Alberta, Canada)

Surgical management of familial pheochromocytoma is controversial, as the risk of recurrence must be balanced with the risk of development of Addisonian adrenal insufficiency. Options for management include complete bilateral adrenalectomy, unilateral adrenalectomy, and bilateral partial adrenal cortex sparing adrenalectomy.

When Should Preoperative Evaluation Occur?

General consensus suggests initial assessment should take place when adrenergic blockade is commenced 7–14 days prior to surgery [1]. Follow-up with the patient or surgical team 2–3 days prior to surgery to gauge the success of medical preparation is prudent.

What Are the Objectives of Preoperative Evaluation?

End-organ damage secondary to pheochromocytoma-induced hypertension is specifically sought (Table 21.1) [4]. Specific pharmacological agents being used to control blood pressure, heart rate, and subsequent normalization of intravascular volume are ascertained, along with their effects on the goals of treatment.

How Should the Patient with Pheochromocytoma Be Evaluated Preoperatively?

A multidisciplinary approach with contributions from an endocrinologist, surgeon, and anesthesiologist serves to achieve the best possible outcome by seamless implementation of an organized plan of care.

History and Physical Examination

The classic triad of symptoms includes headaches, palpitations, and sweating. Other symptoms reported are tachycardia, anxiety, dyspnea, weakness, orthostatic hypotension, blurred vision, and pallor [4]. Hypertension can be sustained or paroxysmal. Up to 15% of patients are normotensive [5].

The focal point of preoperative assessment is end-organ damage resulting from excess catecholamine secretion. Table 21.1 can be used as a guide to clinical evaluation. Symptoms and signs of ischemic heart disease, congestive

Table 21.1 Organ-specific complications of pheochromocytoma-related hypertension

Organ	Syndrome	Mechanism	Receptor	Receptor action
Heart	Angina Myocardial infarction Cardiomyopathies Myocarditis Acute failure Arrhythmias	Coronary spasm Positive inotropic effect Positive chronotropic effect Unmatched O2 demand Hypoperfusion	Coronary $\alpha 1$, β2 Conducting system β1, β2 Conducting system β1, β2 Cardiomyocyte β1, β2	Constriction Increased conduction Increased automaticity Increased contractility
Brain	Stroke Encephalopathy	Vasoconstriction Unmatched O2 demand Hypoperfusion	Cerebral arterioles $\alpha 1$	Mild constriction Most effects related to system hypertension
Vascular	Shock Postural hypotension Aortic dissection Organ ischemia Limb ischemia	Vasoconstriction Unmatched O2 demand Hypoperfusion	Skeletal muscle $\alpha 1$, $\alpha 2$, β2	Arteriolar constriction Arteriolar dilation Venous dilation
Kidneys	Acute renal failure Hematuria	Vasoconstriction Unmatched O2 demand Hypoperfusion	Vascular $\alpha 1$, $\alpha 2$, β1, β2	Dilation > constriction renin secretion
Lungs	Pulmonary edema Acute respiratory distress syndrome (ARDS) Fibrosis Pulmonary hypertension	Cardiac decompensation Increased permeability	Vascular $\alpha 1$, β2 Smooth muscle β2	Dilation > constriction bronchodilation
GI tract	Intestinal ischemia (necrosis, peritonitis)	Vasoconstriction Unmatched O2 demand Hypoperfusion	Visceral arterioles $\alpha 1$, β2	Constriction
Ocular	Acute blindness Retinopathy	Vasoconstriction	–	–
Acute multiorgan failure	All of the above	–	–	–

From Zuber et al. [4], with permission from Elsevier

cardiac failure, and arrhythmia suggestive of an underlying cardiomyopathy are of immediate relevance. Cerebrovascular disease, peripheral ischemia, and acute renal failure indicate more widespread secondary end-organ complications.

A family history of hereditary conditions associated with pheochromocytoma may be evident, e.g., MEN2, von Hippel-Lindau, and neurofibromatosis.

Investigations

- Baseline laboratory testing includes complete blood count, electrolytes and creatinine, and blood glucose
- Type and screen.
- Chest radiograph, looking specifically for cardiomegaly and pulmonary edema.
- 12-lead ECG; echocardiography is indicated to assess left and right systolic and diastolic function, and to rule out catecholamine induced cardiomyopathy in patients with long-standing disease.
- Patients presenting with pheochromocytoma should be further investigated for other neoplasia (e.g., thyroid carcinomas, parathyroid hyperplasia, central and peripheral nervous tumors) [2].

What Are the Goals of Medical Optimization Prior to Surgery?

- The primary objectives of preoperative optimization are control of blood pressure, heart rate, arrhythmias, and restoration of intravascular fluid volume [1].
- The Roizen criteria aim to assess the adequacy of preoperative alpha blockade (Table 21.2) [6, 7].
- Patient counselling and education should include information on avoidance of certain drugs and foods that may stimulate catecholamine release or decrease reuptake:
  - Sympathomimetic drugs, e.g., methamphetamine, pseudoephedrine
  - Tricyclic antidepressants, monoamine oxidase inhibitors, and serotonin reuptake inhibitors
  - Dopaminergic agents such as antipsychotics and antiemetics, e.g., prochlorperazine
  - Corticosteroids
  - Tyramine-containing food, e.g., cheese, wine
- Lifestyle advice on avoidance of strenuous physical activity, tobacco, and alcohol [5].
- Strict glucose control in diabetics in order to avoid glycemic diuresis induced volume depletion.

Table 21.2 The Roizen criteria reflecting adequacy of preoperative alpha blockade

No in-hospital blood pressure >160/90 mmHg for 24 h prior to surgery
No orthostatic hypotension with blood pressure <80/45 mmHg
No ST or T wave changes for 1 week prior to surgery
No more than 5 premature ventricular contractions per minute

From Azadeh et al. [6, 7] with permission Springer Nature © 2016

What Options Are Available for Medical Preparation for Surgery?

The currently accepted consensus focuses on α-adrenoreceptor antagonists as the mainstay of management, with β-adrenoreceptor antagonists and calcium channel antagonists as adjuncts, when needed, to achieve additional blood pressure and heart rate control. Metyrosine, or similar agents, can be indicated in rare cases of widespread metastatic or highly active disease [7].

α-adrenoreceptor antagonists counteract the vasoconstrictive effects of catecholamines and restore intravascular plasma volume [5]. Historically, the non-competitive $\alpha 1$- and $\alpha 2$-adrenoreceptor antagonist, phenoxybenzamine (PBZ), was the most widely used agent. PBZ is nonselective and irreversible (the effect diminishes only after de novo α-adrenoreceptor synthesis) with a long duration of action and may contribute significantly to postoperative hypotension [1]. Reduction of symptoms (especially sweating) and reduction of blood pressure reflect the efficacy of therapy. Patients should be counselled on side effects: orthostatic hypotension with reflex tachycardia, nasal congestion, possible sedation, and at higher doses, paradoxical hypertension. Titration may be necessary to alleviate these side effects. A high sodium and fluid diet can correct the preexisting volume contraction in this patient population and counteract hypotensive episodes related to initiation of alpha receptor blockade.

Selective $\alpha 1$-adrenoreceptors such as prazosin and terazosin have shorter half-lives, as they are competitive inhibitors. This results in less reflex tachycardia and a shorter postoperative hypotensive period [1]. Disadvantages of using shorter acting agents include incomplete α-adrenergic blockade that contributes to more episodes of intraoperative hypertension. Conversely, PBZ is associated with hypotension lasting for several hours post-resection and requires ICU admission on occasion for stabilization of intravascular volume.

β-adrenoreceptor antagonists: The use of these agents is indicated for patients who have persistent tachycardia or

tachyarrhythmias [1]. β-adrenoreceptor antagonists should never be given without prior α-adrenoreceptor blockade due to the potential for unopposed vasoconstrictive effects that can lead to malignant hypertension and end-organ damage. When adequate α-adrenoreceptor blockade is achieved, β-adrenoreceptor antagonists can be initiated Suggested regimes include the use of short-acting agents such as propranolol (6 mg every 6 hours) and after a period of 24–48 hours, if tolerated, the patient can be started on a long-acting preparation (e.g., metoprolol, atenolol) titrated to achieve a resting heart rate of 60–80 beats per minute.

Calcium channel antagonists: These drugs control hypertension, tachyarrhythmias, and coronary vasospasm by the inhibition of norepinephrine-mediated calcium influx into vascular smooth muscle. Nicardipine, a dihydropyridine, is the most commonly used agent for pheochromocytoma management, used as a sustained release preparation at a starting dose of 30 mg twice daily. The main role of calcium channel antagonists in this patient population is to supplement α- and β-adrenoreceptor blockade. They may also be used in normotensive patients with paroxysmal hypertension or intolerance to α-adrenoreceptor antagonists [1]. Calcium channel antagonists are unlikely to cause orthostatic hypotension or hypotension during normotensive periods.

Catecholamine synthesis antagonists: Metyrosine competitively inhibits tyrosine hydroxylase. This enzyme governs the rate-limiting step in the biosynthesis of catecholamine. It can be used in conjunction with α-adrenoreceptor antagonists. The consideration of add-on therapy should be guided by intolerance of side effects of escalating doses of monotherapy as well as inadequate control of blood pressure by monotherapy [1].

What Complications Are Associated with Medical Management of Pheochromocytoma-Induced Hypertension?

- Preoperative medical optimization with α-adrenoreceptor antagonists can result in patients experiencing side effects such as postural hypotension with reflex tachycardia, syncope, and nasal congestion. This can be ameliorated with careful dose titration.
- Severe refractory hypotension with the acute withdrawal of catecholamine stimulation can occur postoperatively [7].

When Consenting Patients for Anesthesia, What Contingencies for Monitoring Should Be Taken into Consideration?

Continuous blood pressure monitoring, judicious fluid balance management, and administration of vasoactive and anti-arrhythmic drugs in the perioperative period contribute to improved patient outcome. Arterial blood pressure monitoring is a prerequisite. Central venous pressure monitoring and anticipated vasopressor support is the accepted standard of care. Pulmonary artery catheter use and intraoperative TEE monitoring may be indicated in certain cases such as severe hemodynamic instability, pulmonary hypertension, or significant myocardial disease [8].

Repeat echocardiogram 48 hours prior to surgery did not show any new changes with respect to that performed 4 months previously. The patient was requested to continue taking aspirin throughout the perioperative period. A detailed discussion of perioperative management of dual antiplatelet medication in the patient with percutaneous coronary intervention, with or without stent placement, can be found in chapter 2. In view of the patient's hypertension on admission, his terazosin dose was titrated upwards (at a rate of 2 mg/day) for each of the 2 days immediately before surgery. He was adequately blocked on the morning of surgery. He had an awake arterial line inserted but no further invasive monitoring was deemed necessary. He did require a prolonged stay in PACU for intravenous fluid resuscitation for hypotension prior to discharge to a step-down surgical unit. His recovery after PACU discharge was uneventful.

True/False Questions

1. Regarding the clinical presentation of pheochromocytoma
   (a) In approximately 10% of patients, pheochromocytoma is part of a familial disorder
   (b) Familial pheochromocytoma is more likely to be unilateral
   (c) MEN 2, von Hippel-Lindau syndrome and neurofibromatosis type 1 are autosomal recessive disorders associated with pheochromocytoma
   (d) Approximately 50% of patients with a diagnosis of pheochromocytoma are asymptomatic
   (e) 10–15% of pheochromocytomas are found outside the adrenal gland
2. Regarding preoperative optimization of the patient presenting for adrenalectomy for pheochromocytoma
   (a) Normalization of catecholamine induced intravascular volume expansion is a primary objective
   (b) Calcium channel antagonists are a first-line treatment

(c) Alpha receptor blockade must be successfully initiated prior to beta receptor blockade
(d) Phenoxybenzamine is an irreversible, non-competitive alpha receptor antagonist
(e) Preoperative treatment with an alpha receptor antagonist is usually initiated 2–3 days prior to surgery

References

1. Challis BG, Casey RT, Simpson HL, Gurnell M. Is there an optimal preoperative management strategy for phaeochromocytoma/paraganglioma? Clin Endocrinol. 2017;86(2):163–7.
2. Zografos GN, Vasiliadis GK, Zagouri F, Aggeli C, Korkolis D, Vogiaki S, et al. Pheochromocytoma associated with neurofibromatosis type 1: concepts and current trends. World J Surg Oncol. 2010;8:14. https://doi.org/10.1186/1477-7819-8-14.
3. Lairmore TC, Ball DW, Baylin SB, Wells SA Jr. Management of pheochromocytomas in patients with multiple endocrine neoplasia type 2 syndromes. Ann Surg. 1993;217(6):595–601; discussion -3
4. Zuber SM, Kantorovich V, Pacak K. Hypertension in pheochromocytoma: characteristics and treatment. Endocrinol Metab Clin N Am. 2011;40(2):295–311. vii
5. Miller RD, Cohen NH, Eriksson LI, Fleisher LA, Wiener-Krnoish JP, Young WL, editors. Miller's anesthesia. 8th ed. Philadelphia: Elsevier/Saunders; 2015.
6. Roizen M, Koike M, Eger I, Mulroy M. A prospective randomized trial of four anesthetic techniques for resection of pheochromocytoma. Anesthesiology. 1982;5, 57
7. Azadeh N, Ramakrishna H, Bhatia NL, Charles JC, Mookadam F. Therapeutic goals in patients with pheochromocytoma: a guide to perioperative management. Ir J Med Sci. 2016;185(1):43–9.
8. Jakus L, Jacquet LM, Maiter D, Mourad M, Jonas C, Scholtes JL. Pheochromocytoma – when acute medicine comes to the surgeon's rescue and vice versa. Case report of a patient presenting unmanageable haemodynamic instability during elective surgery for pheochromocytoma. Acta Clin Belg. 2016;71(3):182–6.

Part V

Hepatobiliary

Liver Dysfunction

22

Barry A. Finegan

A 60-year-old female presented for assessment prior to elective spinal decompression and two-level fusion at L1-L2. She had a 2-year history of lower limb pain when walking, which was relieved by sitting/bending forward, and tingling/numbness of her buttocks and legs. The diagnosis of spinal stenosis was confirmed by MRI, which demonstrated severe canal narrowing with facet and ligamentum flavum hypertrophy.

Systems review revealed a history of viral cardiomyopathy that had required a 3-week admission to hospital 2 years previously. An automatic implantable cardioverter defibrillator (AICD) had been placed as a prophylactic measure during that admission. The device had never been activated. A follow-up echocardiogram 12 months later indicated that her cardiac function had returned to normal. She had last seen a cardiologist 3 years ago, who indicated that she had fully recovered but should continue to attend for annual device checks and annual echocardiography assessment. Shortly thereafter, she relocated to another city. Because she had no symptoms and was feeling well, she discontinued these annual assessments.

The patient indicated that her ability to walk was limited due to pain but that she had been a daily swimmer up to 6 months ago. She had reduced and then discontinued this activity due to increasing fatigue and breathlessness with exertion. She indicated that she had recently gained weight, although her appetite was diminished. She was experiencing a dull right upper quadrant pain and had noticed that she had increasing swelling of her ankles. She noticed that when she woke in the morning and moved from side to side, "it was like a washing machine," as she could hear fluid shifting around her abdomen.

She admitted to drinking two glasses of wine every day for the last 3 years. Current medications included acetaminophen 500 mg QID and ibuprofen 400 mg TID.

Physical Examination: She was a moderately obese female with florid facies. She had mild scleral icterus. Her jugular veins were prominent and obviously pulsatile. A holosystolic murmur 4/6 was audile at the right midsternal boarder. Her liver was easily palpable and mildly tender. She had obvious ankle edema and shifting dullness on abdominal examination.

Investigations: Review of available routine laboratory examinations revealed a normal hemoglobin and electrolytes. Platelet count was 225 × 10^9/L. Liver functions tests were not available. Her electrocardiogram (ECG) was normal. A liver panel, echocardiogram, and abdominal ultrasound were ordered. Surgery was deferred.

There were mild elevations of serum aminotransferases (twice the upper limit of normal). Bilirubin was 51.3 μmol/L (normal <20 μmol/L) and albumin was low normal. Prothrombin time was normal. The echocardiogram demonstrated severe tricuspid regurgitation with encapsulation of the AICD lead by the posterior leaflet of the tricuspid valve. The abdominal ultrasound revealed dilatation of the inferior vena cava and hepatic veins, compatible with a diagnosis of congestive hepatopathy. The patient was urgently referred to cardiology for further management.

What Laboratory Tests Are Helpful in Screening for Undiagnosed Liver Disease Preoperatively?

Bilirubin is a product of the normal catabolism of heme during the clearance of senescent or abnormal red blood cells. Albumin-bound bilirubin (unconjugated bilirubin sometimes termed indirect-reacting) is transported to the liver, conjugated by the liver, and rapidly excreted into bile.

B. A. Finegan (✉)
Department of Anesthesiology & Pain Medicine, University of Alberta, Edmonton, AB, Canada
e-mail: bfinegan@ualberta.ca

D. Dillane, B. A. Finegan (eds.), *Preoperative Assessment*, https://doi.org/10.1007/978-3-030-58842-7_22

The excretion process in a healthy individual is very efficient so that normally <10% of measured total bilirubin in the plasma will be in the conjugated (sometimes termed direct-reacting) form.

In liver disease, conjugated bilirubin will be elevated and unconjugated bilirubin may be elevated or normal.

In hemolysis, conjugated bilirubin will be normal and unconjugated will be elevated.

In Gilberts syndrome, conjugated bilirubin will normal and unconjugated bilirubin will be elevated.

Gilberts syndrome in an inherited disorder of disrupted ability to conjugate bilirubin. It is a relatively benign condition. Gilberts syndrome is found in about 5% of the population. Jaundice is not uncommon particularly at times of stress or during an illness. A sub-set of Gilberts syndrome patients are at increased risk of paracetamol toxicity.

The commonly measured enzymes are alanine aminotransferase (ALT), aspartate aminotransferase (AST), and alkaline phosphatase (ALP).

ALT is present primarily in the liver and is a more specific marker of liver injury than AST which can be elevated in the absence of hepatic damage. Isolated AST elevations may be a reflection of cardiac/skeletal muscle damage, kidney, brain, or lung injury.

ALP is found in all tissues but especially in the liver and bone.

ALP may be elevated in hepatic-related disease including biliary obstruction and hepatitis and in bone-related pathology including osteoporosis, osteoblastic bone lesions, and osteomalacia.

If the AST and ALT are higher of than the ALP, this is typical of hepatocellular injury.

If the ALP is higher than the AST and ALT, this is typical of cholestatic disease.

If the ALP is elevated and the AST and ALT are near normal, this is typical of cholestatic/infiltrative liver disease.

Further reading on this subject is available in an excellent guide to liver test interpretation [1].

Tests of *liver function* include albumin and prothrombin time (PT).

In the setting of preoperative assessment, a history indicative of the potential for liver injury and/or symptoms should prompt a requisition for liver enzymes and indices of liver function.

Mild elevations of ALT and AST (<5X upper limit of normal) in the absence of symptoms of liver dysfunction are common, being present in up to 10% of the adult population of the United States [2]. Most are caused by non-alcoholic fatty liver (a non-aggressive subtype of non-alcoholic fatty liver disease [NAFLD]) and chronic alcohol intake. These transaminase elevations are not a reason to postpone an elective surgical procedure.

However, if the patient has not been previously investigated for liver disease while showing symptoms or signs suggestive of severe liver dysfunction (or if there are significant accompanying abnormalities of PT, albumin, or bilirubin), then referral for further assessment is indicated [3].

What Commonly Used Drugs Can Be Associated with Elevated Liver Transaminases?

Clincally significant drug-induced liver injury is uncommon. Many commonly used drugs, including acetaminophen in therapeutic doses, can cause elevated transaminases. Other medications that can have a similar effect on hepatic transaminases include lisinopril, losartan, ciprofloxacin, methotrexate, allopurinol, NSAIDs, bupropion, risperidone, SSRIs, and herbal medications [2].

What Is Cirrhosis?

Chronic liver inflammation leads to replacement of functioning hepatocytes with fibrotic tissue, the latter leading to portal hypertension and eventually the development of collateral portosystemic shunts in the form of varices. The progression and consequences of the chronic liver inflammation are highly variable among individuals. Cirrhosis is the late stage of this process and is diagnosed definitively by liver biopsy.

What Are the Common Causes of Cirrhosis?

In North America and Europe, by far the most common causes of cirrhosis are alcoholic liver disease, chronic viral hepatitis, and non-alcoholic steatohepatitis (NASH), the aggressive subtype of NAFLD. Less common causes include drug-induced liver damage, autoimmune hepatitis, primary and secondary biliary cirrhosis, and right-sided heart failure.

How Important Is It to Identify the Cirrhotic Patient Prior to Elective Surgery?

Cirrhosis markedly increases the risk of elective surgery. In a review of over 400,000 open aortic valvular procedures included in the U.S. National Inpatient Sample Healthcare Cost Utilization Project database, Steffen et al. [4] found in a propensity matched analysis that the presence of cirrhosis more than tripled the mortality rate, doubled the rate of acute renal failure postoperatively, and prolonged the risk-adjusted length of stay. A similar effect has been observed in much less invasive procedures. Querying the American College of Surgeons National Surgical Quality Improvement database of over 21,000 patients undergoing surgery for degenerative disease of the spine between 2006 and 2015, Goel et al. [5] found that, based on preoperative laboratory values, mild and severe liver disease was present in 2.2% and 1.6% of patients, respectively. The 30-day mortality rates in those with mild and severe liver disease was 1.7% and 5.1%, respectively, whereas it was 0.6% in those without liver disease.

Are There Any Simple Non-invasive Scoring Systems to Assist in Reaching a Probable Diagnosis of Cirrhosis?

The modified Bonacini cirrhosis discriminant score (BDS) is calculated using the platelet count, the ALT:AST ratio, and INR. A higher score makes cirrhosis more likely (Table 22.1) [6].

Table 22.1 The modified Bonacini cirrhosis discriminant score (BDS) is calculated using the platelet count, the alanine aminotransferase (ALT): aspartate aminotransferase (AST) ratio and the INR

Score	Platelets (x103/μL)	ALT:AST ratio	INR
0	>340	>1.7	<1.1
1	280–340	1.2–1.7	1.1–1.4
2	220–279	0.6–1.19	>1.4
3	160–219	<0.6	
4	100–159		
5	40–99		
6	<40		

A higher score makes cirrhosis more likely [6]

Table 22.2 Calculating the CTP and MELD scores for patients with liver disease

Child-Turcotte-Pugh (CTP) score: sum of the assigned point values for each of the clinical parameters			
Clinical parameter	1 point	2 points	3 points
Total bilirubin (mg/dL)	<2	2–3	>3
Serum albumin (g/dL	>3.5	2.8–3.5	<2.8
INR	<1.7	–	>2.3
Ascites	None	Mild	Moderate to severe
Hepatic encephalopathy	None	Grade I or II (suppressed with medication)	Grade II or IV (refractory)

From Hickman et al. [7], with permission from Springer Nature

Model for end-stage liver disease (MELD): 3.78 × $\log_e$[serum bilirubin (mg/dL)] + 11.2 × $\log_e$ [INR] + 9.57 × $\log_e$ [serum creatinine (mg/dL)] + 6.43

INR international normalized ratio

How Is the Severity of Cirrhosis Estimated?

A validated tool in estimating cirrhosis severity in chronic liver disease is the Child-Turcotte-Pugh (CTP) score. The Model for End-Stage Liver Disease (MELD) score stratifies severity of end-stage liver disease for transplant planning (Table 22.2) [7] .

Can Perioperative Mortality Risk in Cirrhotic Patients Be Predicted?

The data derived from the CTP and MELD scores are helpful in risk estimation but may overestimate risk for individual surgical procedures such as umbilical hernia repair [8]. In general, it appears that the laparoscopic approach is preferable in cirrhotic patients if feasible [7]. Patients at very high risk (CTP Class C; MELD >20) are often on a liver transplant list, and elective surgery should be postponed if possible, pending this intervention. The latest clinical practice update from the American Society of Gastroenterology emphasizes the paucity of data available to support definitive individual surgical risk stratification in patients with cirrhosis and stresses the importance of referral to, and management by, teams skilled in treating patients with advanced liver disease [9].

What Was the Etiology of Liver Dysfunction in This Case?

Congestive hepatopathy is a relatively uncommon complication of right heart failure and occurs because of decreased liver blood flow, arterial oxygen desaturation, and increased hepatic venous pressures.

Tricuspid valve dysfunction/damage is increasingly being recognized as a serious complication of pacemaker or AICD lead insertion into the right ventricle [10]. Management options include lead extraction and/or valve repair or replacement.

The patient underwent uneventful lead extraction, tricuspid repair, and AICD removal. Her heart failure and liver dysfunction resolved, and elective spinal decompression surgery proceeded 6 months later without incident.

True/False Questions

1. Elevated liver transaminases are indicative of
   (a) Subsequent surgical morbidity
   (b) Hepatocellular injury if AST elevation is predominant

(c) Cholestatic injury if ALP elevation is predominant
(d) Recent alcohol intake
(e) Poor liver function

2. Cirrhosis
(a) Is a consequence of chronic liver inflammation
(b) Involves replacement of liver cells with fat cells
(c) Is easy to diagnose
(d) If present, increases the risk of elective surgery
(e) Is associated with renal failure

References

1. Mruali AR, Carey WD. Liver test interpretation – approach to the patient with liver disease: a guide to commonly used liver tests. https://www.clevelandclinicmeded.com/medicalpubs/diseasemanagement/hepatology/guide-to-common-liver-tests/. Accessed 28 Jun 2020.
2. Oh RC, Hustead TR, Ali SM, Pantsari MW. Mildly elevated liver transaminase levels: causes and evaluation. Am Fam Physician. 2017;96(11):709–15.
3. Agrawal S, Dhiman RK, Limdi JK. Evaluation of abnormal liver function tests. Postgrad Med J. 2016;79:92(1086):223–34.
4. Steffen RJ, Bakaeen FG, Vargo PR, Kindzelski BA, Johnston DR, Roselli EE, et al. Impact of cirrhosis in patients who underwent surgical aortic valve replacement. Am J Cardiol. 2017;120(4):648–54.
5. Goel NJ, Agarwal P, Mallela AN, Abdullah KG, Ali ZS, Ozturk AK, et al. Liver disease is an independent predictor of poor 30-day outcomes following surgery for degenerative disease of the cervical spine. Spine J. 2019;19(3):448–60.
6. Udell JA, Wang CS, Tinmouth J, FitzGerald JM, Ayas NT, Simel DL, et al. Does this patient with liver disease have cirrhosis? JAMA. 2012;307(8):832–42.
7. Hickman L, Tanner L, Christein J, Vickers S. Non-hepatic abdominal surgery in patients with cirrhotic liver disease. J Gastrointest Surg. 2019;23(3):634–42.
8. Hew S, Yu W, Robson S, Starkey G, Testro A, Fink M, et al. Safety and effectiveness of umbilical hernia repair in patients with cirrhosis. Hernia. 2018;22(5):759–65.
9. Northup PG, Friedman LS, Kamath PS. AGA clinical practice update on surgical risk assessment and perioperative management in cirrhosis: expert review. Clin Gastroenterol Hepatol. 2019;17:595–06.
10. Chang JD, Manning WJ, Ebrille E, Zimetbaum PJ. Tricuspid valve dysfunction following pacemaker or cardioverter-defibrillator implantation. J Am Coll Cardiol. 2017;69(18):2331–41.

23 The Patient Presenting for Liver Transplantation

Ciaran Twomey

A 43-year-old woman presented to the preoperative clinic for review. She had end-stage liver disease (ESLD) and had undergone assessment for liver transplantation by her hepatologist and transplant surgical team. She had a history of alcoholic liver disease that had been complicated by portal hypertension, encephalopathy, and hyponatremia. The portal hypertension had resulted in esophageal varies that required banding, and ascites that needed paracentesis. Her MELD-Na score was 19. Comorbidities were gastroesophageal reflux disease (GERD), asthma, and depression. She had prior uneventful anesthesia for dental surgery (general) and caesarian section (neuroaxial).

Medications: Salbutamol, pantoprazole, lactulose, furosemide, and spironolactone. She had no drug allergies.

She was a non-smoker and had an exercise tolerance greater than four METS. Her GERD symptoms were controlled.

Physical Examination: She had signs of liver disease, including spider nevi, palmar erythema, a distended abdomen, and leg edema. Her airway appeared favorable for intubation.

Investigations: Laboratory investigations are shown in Table 23.1.

A recent transthoracic ECHO demonstrated normal left and right ventricular size and function. The right ventricular systolic pressure was estimated to be 35–40 mmHg

Table 23.1 Laboratory values at the time of preoperative evaluation

Hemoglobin	11 g/dl
Platelet count	65 × 10^9/L
INR	1.4
Sodium	130 mmol/L
Potassium	4.8 mmol/L
Creatinine	108 umol/L

What Are the Common Reasons for Transplantation?

Hepatocellular carcinoma and hepatitis C virus cirrhosis are the most common diseases leading to liver transplantation, followed by patients with alcoholic cirrhosis and non-alcoholic steatohepatitis. Other causes of cirrhosis that may require transplantation include hepatitis B, hemochromatosis, Wilson disease, and autoimmune hepatitis [1]. Diseases of the bile ducts—primary biliary cirrhosis, primary sclerosing cholangitis, and biliary atresia (in children)—are also conditions that can lead to transplantation. Acute liver failure is an indication in less than 10% of liver transplants [2]. This is a decline in liver function with encephalopathy within 26 weeks of jaundice in a patient with no prior liver disease. Etiologies are mostly viral (hepatitis A, B) or drug-induced (acetaminophen overdose).

What Is a MELD Score?

With the diverse range of causes of liver diseases, a way to prioritize patients for transplantation was developed based on laboratory data. Model for End-stage Liver Disease (MELD) is a prognostic model that in its original form was a scoring system to predict 3-month mortality in patients with chronic liver disease undergoing transjugular intrahepatic portosystemic shunt (TIPS) [3]. Variables used to calculate the original MELD score were serum bilirubin, serum creatinine, INR, and cause of the liver disease. It was later modified (MELD-Na) to include serum sodium; the etiology contribution was dropped [4]. Serum sodium is a predictor of mortality in end-stage liver disease [5–7]. MELD-Na is used to allocate donor organs to the sickest patient. In patient populations where there is no, or little liver cirrhosis, MELD-Na will not predict the un-transplanted mortality rate. These conditions—called MELD exceptions—are

C. Twomey (✉)
Department of Anesthesiology & Pain Medicine, University of Alberta Hospital, Edmonton, AB, Canada
e-mail: ctwomey@ualberta.ca

D. Dillane, B. A. Finegan (eds.), *Preoperative Assessment*, https://doi.org/10.1007/978-3-030-58842-7_23

awarded additional points [8]. They include hepatocellular carcinoma, portopulmonary hypertension, hepatopulmonary syndrome, and hepatic artery thrombosis within 14 days of hepatic surgery.

Is This Patient's Hyponatremia a Concern?

About 20% of prospective liver transplant patients are hyponatremic (serum sodium ≤130 mmol/L) [9]. A number of factors contribute to hyponatremia, the most prominent being the systemic vasodilation of ESLD and subsequent release of antidiuretic hormone, resulting in excessive renal water retention relative to sodium [10]. Some medications (e.g., beta-blockade used for the treatment of variceal hemorrhage and some anti-hypertensive medications) are also contributing factors.

Serum sodium as a predictor of mortality in the pretransplantation population is well established. It is also a concern during the intra- and postoperative setting. Patients with severe hyponatremia (<125 mmol/l) have a longer ICU stay compared to those with normal levels [11]. Rapid shifts (>10 mmol/l rise in 24 h) in serum sodium are associated with worse outcomes, including neurological deficits and increased 6-month mortality [12]. Central pontine myelinolysis is an obvious concern, but increased risk of infectious complications, transfusion, and renal impairment have also been demonstrated [13, 14]. Intraoperative sodium <130 mmol/L is independently associated with a significantly higher 1-year mortality [15]. Liver transplantation can involve significant blood loss with massive transfusion, hemodynamic derangements, fluid shifts, and administration of large volumes of colloid and crystalloid solutions. For the anesthesia practitioner, preventing rapid intraoperative sodium changes can be challenging. Having a normal or close-to-normal serum sodium at the time of transplantation is an advantage.

What Can Be Done to Correct the Hyponatremia?

There are two windows of opportunity available to the practitioner where correction can be attempted—in the few weeks or months prior to transplantation, and also in the few hours available after hospital admission when an organ becomes available.

In the outpatient setting, the aim is to remove contributory factors where possible, e.g., beta-blockers, antihypertensive medication. Water restriction (1–1.5 L/day) should be considered [10]. Hypokalemia should be addressed, as potassium will raise the serum sodium concentration when corrected [16]. Vasopressin receptor antagonists produce a solute-free increase in urine production. Thirst is a major side effect that can limit the serum sodium rise. Where the ESLD vasodilatation causes hypotension, midodrine (an alpha-1-antagonist) can be used to maintain blood pressure and reduce water retention [17].

In the hospital setting, there may be sufficient time following admission for a slow controlled correction of low sodium levels prior to transplantation. Strategies include use of hypertonic saline, albumin infusion, and hemodialysis if there is significant renal impairment. Expert advice should be sought, as these actions if improperly executed can cause more harm than good, i.e., when a rapid rise in sodium level occurs [18] .

This Patient's RVSP Is Higher Than Normal—Is This a Concern?

Portopulmonary hypertension (POPH) is a serious complication of portal hypertension that occurs in 6–10% of prospective transplant patients [19, 20]. Pulmonary hypertension is a well-recognized complication of portal hypertension due to chronic liver disease. All prospective transplant patients are evaluated for this condition, as it carries significant risk and can, if severe enough, be a barrier to transplantation.

Screening for POPH starts with a transthoracic ECHO. The RVSP is estimated using the modified Bernoulli equation, with data based on the tricuspid regurgitant jet (TRJ) and estimated mean right atrial pressure (mRAP).

$$\text{RVSP} = 4 \times (\text{Maximum velocity TRJ})^2 + (\text{mRAP})$$

The mRAP is dependent on the collapsibility pattern of the inferior vena cava [20].

While there are guidelines regarding the RVSP threshold at which further investigation of right-sided pressures is triggered, there is no consensus, and it is often institution dependent [21, 22]. Usually if the RVSP is greater than 45–50 mmHg, then a right heart catheterization (RHC) is advisable. This allows direct pressure measurements of the right ventricle and pulmonary artery. Patients can subsequently be stratified according to POPH severity. Raevens et al. investigated where the RSVP cutoff for maximum sensitivity and specificity for the presence of POPH lay [23]. They recommended that a RHC be done at a RVSP of 38 mmHg or greater, where sensitivity and specificity are 100% and 93%, respectively. Irrespective of the preoperative POPH evaluation, a RHC is often routinely placed at the time of anesthesia induction immediately prior to abdominal incision, so that any progression in the condition may be determined and consideration given to interventions that might improve the patient's right-sided hemodynamic profile [21]. As liver transplantation is not a planned procedure, preoperative anesthesia assessment may occur several months before an organ becomes available—adequate time for a patient's condition to deteriorate.

POPH severity is classified according to mean pulmonary artery pressure (mPAP)—mild (25≤ mPAP <35 mmHg), moderate (35≤ mPAP <45 mmHg), and severe (mPAP ≥45 mmHg). Additional criteria necessary for confirmation of a diagnosis of POPH include a normal or low pulmonary capillary wedge pressure (PCWP ≤15 mmHg), and an elevated pulmonary vascular resistance (PVR ≥3 Wood units [240 dynes/sec/cm^{-5}] [24]. The transpulmonary gradient (TPG—the difference between the mPAP mean pressure and the PCWP) should be greater than 12 mmHg. A high mPAP in this patient population can commonly be due to fluid overload (where the TPG would be low), and this should be excluded in order to be confident of the POPH diagnosis.

No single cause of POPH has been identified; factors that contribute—some of which are speculative—are as follows: genetic predisposition, circulating vasoconstrictive mediators that are ordinarily removed by the liver but reach the pulmonary circulation via collateral portosytemic blood vessels, thromboembolic phenomena, shear forces of the hyperdynamic circulation of ESLD, and inflammation. Patients with moderate or greater POPH have a higher mortality and morbidity rate. A mPAP greater than 50 mmHg is a contraindication to transplantation [25].

Treatment of mPAP greater than 35 mmHg with endothelin antagonists, phosphodiesterase inhibitors, prostinoids, or a combination of the above should be considered [24]. The goal is to lower the mPAP, PVR, and improve right ventricular function. The dividend is that during liver transplantation, right ventricular failure precipitated by the rise in right-sided pressures associated with organ reperfusion can be avoided.

Does This Patient Need a Cardiac Stress Test?

Liver transplantation exposes a patient to extreme hemodynamic challenges. Large blood losses, manipulation of the native liver prior to explant, and vascular clamping of caval and portal venous systems can result in periods of resuscitation where organ perfusion is heavily pressor-dependent. Patients compensate with tachycardia, at rates not encountered in pre-transplant life. They need a degree of cardiac reserve to endure these stresses. For these reasons, the presence of coronary artery disease (CAD) can be a burden for the patient during liver transplantation, and is associated with poor outcomes [26, 27]. The prevalence of CAD with >50% stenosis can be up to 25% [28]. Patients are often asymptomatic due to a sedentary lifestyle and may be unable to achieve the target heart rate using a standard treadmill stress test. Screening with a pharmacological stress test using adenosine, dipyridamole, or dobutamine is an alternative [22]. At our institution in patients over 50 years of age, or those who are younger but have risk factors such as diabetes, hypertension, or obesity, a positron emission tomography computed tomography (PET/CT) scan in conjunction with a dobutamine stress test is done. This test provides information on whether ventricular function was preserved under stress, and how well the maximum heart rate achieved was tolerated. Patients with findings suspicious of CAD are sent for cardiac catheterization.

At 43 years, with no risk factors for CAD, this patient was not stress tested.

True/False Questions

1. (a) Hepatocellular carcinoma and alcoholic cirrhosis are the most common indications for liver transplantation.
   (b) The MELD score is a prognostic model intended to predict 3-month mortality after transjugular intrahepatic portosystemic shunt (TIPS).
   (c) MELD-Na score is a modification of the original MELD scoring system that takes into account the etiology of the liver disease.
   (d) MELD-Na is most useful for predicting mortality rate in patient populations where there is a low incidence of cirrhosis.
   (e) MELD-Na is used in the decision-making process for deceased donor liver allocation.
2. (a) Up to 20% of liver transplant patients are hyponatremic.
   (b) Serum sodium should not be corrected in the hours immediately preceding the transplant procedure.
   (c) Portopulmonary hypertension is commonly seen in up to 35% of liver transplant patients.
   (d) A normal or low pulmonary capillary wedge pressure is a requirement for a diagnosis of portopulmonary hypertension to be made.
   (e) A dipyridamole or dobutamine stress test is recommended prior to liver transplantation in patients with, or at risk of, coronary artery disease.

References

1. Neuberger J. An update on liver transplantation: a critical review. J Autoimmun. 2016;66:51–9.
2. Mendizabal M, Silva MO. Liver transplantation in acute liver failure: a challenging scenario. World J Gastroenterol. 2016;22(4):1523–31.
3. Malinchoc M, Kamath PS, Gordon FD, Peine CJ, Rank J, ter Borg PC. A model to predict poor survival in patients undergoing transjugular intrahepatic portosystemic shunts. Hepatology. 2000;31(4):864–71.
4. Biggins SW, Kim WR, Terrault NA, Saab S, Balan V, Schiano T, et al. Evidence-based incorporation of serum sodium concentration into MELD. Gastroenterology. 2006;130(6):1652–60.

5. Ruf AE, Kremers WK, Chavez LL, Descalzi VI, Podesta LG, Villamil FG. Addition of serum sodium into the MELD score predicts waiting list mortality better than MELD alone. Liver Transpl. 2005;11(3):336–43.
6. Biggins SW, Rodriguez HJ, Bacchetti P, Bass NM, Roberts JP, Terrault NA. Serum sodium predicts mortality in patients listed for liver transplantation. Hepatology. 2005;41(1):32–9.
7. Heuman DM, Abou-Assi SG, Habib A, Williams LM, Stravitz RT, Sanyal AJ, et al. Persistent ascites and low serum sodium identify patients with cirrhosis and low MELD scores who are at high risk for early death. Hepatology. 2004;40(4):802–10.
8. Goldberg DS, Fallon MB. Model for end-stage liver disease-based organ allocation: managing the exceptions to the rules. Clin Gastroenterol Hepatol. 2013;11(5):452–3.
9. Angeli P, Wong F, Watson H, Ginès P, Investigators CAPPS. Hyponatremia in cirrhosis: results of a patient population survey. Hepatology. 2006;44(6):1535–42.
10. John S, Thuluvath PJ. Hyponatremia in cirrhosis: pathophysiology and management. World J Gastroenterol. 2015;21(11):3197–205.
11. Yun BC, Kim WR, Benson JT, Biggins SW, Therneau TM, Kremers WK, et al. Impact of pretransplant hyponatremia on outcome following liver transplantation. Hepatology. 2009;49(5):1610–5.
12. Romanovsky A, Azevedo LC, Meeberg G, Zibdawi R, Bigam D, Bagshaw SM. Serum sodium shift in hyponatremic patients undergoing liver transplantation: a retrospective cohort study. Ren Fail. 2015;37(1):37–44.
13. Dawwas MF, Lewsey JD, Neuberger JM, Gimson AE. The impact of serum sodium concentration on mortality after liver transplantation: a cohort multicenter study. Liver Transpl. 2007;13(8):1115–24.
14. Londoño MC, Guevara M, Rimola A, Navasa M, Taurà P, Mas A, et al. Hyponatremia impairs early posttransplantation outcome in patients with cirrhosis undergoing liver transplantation. Gastroenterology. 2006;130(4):1135–43.
15. Yang SM, Choi SN, Yu JH, Yoon HK, Kim WH, Jung CW, et al. Intraoperative hyponatremia is an independent predictor of one-year mortality after liver transplantation. Sci Rep. 2018;8(1):18023.
16. Sterns RH, Nigwekar SU, Hix JK. The treatment of hyponatremia. Semin Nephrol. 2009;29(3):282–99.
17. Patel S, Nguyen DS, Rastogi A, Nguyen MK, Nguyen MK. Treatment of cirrhosis-associated hyponatremia with midodrine and octreotide. Front Med (Lausanne). 2017;4:17.
18. Sterns RH, Hix JK. Overcorrection of hyponatremia is a medical emergency. Kidney Int. 2009;76(6):587–9.
19. Simonneau G, Robbins IM, Beghetti M, Channick RN, Delcroix M, Denton CP, et al. Updated clinical classification of pulmonary hypertension. J Am Coll Cardiol. 2009;54(1 Suppl):S43–54.
20. Humbert M, Sitbon O, Chaouat A, Bertocchi M, Habib G, Gressin V, et al. Pulmonary arterial hypertension in France: results from a national registry. Am J Respir Crit Care Med. 2006;173(9): 1023–30.
21. Krowka MJ, Fallon MB, Kawut SM, Fuhrmann V, Heimbach JK, Ramsay MA, et al. International liver transplant society practice guidelines: diagnosis and management of hepatopulmonary syndrome and portopulmonary hypertension. Transplantation. 2016;100(7):1440–52.
22. Martin P, DiMartini A, Feng S, Brown R, Fallon M. Evaluation for liver transplantation in adults: 2013 practice guideline by the American Association for the Study of Liver Diseases and the American Society of Transplantation. Hepatology. 2014;59(3):1144–65.
23. Raevens S, Colle I, Reyntjens K, Geerts A, Berrevoet F, Rogiers X, et al. Echocardiography for the detection of portopulmonary hypertension in liver transplant candidates: an analysis of cutoff values. Liver Transpl. 2013;19(6):602–10.
24. Cartin-Ceba R, Krowka MJ. Portopulmonary hypertension. Clin Liver Dis. 2014;18(2):421–38.
25. Krowka MJ, Plevak DJ, Findlay JY, Rosen CB, Wiesner RH, Krom RA. Pulmonary hemodynamics and perioperative cardiopulmonary-related mortality in patients with portopulmonary hypertension undergoing liver transplantation. Liver Transpl. 2000;6(4): 443–50.
26. Plotkin JS, Scott VL, Pinna A, Dobsch BP, De Wolf AM, Kang Y. Morbidity and mortality in patients with coronary artery disease undergoing orthotopic liver transplantation. Liver Transpl Surg. 1996;2(6):426–30.
27. Diedrich DA, Findlay JY, Harrison BA, Rosen CB. Influence of coronary artery disease on outcomes after liver transplantation. Transplant Proc. 2008;40(10):3554–7.
28. Lee BC, Li F, Hanje AJ, Mumtaz K, Boudoulas KD, Lilly SM. Effectively screening for coronary artery disease in patients undergoing orthotopic liver transplant evaluation. J Transp Secur. 2016;2016:7187206.

Part VI

Gastrointestinal

Crohn's Disease

24

Derek Dillane and Ryan Snelgrove

A 57-year-old female patient with longstanding Crohn's disease presented at the anesthesia preadmission clinic the day before laparotomy and possible adhesiolysis.

Past surgical history was remarkable for total abdominal hysterectomy, femoral hernia repair, laparoscopic cholecystectomy, multiple bowel resections, and appendectomy. She did not describe any previous problems with anesthesia but recounted that pain control had previously been suboptimal. She had a history of chronic pain, a 40-pack year history of cigarette smoking, and smoked cannabis on a daily basis.

Medications: Azathioprine 100 mg daily, ustekinumab 90 mg subcutaneously monthly, duloxetine delayed release 30 mg daily, fentanyl patch 50mcg/hour, Percocet 1–2 tablets as required, pregabalin 100 mg twice daily, lorazepam 0.5 mg sublingually as needed for sleep, trazodone 50 mg at bedtime, and venlafaxine 75 mg daily.

Physical Examination: On examination, she weighed 45.4 kg and her BMI was 19.7. Cardiovascular and respiratory examinations were normal. Airway exam was reassuring.

Investigations: Hemoglobin 118, WCC 6.3, platelets 248, creatinine 80, sodium 138, potassium 4.0, BNP 11 ng/L.

What Is Crohn's Disease?

Crohn's disease is one of two chronic inflammatory bowel diseases (IBDs), the other being ulcerative colitis. It follows a relapsing, remitting course, usually over many years. Unlike ulcerative colitis, which only involves the colon, Crohn's disease can affect any part of the gastrointestinal tract from the mouth to the anus. Fifty percent of patients have both terminal ileum and colon involvement, 20% have colonic involvement only, and 30% have disease confined to the small bowel. The rectum is typically spared, but 25% of patients have perianal disease [1]. Crohn's disease is characterized by a patchy distribution of skip lesions, i.e., diseased sections of the gastrointestinal tract are interrupted by uninvolved areas.

Extraintestinal manifestations of Crohn's disease are common and not necessarily related to relapses of intestinal disease. Crohn's disease has a slight female preponderance, is more common in smokers, and usually starts in the second or third decade of life. Its incidence is increasing – currently it is 3–20 per 100,000 [2, 3]. It has both environmental and genetic components, e.g., 10% of Crohn's disease sufferers have a first-degree relative with the condition, and there is a 40–50% rate of concordance among identical twins [4].

The histological features account for many of the clinical sequelae seen in Crohn's disease patients. The first thing to note is that in addition to its variable location, inflammation is transmural. Three phenotypic subtypes are described: inflammatory, stricturizing, and fistulizing. Initial inflammation can progress to fibrosis and narrowing of the bowel lumen, which may result in bowel obstruction. Deep ulcers, which appear as linear fissures, can penetrate the bowel wall leading to abscess formation or development of fistulae between the bowel, bladder, vagina, uterus, or perineal skin; 50–80% of patients will eventually require surgery for complications of Crohn's disease.

What Are the Common Classifications of Crohn's Disease?

Clinically, the disease is classified according to severity (mild, moderate, or severe), location (upper gastrointestinal, ileocolic, ileal, colonic, or perianal), and phenotype (inflammatory, stricturizing, and fistulizing). The Crohn's

D. Dillane (✉)
Department of Anesthesiology & Pain Medicine, University of Alberta, Edmonton, AB, Canada

R. Snelgrove
Department of Surgery, University of Alberta, Edmonton, AB, Canada

D. Dillane, B. A. Finegan (eds.), *Preoperative Assessment*, https://doi.org/10.1007/978-3-030-58842-7_24

Table 24.1 Crohn's Disease Activity Index used to define severity of disease activity and as a research tool [5]

Clinical or laboratory variable	Weighting factor
Number of liquid or soft stools each day for 7 days	×2
Abdominal pain rating (0 = none, 1 = mild, 2 = moderate, 3 = severe) each day for 7 days	×5
General wellbeing from 0(well) to terrible (4) each day for 7 days	×7
Presence of complications[a]	×20
Hematocrit<0.47 in males and <0.42 in females	×6
Presence of abdominal mass (0 = none, 2 = questionable, 5 = definite)	×10
Percentage deviation from standard weight	×1

[a]One point added for each set of complications: arthralgia or arthritis; uveitis or iritis; erythema nodosum, pyoderma gangrenosum, or mouth ulcers; anal fistulas, fissures, or abscesses; other fistula, fever >100 °F in previous 7 days

Disease Activity Index (CDAI) (Table 24.1) is used for defining severity of disease activity, defining whether or not a patient is in remission, and response to treatment [1, 5]. Crohn's disease is deemed to be in clinical remission when CDAI <150, mild when CDAI is 150–220, moderate to severe when CDAI is 220–450, and severe-fulminant when CDAI >450. A simplified variant of the CDAI, the Harvey-Bradshaw index (Fig. 24.1) can also be used to grade disease activity [6].

What Are the Risk Factors for Aggressive Disease Activity?

The natural course of Crohn's disease ranges from that of an indolent course with long periods of remission to aggressive and incapacitating disease [7]. Aggressive disease is considered to be that which has a high relapse rate with penetrating disease requiring repeat surgeries or multiple admissions for flare-ups. Age of diagnosis less than 30 years, involvement of the upper gastrointestinal tract and ileum, perianal disease, deep ulceration, prior surgery, and stricturizing or penetrating disease are risk factors for aggressive disease activity [2].

What Extraintestinal Manifestations of Crohn's Disease Are of Perioperative Concern?

Extraintestinal manifestations (EIMs) of Crohn's disease occur with a prevalence ranging from 6% to 36% [8]. The commonest EIM is arthritis. It can involve the peripheral large joints and the axial skeleton. Large joint arthritis is by far the commonest type of arthritis seen in IBD (approximately 60–70% of the arthritis seen in these patients) [9]. Up to 6% of all IBD patients develop ankylosing spondylitis affecting the sacroiliac joints and spine. Patients with ankylosing spondylitis develop gradual fusion of the cervical spine over time.

Other EIMs of Crohn's disease include fatty liver, hepatomegaly, primary sclerosing cholangitis with subsequent cirrhosis and liver failure, venous thrombosis, conjunctivitis, iritis, and anterior uveitis.

What Medications Can We Expect to See Prescribed for the Crohn's Disease Patient?

This is not meant to be an exhaustive manual on how to treat the patient with Crohn's disease but, rather, a primer for the anesthesiologist faced preoperatively with the occasionally confusing array of immunomodulatory medications prescribed for these patients. Medical treatment is dependent on disease location, severity and phenotype, i.e., inflammatory, stricturizing, or fistulizing. The main drug categories used in the treatment of Crohn's disease are 5-aminosalicylates, antibiotics, corticosteroids, immunosuppressants, anti-TNF agents, and interleukin inhibitors. The goal of treatment is to achieve clinical, endoscopic, and histologic remission followed by maintenance of remission.

Glucocorticoids

Enteric-coated budesonide is considered the treatment of choice for inducing remission in patients with low-risk disease of the ileum and proximal colon [10]. The aim of treatment with budesonide is induction of remission within a 12-week period followed by tapering and discontinuation. Glucocorticoids are also used as first-line therapy in patients with moderate to severe disease who require a fast treatment response prior to maintenance treatment with azathioprine or an anti-TNF agent [10].

5-Aminosalicylates (5-ASA): Sulfasalazine, Mesalamine

5-ASA formulations can be used for the treatment of mild to moderate disease when glucocorticoid avoidance is preferable. It decreases cyclooxygenase enzyme activity and subsequently decreases the formation of pro-inflammatory prostaglandins. Sulfasalazine was developed to deliver both an anti-inflammatory agent, 5-ASA, and anti-bacterial agent, sulfapyridine [11]. Up to 25% of patients taking sulfasalazine discontinue taking it due to unwanted effects, e.g.,

Modified Harvey Bradshaw Index Assessment for Crohn's Disease Activity

Date: ______________________
Patient Name: ______________________
Date of Birth: ______________________
PHN/ULI: ______________________

Patient, please complete Questions 1, 2 & 3.

Base your answers on how you felt yesterday.

1. General Well-being (see descriptors)

☐ Very well = 0
☐ Slightly below Par = 1
☐ Poor = 2
☐ Very Poor = 3
☐ Terrible = 4

☐

2. Abdominal Pain (see descriptors)

☐ None = 0
☐ Mild = 1
☐ Moderate = 2
☐ Severe = 3

☐

3. Number of Liquid or Soft Stools per day (Yesterday)

☐

Physician, please complete Question 4

4. Additional Manifestations

☐ None = 0
☐ Arthalgia = 1
☐ Uveitis = 1
☐ Erythema Nodosum = 1
☐ Aphthous ulcer = 1
☐ Pyoderma gangrenosum = 1
☐ Anal Fissure = 1
☐ New Fistula = 1
☐ Abscess = 1

☐

Total Harvey Bradshaw Index score: [sum of all above items]

☐

Remission = <5
Mild Disease = 5-7
Moderate Disease = 8-16
Severe Disease >16

1. General Well-being Descriptors

General well being includes fatigue in the overall rating and how you feel today. Record the worst you have felt today. Compare yourself to someone else of your age, how would they rank their general wellbeing? Below are some descriptors to help you rank your category of general well being.

- **Very Well:** General health is not generally a problem. You're feeling very good or great and under control.
- **Slightly Below Par:** You're getting through things but feeling below par and not normal. Something overall is preventing you from saying " I feel wonderful ". You're feeling good but not great. You can work, socialize, and function on a day to day basis.
- **Poor:** Your symptoms bother you. You occasionally miss work, school, or social activities. You have some embarrassing moments with fecal incontinence. You have diarrhea, abdominal pain, fatigue, and basically just feeling unwell, but you are still able to function. You're getting through the day, doing all your normal stuff but it is a struggle.
- **Very Poor:** Your getting through a part of the day, but can't do you're your normal stuff. You can't attend social events in evening. You sometime leave home from work early. You feel pretty bad and are not doing much activity – only those absolutely necessary. Your symptoms interfere with life considerably, you don't go out or are fearful when out, you miss a lot of school or work. Fecal incontinence happens several times per week.
- **Terrible:** You're unable to function. You can't manage the basics and you're almost bedridden. This is the worse you have ever been. You're not working.

2. Abdominal Pain Descriptors

Abdominal pain may include cramping and discomfort. It does not have to be just "pain" as we know it. Below are some descriptors to help you rank your category of abdominal pain.

- **Mild:** You're aware that the abdominal pain is there but it does not interfere with your life and you continue with activities such as work and pleasure. You feel and hear rumbles, gurgles and cramps.
- **Moderate:** You're aware of your abdominal pain and must alter your activities to manage the pain (ie. lie down to rest, postpone shopping trips until later, and take Tylenol). The pain interferes with your life and daily activities. You may have to miss work or pleasure activities on occasion.
- **Severe:** Your abdominal pain causes you to stop all activity. You are frequently in bed because of the pain, you call in sick to work and cancel all activities.

Page 1 of 1
Version 1 – Sep 15. 2016

Fig. 24.1 Harvey Bradshaw index of Crohn disease activity [6]. (Courtesy of, and with permission from, the IBD Clinic, University of Alberta)

hypersensitivity reactions, bone marrow suppression, pancreatitis, and pneumonitis [12, 13]. Sulfapyridine is responsible for many of the unwanted effects of sulfasalazine. A 5-ASA formulation without the sulfa group, mesalamine, is tolerated by most patients with sulfasalazine intolerance. Unlike sulfasalazine, which is only partially absorbed in the jejunum, mesalamine is rapidly absorbed in the jejunum with only 20% of drug reaching the terminal ileum and colon [12]. A number of enterically coated mesalamine formulations have subsequently been developed to increase delivery to affected areas.

Immunomodulators

The thiopurines (azathioprine and 6-mercaptopurine) are the most commonly used agents in this category for the management of Crohn's disease. They are typically used for patients who require glucocorticoids to maintain remission, i.e., they are glucocorticoid-sparing agents.

Methotrexate

This may be a useful choice for maintenance therapy in patients who cannot tolerate thiopurines. A clinical response is usually seen within 3 months and patients are maintained on glucocorticoid agents with an eventual tapering dose until this response is achieved.

Antibiotics

The use of antibiotics for the treatment of active Crohn's disease is controversial, relating to inconsistencies in the supporting evidence. A systematic review and meta-analysis of 10 studies involving 1160 patients found a modest benefit over placebo for inducing remission [14]. However, the wide range of antibiotics used made the data difficult to interpret. The commonest antibiotics used in the treatment of Crohn's disease are metronidazole and ciprofloxacin.

Anti-TNF Agents

Sometimes called biologic agents, the commonest anti-TNF therapies used in Crohn's disease are the monoclonal antibodies infliximab (Remicade®) and adalimumab (Humira®). These are usually used in combination with an immunomodulator, e.g., azathioprine, to induce and maintain remission in patients with moderate to severe disease.

Ustekinumab (Stelara)

This is a monoclonal antibody which is used as a second-line therapy if anti-TNF agents have been tried unsuccessfully. It is an interleukin-12 and interleukin-23 antagonist. Unwanted effects include increased risk of infection, upper respiratory infection being of particular relevance perioperatively.

What Instructions Should Be Given to Patients with Regard to Discontinuation of Medications Prescribed for Management of Crohn's Disease?

5-ASA is primarily excreted renally. It is reasonable to discontinue 1 day before surgery in patients with, or at risk of, decreased glomerular filtration rate.

Immunosuppressive and immune modulating agents, e.g., azathioprine, methotrexate, glucocorticoids and the biologic agents have been implicated in causing postoperative infection and septic complications [15]. A preoperative drug-free interval has been proposed as being advisable if feasible [15]. The following paragraphs will discuss each drug separately.

For patients taking glucocorticoids preoperatively, it is preferable that these be discontinued prior to surgery to minimize complications associated with chronic use. However, this is rarely possible as it is usually patients with disease refractory to other medications, and are steroid dependent, who require surgery. Stopping steroid therapy in this population may lead to more severe symptoms such as complete obstruction. Subsequently, many patients are likely to be on chronic glucocorticoid therapy and may require surgical stress dosing. This topic has been explored in detail in Chap. 19. A recent review on this subject suggests that the patient taking any dose of glucocorticoid for less than 3 weeks or those taking prednisone 5 mg daily for any period of time do not need steroid stress dose administration [16]. There are numerous practical approaches towards the patient with potential hypothalamic-pituitary-adrenalaxis (HPAA) suppression in the perioperative period. This includes that which calls for maintenance of the usual steroid dose throughout the surgical period and treating hypotension with rescue dose steroid [16, 17]. A more nuanced approach assesses the risk of HPAA suppression based on the clinical picture and/or the ACTH stimulation test. Patients at high risk of HPAA, e.g., presence of Cushingoid features, use of prednisone 20 mg/day or greater, are treated with stress dose steroids; patients at low risk, e.g., < prednisone 5 mg/day, do not require stress dosing [16]. An approach to the dosing required according to surgical type, as adapted from Liu et al., is provided in Table 24.2 [16].

Table 24.2 Recommended dosing by surgery type for patients who may have secondary adrenal insufficiency secondary to steroid use

Surgery type	Endogenous cortisol secretion rate	Examples	Recommended steroid dosing
Superficial	8–10 mg per day (baseline)	Dental surgery Biopsy	Usual daily dose
Minor	50 mg per day	Inguinal hernia repair Colonoscopy Uterine curettage Hand surgery	Usual daily dose *Plus* Hydrocortisone 50 mg IV before incision Hydrocortisone 25 mg IV every 8 h × 24 h Then usual daily dose
Moderate	75–150 mg per day	Lower extremity revascularization Total joint replacement Cholecystectomy Colon resection Abdominal hysterectomy	Usual daily dose *Plus* Hydrocortisone 50 mg IV before incision Hydrocortisone 25 mg IV every 8 h × 24 h Then usual daily dose
Major	75–150 mg per day	Esophagectomy Total proctocolectomy Major cardiac/vascular Hepaticojejunostomy Delivery Trauma	Usual daily dose *Plus* Hydrocortisone 100 mg IV before incision Followed by continuous IV infusion of 200 mg of hydrocortisone more than 24 h *Or* Hydrocortisone 50 mg IV every 8 h × 24 h Taper dose by half per day until usual daily dose reached *Plus* Continuous IV fluids with 5% dextrose and 0.2–0.45% NaCl (based on degree of hypoglycemia)

From Liu et al. [16], with permission from Wolters Kluwer

Azathioprine has been associated with antagonism of neuromuscular blocking agents [11, 18]. There is also a theoretical risk of perioperative bone marrow suppression especially in patients with renal impairment. A cautious approach in patients with compromised renal function would be to hold azathioprine on the day of surgery and resume once renal function does not deteriorate further in the post-operative period [11].

Continuation of anti-TNF agents is contentious [19]. Some single-center studies have found an increased risk of infectious complications with preoperative use of anti-TNFα medications. A meta-analysis of 18 studies found that they significantly increased postoperative infectious complications (OR = 1.93) [19, 20]. However, the overall consensus from retrospective reviews, prospective studies, and meta-analyses points towards a lack of convincing evidence for postoperative complications with the preoperative use of anti-TNFα medications [19].

There are no definitive guidelines regarding perioperative use of ustekinumab. A small cohort study looked at postoperative complications in patients who had been treated with ustekinumab within 4 months of surgery compared with a control cohort of anti-TNF-treated patients [21]. There were no significant differences in early or late wound infections, anastomotic leak, or postoperative ileus between the groups.

What Are the Indications for Surgery in Crohn's Disease?

Most patients with Crohn's disease will require surgery at least once, and some patients require multiple surgical procedures. Surgery is not curative but may be required for some of the complications associated with the disease. It is usually performed for obstructive complications due to strictures or for complications related to fistulae. Patients unresponsive to medical therapy or those who are steroid dependent also require surgery [1]. Urgent/semi-urgent indications for surgery include uncontrolled bleeding, toxic megacolon, and dysplasia.

Are There Any Specific Concerns That Need to Be Addressed Preoperatively in This Patient Population?

Patients undergoing open abdominal surgery are at increased risk for postoperative pulmonary complications, e.g., atelectasis, pneumonia, respiratory failure, and prolonged mechanical ventilation. Patients with chronic obstructive pulmonary disease should be assessed and optimized as outlined in Chap. 14 and patients who smoke should be offered counseling on stopping. The preoperative visit may also be an opportune time for patient education on breathing exercises such as incentive spirometry.

Patients with IBD may have chronic anemia from persistent gastrointestinal bleeding, may have active infection, or can be immunosuppressed from medication. Laboratory investigations should be directed accordingly.

Patients with ankylosing spondylitis require a thorough airway assessment, including range of neck motion evaluation. The plan for intubation should be discussed with the patient.

Patients requiring a stoma will require counseling and education. Preoperative education is associated with fewer stoma-related postoperative complications and earlier hospital discharge [22, 23]. Stoma site selection can also be performed at the preoperative anesthesia visit, ideally in collaboration between the patient, the stoma nurse, and the surgeon.

How Is Nutritional Status Assessed Preoperatively?

Malnutrition is an independent risk factor for postoperative complications including poor surgical wound healing and prolonged ventilation. It is seen in up to 70% of patients with inflammatory bowel disease [24, 25]. Body mass index (BMI), unintentional weight loss, body fat percentage, and reduced dietary intake are commonly used clinical measures of nutritional status. Serum albumin (<30 g/L), prealbumin, transferrin, total cholesterol, and triiodothyronine (T3) can be used as surrogate serologic markers of nutritional status [25]. Oral nutritional supplements may be required preoperatively and if the patient's caloric needs (which are typically high due to malnutrition and the need to boost nutritional status before surgery) cannot be met using oral supplementation, enteral nutrition through a nasogastric or nasoenteric tube may be indicated. Guidelines issued by the European Society for Clinical Nutrition and Metabolism (ESPEN) recommend delaying surgery for 1–2 weeks if malnutrition is identified in IBD patients to allow enteral nutrition to be commenced [26]. Our approach is to screen patients with the Canadian Nutrition Screening Tool [27]. A dietician is consulted if the patient is flagged with this tool. If there is no weight gain with outpatient dietician support, enteral nutrition is commenced. The enteral route is preferred unless there is a strong indication for parenteral feeding, e.g., complete obstruction.

What Perioperative Precautions Should Be Taken for Venous Thromboembolism Prophylaxis in the Patient with Crohn's Disease?

Patients with IBD having intra-abdominal surgery are at increased of thromboembolism compared with patients without IBD and that includes patients having surgery for abdominal neoplasms. No guidelines have been published for VTE prophylaxis in this specific population. It is recommended that patients with Crohn's disease receive VTE prophylaxis based on American College of Chest Physicians Evidence-Based Clinical Practice Guidelines (eighth Edition), i.e., for laparotomy, 5000u subcutaneous unfractionated heparin three times daily or 40 mg subcutaneous enoxaparin once daily [11, 28].

How Should This Patient Be Educated Regarding Postoperative Pain Control?

This patient uses opioid analgesia on a regular basis preoperatively. Postoperative opioid requirements will likely be higher than in the opioid naïve patient and she is at risk for chronic postsurgical pain and chronic postsurgical opioid use [29, 30]. As a regular cannabis smoker, she may have more difficulty with postoperative analgesia and may have increased opioid requirements [31, 32].

A thorough history of opioid consumption is required including average consumption of "as required" opioids taken daily, in this case oxycodone. She should be advised to continue using her fentanyl patch throughout the perioperative period. For more complex surgeries with large fluid shifts, contingencies need to be made for incomplete absorption. If this is the case, transdermal fentanyl should be replaced with equipotent morphine or hydromorphone. There is evidence to suggest that opioid-tolerant patients are resistant to local anesthetic nerve blockade [33, 34]. Dosing of adjunctive opioid and non-opioid analgesia will need to be adjusted accordingly if a regional anesthesia technique is used, e.g., epidural analgesia or continuous transversus abdominis plane nerve blockade.

Is There Evidence That NSAID Use Is a Risk Factor for Disease Exacerbation?

NSAIDs are usually associated with aggravation of preexisting disease and are occasionally implicated in the development of new-onset colitis [35, 36]. A number of studies and reports examine the association between NSAID use and worsening of Crohn's disease, the mechanism likely being related to cyclooxygenase inhibition and disruption of the gut epithelium [35, 37]. Results are conflicting; there is some evidence than infrequent use, i.e., less than 5 times per month is not associated with disease exacerbation [38, 39]. Conversely, a number of studies find that NSAIDs provoke existing Crohn's disease [40, 41]. Unfortunately, most studies have small subject numbers, are of mediocre quality, and do not make a meaningful contribution to the dialogue. Given this paucity of evidence in favor of NSAID use, it may be prudent to avoid their use when possible. If recourse to

NSAID use is deemed necessary, a low dose of drug for a short period of time is recommended. This should also be discussed with the colorectal surgery team.

What Are the Preoperative Considerations in a Patient Who Smokes Marijuana on a Daily Basis?

The chronic effects of smoking marijuana on a daily basis include cough and chronic obstructive pulmonary disease, similar to that seen in chronic tobacco smokers (Table 24.3) [42]. Chronic marijuana smokers may be at higher risk of developing atheromatous disease due to the relatively high amount of carbon monoxide in marijuana cigarettes [43]. Risk of myocardial infarction has been shown to be elevated 4.8 times over baseline in the 60 minutes after marijuana use [44]. Consideration should be given to delaying elective surgery for over 1 hour if this becomes evident.

Cannabis withdrawal syndrome can develop within 24 hours of cessation for high-dose chronic users and can takes weeks to fully resolve [45]. Symptoms of withdrawal include irritability, anger, anxiety, aggression, insomnia, restlessness, anorexia, and abdominal cramping. Administration of benzodiazepines and synthetic tetrahydrocannabinol (THC) may be useful for improving withdrawal symptoms [42, 46].

Table 24.3 Acute and chronic physiological effects of marijuana use

	Acute effects	Chronic effects
Cardiovascular	Tachycardia Vasodilation Orthostasis	Atheromatous disease
Pulmonary	Bronchodilation Hyperreactivity Airway edema	Chronic bronchitis Emphysema
Central nervous system	Anxiolysis Anxiety Paranoia/psychosis Euphoria Dizziness Headache Memory dysfunction Analgesia	Similar to acute effects, but tolerance develops, requiring higher doses for similar effects
Gastrointestinal	Antinausea Increased appetite Abdominal pain	Hyperemesis
Endocrine	None	Gynecomastia Anovulation Galactorrhea

From Alexander and Joshi [42], with permission Taylor & Francis Ltd., http://www.tandfonline.com

Preoperative evaluation should include obtaining a history of duration, frequency, dose, and route of use. Timing of most recent use should be noted. Patients exhibiting signs of acute intoxication in the immediate preoperative period, e.g., anxiety, paranoia, psychosis may be subject to more violent emergence from anesthesia [42]. Cannabis-induced psychosis resulting from the use of high-potency THC formulations may present with a similar constellation of symptoms (fever, tachycardia, hypertension) to that seen in malignant hyperthermia, serotonin syndrome, neuroleptic malignant syndrome, or thyrotoxicosis and may be mistaken for these conditions.

Should Surgery Be Performed Laparoscopically When Feasible? Is There Any Difference in Outcomes for Laparoscopic Versus Robot-Assisted Approaches?

Technically, these approaches are more challenging in IBD than other bowel resections such as that for cancer. This is due to the inflammatory process creating phlegmons and fistulas within the mesentery. However, minimally invasive surgical approaches are recommended when possible. Laparoscopic resections are associated with significantly reduced rates of minor complications such as ileus and wound infection. They also have a markedly reduced length of hospital stay and postoperative recovery. They are associated with slightly longer operative duration – on average 30 minutes. Robotic surgery for inflammatory bowel disease is less common in Canada due to financial constraints. However, it is associated with less blood loss and fewer conversions to open procedures.

True/False Questions

1. (a) Crohn's disease is a relapsing, remitting chronic inflammatory disease which only involves the colon
   (b) Extraintestinal manifestations are rare in Crohn's disease
   (c) Ankylosing spondylitis is an extraintestinal manifestation of Crohn's disease
   (d) At least 50% of patients with Crohn's disease will eventually require surgery for associated complications
   (e) NSAID use is not a risk factor for disease exacerbation
2. (a) Glucocorticoids are frequently used as first line therapy in Crohn's disease
   (b) Glucocorticoids should never be discontinued before surgery
   (c) Azathioprine is used as a steroid-sparing agent in patients who require glucocorticoids to maintain remission

(d) Perioperative continuation of anti-TNF agents is strongly associated with postoperative complications
(e) One of the main indications for surgery in Crohn's disease is steroid dependency

References

1. Cheifetz AS. Management of active Crohn disease. JAMA. 2013;309(20):2150–8.
2. Feuerstein JD, Cheifetz AS. Crohn disease: epidemiology, diagnosis, and management. Mayo Clin Proc. 2017;92(7):1088–103.
3. Molodecky NA, Soon IS, Rabi DM, Ghali WA, Ferris M, Chernoff G, et al. Increasing incidence and prevalence of the inflammatory bowel diseases with time, based on systematic review. Gastroenterology. 2012;142(1):46–54 e42; quiz e30.
4. El-Omar E, McLean M. Gastroenterology. In: Ralston S, Penman I, Strachan M, Hobson R, editors. Davidson's principles and practice of medicine. 23rd ed. Canada: Elsevier; 2018.
5. Best WR, Becktel JM, Singleton JW, Kern F Jr. Development of a Crohn's disease activity index. National Cooperative Crohn's Disease Study. Gastroenterology. 1976;70(3):439–44.
6. Harvey RF, Bradshaw JM. A simple index of Crohn's-disease activity. Lancet. 1980;1(8167):514.
7. Yarur AJ, Strobel SG, Deshpande AR, Abreu MT. Predictors of aggressive inflammatory bowel disease. Gastroenterol Hepatol (N Y). 2011;7(10):652–9.
8. Wojcik B, Loga K, Wlodarczyk M, Sobolewska-Wlodarczyk A, Padysz M, Wisniewska-Jarosinska M. Extraintestinal manifestations of Crohn's disease. Prz Gastroenterol. 2016;11(3):218–21.
9. Orchard TR. Management of arthritis in patients with inflammatory bowel disease. Gastroenterol Hepatol (NY). 2012;8(5):327–9.
10. Regueiro M, Al HJ. Overview of the medical management of mild (low risk) Crohn disease in adults. In: Post TW, editor. UpToDate. Waltham MA: UpToDate; 2020.
11. Kumar A, Auron M, Aneja A, Mohr F, Jain A, Shen B. Inflammatory bowel disease: perioperative pharmacological considerations. Mayo Clin Proc. 2011;86(8):748–57.
12. Cheifetz A, Cullen G. Sulfasalazine and 5-aminosalicylates in the treatment of inflammatory bowel disease. In: Post TW, editor. UpToDate. Waltham, MA: UpToDate; 2020.
13. Box SA, Pullar T. Sulphasalazine in the treatment of rheumatoid arthritis. Br J Rheumatol. 1997;36(3):382–6.
14. Khan KJ, Ullman TA, Ford AC, Abreu MT, Abadir A, Marshall JK, et al. Antibiotic therapy in inflammatory bowel disease: a systematic review and meta-analysis. Am J Gastroenterol. 2011;106(4):661–73.
15. Ahmed Ali U, Martin ST, Rao AD, Kiran RP. Impact of preoperative immunosuppressive agents on postoperative outcomes in Crohn's disease. Dis Colon Rectum. 2014;57(5):663–74.
16. Liu MM, Reidy AB, Saatee S, Collard CD. Perioperative steroid management: approaches based on current evidence. Anesthesiology. 2017;127(1):166–72. https://anesthesiology.pubs.asahq.org/article.aspx?articleid=2626031.
17. Glowniak JV, Loriaux DL. A double-blind study of perioperative steroid requirements in secondary adrenal insufficiency. Surgery. 1997;121(2):123–9.
18. Gramstad L. Atracurium, vecuronium and pancuronium in end-stage renal failure. Dose-response properties and interactions with azathioprine. Br J Anaesth. 1987;59(8):995–1003.
19. Lightner AL, Shen B. Perioperative use of immunosuppressive medications in patients with Crohn's disease in the new "biological era". Gastroenterol Rep (Oxf). 2017;5(3):165–77.
20. Yang ZP, Hong L, Wu Q, Wu KC, Fan DM. Preoperative infliximab use and postoperative complications in Crohn's disease: a systematic review and meta-analysis. Int J Surg. 2014;12(3):224–30.
21. Shim HH, Ma C, Kotze PG, Seow CH, Al-Farhan H, Al-Darmaki AK, et al. Preoperative ustekinumab treatment is not associated with increased postoperative complications in Crohn's Disease: a Canadian multi-centre observational cohort study. J Can Assoc Gastroenterol. 2018;1(3):115–23.
22. Chaudhri S, Brown L, Hassan I, Horgan AF. Preoperative intensive, community-based vs. traditional stoma education: a randomized, controlled trial. Dis Colon Rectum. 2005;48(3):504–9.
23. Nagle D, Pare T, Keenan E, Marcet K, Tizio S, Poylin V. Ileostomy pathway virtually eliminates readmissions for dehydration in new ostomates. Dis Colon Rectum. 2012;55(12):1266–72.
24. Grass F, Pache B, Martin D, Hahnloser D, Demartines N, Hubner M. Preoperative nutritional conditioning of Crohn's patients-systematic review of current evidence and practice. Nutrients. 2017;9(6)
25. Stoner PL, Kamel A, Ayoub F, Tan S, Iqbal A, Glover SC, et al. Perioperative care of patients with inflammatory bowel disease: focus on nutritional support. Gastroenterol Res Pract. 2018;2018:7890161.
26. Forbes A, Escher J, Hebuterne X, Klek S, Krznaric Z, Schneider S, et al. ESPEN guideline: clinical nutrition in inflammatory bowel disease. Clin Nutr. 2017;36(2):321–47.
27. Canadian Nutrition Society. Canadian Nutrition Screening Tool 2014. Available from: https://nutritioncareincanada.ca/sites/default/uploads/files/CNST.pdf. Accessed 8 Jun 2020.
28. Douketis JD, Spyropoulos AC, Spencer FA, Mayr M, Jaffer AK, Eckman MH, et al. Perioperative management of antithrombotic therapy: antithrombotic therapy and prevention of thrombosis, 9th ed: American College of Chest Physicians Evidence-Based Clinical Practice Guidelines. Chest. 2012;141(2 Suppl):e326S–e50S.
29. Huang A, Azam A, Segal S, Pivovarov K, Katznelson G, Ladak SS, et al. Chronic postsurgical pain and persistent opioid use following surgery: the need for a transitional pain service. Pain Manag. 2016;6(5):435–43.
30. Clarke H, Soneji N, Ko DT, Yun L, Wijeysundera DN. Rates and risk factors for prolonged opioid use after major surgery: population based cohort study. BMJ. 2014;348:g1251.
31. Jamal N, Korman J, Musing M, Malavade A, Coleman BL, Siddiqui N, et al. Effects of pre-operative recreational smoked cannabis use on opioid consumption following inflammatory bowel disease surgery: a historical cohort study. Eur J Anaesthesiol. 2019;36(9):705–6.
32. Jefferson DA, Harding HE, Cawich SO, Jackson-Gibson A. Postoperative analgesia in the Jamaican cannabis user. J Psychoactive Drugs. 2013;45(3):227–32.
33. Vosoughian M, Dabbagh A, Rajaei S, Maftuh H. The duration of spinal anesthesia with 5% lidocaine in chronic opium abusers compared with nonabusers. Anesth Analg. 2007;105(2):531–3.
34. Brennan TJ, Lennertz RC, Kang S. Are opioid-tolerant patients resistant to local anesthetic nerve blockade?: we need more information. Anesthesiology. 2016;125(4):625–6.
35. Takeuchi K, Smale S, Premchand P, Maiden L, Sherwood R, Thjodleifsson B, et al. Prevalence and mechanism of nonsteroidal anti-inflammatory drug-induced clinical relapse in patients with inflammatory bowel disease. Clin Gastroenterol Hepatol. 2006;4(2):196–202.
36. Puspok A, Kiener HP, Oberhuber G. Clinical, endoscopic, and histologic spectrum of nonsteroidal anti-inflammatory drug-induced lesions in the colon. Dis Colon Rectum. 2000;43(5):685–91.
37. Singh S, Graff LA, Bernstein CN. Do NSAIDs, antibiotics, infections, or stress trigger flares in IBD? Am J Gastroenterol. 2009;104(5):1298–313; quiz 314.

38. Long MD, Kappelman MD, Martin CF, Chen W, Anton K, Sandler RS. Role of nonsteroidal anti-inflammatory drugs in exacerbations of inflammatory bowel disease. J Clin Gastroenterol. 2016;50(2):152–6.
39. Bernstein CN, Singh S, Graff LA, Walker JR, Miller N, Cheang M. A prospective population-based study of triggers of symptomatic flares in IBD. Am J Gastroenterol. 2010;105(9) 1994–2002.
40. Felder JB, Korelitz BI, Rajapakse R, Schwarz S, Horatagis AP, Gleim G. Effects of nonsteroidal antiinflammatory drugs on inflammatory bowel disease: a case-control study. Am J Gastroenterol. 2000;95(8):1949–54.
41. Evans JM, McMahon AD, Murray FE, McDevitt DG, MacDonald TM. Non-steroidal anti-inflammatory drugs are associated with emergency admission to hospital for colitis due to inflammatory bowel disease. Gut. 1997;40(5):619–22.
42. Alexander JC, Joshi GP. A review of the anesthetic implications of marijuana use. Proc (Bayl Univ Med Cent). 2019;32(3):364–71.
43. Ashton CH. Adverse effects of cannabis and cannabinoids. Br J Anaesth. 1999;83(4):637–49.
44. Mittleman MA, Lewis RA, Maclure M, Sherwood JB, Muller JE. Triggering myocardial infarction by marijuana. Circulation. 2001;103(23):2805–9.
45. Budney AJ, Hughes JR, Moore BA, Vandrey R. Review of the validity and significance of cannabis withdrawal syndrome. Am J Psychiatry. 2004;161(11):1967–77.
46. Allsop DJ, Copeland J, Lintzeris N, Dunlop AJ, Montebello M, Sadler C, et al. Nabiximols as an agonist replacement therapy during cannabis withdrawal: a randomized clinical trial. JAMA Psychiat. 2014;71(3):281–91.

Carcinoid Tumor

25

Derek Dillane and Ryan Snelgrove

A 62-year-old male scheduled for ileocolic resection presented for preoperative optimization. He had a history of several months of crampy abdominal pain and obstructive symptoms. CT abdomen identified a desmoplastic mass in the small bowel mesentery encasing the major blood vessels to the right colon. Recent colonoscopy showed mild right-sided ischemic colitis and a stricture of the ileum. Biopsy of the ileal lesion identified a carcinoid tumor. A surgical approach to management was decided upon because of obstructive symptoms and worry for progressive ischemia.

He had a background history of hypertension, diabetes mellitus type 2, and COPD.

Medications: Fluticasone/salmeterol inhaler, ramipril, aspirin, atorvastatin, furosemide, metformin, and gliclazide.

Physical Examination: The patient weighed 68 kg. His vital signs and oxygen saturation were normal. Physical examination was otherwise unremarkable.

What Are Carcinoid Tumors?

Carcinoid tumors are relatively rare neuroendocrine tumors most commonly arising from the gastrointestinal (GI) tract (60% of carcinoid tumors) followed by the bronchopulmonary system (27%) and most infrequently the kidneys and ovaries [1, 2]. The breakdown according to location for carcinoid tumors within the GI tract is as follows: small intestine (34%), rectum (23%), colon (19%), stomach (8%), and appendix (7%) [3]. The incidence of carcinoid tumor is approximately 2.5–5 per 100,000—this represents 0.49% of all malignancies [1].

Do All Patients with a Carcinoid Tumor Have Carcinoid Syndrome?

No. Carcinoid tumors are capable of secreting a range of GI peptides, e.g., insulin, somatostatin, glucagon, and gastrin as well as vasoactive substances such as serotonin, bradykinin, histamine, and tachykinins. Carcinoid syndrome results from systemic secretion of these vasoactive substances.

About 10–20% of patients with a carcinoid tumor display symptoms and signs of carcinoid syndrome, i.e., flushing, diarrhea, hypotension, hypertension, and bronchoconstriction [4, 5]. Flushing and diarrhea are the most common symptoms. Flushing is characterized by being of sudden onset, and can be precipitated by stress, exercise, alcohol, and certain foods or medications (discussed in detail below). Most patients with carcinoid syndrome have liver metastases in addition to a primary carcinoid tumor. Normally, serotonin is metabolized to 5-hydroxyindolacetic acid (5-HIAA) for renal excretion. In the presence of hepatic carcinoid metastases, this metabolic pathway is saturated by the large quantities of serotonin produced. More infrequently, a primary neuroendocrine tumor in the lung gives rise to carcinoid syndrome without liver metastases. In this instance, the vasoactive products produced by the tumor bypass the liver and thus are not inactivated.

How Do Carcinoid Tumors Present?

Patients may present with the typical symptoms of carcinoid syndrome, symptoms related to the mechanical effects of a tumor mass, e.g., bowel obstruction or hepatomegaly, or symptoms of carcinoid heart disease. Occasionally carcinoid tumors are discovered incidentally during investigation and work-up for other conditions.

D. Dillane (✉)
Department of Anesthesiology & Pain Medicine, University of Alberta, Edmonton, AB, Canada

R. Snelgrove
Department of Surgery, University of Alberta, Edmonton, AB, Canada

D. Dillane, B. A. Finegan (eds.), *Preoperative Assessment*, https://doi.org/10.1007/978-3-030-58842-7_25

How Is a Diagnosis of Carcinoid Syndrome Confirmed?

24-hour urinary excretion of 5-HIAA, the end-product of serotonin metabolism, has a sensitivity and specificity of over 90% for diagnosis of carcinoid syndrome.

What Is Carcinoid Heart Disease?

Carcinoid tumors can affect the heart in several ways. Twenty percent of carcinoid syndrome patients will initially *present* with cardiac symptoms. Carcinoid heart disease occurs in up to 50% of patients with carcinoid syndrome [6]. Most patients with cardiac manifestations have hepatic carcinoid metastases. Elevated levels of serotonin and other vasoactive amines can precipitate vasovagal syncope, arrhythmias, and pulmonary hypertension. Endocardial deposition of plaque-like fibrous tissue in the valves and myocardium of the right side of the heart causes myocardial fibrosis, and tricuspid and pulmonary valve dysfunction. Valvular regurgitation is the most common manifestation. The left side of the heart is normally spared due to metabolism of excess circulating serotonin by pulmonary monoamine oxidase. Left-sided cardiac involvement may indicate an intracardiac shunt, severe or poorly controlled carcinoid activity overwhelming pulmonary metabolism capability, or an endobronchial tumor. The incidence of left-sided heart involvement is 5–10% of carcinoid heart disease [1, 6].

What Are the Clinical Manifestations of Carcinoid Heart Disease?

Cardiac-specific symptoms are frequently related to tricuspid and pulmonary regurgitation. Mild to moderate tricuspid regurgitation is usually asymptomatic. Patients with severe disease may display symptoms of right heart failure, e.g., peripheral edema, ascites, or painful hepatosplenomegaly. Similarly, patients with pulmonary regurgitation can be asymptomatic until the onset of right ventricular dysfunction at which time patients may display exertional dyspnea and fatigue, as well as atrial or ventricular arrhythmias giving rise to palpitations or syncope. Enlargement of the right ventricle can cause tricuspid regurgitation, if not already present, due to carcinoid fibrous deposits.

Though valvular involvement is the dominant clinical presentation, atypical presentations of carcinoid heart disease have been reported; coronary artery vasospasm with ST segment elevation, atrial fibrillation, ventricular tachycardia and fibrillation, and cardiac arrest have all been reported as the primary presenting feature [7–10].

What Is a Carcinoid Crisis?

This is a potentially fatal exacerbation of carcinoid syndrome that arises from the uncontrolled release of an overwhelming number of vasoactive hormones. This can be spontaneous or secondary to tumor handling, stress, administration of certain anesthetic agents (Boxes 25.1 and 25.2), or tumor necrosis caused by chemotherapy [1]. It is manifest clinically as intense flushing, edema, severe bronchospasm, and significant hemodynamic instability, including tachycardia, hypotension, or hypertension, which may be refractory to treatment.

How Are Carcinoid Tumors Treated?

Definitive treatment will depend on whether the disease is localized or metastatic. The presence of liver metastases is the most important factor affecting survival in patients with GI or pancreatic neuroendocrine tumors [11]. The liver is the most common site for metastasis due to hematogenous spread via the portal venous drainage of the GI tract and pancreas [12]. Liver metastases have been reported in up to 85% of patients with a primary neuroendocrine tumor, although a more conservative estimate puts the incidence closer to 40% [13, 14]. Radiographic staging is commonly performed using CT, MRI, or somatostatin receptor imaging. Localized GI and bronchial carcinoid tumors are surgically resected even

Box 25.1 Drugs associated with carcinoid crisis

- Succinylcholine
- Atracurium
- Mivacurium
- Thiopental
- Epinephrine
- Norepinephrine
- Dopamine
- Isoproterenol

Box 25.2 Drugs thought to be safe in patients with carcinoid syndrome

- Propofol
- Etomidate
- Vecuronium
- Cisatracurium
- Rocuronium
- Fentanyl/remifentanil/alfentanil/sufentanil
- All inhalation agents

in the presence of liver metastases If possible, surgical resection of liver metastases provides the best opportunity for long-term survival. However, fewer than 20% of patients with metastatic liver disease are eligible for metastasectomy or partial liver resection, due to wide dissemination of metastases or the expectation that liver volume after resection will be inadequate [11]. Somatostatin analogs can be used for symptomatic treatment in patients with unresectable liver metastases. A variety of liver-directed therapies can be explored when liver disease is unresectable, e.g., thermal ablation, embolization, and cytotoxic chemotherapy [11].

How Are Patients with Carcinoid Tumors Optimized for Surgery?

Preoperative evaluation should consist of (1) determining the presence and/or extent of carcinoid syndrome, i.e., severity of symptoms related to vasoactive peptide release, and (2) presence and/or extent of cardiac disease. Patients with persistent diarrhea require electrolyte and creatinine measurement with subsequent volume resuscitation and correction of electrolyte abnormalities [15]. The presence of hypoalbuminemia may require nutritional supplementation.

Abnormally elevated levels of serotonin and other vasoactive amines are surrogates of tumor burden [1]. Preoperative optimization aims to antagonize these mediators of carcinoid syndrome. The somatostatin analogs octreotide and lanreotide inhibit a wide range of vasoactive hormones by binding to the somatostatin receptors that are expressed in the majority of neuroendocrine tumors [16]. Somatostatin is a peptide hormone that regulates the endocrine system by inhibiting hormone secretion. These somatostatin analogs can control symptoms in more than 80% of patients with a carcinoid tumor [4]. Monthly depot injections of both octreotide and lanreotide are available and can be titrated for optimal symptom control. In addition to controlling vasoactive mediator release, somastatin analogs have also been shown to control tumor growth of pancreatic and GI neuroendocrine tumors [17].

Echocardiographic evaluation of valvular and ventricular dysfunction is recommended even in the absence of symptoms. As outlined above, moderate to severe carcinoid cardiac disease can be asymptomatic.

How Is Carcinoid Crisis Managed? Can Any Measures Be Taken Preoperatively to Prevent the Intraoperative Occurrence of a Carcinoid Crisis?

Octreotide can be used prophylactically and for the management of an evolving carcinoid crisis. Patients with a history of carcinoid syndrome can be given up to 500 mcg intravenously, as a bolus or by infusion, prior to surgical resection, and this can be repeated intraoperatively if required. Octreotide, 100–500 mcg intravenously can also be used to treat carcinoid crisis. Higher doses may be required in patients with previous exposure to octreotide and in patients with carcinoid heart disease [18].

Despite the lack of signs and symptoms indicative of the presence of carcinoid heart disease, an echocardiogram was obtained, as recommended. This did not show any valvular disease. The patient continued not to exhibit any symptoms or signs of carcinoid syndrome. An electrolyte screen, creatinine and liver function tests were normal on day before surgery. The patient proceeded to have an uneventful ileocolic resection.

True-False Questions

1. (a) Most carcinoid tumors originate in the gastrointestinal tract
   (b) The stomach is the commonest location in the gastrointestinal tract for a carcinoid tumor to occur
   (c) The majority of patients with a carcinoid tumor display symptoms of carcinoid syndrome
   (d) Carcinoid syndrome can be diagnosed using 24-hour urinary excretion of 5-HIAA
   (e) Octreotide can be used to prevent the occurrence of an intraoperative carcinoid crisis
2. (a) Carcinoid heart disease is commonly associated with carcinoid syndrome
   (b) Pulmonary and tricuspid valvular stenosis are the commonest valvular manifestations of carcinoid heart disease
   (c) The left and right sides of the heart are equally affected in carcinoid heart disease
   (d) Patients with severe carcinoid heart disease display symptoms of right heart failure
   (e) Most patients with carcinoid heart disease have hepatic carcinoid metastases

References

1. Castillo J, Silvay G, Weiner M. Anesthetic management of patients with carcinoid syndrome and carcinoid heart disease: the Mount Sinai Algorithm. J Cardiothorac Vasc Anesth. 2018;32(2):1023–31.
2. Bhosale P, Shah A, Wei W, Varadhachary G, Johnson V Shah V, et al. Carcinoid tumours: predicting the location of the primary neoplasm based on the sites of metastases. Eur Radiol. 2013;23(2):400–7.
3. Modlin IM, Oberg K, Chung DC, Jensen RT, de Herder WW, Thakker RV, et al. Gastroenteropancreatic neuroendocrine tumours. Lancet Oncol. 2008;9(1):61–72.
4. Tantawy H, Myslajek T. Diseases of the gastrointestinal system. In: Hines R, Marschall K, editors. Stoelting's anesthesia and co-existing disease. 7th ed. Philadelphia: Elsevier; 2017.
5. Connolly HM. Carcinoid heart disease. In: Post TW, editor. UpToDate. Waltham, MA: UpToDate; 2020.
6. Pellikka PA, Tajik AJ, Khandheria BK, Seward JB, Callahan JA, Pitot HC, et al. Carcinoid heart disease. Clinical and echocardiographic spectrum in 74 patients. Circulation. 1993;87(4):1188–96.

7. Eapen DJ, Clements S Jr, Block P, Sperling L. Metastatic carcinoid disease inducing coronary vasospasm. Tex Heart Inst J. 2012;39(1):76–8.
8. Langer C, Piper C, Vogt J, Heintze J, Butz T, Lindner O, et al. Atrial fibrillation in carcinoid heart disease: the role of serotonin. A review of the literature. Clin Res Cardiol. 2007;96(2):114–8.
9. Rupp AB, Ahmadjee A, Morshedzadeh JH, Ranjan R. Carcinoid syndrome-induced ventricular tachycardia. Case Rep Cardiol. 2016;2016:9142598.
10. Topol EJ, Fortuin NJ. Coronary artery spasm and cardiac arrest in carcinoid heart disease. Am J Med. 1984;77(5):950–2.
11. Lewis MA, Hobday TJ. Treatment of neuroendocrine tumor liver metastases. Int J Hepatol. 2012;2012:973946.
12. Riihimaki M, Hemminki A, Sundquist K, Sundquist J, Hemminki K. The epidemiology of metastases in neuroendocrine tumors. Int J Cancer. 2016;139(12):2679–86.
13. John BJ, Davidson BR. Treatment options for unresectable neuroendocrine liver metastases. Expert Rev Gastroenterol Hepatol. 2012;6(3):357–69.
14. Mayo SC, de Jong MC, Pulitano C, Clary BM, Reddy SK, Gamblin TC, et al. Surgical management of hepatic neuroendocrine tumor metastasis: results from an international multi-institutional analysis. Ann Surg Oncol. 2010;17(12):3129–36.
15. Wijeysundera DN, Finlayson E. Preoperative evaluation. In: Gropper MA, editor. Miller's anesthesia. 9th ed. Philadelphia: Elsevier; 2020. p. 918–98.
16. Reubi JC, Kvols LK, Waser B, Nagorney DM, Heitz PU, Charboneau JW, et al. Detection of somatostatin receptors in surgical and percutaneous needle biopsy samples of carcinoids and islet cell carcinomas. Cancer Res. 1990;50(18):5969–77.
17. Ang Chan J, Kulke M, Clancy T. Metastatic well-differentiated pancreatic neuroendocrine tumors: systemic therapy options to control tumor growth and symptoms of hormone hypersecretion. In: Post TW, editor. UpToDate. Waltham, MA: UpToDate; 2020.
18. Seymour N, Sawh SC. Mega-dose intravenous octreotide for the treatment of carcinoid crisis: a systematic review. Can J Anaesth. 2013;60(5):492–9.

Part VII

Renal

Chronic Kidney Disease and the Dialysis Patient

26

Stephen Young

A 64-year-old male with chronic hypercalcemia presented for elective four-gland parathyroidectomy with auto-transplantation. He had a history of end-stage kidney disease and was intermittently hemodialyzed at home via a tunnelled central venous catheter in his right internal jugular vein. Other past medical history included diabetes mellitus (DM) (type two) for the preceding 16 years, longstanding essential hypertension, four myocardial infarctions with subsequent coronary artery bypass grafting 2 years prior to this visit, gastroesophageal reflux disease, and obstructive sleep apnea requiring continuous positive airway pressure support at night. He was a non-smoker and had a body mass index of 35 kg/m². He reported good functional capacity with no exertional angina.

Medications: Novolin 70/30® insulin twice daily, Novorapid® insulin with meals, aspirin, atorvastatin, metoprolol, pantoprazole, calcitriol, sevelamer, vitamin B, vitamin C, folic acid, and iron supplementation.

Investigations: Laboratory blood results are shown in Table 26.1. *Chest radiograph showed evidence of sternotomy, tunnelled central venous catheter, and no pulmonary edema. Electrocardiogram (ECG) revealed sinus rhythm, first-degree heart block, and old anterior Q waves.*

What Is the Definition of Chronic Kidney Disease (CKD) and What Are the Common Causes?

Kidney Disease Improving Global Outcomes (KDIGO) [1] defines CKD as abnormalities of kidney structure or function, present for greater than 3 months, with implications for health (Table 26.2). CKD is classified based on cause, glomerular filtration rate (GFR), and albuminuria category. These factors also determine prognosis (Fig. 26.1).

DM and hypertension are two of the most common causes of CKD in the United States [2] and the developed world.

Table 26.1 Laboratory values at preadmission clinic visit

Test	Result	Reference range (units)
Sodium	139	134–146 (mmol/L)
Potassium	5.1	3.6–5.0 (mmol/L)
Urea	23.7	2.8–7.5 (mmol/L)
Creatinine	871	50–120 (μmol/L)
Estimated GFR	5	>59 (mL/min/1.73m²)
Calcium	2.53	2.10–2.60 (mmol/L)
Ionized Ca^{2+}	1.40	1.10–1.35 (mmol/L)
Phosphate	1.22	0.80–1.50 (mmol/L)
Magnesium	1.13	0.65–1.05 (mmol/L)
Chloride	103	98–108 (mmol/L)
Bicarbonate	24	23–29 (mmol/L)
Albumin	37	33–48 (g/L)
Intact PTH	117.0	1.4–6.8 (pmol/L)
HbA1c	6.9%	4.3–6.1 (%)
Hemoglobin	118	140–175 (g/L)
Platelet count	219	145–400 (×10⁹/L)
WBC count	5.1	4.0–10.0 (×10⁹/L)

GFR Glomerular filtration rate, *PTH* Parathyroid hormone, *WBC* white blood cell

Table 26.2 Definition of chronic kidney disease

Criteria for CKD (either of the following present for >3 months	
Markers of kidney damage (one or more)	Albuminuria (AER ≥30 mg/24 hours; ACR ≥30 mg/g [≥3 mg/mmol]) Urine sediment abnormalities Electrolyte and other abnormalities due to tubular disorders Abnormalities detected by histology Structural abnormalities detected by imaging History of kidney transplantation
Decreased GFR	GFR <60 ml/min/1.73 m² (GFR categories G3a-G5)

From Kidney Disease: Improving Global Outcomes (KDIGO) CKD Work Group [1], with permission
AER Albumin excretion rate, *ACR* Albumin-to-creatinine ratio, *GFR* Glomerular filtration rate

S. Young (✉)
Department of Anaesthesia, Hawke's Bay Fallen Soldiers' Memorial Hospital, Hastings, New Zealand

D. Dillane, B. A. Finegan (eds.), *Preoperative Assessment*, https://doi.org/10.1007/978-3-030-58842-7_26

Fig. 26.1 Prognosis of chronic kidney disease by glomerular filtration rate and albuminuria categories. Green: low risk (if no other markers of kidney disease, no CKD). Yellow: moderately increased risk. Orange: high risk. Red: very high risk. (From Kidney Disease: Improving Global Outcomes (KDIGO) CKD Work Group [1], with permission)

Prognosis of CKD by GFR and Albuminuria Categories: KDIGO 2012

				Persistent albuminuria categories Description and range		
				A1	A2	A3
				Normal to mildly increased	Moderately increased	Severely increased
				<30 mg/g <3 mg/mmol	30-300 mg/g 3-30 mg/mmol	>300 mg/g >30 mg/mmol
GFR categories (ml/min/ 1.73m^2) Description and range	G1	Normal or high	≥90			
	G2	Mildly decreased	60-89			
	G3a	Mildly to moderately decreased	45-59			
	G3b	Moderately to severely decreased	30-44			
	G4	Severely decreased	15-29			
	G5	Kidney failure	<15			

Other causes include chronic glomerulonephritis (e.g., IgA nephropathy); autoimmune diseases (e.g., systemic lupus erythematosus); genetic disorders (e.g., polycystic kidney disease); urinary tract diseases (e.g., infection, obstruction); toxin exposure (e.g., heavy metals, drugs); and infectious diseases (e.g., tuberculosis, human immunodeficiency virus, hepatitis B and C).

When Is Dialysis Indicated in CKD Patients?

KDIGO guidelines [1] and the Canadian Society of Nephrology [3] are largely in agreement in recommending that the decision to initiate renal replacement therapy (RRT) is based on signs and symptoms of CKD and the GFR. Clinical indications to commence dialysis include symptomatic uremia, fluid overload, and refractory hyperkalemia or acidemia. Asymptomatic patients with GFR of 5–15 mL/min/1.73m^2 are closely followed on a monthly basis, and dialysis is not initiated until symptoms develop that are refractory to medical therapy. Dialysis is initiated in patients with a GFR <5 mL/min/1.73m^2 irrespective of the clinical status.

What Complications Is the Patient with CKD Subject to in the Perioperative Period?

In general, morbidity and mortality are increased compared to patients without CKD.

- Cardiovascular events are increased as a result of CKD, independent of other commonly associated cardiovascular risk factors. These represent the leading cause of mortality, which increases with declining GFR [4].
- Worsening electrolyte disturbance, particularly hyperkalemia. Blood calcium levels can become high or low.
- Worsening metabolic acidosis with reduced capacity for further respiratory compensation. Work of breathing and hypoxia are further increased if pulmonary edema is present.
- Impaired sodium and water excretion can lead to hypervolemia if there is excess intravenous (IV) fluid administration. Issues with fluid and electrolyte disturbances are further worsened by sub-optimal dialysis planning.
- Acute on chronic kidney injury from multiple causes, such as ischemia (e.g., intra-operative hypotension [5], aortic cross-clamping) and known nephrotoxic drugs (e.g., non-steroidal anti-inflammatories, aminoglycoside antibiotics, IV contrast). Fluorinated volatile anesthetics such as methoxyflurane and enflurane can cause nephrotoxicity. Sevoflurane appears to be safe despite concerns with compound A production, as are isoflurane and desflurane [6].
- Bleeding due to platelet dysfunction caused by uremic toxins. Blood transfusion is more likely in the presence of pre-existing chronic anemia secondary to erythropoietin insufficiency and decreased red cell survival.

- Cognitive dysfunction and encephalopathy become more apparent in late-stage CKD [7]. Delayed emergence from anesthesia and postoperative delirium are more common than in the general population.
- Autonomic neuropathy as a result of CKD can lead to delayed gastric emptying and cardiovascular instability.
- Pain management may be difficult, as chronic pain may be present secondary to calciphylaxis (calcification of the small blood vessels of the skin and subcutaneous fat) or peripheral neuropathy due to CKD.
- Undesired or serious adverse effects from common anesthesia drugs can occur due to altered pharmacokinetics such as varied protein binding and impaired renal clearance.
- Impaired wound healing and risk of infection are increased due to impaired immunity [8].
- Complications associated with the underlying cause of CKD [9].

What Specific Considerations Should Be Evaluated During the Preoperative Assessment of CKD Patients?

Relevant history, physical examination, and investigations pertaining to the CKD illness, treatment, and associated conditions will be considered in the following sections.

Chronic Kidney Disease

The disease processes and complications due to the underlying cause of the CKD should be explored, such as the commonly associated diagnoses of DM and hypertension (see Chaps. 8 and 21).The onset, duration, and severity of CKD should be elicited, as well its complications in all other organ systems (Table 26.3) [9]. Blood urea nitrogen and creatinine

Table 26.3 Systemic complications of chronic kidney disease and cross-link

System	Common manifestations	Cardiovascular	Endocrine and metabolic	Gastrointestinal	Hematologic	Neurologic	Musculoskeletal	Integument
Cardiovascular	Atherosclerosis, hypertension, cardiomyopathy		X		X	X		
Endocrine and metabolic	Menstrual disorders, sexual dysfunction, infertility, pregnancy disorders, electrolytes, and MBD	X		X	X	X		X
Gastrointestinal	Anorexia, nausea, emesis, weight loss		X					
Hematologic	Anemia, platelets disorders, coagulopathy, low cell count, and infection risk	X		X				X
Neurologic	Neuropathy, seizures (with severe uremia), strokes	X	X					X
Musculoskeletal	MBD, fractures, myopathy	x	x			x		x
Integument	Dry skin, dermatitis, pruritis		X		X	X		
Complex symptoms[a]	Fatigue, insomnia, impotence, cachexia	X	X	X	X	X		X

From Bello et al. [9], with permission from Elsevier

HTN Hypertension, *MBD* Mineral bone disorder

X denotes a crosslink between systems, e.g., MBD contributing to cardiovascular system, anemia contributing to cardiovascular system, and interplay of all system features causing complex systems

[a]Poorly defined disorders associated with advanced chronic kidney disease

are usually ordered, as their trends are used to monitor renal function.

For pre-dialysis patients, first determine whether they have an indication for dialysis preoperatively as above. Discuss with renal medicine and postpone surgery if appropriate. For patients who need an upper limb arteriovenous fistula (AVF) formed in the future to allow for hemodialysis (HD), vessels at the wrist (radio-cephalic) or antecubital fossa (brachio-cephalic) are the most commonly chosen AVF sites. In order to preserve these veins for an AVF, dorsal veins of the hands are preferred for IV cannulation.

Establish whether the patient is being considered for kidney transplantation. Avoiding allogenic blood transfusions is particularly important, as alloimmunization of human leukocyte antigens affects future graft success [10].

In addition to the presence of poor physical health and nutrition, CKD is a chronic illness with a significant psychosocial impact on the patient. Ensure that these are also evaluated.

Dialysis

Obtain history regarding the commencement of dialysis, complications, and previous and current treatment regimes. Usual routes are either HD through an AVF or a central venous catheter (CVC), or peritoneal dialysis through an intra-peritoneal catheter. IV cannula insertion, phlebotomy, and blood pressure cuff placement should be avoided on the ipsilateral limb with an AVF. Superior vena cava or subclavian vein stenosis may be present due to previous repeated CVC insertions [11].

Determine the patient's weekly dialysis schedule in order to plan perioperative dialysis effectively. Discuss with renal medicine if required.

Electrolyte and Metabolic Abnormalities

Laboratory blood testing to check for any electrolyte disturbances is necessary, even for minor surgery. Hyperkalemia is common and can be life threatening because blood potassium (K^+) excretion is decreased due to impaired renal tubular function. Previous hyperkalemic events should be noted, as some patients may be more prone than others. Symptoms and signs of severe hyperkalemia include dyspnea, palpitations, paresthesias, nausea, bradycardia, muscle weakness, and depressed tendon reflexes. Early ECG changes include narrow peaked T waves, short QT interval, and ST depression. With worsening hyperkalemia, P waves become absent, QRS interval widens, and conduction block develops. Terminally, the QRS complex and T wave merge into a sine wave, culminating in cardiac arrest. Hypermagnesemia usually coincides with a rise in blood potassium.

Reduced production of active vitamin D_3 (calcitriol) leads to hypocalcemia, hyperphosphatemia, secondary hyperparathyroidism, and renal osteodystrophy. Tertiary hyperparathyroidism and hypercalcemia develop after longstanding secondary hyperparathyroidism. Although hypercalcemia may be managed by dialysis and medications in this setting, parathyroidectomy is the treatment of choice for long-term control, as the hyperparathyroidism itself continues to contribute to renal osteodystrophy.

Symptoms and signs of hypercalcemia include lethargy, confusion, abdominal pain, nausea, constipation, and hypotonia. Severe complications include coma and cardiac arrhythmias (from shortened QT interval to complete heart block). Sodium and chloride levels are usually within the normal range. Hyponatremia may coincide with hypervolemia.

Arterial blood gases may show chronic metabolic acidosis with respiratory compensation. Blood albumin level may be low due to proteinuria, malnutrition, inflammation, or other concurrent diseases. Hypoalbuminemia will produce a higher ionized blood calcium for a given total blood calcium. Low albumin is a predictor for poor postoperative outcomes [12].

Fluid Status

Patients on dialysis usually have a target or dry weight (baseline euvolemic weight) to which they are dialyzed. Any acute and significant weight gain preoperatively most likely indicates an increase in total body water. Other symptoms and signs of fluid overload include increased dyspnea, hypertension, elevated jugular venous pressure (JVP), and peripheral and pulmonary edema.

Chest radiograph may show signs of cardiac failure, e.g., cardiomegaly, pleural effusions, and pulmonary vascular congestion.

The ability to concentrate or dilute urine is impaired. Some patients, even while on dialysis, can still produce a "normal" amount of urine per day. This may mean a urinary catheter is required perioperatively. Caution is needed when interpreting urine output as marker of intravascular fluid status.

Cardiovascular System

With accelerated atherosclerosis and associated cardiovascular diseases (e.g., hypertension, DM) being major underlying causes of CKD, a thorough cardiovascular and respiratory assessment is required. Importantly, the severity and stability of cardiopulmonary pathologies need to be established, along with functional status. The latest American College of

Cardiology/American Heart Association guidelines should be employed (discussed in Chap. 2) [13].

Symptoms and signs such as angina, dyspnea, orthopnea, palpitations, syncope, peripheral edema, lethargy, postural hypotension, elevated JVP, displaced apex beat, cardiac murmurs, extra heart sounds, and pulmonary edema should be explored at a minimum.

Plasma cardiac troponin and brain-natriuretic peptide levels help to assess dyspnea, ischemic heart disease (IHD), left ventricular (LV) strain, and perioperative risk stratification. However, levels need to be interpreted carefully in the setting of declining GFR and dialysis [14]. Obtaining preoperative baseline levels assists with interpreting postoperative trends.

Baseline ECG without hyperkalemia may show pre-existing conduction abnormalities (e.g., arrhythmias, heart block), decreased R-R variability (from autonomic dysfunction), and left ventricular hypertrophy (LVH).

Bedside echocardiography is useful to assess patients with valvular heart disease and cardiac failure. LVH is common [4] and its extent can be quantified. LV ejection fraction can be calculated, along with evidence of any diastolic dysfunction. Rarely, uremic pericarditis may be present [15].

Bleeding and Blood Loss

Any history of bleeding diathesis should be sought, and a complete blood count ordered as a minimum. Chronic anemia is ubiquitous and usually physiologically compensated. Blood transfusion may be required, depending on the surgery. A blood group and screen should be considered.

Platelet levels are typically within the normal range, but platelet dysfunction occurs due to the presence of uremic toxins. In vitro laboratory tests such as partial thromboplastin time and international normalized ratio are usually within normal limits. The effects of CKD on in vivo coagulation and fibrinolytic pathways are complex. Patients are usually considered to be in a prothrombotic state [6].

Neuraxial anesthesia techniques are generally considered safe in uremic patients with no other coagulopathy. Benefits and risks should be tailored to each patient.

Surgical Factors

If a pre-dialysis patient is due to undergo major surgery with a high likelihood of requiring RRT postoperatively (e.g., supra-inguinal vascular surgery), the patient may benefit from a dialysis CVC inserted before surgery. This possibility should be discussed with relevant specialties, such as renal and intensive care medicine.

For peritoneal dialysis patients undergoing intra-abdominal surgery, an alternative route of dialysis is required postoperatively. For patients needing bowel preparation preoperatively, phosphate-based preparations may cause acute phosphate nephropathy and are not recommended [1]. If surgery is for AVF formation, assess the patient's suitability for regional anesthesia, as it may provide better fistula outcomes [16].

What Medications Should We Expect to See in the Preoperative CKD Patient?

- Angiotensin-converting enzyme (ACE) inhibitors and angiotensin II receptor blockers (ARBs) slow the progression of CKD, particularly in patients with proteinuria [4]. They are also used as anti-hypertensives. However, they can contribute to nephrotoxicity and may cause potassium retention.
- Loop diuretics are used to prevent hypervolemia and hypertension, as well as to promote the urinary excretion of potassium.
- Statins are used for treatment of dyslipidemia and to lower cardiovascular risk, especially in patients with established IHD. They may decrease proteinuria [4].
- Erythropoiesis-stimulating agents (ESA), iron, folate, and vitamin B12 can be used to treat anemia once hemoglobin level drops below 100 g/L. Over-treatment of hemoglobin back to the normal range is paradoxically detrimental due to the increased risk of thrombotic events [10]. ESA and the improvement in red cell mass help to reduce uremic bleeding [17].
- Vitamin D_3 and calcium for treatment of hypocalcemia and secondary hyperparathyroidism.
- Dietary phosphate binders for treatment of hyperphosphatemia. Older preparations containing aluminum hydroxide should not be given with sodium citrate. Increased aluminum absorption can occur when they are given together, causing neuro-toxicity [18].
- Bicarbonate for treatment of metabolic acidosis when blood bicarbonate levels reach <22 mmol/L [1].

How Should CKD Patients Be Optimized Prior to Elective Surgery?

Optimization of associated cardiovascular risk factors such as hypertension and DM is advisable. Cases involving symptomatic and unstable IHD, arrhythmias, valvular lesions, and cardiac failure should be discussed with the cardiology service.

Ensure the patient is euvolemic and has no significant electrolyte abnormalities. Dialysis patients should be close to their dry weight. A repeat check of blood electrolyte levels on the day of surgery should be considered in all patients.

Patients normally on HD should be dialyzed within 24 hours before elective surgery but not immediately before. Hypotension, hypoxemia, neutropenia, coagulopathy, and dialysis disequilibrium syndrome [19] are possible immediately after HD.

Guidance from renal medicine should be sought regarding the need for additional treatments for peritoneal dialysis patients prior to surgery [20]. Dialysate should be drained to decrease intra-abdominal pressure on the day of surgery.

Other causes of chronic anemia, e.g., iron deficiency anemia, should be identified and managed to ensure optimal red cell mass, thus reducing the need for blood transfusion.

Minimization of perioperative blood loss is paramount. Any coexisting coagulopathy should be identified and corrected. In addition to ESA and dialysis, specific treatments to reduce uremic bleeding include desmopressin, cryoprecipitate, and conjugated estrogens [17].

The risk of perioperative thrombosis versus bleeding should be considered when deciding whether to cease aspirin therapy preoperatively. It would be safe to withhold aspirin preoperatively in CKD patients with low risk of thrombosis. The continued administration of aspirin perioperatively has been associated with increased bleeding, while having no benefit in reducing a composite of death and non-fatal myocardial infarction [21].

Diuretic medications are normally withheld on the day of surgery. However, if the patient is due to undergo minor day surgery, diuretics may be continued to help maintain euvolemia and potassium excretion postoperatively.

ACE inhibitors and ARBs should be withheld on the day of surgery to prevent intra-operative hypotension.

Pharmacological kidney protection such as the administration of N-acetyl cysteine, sodium bicarbonate, loop diuretics, mannitol, and dopamine have been studied. No clear benefit has been shown for these therapies [22].

Appropriate antibiotic prophylaxis should be prescribed to prevent surgical site infections.

Patients with suspected delayed gastric emptying should be treated with aspiration prophylaxis.

A CKD Patient on Dialysis Presents for Surgery with a K+ of 6.2 mmol/L. How Would You Proceed?

Ensure that this result is from a recent sample. Blood K^+ level may have increased further with elapsed time. Check whether the blood sample is hemolyzed — release of potassium from red blood cells will give a falsely high K^+. Concurrent 12-lead ECG should be reviewed and compared to the patient's baseline ECG.

There is currently no established consensus as to what constitutes a safe level of K^+ prior to elective surgery. The decision will mainly be based on the chronicity of the hyperkalemia for the particular patient (increased tolerance to ECG changes) and the type of surgery (anticipated tissue damage and metabolic impact). Generally, a K^+ of ≤5.5 mmol/L would be acceptable to proceed with elective surgery. Consider postponing surgery if K^+ is >6.0 mmol/L with ECG changes where urgent preoperative dialysis is not feasible. A multidisciplinary discussion is vital. Ensure improved preoperative optimization prior to rescheduled surgery.

Similar considerations apply for emergency surgery. The urgency of surgery largely dictates the preoperative management. Surgery can proceed if K^+ is ≤6.0 mmol/L with no ECG changes, as this should be tolerated well by most patients. Patients with a K^+ >6.0 mmol/L and ECG changes should be dialyzed preoperatively if possible. Dialysis for 2 hours can sufficiently improve hyperkalemia and reverse ECG changes [20]. Ensure that anticoagulation is not used or that it has been reversed to prevent subsequent surgical bleeding. If dialysis before emergency surgery is not feasible or if the hyperkalemia worsens intra-operatively, pharmacological treatment and physiological manipulation are required until the patient can receive RRT postoperatively. It may be possible to provide continuous RRT intra-operatively in exceptional cases.

The acute management of severe hyperkalemia is summarized in Table 26.4 [23]. In addition, mechanical hyperventilation in intubated patients can help temporize hyperkalemia by compensating for metabolic acidosis, shifting K^+ back into cells.

True/False Questions

1. (a) Perioperative risk of cardiovascular events is increased in CKD patients.
   (b) Tertiary hyperparathyroidism causes hypocalcemia and hypophosphatemia.
   (c) Indications for dialysis in CKD patients include refractory hyperkalemia and fluid overload.
   (d) Daily urine production reduces in proportion to declining GFR.
   (e) ACE inhibitor therapy helps decrease proteinuria in CKD patients.
2. (a) Treatment of anemia in CKD patients should aim for a target hemoglobin level back in the normal reference range.
   (b) For elective surgery, end-stage CKD patients should be dialyzed immediately before surgery to achieve optimal fluid and electrolyte status.
   (c) CKD patients with a preoperative K^+ level of 6.0 mmol/L should always have their surgery postponed.
   (d) ECG signs of severe hyperkalemia include absent P waves, QRS interval widening, and conduction block.
   (e) The prevention of uremic bleeding involves the infusion of functional allogenic platelets.

Table 26.4 Management of acute hyperkalemia

Medication	Response type	Onset of action	Duration of action	Mechanism of action	Expected decrease in potassium level
Calcium gluconate	Rapid	1–2 min	30–60 min	Protect cardiomyocytes	
Glucose + insulin	Intermediate	10–20 min	2–6 h	Shift potassium intracellularly	0.5–1.5 mEq/L (dose dependent)
Beta-agonists	Intermediate	3–5 min	1–4 h	Shift potassium intracellularly	0.5–1.5 mEq/L (dose dependent)
Sodium bicarbonate (only in patients with metabolic acidosis, bicarbonate <22 mEq/L	Intermediate	30–60 min	2–6 h	Shift potassium intracellularly (questionable effect)	
Exchange resin	Delayed	2–6 h	4–6 h	Elimination of potassium from the body	
Furosemide	Delayed	5–30 min	2–6 h	Elimination of potassium from the body	
Hemodialysis	Delayed	Immediate		Elimination of potassium from the body	1 mmol/L in the first 60 min and total of 2 mmol/L by 180 min

Modified from Mushiyakh et al. [22]), with permission. © Yelena Mushiyakh et al. taken from the *Journal of Community Hospital Internal Medicine Perspectives*. Published by Informa UK Limited, trading as Taylor & Francis Group on behalf of Greater Baltimore Medical Center

References

1. Kidney Disease: Improving Global Outcomes (KDIGO) CKD Work Group. KDIGO 2012 Clinical practice guideline for the evaluation and management of chronic kidney disease. Kidney Int. 2013;3(Suppl):1–150.
2. Centers for Disease Control and Prevention. Chronic kidney disease Initiative website. https://www.cdc.gov/kidneydisease/basics.html. Accessed 13 Feb 2019.
3. Nesrallah GE, Mustafa RA, Clark WF, Bass A, Barnieh L, Hemmelgarn BR, et al.; Canadian Society of Nephrology. Canadian Society of Nephrology 2014 clinical practice guideline for timing the initiation of chronic dialysis. CMAJ. 2014;186(2):112–7.
4. Gansevoort RT, Correa-Rotter R, Hemmelgarn BR, Jafar TH, Heerspink HJ, Mann JF, et al. Chronic kidney disease and cardiovascular risk: epidemiology, mechanisms, and prevention. Lancet. 2013;382(9889):339–52.
5. Sun LY, Wijeysundera DN, Tait GA, Beattie WS. Association of intraoperative hypotension with acute kidney injury after elective noncardiac surgery. Anesthesiology. 2015;123(3):515–23.
6. Craig RG, Hunter JM. Recent developments in the perioperative management of adult patients with chronic kidney disease. Br J Anaesth. 2008;101(3):296–310.
7. Arnold R, Issar T, Krishnan AV, Pussell BA. Neurological complications in chronic kidney disease. JRSM Cardiovasc Dis. 2016;5:2048004016677687.
8. Maroz N, Simman R. Wound healing in patients with impaired kidney function. J Am Coll Clin Wound Spec. 2013;5(1):2–7.
9. Bello AK, Alrukhaimi M, Ashuntantang GE, Basnet S, Rotter RC, Douthat WG, et al. Complications of chronic kidney disease: current state, knowledge gaps, and strategy for action. Kidney Int Suppl (2011). 2017;7(2):122–9.
10. KDIGO. Clinical practice guideline for anemia in chronic kidney disease. Kidney Int Suppl. 2012;2(4):288–335.
11. Khanna S, Sniderman K, Simons M, et al. Superior vena cava stenosis associated with hemodialysis catheter. Am J Kidney Dis. 1993;21(3):278–81.
12. Oh TK, Lee J, Hwang JW, Do SH, Jeon YT, Kim JH, et al. Value of preoperative modified body mass index in predicting postoperative 1-year mortality. Sci Rep. 2018;8(1):4614.
13. Fleisher LA, Fleischmann KE, Auerbach AD, Barnason SA, Beckman JA, Bozkurt B, et al. ACC/AHA guideline on perioperative cardiovascular evaluation and management of patients undergoing noncardiac surgery: a report of the American College of Cardiology/American Heart Association Task Force on Practice Guidelines. Circulation. 2014;9:130(24):e278–333.
14. Wang AY, Lai KN. Use of cardiac biomarkers in end-stage renal disease. J Am Soc Nephrol. 2008;19(9):1643–52.
15. Rehman KA, Betancor J, Xu B, Kumar A, Rivas CG, Sato K, et al. Uremic pericarditis, pericardial effusion, and constrictive pericarditis in end-stage renal disease: insights and pathophysiology. Clin Cardiol. 2017;40(10):839–46.
16. Cerneviciute R, Sahebally SM, Ahmed K, Murphy M, Mahmood W, Walsh SR. Regional versus local anaesthesia for haemodialysis arteriovenous fistula formation: a systematic review and meta-analysis. Eur J Vasc Endovasc Surg. 2017;53(5):734–42.
17. Hedges SJ, Dehoney SB, Hooper JS, Amanzadeh J, Busti AJ. Evidence-based treatment recommendations for uremic bleeding. Nat Clin Pract Nephrol. 2007;3(3):138–53. Review.
18. Rudy D, Sica DA, Comstock T, Davis J, Savory J, Schoolwerth AC. Aluminum-citrate interaction in end-stage renal disease. Int J Artif Organs. 1991;14(10):625–9.
19. Mailloux LU. Dialysis disequilibrium syndrome. In: Post TW, editor. UpToDate. Waltham, MA: UpToDate; 2020.
20. Sanghani NS, Soundararajan R, Golper TA. Medical management of the dialysis patient undergoing surgery. In: Post TW, editor. UpToDate. Waltham, MA: UpToDate; 2020.
21. Devereaux PJ, POISE-2 investigators. Aspirin in patients undergoing noncardiac surgery. N Engl J Med. 2014;370:1494–503.
22. Zacharias M, Mugawar M, Herbison GP, Walker RJ, Hovhannisyan K, Sivalingam P, Conlon NP. Interventions for protecting renal function in the perioperative period. Cochrane Database Syst Rev. 2013;11(9):CD003590.
23. Mushiyakh Y, Dangaria H, Qavi S, Ali N, Pannone J, Tompkins D. Treatment and pathogenesis of acute hyperkalemia. J Community Hosp Intern Med Perspect. 2011;1(4) https //doi.org/10.3402/jchimp.v1i4.7372.

Non-transplant Surgery for the Transplant Patient

27

Michael J. Jacka

A 48-year-old male presented for urgent surgery for repair of a fractured hip. He sustained a fall on an icy sidewalk. Of note, he received a heart transplant 2 years previously after developing life-threatening heart failure due to a viral myocarditis that had required prolonged support with a left ventricular assist device. Since then, he had returned to work as an engineer and maintained a modest but persistent exercise program under the supervision of the cardiac rehabilitation outreach program.

Medications: Prednisone, tacrolimus, and mycophenolate. He had no medical allergies.

He indicated that he was compliant with his immunosuppressive therapy. He denied use of tobacco, alcohol, cannabis, and other non-prescribed medications.

Physical Examination: Revealed a heart rate of 92, blood pressure of 130/70, and respiratory rate of 16 breaths per minute. He had a midline sternotomy scar. The BMI was 29.

Investigations: His ECG was unremarkable apart from double P waves and mild right ventricular conduction delay. An ECHO from 3 months previously was available and demonstrated an LV ejection fraction of 50% and normal valvular function. His most recent myocardial biopsy was not suggestive of rejection and was performed 2 weeks prior to his accident.

Does This Patient Need to Be Referred to a Center That Does Transplant Surgery to Have His Hip Surgery?

This is not essential but the patient needs to be reviewed and treated by a perioperative medical team who are experienced in managing post-heart transplant patients. In particular, the team should have expertise in the assessment of cardiac and immunosuppressive status preoperatively and of supervising anti-rejection therapy postoperatively.

Which Surgical Post-transplant Patients Should Be Referred to a Transplant Surgery Center to Have Non-transplant Surgery?

If the non-transplant surgery involves the transplanted organ, may significantly affect the function of the transplanted organ, or if the patient appears unstable, referral to a transplant center is advisable.

In the case described, the patient has a complication that is common in the general population, likely has no relationship to the transplanted organ, and the surgery will be unlikely to affect the transplanted organ directly. It should be possible to perform the orthopedic intervention in a non-transplant center, assuming appropriate team expertise in post-transplant management.

Is This Patient at Increased Risk for Traumatic Hip Fracture?

Long-term immunosuppressive therapy is required following organ transplantation and is associated with the development of osteoporosis and bone demineralization, which increase the risk of fractures and avascular necrosis of the femoral head.

M. J. Jacka (✉)
Department of Anesthesiology & Pain Medicine/Department of Critical Care, University of Alberta, Edmonton, AB, Canada
e-mail: mjacka@ualberta.ca

D. Dillane, B. A. Finegan (eds.), *Preoperative Assessment*, https://doi.org/10.1007/978-3-030-58842-7_27

What Are the Physiological Features of the Transplanted Heart?

Transplant surgery requires removal of all neural and vascular connections from the donor organ and restoring the vascular connections but not the neural connections [1–5]. Partial cardiac reinnervation may occur in many patients and the higher resting rate of the transplanted heart may trend downward with time. The transplanted heart is preload-dependent to maintain cardiac output and blood pressure. Hemodynamics are very sensitive to vasodilated conditions such as septic shock and neuraxial anesthesia.

Are There Any Unique ECG Features That May Be Seen Following Orthotopic Heart Transplant?

If a biatrial surgical approach has been used, there will be two P waves visible on the ECG. With the biatrial technique, remnants of the native atria, including tissue that contains the native sinus node and the pulmonary venous ostia remain in situ and are anastomosed to parts of the donor atria including on the right side, tissue containing the donor sinus node. Both sinus nodes retain automaticity and excite the surrounding tissue, hence the two P waves. Propagation of conduction of the native node is impeded by the suture line; consequently, the resting heart rate is determined by the donor node. The bicaval surgical technique, where the recipient atria are excised, is more popular today and under these circumstances there will be only one P wave.

It is common to observe right bundle branch block and/or right intraventricular delay on the ECG of a recently transplanted patient, this is a benign finding.

Acute rejection is usually manifest on an ECG as low QRS voltage and concomitant atrial fibrillation/flutter.

Describe a General Approach to Preoperative Evaluation of this Patient

Preoperative evaluation of transplant patients undergoing non-transplant surgery includes assessment of graft function, indicators of rejection, presence of infection, and other organ function. Solid organ transplant recipients may be at increased risk for atherosclerotic coronary artery disease and should be assessed accordingly [6]. Changes in immunosuppressive medication and a history of rejection episodes requiring rescue immunosuppressive therapy should be noted [7]. During the preoperative workup, the perioperative team must be mindful that patients on chronic immunosuppressive therapy are predisposed to diabetes, epilepsy, hypertension, renal insufficiency, hyperkalemia, hypomagnesemia, pancytopenia, and poor wound healing.

What Blood Tests Should He Have Before Surgery?

In general, testing should be directed by the likelihood of detecting abnormalities that affect management either preoperatively or in anticipation of postoperative abnormalities for which a baseline comparison may be useful [1–5].

In this case, most testing can be guided by the probability of abnormalities caused by the immune-modulating drugs. Since this immune regimen can affect renal function, and steroids have been associated with gastric ulcerations, evaluation of the complete blood count, electrolytes, and creatinine are appropriate.

Should This Patient Have an Echocardiogram or Chest Radiograph?

These tests are not likely to be useful in the absence of specific symptoms suggestive of an acute change in the status of the patient, but review of the most recent echocardiogram findings is appropriate. It is helpful to be aware of the ventricular and valvular function.

Do Other Transplanted Solid Organs Differ from Native Organs?

Transplanted organs, other than the heart in some cases, remain denervated. In the lung transplant patient, normal sensation is present at the glottis but is lost below the level of the tracheal or bronchial anastomoses. The cough reflex is lost below the level of the anastomosis. Mild airway hyperactivity and impaired mucociliary clearance are features of the transplanted lung [7]. Pulmonary function tests (PFTs) return to near normal in double lung transplant patients at 6–12 months, and single lung transplant patients with obstructive disease undergo a 50–60% improvement in PFTs [8, 9].

Neither the transplanted liver nor kidney are significantly affected by denervation. The transplanted kidney is usually placed in the iliac fossa. The anesthesiologist delivering a nerve block to a patient with a transplanted kidney should be cognizant of the specific location of the transplanted kidney.

Do the Systemic Effects of the Condition Leading to the Organ Failure and Transplant Persist?

This applies in many cases. For example, diabetes is a common condition leading to end-stage renal failure. Unless the diabetic patient has had a pancreas transplant, the diabetes persists. This affects preoperative testing and the probability of perioperative complications, and investigations should be directed as appropriate.

Some conditions leading to organ failure are non-systemic and may be largely resolved with a transplant, while others are mixed. Primary biliary cirrhosis and progressive sclerosing cholangitis are conditions that often lead to liver failure but are usually non-systemic unless associated with another condition such as ulcerative colitis. An example of a mixed condition is cystic fibrosis. Cystic fibrosis can affect primarily the lung, primarily the intestine, or both. When cystic fibrosis leads to pulmonary failure and transplant, the pre-existing intestinal effects persist.

What Complications Are Common Among Organ Transplant Patients?

Several complications can commonly occur. Rejection of the transplanted organ may be a chronic condition of varying intensity, requiring periodic adjustment of the immunosuppressive therapy. Hypertension, diabetes, anemia, thrombocytopenia, leukopenia, neurotoxicity, renal insufficiency, and episodic fever, among others, occur periodically. The patient may be receiving corrective medications, and these do not usually need perioperative adjustment.

Are There Any Special Considerations for Liver Transplant Recipients?

- Liver transplant recipients recover the capacity for drug metabolism after reperfusion of the transplanted liver [6].
- Liver transplant patients are at high risk for development of post-transplant hypertension, acute coronary syndrome, and cardiac failure even when cardiac disease is not present pre-transplant [10, 11].
- There is a significant risk of chronic renal failure after liver transplant—the 5-year cumulative incidence of end-stage renal disease is 18–22% [6, 12].
- Hyperlipidemia and diabetes mellitus are more common in liver transplant patients, and those who develop diabetes are at increased risk of cardiac disease and graft dysfunction [13].

Does This Patient Need a Cardiology Consult Before Surgery?

This is not necessary in the case described. This patient has been medically stable, is followed regularly, and fit for the planned surgery. However, should the patient not be followed carefully, or should another complicating condition be suspected, consultation is appropriate. For example, had this patient's fall occurred after a loss of consciousness and particularly if faints had become a problem for the patient, further investigation to determine the cause of loss of consciousness would be appropriate.

What Immunosuppression Protocols Are Typically Seen in Transplant Patients?

Rejection is one of the major barriers to long-term transplant survival. Solid organ transplant recipients take immunosuppressive agents for life. Chronic exposure to immunosuppressants is associated with infection, lymphoproliferative diseases, and organ dysfunction [14].

A usual regimen consists of initial administration of intense, short-term immunosuppression during the perioperative and immediate postoperative period followed by lifelong maintenance. One of the most common induction immunosuppressive agents is basiliximab. It is an interleukin-2 receptor antagonist that decreases the incidence of acute rejection when used as induction therapy when combined with maintenance immunosuppression. No significant drug interactions have been reported for basiliximab.

Maintenance immunosuppression makes use of multiple medications that target different parts of the immune system. A triple therapy regimen is commonly used, consisting of the second-generation calcineurin inhibitor tacrolimus, the antiproliferative agent mycophenolic acid, and a corticosteroid. The most commonly used corticosteroid agents are prednisone, prednisolone, and methylprednisolone. As with other immunosuppressive agents, tacrolimus can cause nephrotoxicity and neurotoxicity and can increase the risk of infection [14].

How Do the Immune System-Modifying Drugs Affect Anesthetic Management?

There are multiple perioperative effects to consider. Common to many of these medications is induction of liver enzyme metabolism e.g., prednisone induces cytochrome P450. This can lead to an interaction with other drugs metabolized by the cytochrome P450 system, e.g., opioid analgesics, antibiotics, and muscle relaxants, and may lead to a reduction in the half-life of these medications [4, 5, 15–18].

All immune modifiers suppress the immune system, necessitating meticulous attention to sterile technique in order to minimize risk to the patient.

Steroids are associated with glucose intolerance, and the patient may require an insulin infusion perioperatively. Moreover, any steroid exposure within the year prior to surgery leads to the risk of adrenal suppression and requires steroid supplementation to respond to the surgical stress. The specific amount of steroid supplementation is controversial. Further discussion regarding perioperative steroid management and stress dosing can be found in Chap. 19. Awareness of the possibility of Addisonian phenomena due to steroid deficiency and the ability to recognize them are vital [15–18].

Tacrolimus can occasionally produce central and peripheral nervous system effects characterized by denervation or dysesthesias. If these are present, they should be documented preoperatively so that their recognition postoperatively is not attributed to intraoperative events [16, 17].

Cyclosporine has been associated with prolonged effects of neuromuscular relaxants. Limitation of the dose of neuromuscular relaxants is prudent.

How Should the Immune System-Modifying Drugs Be Managed?

Maintenance of immune suppression is vital to organ survival. Most are available for intravenous administration, and this substitution is advisable perioperatively to ensure adequate drug levels [15–18]. It is prudent to measure blood levels of immune suppressants to guide dosing. Prednisone dosing may need to be adjusted to accommodate for the stress of the perioperative period, as discussed above.

Can This Patient Have a Regional Anesthetic, or Should He Have a General Anesthetic?

In this case, regional anesthesia is an option; however, the merits of regional anesthesia are few, while the situational risks are notable [19]. In this patient, the transplanted heart has been denervated and does not respond to the neural component of the patient's sympathetic nervous system. As well, the heart is preload dependent to maintain cardiac output and blood pressure. Consequently, the patient is not well positioned to respond to the usual hemodynamic changes of a central neuraxial block. Also, the decision to employ a central or peripheral block in a patient with documented neuropathy should be taken carefully.

By comparison, the use of general anesthesia does not present the same concerns and may be both simpler and safer.

Does the Patient Need a Pacemaker Available Perioperatively?

This is not required as this patient has an intact conduction system and his heart has a normal rhythm.

Are There Any Concerns Perioperatively with Regard to Other Solid Organ Recipients, for Example, Liver, Kidney, Lung?

The transplanted lung is affected by denervation, and patients will not have the normal sensitivity to react to foreign material in the airway and will not have a reflex cough in response.

Patients with kidney transplants are often affected by the same systemic condition that led to the kidney failure, e.g., diabetes, and attention to these possible effects is appropriate.

True-False Questions

1. (a) The transplanted heart does not respond to the autonomic nervous system of the recipient.
   (b) The resting heart rate of the transplanted heart is lower than in the non-transplanted heart.
   (c) Two P waves are usually seen in the ECG of the heart transplant recipient.
   (d) Pulmonary function tests do not return to normal after a double lung transplant.
   (e) Liver transplant recipients completely recover the capacity for drug metabolism.
2. (a) Solid organ transplant recipients usually discontinue immunosuppressive medications within 5 years of transplant.
   (b) Basiliximab is a common induction immunosuppressive agent used perioperatively.
   (c) A corticosteroid agent is normally part of the triple agent anti-rejection regimen administered to solid organ transplant recipients.
   (d) Tacrolimus is commonly associated with neurotoxic adverse events.
   (e) Patients who take cyclosporine may need a larger dose of neuromuscular relaxants for effective paralysis.

References

1. Kostopanagiotou G, Smyrniotis V, Arkadopoulos N, Theodoraki K, Papadimitriou L, Papadimitriou J. Anesthetic and perioperative management of adult transplant recipients in nontransplant surgery. Anesth Analg. 1999;89(3):613–22.
2. Ashary N, Kaye AD, Hegazi AR, M'Frost EA. Anesthetic considerations in the patient with a heart transplant. Heart Dis. 2002;4(3):191–8.
3. Herborn J, Parulkar S. Anesthetic considerations in transplant recipients for nontransplant surgery. Anesth Clin. 2017;35(3):539–53.
4. De Hert S, Imberger G, Carlisle J, Diemunsch P, Fritsch G, Moppett I, et al. Task force on preoperative evaluation of the adult noncardiac surgery patient of the European Society of Anaesthesiology. Preoperative evaluation of the adult patient undergoing non-cardiac surgery: guidelines from the European Society of Anaesthesiology. Eur J Anaesthesiol. 2011;28(10):684–722.
5. Bristow MR. The surgically denervated, transplanted human heart. Circulation. 1990;82:658–60.
6. Pisano G, Fracanzani AL, Caccamo L, Donato MF, Fargion S. Cardiovascular risk after orthotopic liver transplantation, a review of the literature and preliminary results of a prospective study. World J Gastroenterol. 2016;22(40):8869–82.
7. Herborn J, Parulkar S. Anesthetic considerations in transplant recipients for nontransplant surgery. Anesthesiol Clin. 2017;35(3):539–53.
8. Pochettino A, Kotloff RM, Rosengard BR, Arcasoy SM, Blumenthal NP, Kaiser LR, et al. Bilateral versus single lung transplantation for chronic obstructive pulmonary disease: intermediate-term results. Ann Thorac Surg. 2000;70(6):1813–8. discussion 8-9
9. Pego-Fernandes PM, Abrao FC, Fernandes FL, Caramori ML, Samano MN, Jatene FB. Spirometric assessment of lung transplant patients: one year follow-up. Clinics (Sao Paulo). 2009;64(5):519–25.
10. Albeldawi M, Aggarwal A, Madhwal S, Cywinski J, Lopez R, Eghtesad B, et al. Cumulative risk of cardiovascular events after orthotopic liver transplantation. Liver Transpl. 2012;18(3):370–5.
11. Watt KD, Pedersen RA, Kremers WK, Heimbach JK, Charlton MR. Evolution of causes and risk factors for mortality post-liver transplant: results of the NIDDK long-term follow-up study. Am J Transplant. 2010;10(6):1420–7.
12. Kida Y. Chronic renal failure after transplantation of a nonrenal organ. N Engl J Med. 2003;349(26):2563–5; author reply –5.
13. Bodziak KA, Hricik DE. New-onset diabetes mellitus after solid organ transplantation. Transpl Int. 2009;22(5):519–30.
14. Holt CD. Overview of immunosuppressive therapy in solid organ transplantation. Anesthesiol Clin. 2017;35(3):365–80.
15. Bornstein SR, Allolio B, Arlt W, Barthel A, Don-Wauchope A, Hammer GD, et al. Diagnosis and treatment of primary adrenal insufficiency: an Endocrine Society clinical practice guideline. J Clin Endocrinol Metab. 2016;101(2):364–89.
16. Greig P, Lilly L, Scudamore C, Erb S, Yoshida E, Kneteman N, et al. Early steroid withdrawal after liver transplantation: the Canadian tacrolimus versus microemulsion cyclosporin a trial: 1-year follow-up. Liver Transpl. 2003;9(6):587–95.
17. Liu MM, Reidy AB, Saatee S, Collard CD. Perioperative steroid management: approaches based on current evidence. Anesthesiology. 2017;127(1):166–72.
18. Fleisher LA, Mythen M. Anesthetic implications of concurrent diseases. In: Miller RD, Eriksson LI, Fleisher LA Wiener-Kronish JP, Cohen NH, Young WL, editors. Miller's anesthesia. 8th ed. Philadelphia: Saunders; 2015. p. 1156–225.
19. Wall R. Endocrine disease. In: Hines RL, Marschall K, editors. Stoelting's anesthesia and co-existing disease. 7th ed. Philadelphia: Elsevier; 2018. p. 449–75.

Part VIII

Musculoskeletal

28 Systemic Sclerosis

Derek Dillane

A 46-year-old female presented to the anesthesia preadmission clinic 1 week prior to esophageal dilatation. She had been diagnosed with systemic sclerosis 18 months prior to this presentation. She had thickening and tightening of the skin of the face and hands, Raynaud's disease, and arthralgia. She had a year-long history of exertional dyspnea and poor exercise tolerance prior to being formally diagnosed with scleroderma. This had improved after starting treatment and undergoing cardiac rehabilitation; 6-minute walk distance improved from 325 to 400 meters.

Medications: Bisoprolol, omeprazole, ramipril, frusemide, amitriptyline, salbutamol inhaler, spironolactone, prednisone 20 mg daily for 6 months, mycophenolate, vitamin D, and calcium supplements.

Physical Examination: In addition to the classic skin changes described above, revealed a grade 2/6 early systolic murmur at the left sternal border, raised jugular venous pressure at 5 cm above the sternal angle, and faint crackles at the lung bases.

Investigations: Electrocardiogram (ECG) (Fig. 28.1) showed sinus tachycardia, left atrial enlargement, and left anterior hemiblock; 24-hour Holter monitoring showed sinus rhythm with premature atrial complexes, frequent runs of supraventricular tachycardia varying between 3 and 18 beats per minute, and multiple premature ventricular complexes. A non-ischemic dilated cardiomyopathy with left ventricular ejection fraction of 39% was diagnosed by cardiac MRI. The echocardiogram showed a moderately dilated left ventricle, global hypokinesis including right ventricle hypokinesis, moderate mitral regurgitation, increase in left atrial size, and right ventricular systolic pressure of 43 mmHg.

She had interstitial lung disease (ILD) with a total lung capacity (TLC) and DLco of 73% and 57% of predicted reference values respectively on pulmonary function testing (Fig. 28.2). Chest CT 6 months prior to preadmission clinic consultation (Fig. 28.3) revealed basal peripheral ground-glass change and subpleural reticulation. This was most pronounced in the right lower lobe posterior segment where there was also evidence of minimal bronchiectasis. These basal predominant findings were reported as being consistent with the nonspecific interstitial pneumonic type pattern associated with scleroderma. (The chest radiograph from the same time period was completely normal). In addition, the esophagus was noted to be distended and containing secretions and food.

What Is Systemic Sclerosis?

Systemic sclerosis is an autoimmune condition of connective tissue that is characterized by autoantibody production, fibrosis and matrix deposition in the skin, vasculature, and internal organs [1]. Small-vessel vasculopathy with endothelial cell injury results in diffuse capillary loss and leakage into the interstitial space. It is a systemic multi-organ disease with skin, cardiac, pulmonary, renal, gastrointestinal, and musculoskeletal lesions. Two clinical patterns of systemic sclerosis are recognized based on the extent of cutaneous involvement: (a) limited cutaneous systemic sclerosis (lcSSc) with skin involvement usually limited to the hands (occasionally face and neck) and possible manifestations of CREST syndrome (calcinosis, Raynaud's phenomenon, esophageal hypomotility, sclerodactyly, and telangiectasia), and (b) diffuse cutaneous systemic sclerosis (dcSSc) with skin involvement proximal to the wrists and the trunk (Fig. 28.4) [2, 3].

What Is the Difference Between Scleroderma and Systemic Sclerosis?

Sclerosis that is limited to the skin and subcutaneous tissue of the hands and/or face is known as scleroderma.

D. Dillane (✉)
Department of Anesthesiology & Pain Medicine, University of Alberta, Edmonton, AB, Canada

D. Dillane, B. A. Finegan (eds.), *Preoperative Assessment*, https://doi.org/10.1007/978-3-030-58842-7_28

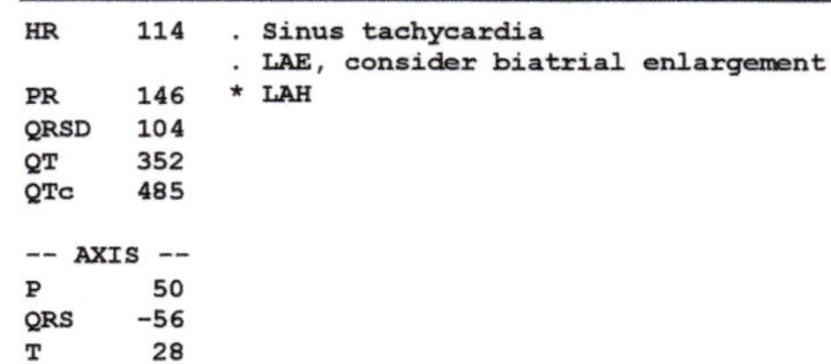

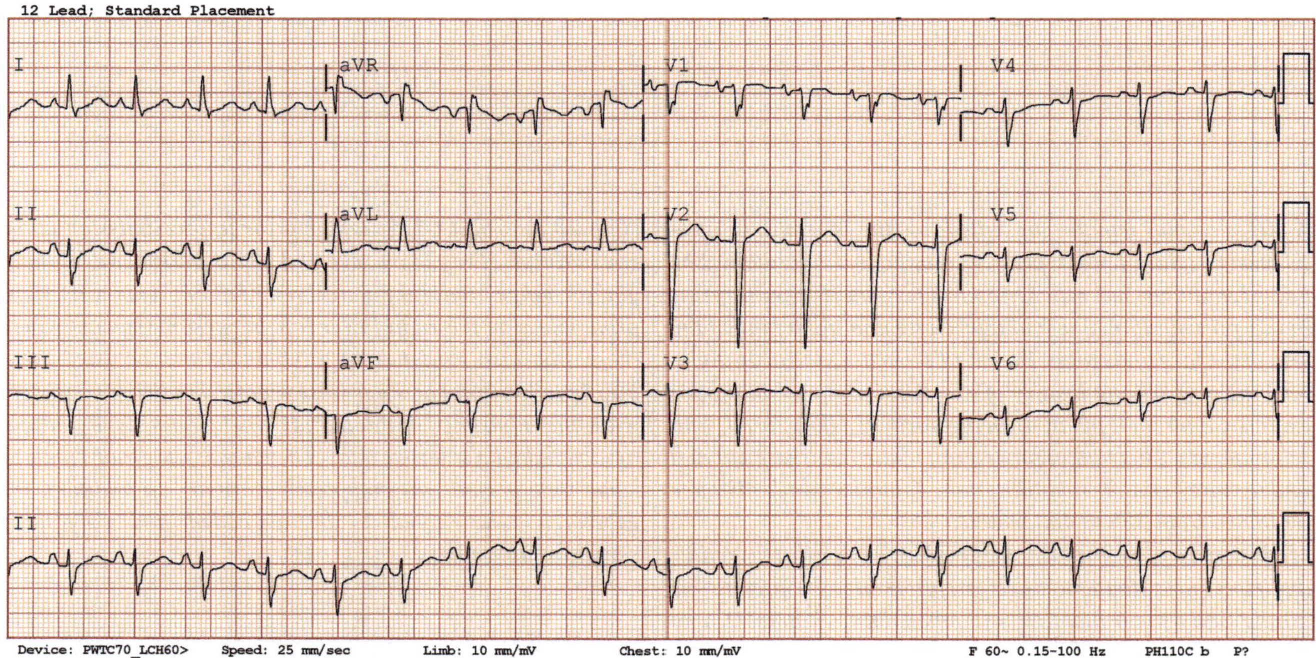

Fig. 28.1 Electrocardiogram showing sinus tachycardia, left atrial enlargement, and incomplete left bundle branch block

What Specific Surgeries Is the Scleroderma Patient Likely to Present For?

- Debridement of digital gangrene
- Amputation of digits
- Periarterial, cervical, or lumbar sympathectomy to improve blood flow
- Repeated esophageal dilatation
- Laparotomy for intestinal pseudo-obstruction
- Lung transplantation due to pulmonary artery hypertension or ILD

What Systemic Complications Is the Patient with Systemic Sclerosis Subject To?

Systemic sclerosis is associated with a significant increase in mortality, most deaths are related to pulmonary fibrosis or pulmonary hypertension.

- Pulmonary disease is seen in over 70% of patients with systemic sclerosis and is the main cause of death in these patients [4]. This is manifest as pulmonary hypertension or ILD. In the perioperative period, patients with pulmonary hypertension are at risk of acute right heart failure, congestive heart failure, arrhythmias, and respiratory failure. ILD develops due to interstitial and peri-bronchial fibrosis and bronchial epithelial proliferation [2]. Patients with ILD are susceptible to an acute exacerbation of this condition, pneumonia, acute lung injury, and prolonged mechanical ventilation (see Chap. 16 for detailed discussion on ILD).
- Cardiovascular disease is due to sclerosis of small coronary arteries and to myocardial fibrosis. It is frequently secondary to systemic or pulmonary hypertension. The pericardium and/or myocardium may be affected. Pericardial disease may be present in the form of acute or chronic pericarditis and pericardial effusion. Myocardial disease results in myocardial fibrosis and ischemia, cardiomegaly, or cardiomyopathy. Left ventricular diastolic dysfunction is more common than systolic dysfunction [5]. Arrhythmias, conduction defects, and congestive heart failure are frequently seen in patients with cardiac involvement. Systemic sclerosis is an independent risk

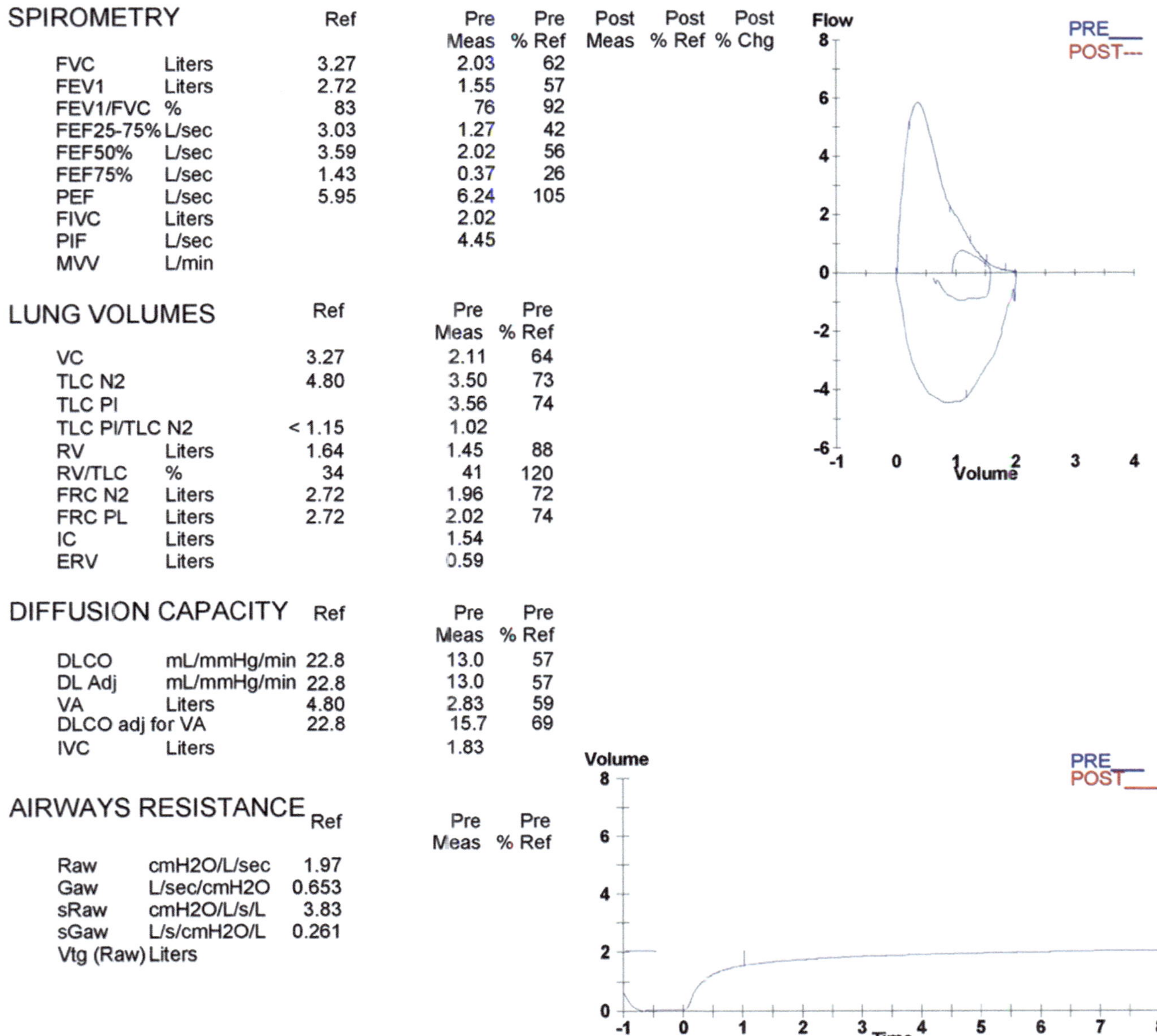

SPIROMETRY

		Ref	Pre Meas	Pre % Ref	Post Meas	Post % Ref	Post % Chg
FVC	Liters	3.27	2.03	62			
FEV1	Liters	2.72	1.55	57			
FEV1/FVC	%	83	76	92			
FEF25-75%	L/sec	3.03	1.27	42			
FEF50%	L/sec	3.59	2.02	56			
FEF75%	L/sec	1.43	0.37	26			
PEF	L/sec	5.95	6.24	105			
FIVC	Liters		2.02				
PIF	L/sec		4.45				
MVV	L/min						

LUNG VOLUMES

		Ref	Pre Meas	Pre % Ref
VC		3.27	2.11	64
TLC N2		4.80	3.50	73
TLC PI			3.56	74
TLC PI/TLC N2		< 1.15	1.02	
RV	Liters	1.64	1.45	88
RV/TLC	%	34	41	120
FRC N2	Liters	2.72	1.96	72
FRC PL	Liters	2.72	2.02	74
IC	Liters		1.54	
ERV	Liters		0.59	

DIFFUSION CAPACITY

		Ref	Pre Meas	Pre % Ref
DLCO	mL/mmHg/min	22.8	13.0	57
DL Adj	mL/mmHg/min	22.8	13.0	57
VA	Liters	4.80	2.83	59
DLCO adj for VA		22.8	15.7	69
IVC	Liters		1.83	

AIRWAYS RESISTANCE

		Ref	Pre Meas	Pre % Ref
Raw	cmH2O/L/sec	1.97		
Gaw	L/sec/cmH2O	0.653		
sRaw	cmH2O/L/s/L	3.83		
sGaw	L/s/cmH2O/L	0.261		
Vtg (Raw)	Liters			

Fig. 28.2 Most recent pulmonary function tests available at time of preoperative assessment

factor for acute myocardial infarction [6]. The incidence and range of cardiac complications seen in systemic sclerosis can be gauged from a large international study involving 3656 systemic sclerosis patients [7]. The study reported complications separately for lcSSc and dcSSc: palpitations were seen in 22.6% of patients with lcSSc and 27.3% of dcSSc patients, conduction block in 10.4% of patients with lcSSc and 12.7% of dcSSc patients, diastolic dysfunction in 15.4% of patients with lcSSc and 16.6% of dcSSc patients, and reduced left ventricular ejection fraction in 5% of patients with lcSSc and 7.2% of dcSSc patients. Patients with clinically apparent cardiac involvement have a poor prognosis with a 5-year mortality rate of 75% [8].

- Patients may be hemodynamically unstable as a result of systemic hypertension, vasomotor instability, and subsequent intravascular volume contraction. Finally, most patients have Raynaud's disease, and this can be exacerbated perioperatively due to exposure to cold temperatures and sympathomimetic or vasopressor agents. Pulse oximetry from the finger may be unreliable.
- Gastrointestinal disease is present in up to 90% of patients, and any part of the gastrointestinal tract may be affected [2]. The esophagus is most commonly involved. Chronic gastroesophageal reflux, esophagitis, and recurrent strictures are seen. Frequent aspiration of gastric contents may either cause ILD or worsen pre-existing ILD. Patients may present for surgery with malnutrition secondary to

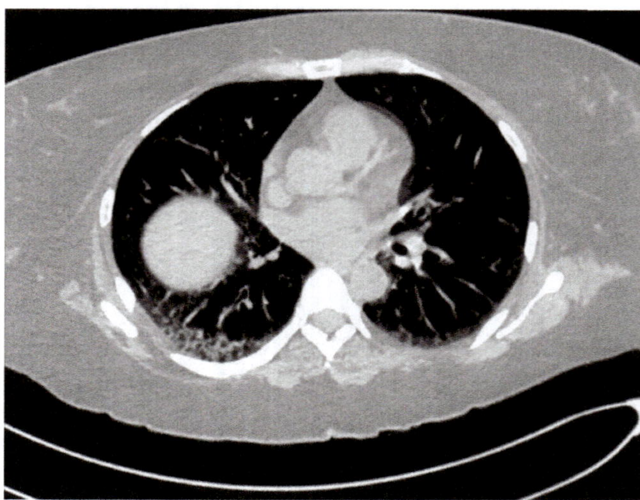

Fig. 28.3 Computed tomography of the chest 6 months prior to preadmission clinic consultation, revealed basal peripheral groundglass change and subpleural reticulation. Most pronounced in the right lower lobe posterior segment where there was minimal bronchiectasis. These basal predominant findings are consistent with nonspecific interstitial pneumonia-type pattern associated with scleroderma

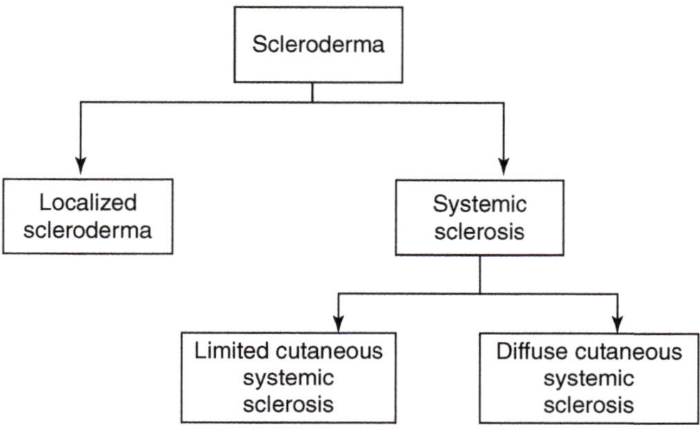

Fig. 28.4 Spectrum of sclerodermal disease [2]

gastrointestinal disease. Enteral absorption of oral medication may be delayed due to impaired motility. Malabsorption of vitamin K may lead to coagulation disorders.

- Renal involvement as a consequence of sclerosis is usually manifest as mild proteinuria or elevated serum creatinine, which does not progress to more advanced disease. A more serious presentation, scleroderma renal crisis, can occur in up to 5–20% of diffuse cutaneous systemic sclerosis patients [9]. Scleroderma renal crisis is defined by severe or worsening arterial hypertension and rapidly progressive renal failure. In the past, this was a common cause of death in patients with systemic sclerosis. It is now effectively treated with angiotensin-converting enzyme (ACE) inhibitors.
- The airway can be especially challenging secondary to restricted mouth opening, temporomandibular joint fibrosis, atrophied nasal alae, and oral or nasal telangiectasias that can bleed profusely if traumatized during intubation [2, 10].

How Should the Patient with Scleroderma Be Evaluated Preoperatively?

Preoperative evaluation focuses on the affected organs. A history and physical examination are required to establish the extent and severity of systemic disease. The following are investigations for consideration preoperatively (*) or may be available as part of routine monitoring of these patients.

Cardiac

- *ECG.
- 24-hour Holter monitoring is part of the standard cardiac diagnostic work-up for systemic sclerosis patients and repeat Holter monitoring has been recommended every 1–2 years even in asymptomatic patients.
- Echocardiogram is performed annually for evaluation of systolic and diastolic dysfunction, pulmonary hypertension, and pericardial effusion [11].
- Doppler echocardiogram is performed for initial assessment of pulmonary hypertension. If found, right heart catheterization may follow.
- Tissue Doppler echocardiography may be performed to provide a fuller extent of myocardial dysfunction in patients with subclinical cardiac involvement [12].
- Cardiac MRI may be used for early assessment of subclinical cardiac involvement [13].
- * Test for brain natriuretic peptide (BNP) or N-terminal pro-brain natriuretic peptide (NT-ProBNP) biomarkers, which may be elevated in LV or RV dysfunction and myocardial ischemia.

Pulmonary

- *Chest radiograph if acute disease suspected.
- Arterial blood gases.
- *Spirometry.
- Pulmonary function tests are carried out every 1–2 years. FVC, DLCO, and TLC are the most common PFT measures used to monitor the progress of pulmonary involvement [14].
- Chest CT based on clinical findings.

Gastrointestinal

- *Complete blood count, electrolyte screen, liver function tests, coagulation screen

Renal

- *Serum urea and creatinine
- Estimated glomerular filtration rate (eGFR)/creatinine clearance
- Urinary protein
- Renal artery Doppler
- Renal biopsy

What Is the Significance of the Improvement in 6-Minute Walk Test After Cardiac Rehabilitation?

The 6-minute walk test (6MWT) is a simple, practical evaluation of functional exercise capacity. One of the strongest indications for the 6MWT is for measuring response to medical therapy and rehabilitation. It is useful in patients with chronic pulmonary disease, e.g., ILD [15]. It needs to be conducted according to a standard set of guidelines [16]. Healthy subjects walk an average of 571 +/− 90 m (range 380–782 m) [17]. The minimal clinically important distance for improvement is approximately 25–50 m [18, 19].

Are There Any Other Tests of Functional Ability That Could Be Used for This Patient?

Recent evidence suggests that subjective assessment of functional capacity, e.g., metabolic equivalent score (Table 28.1) is a poor predictor of postoperative morbidity and mortality [20]. Suggested alternatives with better accuracy include cardiopulmonary exercise testing and the Duke Activity Status Index (Table 28.2) [21].

What Medical Therapies Can We Expect to See in Patients with a Diagnosis of Systemic Sclerosis?

There is no curative treatment available for the underlying disease process. Precipitating or aggravating factors should be stopped, e.g., smoking, vasoconstrictor drugs.

Table 28.1 Metabolic equivalent score for subjective assessment of functional ability

Physical activity	METs
Watching television	1
Light housework, e.g., cooking, ironing, dishes	2–3
Walking, slow stroll	4.7
Walking upstairs	5
Shoveling snow	5–7
Mowing lawn	7
Playing soccer	10

METs Metabolic equivalent of task

Table 28.2 Duke Activity Status Index, a brief self-administered questionnaire to determine functional capacity

Activity	Weight
Can you …	
1. Take care of yourself, that is, eating, dressing, bathing, or using the toilet?	2.75
2. Walk indoors, such as around your house?	1.75
3. Walk a block or two on level ground?	2.75
4. Climb a flight of stairs or walk up a hill?	5.50
5. Run a short distance?	8.00
6. Do light work around the house like dusting or washing dishes?	2.70
7. Do moderate work around the house like vacuuming, sweeping floors, or carrying in groceries?	3.50
8. Do heavy work around the house like scrubbing floors, or lifting or moving heavy furniture?	8.00
9. Do yardwork like raking leaves, weeding, or pushing a power mover?	4.50
10. Have sexual relations?	5.25
11. Participate in moderate recreational activities like golf, bowling, dancing, doubles tennis, or throwing a baseball or football?	6.00
12. Participate in strenuous sports like swimming, singles tennis, football, basketball, or skiing?	7.50
Total score:	
DASI scoring: Positive responses are summed to get a total score, which ranges from 0 to 58.2. Higher scores indicate higher functional capacity	

From Hlatky et al. [21] with permission from Elsevier

Medical management consists of symptomatic treatment of the various systemic manifestations, e.g., gastroesophageal reflux is treated with proton pump inhibitors, calcium channel blockers are first-line therapy for patients with Raynaud phenomenon, and ACE inhibitors are used to treat patients with scleroderma renal crisis.

Patients with severe or rapidly progressive disease are treated with systemic immunosuppressive therapy, e.g., methotrexate, mycophenolate, cyclophosphamide, and rituximab. The choice of agent depends on how extensive the cutaneous or visceral disease progression is, e.g., cyclophosphamide is usually reserved for patients with complicating ILD.

Glucocorticoids are sometimes used to treat systemic sclerosis complicated by ILD. A number of studies have shown benefit from a combination of cyclophosphamide and prednisone [22]. However, there is an association between glucocorticoid therapy and scleroderma renal crisis, which has limited its use.

Is Steroid Stress Dosing Required?

Patients on chronic steroid therapy may develop secondary adrenal insufficiency due to suppression of the hypothalamic-pituitary-adrenal axis (HPAA). Subsequent low corticotropin-releasing hormone (CRH) and adrenocorticotropic hormone (ACTH) levels lead to adrenal atropy and decreased cortisol production. The adrenal gland normally secretes approximately 10 mg cortisol daily. Surgical stress increases adrenal output of cortisol. This varies from 50 mg/day for minor procedures to 150 mg/day for major surgery [23]. Patients on chronic steroid therapy are therefore at risk for perioperative adrenal crisis. This can be life-threatening and requires treatment with stress-dose steroids, fluid, and vasopressors.

Steroid stress dosing is a complex subject, and available recommendations can be confusing. Administering a supplementary stress steroid dose may prevent perioperative adrenal crisis. However, this is a rare occurrence, and it must be balanced against the risk of unnecessary steroid administration. A recent review by Liu et al. is helpful in this regard [23]. The authors state that patients taking any dose of glucocorticoid for less than 3 weeks, morning doses of prednisone 5 mg/day or less, or prednisone 10 mg/day on alternate days are at low risk for HPAA suppression and do not need stress steroid dosing. However, those taking prednisone 20 mg/day for more than 3 weeks require a steroid stress dose.

It was noted that the patient's LVEF returned to normal after starting steroid treatment. She was deemed to be medically optimized for esophagoscopy and was given instructions to take bisoprolol and omeprazole, only, on the morning of surgery. She was prescribed a salbutamol nebulizer for the immediate pre-procedure period. She proceeded to have a short general anesthetic. For a minor procedure such as esophagoscopy and esophageal dilatation, stress dosing consisted of the usual daily dose plus hydrocortisone 50 mg IV at induction, followed by hydrocortisone 25 mg IV every 8 hours for 24 hours on day 1. She returned to her usual daily prednisone dose on day 2.

True/False Questions

1. Concerning the clinical presentation and progression of systemic sclerosis
   (a) Women are more frequently affected
   (b) Raynaud's phenomenon is present in over 90% patients
   (c) The commonest affected organ is the kidney
   (d) Pulmonary disease is the main cause of death
   (e) Scleroderma renal crisis occurs in up to 20% of patients with dcSSc
2. Preoperative evaluation and optimization
   (a) An echocardiogram is indicated if one has not been performed for a year or longer
   (b) Peak expiratory flow rate (PEFR) is the most useful component of PFTs for the systemic sclerosis patient
   (c) Immunosuppressive therapy is curative
   (d) Cyclophosphamide is a first-line treatment for systemic sclerosis and ILD
   (e) ACE inhibitors have revolutionized the treatment of scleroderma renal crisis

References

1. Elhai M, Avouac J, Kahan A, Allanore Y. Systemic sclerosis: recent insights. Joint Bone Spine. 2015;82(3):148–53.
2. Dempsey ZS, Rowell S, McRobert R. The role of regional and neuroaxial anesthesia in patients with systemic sclerosis. Local Reg Anesth. 2011;4:47–56.
3. Varga J. Clinical manifestations and diagnosis of systemic sclerosis (scleroderma) in adults: In: Post TW, editor. UpToDate. Waltham MA: UpToDate; 2020.
4. Steen VD, Medsger TA. Changes in causes of death in systemic sclerosis, 1972-2002. Ann Rheum Dis. 2007;66(7):940–4.
5. de Groote P, Gressin V, Hachulla E, Carpentier P, Guillevin L, Kahan A, et al. Evaluation of cardiac abnormalities by Doppler echocardiography in a large nationwide multicentric cohort of patients with systemic sclerosis. Ann Rheum Dis. 2008;67(1):31–6.
6. Chu SY, Chen YJ, Liu CJ, Tseng WC, Lin MW, Hwang CY, et al. Increased risk of acute myocardial infarction in systemic sclerosis: a nationwide population-based study. Am J Med. 2013;126(11):982–8.
7. Walker UA, Tyndall A, Czirjak L, Denton C, Farge-Bancel D, Kowal-Bielecka O, et al. Clinical risk assessment of organ manifestations in systemic sclerosis: a report from the EULAR scleroderma trials and research group database. Ann Rheum Dis. 2007;66(6):754–63.
8. Janosik DL, Osborn TG, Moore TL, Shah DG, Kenney RG, Zuckner J. Heart disease in systemic sclerosis. Semin Arthritis Rheum. 1989;19(3):191–200.
9. Varga J, Fenves AZ. Renal disease in systemic sclerosis (scleroderma), including scleroderma renal crisis.In: post TW, editor. UpToDate. UpToDate: Waltham MA; 2020.
10. Orphanet version 5.26.0. Orphananesthesia. Anaesthesia recommendations for patients uffering from system sclerosis, Last modified Aug 2015. Available from: https://www.orphananesthesia.eu/en/rare-diseases/published-guidelines/systemic-sclerosis/234-systemic-sclerosis/file.html. Accesseed 6 Jun 2020.
11. Vacca A, Meune C, Gordon J, Chung L, Proudman S, Assassi S, et al. Cardiac arrhythmias and conduction defects in systemic sclerosis. Rheumatology (Oxford). 2014;53(7):1172–7.
12. Desai CS, Lee DC, Shah SJ. Systemic sclerosis and the heart: current diagnosis and management. Curr Opin Rheumatol. 2011;23(6):545–54.
13. Di Cesare E, Battisti S, Di Sibio A, Cipriani P, Giacomelli R, Liakouli V, et al. Early assessment of sub-clinical cardiac involvement in systemic sclerosis (SSc) using delayed enhancement cardiac magnetic resonance (CE-MRI). Eur J Radiol. 2013;82(6):e268–73.
14. Caron M, Hoa S, Hudson M, Schwartzman K, Steele R. Pulmonary function tests as outcomes for systemic sclerosis interstitial lung disease. Eur Respir Rev. 2018;27(148):170102.
15. Brown AW, Nathan SD. The value and application of the 6-minute-walk test in idiopathic pulmonary fibrosis. Ann Am Thorac Soc. 2018;15(1):3–10.
16. Laboratories ATSCPSCPF. ATS statement: guidelines for the six-minute walk test. Am J Respir Crit Care Med. 2002;166(1):111–7.
17. Casanova C, Celli BR, Barria P, Casas A, Cote C, de Torres JP, et al. The 6-min walk distance in healthy subjects: reference standards from seven countries. Eur Respir J. 2011;37(1):150–6.
18. Swigris JJ, Wamboldt FS, Behr J, du Bois RM, King TE, Raghu G, et al. The 6 minute walk in idiopathic pulmonary fibrosis: longitudinal changes and minimum important difference. Thorax. 2010;65(2):173–7.
19. du Bois RM, Weycker D, Albera C, Bradford WZ, Costabel U, Kartashov A, et al. Six-minute-walk test in idiopathic pulmonary

fibrosis: test validation and minimal clinically important difference. Am J Respir Crit Care Med. 2011;183(9):1231–7.

20. Wijeysundera DN, Pearse RM, Shulman MA, Abbott TEF, Torres E, Ambosta A, et al. Assessment of functional capacity before major non-cardiac surgery: an international, prospective cohort study. Lancet. 2018;391(10140):2631–40.
21. Hlatky MA, Boineau RE, Higginbotham MB, Lee KL, Mark DB, Califf RM, et al. A brief self-administered questionnaire to determine functional capacity (the Duke activity status index). Am J Cardiol. 1989;64(10):651–4.
22. Cappelli S, Guiducci S, Bellando Randone S, Matucci Cerinic M. Immunosuppression for interstitial lung disease in systemic sclerosis. Eur Respir Rev. 2013;22(129):236–43.
23. Liu MM, Reidy AB, Saatee S, Collard CD. Perioperative steroid management: approaches based on current evidence. Anesthesiology. 2017;127(1):166–72.

Rheumatoid Arthritis

29

Barry A. Finegan

A 70-year-old female was assessed preoperatively for elective hip replacement. She had been diagnosed with rheumatoid arthritis (RA) 10 years previously after presenting with gradual onset of swelling, stiffness, and pain in her metacarpal, proximal interphalangeal, and metatarsal joints bilaterally. She was prescribed hydroxychloroquine, which ameliorated her symptoms, but due to financial issues, she stopped taking it after a year of treatment.

Systems review revealed an episode of acute coronary syndrome and consequent heart failure 3 years before presentation, which was treated with percutaneous coronary intervention and stenting of the left anterior descending artery. She denied any symptoms suggestive of current active cardiovascular disease, but her exercise tolerance was very limited (≤4 METs) as she had significant hip pain on ambulation. She had hypothyroidism, mild gastroesophageal reflux disease, type 2 diabetes, and dyslipidemia.

Her electrocardiogram demonstrated first-degree AV block. A recent myocardial perfusion MIBI scan was reassuring in that no reversible ischemia was noted. Her echocardiogram revealed a mildly reduced ejection fraction (45%), moderate aortic sclerosis, and mild mitral regurgitation.

She indicated that she regained insurance coverage on turning 65 years of age and had come under the care of a rheumatologist. She was prescribed methotrexate 25 mg weekly and prednisone 15 mg BID, the latter being tapered off over the course of 2 months. Her last flare of disease has occurred 6 months before her clinic visit and was managed by a three week tapering course of prednisone. She had not had corticosteroid treatment since that time. Current medications included methotrexate 15 mg weekly, oxycodone 2.5 mg/acetaminophen 325 mg TID, ibuprofen 600 mg TID, atorvastatin 20 mg OD, pregabalin 75 mg OD, pantoprazole 40 mg OD, levothyroxine 150 mcg OD, and clopidogrel 75 mg OD.

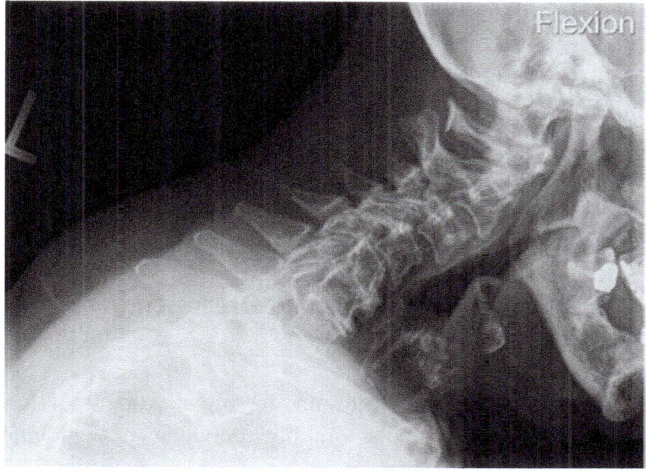

Fig. 29.1 The radiograph demonstrated mild active subluxation at C3-C4 and C4-C5, disc space narrowing, and diffuse facet degeneration

The patient complained of mild tingling and weakness of both upper limbs in the area of the median nerve distribution. A cervical spine radiograph was ordered (Fig. 29.1).

What Is Rheumatoid Arthritis?

RA is an immune-mediated inflammatory disease. RA has a prevalence of ≈ 1% among Caucasians but is far more common in sub-populations (e.g., 5% in some Native American tribes). A family history increases the risk of developing the disease up to fivefold. The *HLA-DRB1* gene is a dominant marker of risk for the development of RA. *HLA-DRB1* encodes cell surface proteins belonging to the major histocompatibility (MHC) class II system and are key components of the immune response system. The MHC class II system presents antigens to T-lymphocytes that stimulate T-helper cells, which in turn evoke B-cells to produce antibodies to the presented antigen. Some B-cells can become

B. A. Finegan (✉)
Department of Anesthesiology & Pain Medicine, University of Alberta, Edmonton, AB, Canada
e-mail: bfinegan@ualberta.ca

D. Dillane, B. A. Finegan (eds.), *Preoperative Assessment*, https://doi.org/10.1007/978-3-030-58842-7_29

autoreactive, i.e., mount an inappropriate response to host tissue. Immune tolerance mechanisms function at several stages of B-cell development to regulate such potentially destructive behavior. It is thought that RA develops in part due to a loss of tolerance in this system in genetically predisposed individuals, perhaps initiated due to exposure to environmental factors [1].

There are no specific diagnostic criteria for RA; it is one of exclusion. The finding of serological markers such as rheumatoid factor (RF) and autoantibodies against citrullinated peptides (ACPA) are suggestive of RA.

The classic extra-articular manifestations of RA including vasculitis, interstitial lung disease, secondary amyloidosis, and cardiovascular disease appear to be reduced if current therapeutic algorithms are instituted early in the disease process.

Modern management involves ongoing assessment and disease monitoring with appropriate adjustment of the therapeutic approach to minimize immune activation and attenuate the inflammatory response.

What Is the Current Approach to Management of a Patient Presenting with RA?

The overarching principles underlying treatment of RA include shared decision-making between patient and rheumatologist. Treatment is based on disease activity, progression of structural damage and safety issues, and recognition of the cost of RA both to the patient and to society [2].

Treatment guidelines suggest therapy should be initiated at time of RA diagnosis.

Prior to initiating treatment, patients are screened for preexisting liver disease (including hepatitis B and C) and tuberculosis, as these conditions can be exacerbated or reactivated by RA drug therapy.

Four main classes of drug [2, 3] are used in the treatment of RA:

1. Conventional synthetic disease-modifying antirheumatic drugs (DMARDs):
   (a) Methotrexate
   (b) Sulfasalazine
   (c) Leflunomide
   (d) Chloroquine
   (e) Hydroxychloroquine
2. Biological disease-modifying antirheumatic drugs (bDMARDs):
   (a) Tumour necrosis factor (TNF)- α inhibitors: adalimumab; golimumab; certolizumab; infliximab; etanercept
   (b) IL-1 receptor antagonist: anakinra
   (c) IL-6 receptor antagonist: tocilizumab
   (d) Anti-CD20 monoclonal antibody: rituximab
3. Biosimilar disease-modifying antirheumatic drugs (bsDMARDs): These are generic versions of the above biologics.
4. Targeted synthetic disease-modifying antirheumatic drugs (tsDMARDs):
   (a) Janus kinase inhibitors: Tofacitinib and baricitinib

The above list is not exhaustive.

Usual initial treatment of RA is with a conventional DMARD, usually methotrexate in combination with low-dose (usually short-term) glucocorticoids. Other DMARDs may be used in combination with methotrexate, although the value of this approach is controversial due to the increased risk of drug-related side effects. The goal of initial treatment is to achieve 80% improvement of disease activity within 3 months of starting treatment.

Failure of this regime calls for the introduction of bDMARDs and thereafter tsDMARDs.

How Should These Medications Be Managed Perioperatively?

Given the forgoing, it is appropriate, time permitting, for the patient's rheumatologist to be informed of planned surgical interventions and advice regarding RA status and perioperative management solicited.

A shared component of all forms of DMARDs is immunosuppression, as the goal of therapy is to reduce inflammation and inhibit joint damage. DMARDs may, in theory, increase the risk of perioperative infection, particularly in the case of elective joint arthroplasty (EJA) procedures. Studies investigating this issue are inconclusive. However, the reality is that perioperative infection rates in patients with immune-mediated inflammatory joint disease are greater than similar patients with osteoarthritis undergoing EJA. Recognizing the paucity of trial data, the College of Rheumatology and the American Association of Hip and Knee Surgeons have jointly developed empirical best practice guidelines on how to manage DMARDs perioperatively [4].

Key recommendations for preoperative management for RA patients undergoing EJA are as follows:

1. Continue conventional DMARDs at current dose
2. Withhold all bDMARDs/bsDMARDs preoperatively and plan surgery at the end of the dosing cycle for the specific medication
3. Withhold tofacitinib 7 days prior to surgery
4. Continue current doses of glucocorticoids (if <16 mg/day prednisone or equivalent) rather than administering supra-physiological doses (stress dosing) on the day of surgery

What Are the Extra-articular Manifestations of RA of Concern Perioperatively?

Patients with RA are at greater risk of suffering a stroke or myocardial infarction than the general population. There are emerging data suggesting that the current treatment paradigm of using DMARDs to target the inflammatory process underlying RA in an aggressive manner may ameliorate the cardiovascular consequences of RA [5]. Symptoms of ischemic heart disease or a history of transient ischemia events should be rigorously investigated preoperatively. Pulmonary nodules, fibrosing alveolitis, and decreased chest wall compliance may occur. Drug-related issues and peripheral neuropathy should be documented.

Should This Patient Receive "Stress Dose" Steroid Treatment?

There is still ambiguity about the role of "stress dose" steroid treatment during the perioperative period. An exhaustive review of the literature by Joseph et al. [6] concludes that there is insufficient evidence to determine the prevalence of, time to recovery from, and influence of glucocorticoid dose and duration on glucocorticoid-induced adrenal insufficiency. The routine administration of standard "stress dose" steroids (typically hydrocortisone 100 mg) prior to surgery is to be carefully considered, given the risks inherent in this approach, which include immunosuppression, bone fracture, and gastrointestinal hemorrhage. A simple way to assess the integrity of the hypothalamic-pituitary-adrenal (HPA) axis is to measure early morning cortisol levels—a patient with a level >10 mcg/dl (275 nmol/L) is unlikely to have HPA axis issues and suggests that the patient does not require supplemental steroid therapy perioperatively. This approach, although optimal, does present practical difficulties in obtaining the appropriate blood specimen. A thoughtful and practical approach has been outlined by Liu et al. [7]. Under these recommendations our patient would be considered to be at "low" risk of HPA suppression and no "stress dose" would be administered.

What Is the Current Approach to Opioid Use in RA?

Chronic opioid use is relatively common among RA patients, although there is little evidence that such treatment is efficacious or safe [8]. It is recommended that a range of non-pharmacological measures be considered prior to initiating opioid therapy [9]. Opioids are best reserved for acute management of pain associated with an RA flare. Nevertheless, many patients with RA have been taking opioids for many years, and it is important to document this and indicate to the patient to take their usual dose of opioid on the morning of surgery.

Are There Any Specific Laboratory Tests That Should Be Ordered Preoperatively in a Patient with RA Being Treated with Any Form of DMARD?

Patients under the care of a rheumatologist will have had scheduled laboratory monitoring of renal, liver, and hematological function. In the absence of available data within 6 months of the date of scheduled surgery, a prudent course would be to obtain a complete blood count, renal panel, and baseline liver function tests. Anemia and drug-induced thrombocytopenia and neutropenia, as well as impaired renal and liver function, are not uncommon in patients with RA.

How Common Is Cervical Spine Disease in the Patient with RA?

Joint and ligament destruction is the hallmark of RA, but early and aggressive use of DMARDs and TNF-α inhibitors may significantly impede if not halt this aspect of the disease,[1] though long-term studies are lacking. However, there are many patients who developed RA prior to the use of current management strategies or who, for whatever reason, are unable to access such therapy. In the latter populations, cervical spine involvement by RA is undoubtedly common.

The occiput-C1 and C1-C2 joints are most prone to RA involvement, as they are synovial joints without cushioning discs (the latter are not affected by RA-induced inflammation) [10]. The occiput-C1 joint is a relatively stable saddle joint, but basilar invagination can occur, so that the odontoid process appears to enter the foramen magnum. The C1-C2 joint has horizontally orientated articulations (no bone barrier to subluxation) and is supported in this plane by ligaments that can be significantly damaged by RA, inducing laxity and instability [10]. It is the cervical joint most commonly affected by RA.

Subluxation of these joints decreases the space available for the spinal cord and can lead to compression of the cord and/or vertebral arteries. Subaxial subluxation, as seen in the patient under discussion, is less common and results from destruction of the facet and uncovertebral joints.

Patients with significant RA-induced cervical spine disease may be asymptomatic, and preoperative radiological assessment of the cervical spine is reasonable in any patient with significant disability and ongoing disease activity. Pain radiating to the occiput, paresthesia in the shoulders and arms on head movement, and/or sensory loss in the dermatomes supplied by brachial plexus are suggestive of cervical spine pathology and warrant radiological examination of the cervical spine, with MRI assessment if significant pathology is found on screening films [11].

Is Regional Anesthesia the "Best" Choice in This Patient?

If acceptable, appropriate, and feasible, regional anesthesia is an excellent choice for anesthetic management of the patient with significant RA-induced pathology undergoing surgery [12]. It is advisable to discuss the possibility of awake fiberoptic intubation if there is any evidence of airway compromise, as it may be difficult, if not impossible, in some cases to perform a regional technique.

Spinal anesthesia was discussed with and agreed to by the patient. She was quite relieved at being offered this option, as she had undergone awake fiberoptic intubation once before, which she found quite distressing. An AM (between 0600 and 0800 hours) cortisol was obtained and was determined to be within the normal range (10–20 mcg/dL). "Stress dose" steroids were not ordered. The patient was told to take her usual oxycodone dose on the morning of surgery and to continue taking her methotrexate without interruption on a weekly basis as she awaited surgery. The latter proceeded uneventfully 4 weeks after her preoperative visit.

True-False Questions

1. In a patient with RA:
   (a) The diagnosis is confirmed if the rheumatoid factor is positive
   (b) Early and consistent use of medication should minimize joint destruction
   (c) All disease-modifying drugs suppress the immune response
   (d) The subaxial cervical spine is most commonly affected by RA
   (e) The risk of stroke is increased
2. In the perioperative management of a patient with RA:
   (a) Methotrexate should be held for 14 days before surgery
   (b) All biological disease-modifying drugs should be held preoperatively
   (c) Liver and renal function should be assessed
   (d) "Stress dose" steroids in the form of hydrocortisone should always be ordered
   (e) A cervical spine radiograph is always mandatory

References

1. Smolen JS, Aletaha D, McInnes I. Rheumatoid arthritis. Lancet. 2017;388(10055):2023–38.
2. Smolen JS, Landewé R, Bijlsma J, Burmester G, Chatzidionysiou K, Dougados M, et al. EULAR recommendations for the management of rheumatoid arthritis with synthetic and biological disease-modifying antirheumatic drugs: 2016 update. Ann Rheum Dis. 2017;76(6):960–77.
3. Singh JA, Saag KG, Bridges SL Jr, Akl EA, Bannuru RR, Sullivan MC, et al. American College of Rheumatology. 2015 American College of Rheumatology guideline for the treatment of rheumatoid arthritis. Arthritis Care Res (Hoboken). 2016;68(1):1–25.
4. Goodman SM, Springer B, Guyatt G, Abdel MP, Dasa V, George M, et al. American College of Rheumatology/American Association of Hip and Knee Surgeons guideline for the perioperative management of antirheumatic medication in patients with rheumatic diseases undergoing elective total hip or Total knee arthroplasty. J Arthroplast. 2017;201732(9):2628–38.
5. Day AL, Singh JA. Cardiovascular disease risk in older adults and elderly patients with rheumatoid arthritis: what role can disease-modifying antirheumatic drugs play in cardiovascular risk reduction? Drugs Aging. 2019;36(6):493–510.
6. Joseph RM, Hunter AL, Ray DW, Dixon WG. Systemic glucocorticoid therapy and adrenal insufficiency in adults: a systematic review. Semin Arthritis Rheum. 2016;46(1):133–41. 5.
7. Liu MM, Reidy AB, Saatee S, Collard CD. Perioperative steroid management: approaches based on current evidence. Anesthesiology. 2017;127(1):166–72.
8. Day AL, Curtis JR. Opioid use in rheumatoid arthritis: trends, efficacy, safety, and best practices. Curr Opin Rheumatol. 2019;31(3):264–70.
9. Geenen R, Overman CL, Christensen R, Åsenlöf P, Capela S, Huisinga KL, et al. EULAR recommendations for the health professional's approach to pain management in inflammatory arthritis and osteoarthritis. Ann Rheum Dis. 2018;77(6):797–807.
10. Kim HJ, Nemani VM, Riew KD, Brasington R. Cervical spine disease in rheumatoid arthritis: incidence, manifestations, and therapy. Curr Rheumatol Rep. 2015;17(2):9.
11. Fombon FN, Thompson JP. Anaesthesia for the adult patient with rheumatoid arthritis. Contin Educ Anaesth Crit Care Pain. 2006;6(6):235–9.
12. Samanta R, Shoukrey K, Griffiths R. Rheumatoid arthritis and anaesthesia. Anaesthesia. 2011;66(12):1146–59.

Systemic Lupus Erythematosus

30

Derek Dillane and Stephanie Keeling

A 56-year-old female was referred to the anesthesia pre-assessment clinic for optimization prior to total knee arthroplasty. She had a 12-year history of systemic lupus erythematosus (SLE). Her SLE-presenting symptoms were malar rash, photosensitivity, arthralgia, and anemia. During the anesthesia consultation, she was also noted to have a history of hypertension and seizure disorder. Three years prior to this visit, she had a frontal lobe ischemic infarct resulting in left-sided hemiparesis which had fully resolved.

Medications: Prednisone 10 mg daily, hydroxychloroquine 200 mg daily, perindopril 8 mg daily, and levetiracetam 500 mg twice daily.

Physical Examination: The patient was noted to have an elevated BMI 38.6. Blood pressure (BP) was 148/92. Radial artery pulse examination revealed a heart rate of 92 bpm with a regular rhythm. Mallampati II mouth opening was documented on examination of the airway along with a full range of cervical spine movement.

Investigations: Hemoglobin was 92 g/L, WCC 4.3 × 10⁹ /L, platelet count 59 × 10⁹ /L, and creatinine 115 umol/L. Chest radiograph and ECG were normal. Echocardiography showed calcified aortic valve leaflets with mild aortic regurgitation, mild mitral regurgitation, no valvular vegetation, global hypokinesia of the left ventricle with an ejection fraction of 40%, and no evidence of pericardial effusion.

What Is SLE?

Systemic lupus erythematosus (SLE) is a chronic autoimmune, multisystem, connective tissue disorder. It affects females more than males (female to male ratio 9:1) and is more common among specific ethnic groups, e.g., East Asian and African American ancestry. Overall prevalence varies from 20 to 150 cases per 100,000 [1]. This is increased in women to as many as 406 per 100,000 [2]. Peak age of onset is late teens to early forties [3]. The spectrum of disease ranges from mild arthritis and rash to life-threatening renal and cardiac dysfunction. The natural history of the disease is one of flare-ups intercepting periods of remission, which result in accrual of disease- and therapy-related damage.

How Is SLE Diagnosed?

There are no definitive diagnostic criteria. A diagnosis of SLE is made based on the presence of characteristic clinical and laboratory features in the context of serologic biomarkers, e.g., antinuclear antibodies or anti-double-stranded DNA antibodies A number of classification criteria have been developed for the purposes of research and disease surveillance (Tables 30.1 and 30.2) [4–7]. Consensus diagnostic

Table 30.1 American College of Rheumatology revised criteria for systemic lupus erythematosus

Criterion	Definition
Malar rash	Fixed erythema, flat or raised, over the malar eminences, tending to spare the nasolabial folds
Discoid rash	Erythematous raised patches with adherent keratotic scaling and follicular plugging; atrophic scarring may occur in older lesions
Photosensitivity	Skin rash as a result of unusual reaction to sunlight, by patient history *or* physician observation

(continued)

D. Dillane (✉)
Department of Anesthesiology & Pain Medicine, University of Alberta, Edmonton, AB, Canada

S. Keeling
Division of Rheumatology, Department of Medicine, University of Alberta, Edmonton, AB, Canada

D. Dillane, B. A. Finegan (eds.), *Preoperative Assessment*, https://doi.org/10.1007/978-3-030-58842-7_30

Table 30.1 (continued)

Criterion	Definition
Oral ulcers	Oral or nasopharyngeal ulceration, usually painless, observed by a physician
Arthritis	Nonerosive arthritis involving two *or* more peripheral joints, characterized by tenderness, swelling, or effusion
Serositis	Pleuritis: convincing history of pleuritic pain or rub heard by a physician or evidence of pleural effusion *or* Pericarditis: documented by ECG or rub or evidence of pericardial effusion
Renal disorder	Persistent proteinuria greater than 0.5 grams per day or greater than *3+* if quantitation not performed *or* Cellular casts: may be red cell, hemoglobin, granular, tubular, or mixed
Neurologic disorder	Seizures: in the absence of offending drugs or known metabolic derangements, e.g., uremia, ketoacidosis, or electrolyte imbalance *or* Psychosis: in the absence of offending drugs or known metabolic derangements, e.g., uremia, ketoacidosis, or electrolyte imbalance
Hematologic disorder	Hemolytic anemia : with reticulocytosis *or* Leukopenia: less than 4000/mm^3 total on 2 or more occasions *or* Lymphopenia- less than 1500/mm^3 total on 2 or more occasions *or* Thrombocytopenia: less than 100,000/mm^3 in the absence of offending drugs
Immunologic disorder	Anti-DNA: antibody to native DNA in abnormal titer *or* Anti-Sm: presence of antibody to Sm nuclear antigen *or* Positive finding of antiphospholipid antibodies based on (1) an abnormal serum level of IgG or IgM anticardiolipin antibodies, (2) a positive test result for lupus anticoagulant using a standard method, or (3) a false-positive serologic test for syphilis known to be positive for at least 6 months and confirmed by *Treponema pallidum* immobilization or fluorescent treponemal antibody absorption test
Antinuclear antibody	An abnormal titer of antinuclear antibody by immunofluorescence or an equivalent assay at any point in time and in the absence of drugs known to be associated with "drug-induced lupus" syndrome

Adapted from Tan et al. [6] with permission John Wiley and Sons
SLE can be diagnosed when 4 or more of the 11 criteria are present, either serially or simultaneously, during any period of observation [5]

Table 30.2 Systemic Lupus International Collaborating Clinics (SLICC) clinical and immunologic criteria for use in SLE clinical care and diagnosis. Patients must have at least 1 of 11 clinical criteria and 1 of 6 immunologic criteria for diagnosis of SLE.

Criteria	Definition
Acute cutaneous lupus	Lupus malar rash (do not count if malar discoid) Bullous lupus Toxic epidermal necrolysis variant of SLE maculopapular lupus rash Photosensitive lupus rash *in the absence of dermatomyositis* *or* subacute cutaneous lupus (nonindurated psoriaform *and/or* annular polycyclic lesions that resolve without scarring, although occasionally with postinflammatory dyspigmentation or telangiectasias)
Chronic cutaneous lupus	Classic discoid rash Localized (above the neck) Generalized (above and below the neck) Hypertrophic (verrucous) lupus Lupus panniculitis (profundus) Mucosal lupus Lupus erythematosus tumidus Chillblains lupus Discoid lupus/lichen planus overlap
Oral ulcers	Palate Buccal Tongue *or* nasal ulcers *in the absence of other causes, such as vasculitis, Behcet's disease, infection (herpesvirus), inflammatory bowel disease, reactive arthritis, and acidic foods*
Alopecia	Nonscarring alopecia (diffuse thinning or hair fragility with visible broken hairs) *in the absence of other causes such as alopecia areata, drugs, iron deficiency, and androgenic alopecia*
Synovitis	Synovitis involving 2 or more joints, characterized by swelling or effusion or tenderness in 2 or more joints and at least 30 minutes of morning stiffness
Serositis	Typical pleurisy for more than 1 day OR pleural effusions OR pleural rub Typical pericardial pain (pain with recumbency improved by sitting forward) for more than 1 day OR pericardial effusion OR pericardial rub OR pericarditis by electrocardiography *in the absence of other causes, such as infection, uremia, and Dressler's pericarditis*
Renal	Urine protein–to-creatinine ratio (or 24-hour urine protein) representing 500 mg protein/24 hours OR red blood cell casts

Table 30.2 (continued)

Criteria	Definition
Neurologic	Seizures Psychosis Mononeuritis multiplex *in the absence of other known causes such as primary vasculitis* Myelitis Peripheral or cranial neuropathy *in the absence of other known causes such as primary vasculitis, infection, and diabetes mellitus* Acute confusional state *in the absence of other causes, including toxic/metabolic, uremia, drugs*
Hemolytic anemia	
Leukopenia	<1000/mm^3 at least once *in the absence of other known causes such as corticosteroids, drugs, and infection*
Thrombocytopenia	<100,000/mm^3 at least once *in the absence of other known causes such as drugs, portal hypertension, and thrombotic thrombocytopenic purpura*
Immunologic criteria	1. ANA level above laboratory reference range 2. Anti-dsDNA antibody level above laboratory reference range (or >2-fold the reference range if tested by ELISA) 3. Anti-Sm: presence of antibody to Sm nuclear antigen 4. Antiphospholipid antibody positivity as determined by any of the following: Positive test result for lupus anticoagulant False-positive test result for rapid plasma reagin Medium- or high-titer anticardiolipin antibody level (IgA, IgG, or IgM) Positive test result for anti–β2-glycoprotein I (IgA, IgG, or IgM) 5. Low complement Low C3 Low C4 Low CH50 6. Direct Coombs' test *in the absence of hemolytic anemia*

From Petri et al. [7] with permission John Wiley and Sons

guidelines from the American College of Rheumatology (ACR) and the Systemic Lupus International Collaborating Clinics (SLICC) criteria are two commonly used tools [5, 7]. Even though these tools were developed to ensure consistency for the purposes of research, they can be useful in clinical practice to differentiate patients with lupus-like clinical features from patients with another systemic autoimmune disease [8].

What Common Clinical Features of SLE Are of Concern During the Perioperative Period?

Common manifestations include arthritis, nephritis, pericarditis, pleuritis, psychosis, and hematologic disorders (Table 30.3) [9]. The stress of surgery may exacerbate the effects of SLE.

Table 30.3 Common clinical manifestations of SLE and estimated lifetime prevalence

Condition	Estimated prevalence (%)
Dermatologic	
Malar rash	50
Chronic discoid lesions	25
Neurologic	
Seizures	7–20
Cardiovascular	
Symptomatic pericarditis	25
Pericardial tamponade	< 2
Myocarditis	5–10
Libman-Sacks endocarditis	10
Valvular dysfunction	3–4
Raynaud's phenomenon	30–40
Pulmonary	
Pleuritis	35
Pneumonitis	1–10
Diffuse alveolar hemorrhage	1–5
Pulmonary arterial hypertension	0.5–14
Renal	
Lupus nephritis	60
End-stage renal disease	3–12
Hematology	
Anemia of chronic disease	40
Autoimmune hemolytic anemia	5–10
Autoimmune thrombocytopenia	10
Gastrointestinal	
Oral ulcers	7–52
Sjogren syndrome	10
Dysphagia	1–13
Acute abdominal pain	40
Abnormal liver function tests	Up to 60
Autoimmune hepatitis	2–5
Musculoskeletal	
Arthritis	15–50
Osteoporosis	23
Fractures	12.5
Asymptomatic atlantoaxial subluxation	8.5

From Ben-Menachem [9], with permission Wolters Kluwer

What Cardiovascular Features of SLE Are of Perioperative Concern?

Cardiac involvement in SLE is common and can involve all components of the heart including the pericardium, myocardium, coronary arteries, valves, and conduction system [10].

SLE is an independent risk factor for the development of coronary artery disease. This is especially true for female patients [3]. Women with SLE aged 35–44 years have been found to be over 50 times more likely to have an MI compared with similarly aged healthy females [11]. Older age at time of diagnosis, longer disease duration, and longer duration of corticosteroid use were associated with greater risk of development of cardiovascular disease in this cohort. Pathogenesis of coronary artery disease in SLE is, in part, likely related to inflammatory activity resulting in vascular endothelial damage and ensuing atherosclerosis. Corticosteroid use with associated glucose intolerance, hypertension, dyslipidemia, and central obesity may also be a contributing etiological factor.

Pericarditis is the commonest cardiac manifestation in SLE. Symptomatic pericarditis is seen in 25% of SLE patients, and more than 50% of patients have asymptomatic pericarditis [12]. Pericarditis is common during disease exacerbation and may be seen together with pleuritis as part of a generalized serositis [9]. Acute pericarditis is diagnosed in the presence of at least two of the following: (1) sharp pleuritic chest pain, (2) pericardial friction rub over left sternal border, (3) pericardial effusion, and (4) widespread ST segment elevation. It is successfully treated medically with NSAIDs, corticosteroids, and colchicine most of the time. Pericardiocentesis may be required for frequent recurrences, large effusions or in the presence of constrictive pericarditis [13].

SLE myocarditis has a lifetime prevalence of 5–10%. It is associated with ventricular dysfunction and reduced ejection fraction, dilated cardiomyopathy, and cardiac failure.

The characteristic valvular abnormality seen in SLE, Libman-Sacks endocarditis, is caused by verrucous noninfective vegetations. It is seen in approximately 10% of SLE patients. Mitral and aortic insufficiency are the commonest clinical manifestations. A longitudinal study over 57 months of 69 SLE patients reported that the combined incidence of stroke, peripheral embolism, heart failure, infective endocarditis, and the need for valve replacement was 22 percent in patients with valvular disease [14].

The commonest rhythm and conduction abnormalities seen in SLE are sinus tachycardia, atrial fibrillation, and atrioventricular block [9, 15].

Vasculitis is seen in SLE patients with a prevalence of between 11% and 36%. Inflammation of all vessel sizes can be present, with small vessel vasculitis manifest as cutaneous lesions (purpura, petechiae) being most common [16]. Medium to large vessel vasculitis is much more serious and presents as mesenteric vasculitis, pulmonary hemorrhage, mononeuritis multiplex, or visceral involvement of the kidney or pancreas.

Raynaud's phenomenon, peripheral arterial vasospasm secondary to triggers such as cold, has been reported in up to 16.3% of lupus patients [17].

What Is the Association Between SLE and Hypertension?

The incidence of hypertension appears to be higher in lupus patients particularly in females under 40 years [18, 19]. As the risk of cardiovascular disease is already high in patients with SLE, it is important to aggressively control blood pressure in addition to other traditional cardiovascular risk factors such as hyperglycemia, smoking, and obesity [10]. The pathogenesis of hypertension in SLE has not been fully elucidated but is thought to involve a combination of traditional risk factors (ethnicity, obesity) and lupus-related factors (renal involvement, immune system dysfunction, steroid therapy [20]).

What Are the Renal Features of SLE?

Lupus nephritis is one of the commonest complications of SLE. It is seen in approximately 60% of patients and commonly presents within the first 3 years of diagnosis [21]. It is a significant cause of morbidity and mortality; therefore, prevention of renal damage has long-term prognostic implications for lupus patients [22]. Clinical manifestations of lupus renal disease vary from asymptomatic proteinuria or hematuria to nephrotic syndrome and glomerulonephritis with progressively deteriorating renal impairment [4]. Approximately 5–20% of patients with lupus nephritis progress to end-stage renal disease [21]. Regular screening is carried out by urinalysis for proteinuria, hematuria, and cellular casts or estimation of glomerular filtration rate. Renal biopsy is performed to confirm diagnosis and to guide treatment by providing a histological subtype.

What Pulmonary Features of SLE Are of Perioperative Concern?

All pulmonary tissue can be affected with pleural disease being the most frequent manifestation. Up to 35% of SLE patients will develop pleuritis. Pleural effusions when present are usually mild, but large and clinically significant effusions can develop [9, 23]. Other pulmonary manifestations include pulmonary embolism, acute lupus pneumonitis, interstitial lung disease, and diffuse alveolar hemorrhage (a rare but serious complication that occurs in up to 5% of patients and has an associated mortality of 50% [23]). Pulmonary artery hypertension has a prevalence of 0.5–14% in lupus patients and is associated with interstitial lung disease, thromboembolism, and pulmonary vasculitis [9]. Even more rare is shrinking lung syndrome, a condition found only in 1–6% of patients with symptoms of pleuritic chest pain. Decreased lung volumes in the absence of pleural or interstitial disease can be seen on pulmonary function testing, which may have implications during ventilation [24]. While the cause is unclear, theories include possible diaphragmatic muscle dysfunction or impaired lung compliance due to chronic pleural inflammation [25, 26].

Are There Any Airway Concerns in SLE Patients?

Laryngeal complications have been described in lupus patients with an incidence ranging from 0.3% to 30% [27, 28]. They are generally considered to occur less frequently than airway complications associated with other connective tissue disorders, e.g., rheumatoid arthritis [29]. Clinical manifestations range from mild inflammation to epiglottitis, vocal cord paralysis, and laryngeal edema with acute obstruction [9, 30]. Post-intubation subglottic stenosis has been described, even after brief (3- to 48-hour) periods of intubation [29].

What Hematologic Features Should We Be Aware Of?

Hematologic abnormalities are common in SLE and affect all three blood cell types. Leukopenia has been reported to occur in 50% of patients. It can be due to either lymphopenia or neutropenia and correlates with clinically active disease [4]. Neutropenia can also occur secondary to immunosuppressive therapy [4]. Anemia is seen in approximately 50% of lupus patients, the commonest type being anemia of chronic disease. Other causes of anemia include autoimmune hemolytic anemia, iron deficiency anemia, and anemia of chronic renal impairment [9]. Autoimmune thrombocytopenia is seen in up to 10% of patients. Most patients respond to immunosuppressive therapy (e.g., rituximab) and intravenous immunoglobulin, but a splenectomy will be required in the 20% of non-responders [31].

What Are the Neuropsychiatric Manifestations of SLE?

Seizures have been reported in 7–20% of patients [32]. Thromboembolic events, frequently associated with the presence of antiphospholipid antibodies (seen in 20% of patients with SLE), cause either focal neurological deficits or more diffuse cognitive defects. Psychosis may occur either as a result of SLE or glucocorticoid therapy. Acute confusional states, depression, anxiety, and demyelinating disease have also been associated with SLE [4, 9].

What Gastrointestinal and Hepatobiliary Features Are Concerning?

Mild abnormalities of liver function tests (LFTs) may be seen in lupus patients. Etiology is multifactorial and includes treatment with NSAIDs, azathioprine, methotrexate, fatty infiltration secondary to corticosteroid therapy, and viral hepatitis [33]. Persistent and severe derangement of LFTs warrants investigation with ultrasonography and/or liver biopsy. Clinically significant liver disease, attributable to causes including steatohepatitis and cirrhosis, was found in 21% of patients with abnormal LFTs in one case series [34]. Lupus and autoimmune hepatitis are rare but possible explanations of transaminitis in lupus patients [35].

The gastrointestinal tract can be affected by lupus complications almost along its entire length, but the commonest abnormalities are oral ulcers, esophagitis, and acute abdominal pain. Up to 50% of SLE patients report heartburn, yet they appear not to be at increased risk of gastroesophageal reflux [36, 37]. Esophageal motility disorder is the usual culprit. Acute abdominal pain has been reported in up to 40% of lupus patients [33]. Though usually attributed to non-SLE causes, the commonest lupus-related cause for acute abdominal pain is intestinal vasculitis [9].

Are Patients with SLE at Increased Risk for Perioperative Thromboembolic Complications?

Patients with lupus are at increased risk for both arterial and venous thromboembolic complications. An observational cohort study of 544 patients who had been diagnosed with SLE within the previous year were followed for a median duration of 6.3 years. The overall incidence of a thrombotic event was 16%: arterial thromboembolism occurred in 11% of patients and venous thromboembolism in the remaining 5%. The estimated 20-year risk was 33% for any thrombotic event [38].

The presence of prothrombotic antiphospholipid antibodies, found in SLE patients at a higher incidence than in the general population, predisposes towards thrombotic complications. A specific syndrome, secondary antiphospholipid antibody syndrome, is seen in a subset of lupus patients. In a study of 1000 patients with antiphospholipid syndrome, 36.2% of patients had antiphospholipid syndrome associated with SLE [39]. Diagnosis requires meeting the revised Sapporo criteria: at least one clinical criterion (e.g., vascular thrombosis or adverse pregnancy outcome) and one or more positive antiphospholipid antibody tests on two or more occasions at least 12 weeks apart.

Thromboembolic complications have been found in 53% of SLE patients with lupus anticoagulant versus 12% without, and 40% of patients with anticardiolipin antibodies versus 18% without [40]. The prothrombotic lupus anticoagulant (the confusing name arises from its in vitro actions) and anticardiolipin antibodies are found with a prevalence of 34% and 44%, respectively, in SLE patients [40]. Lupus anticoagulant may falsely prolong aPTT; lupus anticoagulant measurement is therefore warranted in any lupus patient with a prolonged aPTT.

What Musculoskeletal Complications Occur with SLE?

A symmetrical migratory arthritis involving the hands, wrists, elbows, knees, and ankles is seen in over 90% of patients [41]. The arthritis is not erosive and is usually not deforming, although some develop more ligamentous laxity resulting in reducible deformities (e.g., Jaccoud's arthropathy) [4, 42]. Lupus arthritis is not reported to involve the cervical spine. However, atlantoaxial subluxation has been reported in a number of case reports [43, 44].

Are Patients with SLE More Susceptible to Infection?

As a result of treatment-related immunosuppression and an inherent susceptibility, lupus patients have a higher rate of infection. Indeed, it is one of the leading causes of death during the first 5 years of follow-up [17]. Most infections are bacterial and affect the skin, respiratory system, and urinary tract. Active lupus disease, disease duration, renal involvement, CNS involvement, cytopenia, and immunosuppressive therapy are predictive of infection [9].

How Is SLE Treated?

Treatment is predicated upon individual disease manifestations and is based on regular assessment of disease activity and severity as well as response to existing therapies. Patients with any disease activity are usually prescribed hydroxychloroquine or chloroquine unless contraindicated. Adjunctive treatment is based on the severity of active disease manifestations. Patients with mild disease activity can also be administered NSAIDs or short-term low-dose corticosteroid therapy [45]. Moderate and severe disease activity require high-dose corticosteroid (oral or intravenous) therapy and/or steroid-sparing immunosuppressive agents, e.g., azathioprine, methotrexate, or mycophenolate mofetil. The monoclonal antibodies belimumab and rituximab can be used for patients who fail to respond to standard therapies.

Toxicity resulting from drugs used to manage SLE can have important perioperative implications. Adverse effects secondary to corticosteroid therapy have been detailed in Chap. 19. The antimalarial medications hydroxychloroquine and chloroquine are associated with cardiotoxicity, while azathioprine and methotrexate can cause hepatotoxicity (Table 30.4) [9].

Table 30.4 Drugs used for treatment of SLE and associated toxicity

Drug	Indication	Anesthetic implications
Anti-malarial (hydroxychloroquine)	Cutaneous SLE	Retintoxicity
	Pleuritis/pericarditis	Neuromyotoxicity
	Arthritis	Cardiotoxicity
	Reduced renal flares	
Corticosteroids (prednisone, methylprednisone, topical preparations	Cutaneous SLE	Hyperglycemia
	Arthritis	Hypercholesterolemia
	Nephritis	Hypertension
	Pleuritis/pericarditis	Osteoporosis
	Diffuse alveolar hemorrhage	
	NPSLE	
	Mesenteric vasculitis	
	SLE pancreatitis	
Aspirin/NSAIDs	Antiphospholipid syndrome	Peptic ulceration
	SLE arthritis	Platelet inhibition
		Renal impairment
		Fluid retention/ electrolyte disturbance
		Hepatic dysfunction
		Bronchospasm
Cyclophosphamide	Nephritis	Myelosuppression
	NPSLE	Pseudocholinesterase inhibition
		Cardiotoxicity
		Leucopenia
		Hemorrhagic cystitis
Azathioprine	Arthritis	Myelosuppression
		Hepatotoxicity
Methotrexate	Arthritis	Myelosuppression
	Cutaneous SLE	Hepatic fibrosis/ cirrhosis
		Pulmonary infiltrates/ fibrosis
Mycophenolate mofetil	Nephritis	GI upset
	Hemolytic anemia, thrombocytopenia	Pancytopenia

From Ben-Menachem [9], with permission Wolters Kluwer

How Can the SLE Patient Be Optimized Prior to Surgery?

A complete history and physical examination are fundamental for assessing a patient with lupus. Disease activity and end-organ damage can be assessed using a variety of indices, which integrate components of the history and physical examination (e.g., the SLICC/ACR Damage Index that has been validated to record cumulative damage in 12 organ systems in SLE patients over time) [46]. Current medication use and medication history will also provide an indication of disease severity in well-monitored patients. The patient's rheumatologist will be able to provide valuable information with regard to disease flare-ups, end-organ damage, and drug history [9]. Indeed, patients with moderate and severe disease should be managed throughout the perioperative period in collaboration with a rheumatologist.

Preoperative history and physical examination should focus on cardiorespiratory function, presence of renal disease, prior thromboembolic events, and neurological injury, e.g., prior stroke or seizure activity.

Required laboratory investigations include CBC and differential (for anemia, leukopenia, and thrombocytopenia), and serum electrolytes, creatinine, and urinalysis (looking for proteinuria, red cells, white cells, and cellular casts). Anti-phospholipid antibody measurement in the context of past test results and thromboembolic history can aid in decision-making with regard to assessment of thromboembolic risk and degree of subsequent thromboprophylaxis. This is especially relevant in the patient presented at the beginning of this chapter who will be undergoing major joint replacement and as a result is at increased risk for postoperative venous thromboembolism.

ECG may indicate the presence of clinically silent ischemia, pericarditis, and rhythm and conduction abnormalities. Chest X-ray is warranted to detect the presence of pericardial effusion, interstitial pneumonitis, or pleural effusion [9]. Pulmonary function testing may be required for investigation of worsening dyspnea [47]. Coronary angiography should be performed as part of the preoperative work-up if coronary atherosclerosis is suspected based on clinical evaluation and less invasive cardiac investigations, and if it is expected to alter management.

What Advice Should the Patient Be Given Regarding Continuation of Medications Perioperatively?

Corticosteroid medication should be continued and depending on the dose and duration of treatment, perioperative surgical stress dosing may be required. This is discussed in detail in Chap. 19. A useful guide to continuation of lupus-modifying medication for patients undergoing total hip or knee replacement has been provided by the American College of Rheumatology and American Association of Hip and Knee Surgeons (Table 30.5) [48]. Patients taking long-term anticoagulation may require discontinuation and possible bridging, which can be performed in consultation with a hematologist. For lupus patients with secondary antiphospholipid syndrome, aspirin use and timing during the perioperative period should be reviewed.

Hydroxychloroquine and chloroquine should be continued in most cases unless there are concerns of specific drug interactions with perioperative medications, or organ abnor-

Table 30.5 2017 guideline for the perioperative management of antirheumatic medication in patients undergoing elective total hip or total knee arthroplasty from the American College of Rheumatology/American Association of Hip and Knee Surgeons

DMARDS: Continue these medications through surgery	*Dosing interval*	*Continue/withhold*
Methotrexate	Weekly	Continue
Sulfasalazine	Once or twice daily	Continue
Hydroxychloroquine	Once or twice daily	Continue
Leflunomide (Arava)	Daily	Continue
Doxycycline	Daily	Continue
Biologic agents: Stop these medications prior to surgery and schedule surgery at the end of the dosing cycle. Resume medications at minimum 14 days after surgery in the absence of wound healing problems, surgical site infection, or system infection	*Dosing interval*	*Schedule surgery (relative to last biologic agent dose administered during*
Adalimumab (Humira	Weekly or every 2 weeks	Week 2 or 3
Etanercept (Enbrel)	Weekly or twice weekly	Week2
Golimumab (Simponi)	Every 4 weeks (SQ) or every 8 weeks (IV)	Week 5 Week 9
Infliximab (Remicade)	Every 4, 6, or 8 weeks	Week 5, 7, or 9
Abatacept (Orencia)	Monthly (IV) or weekly (SQ)	Week 5 Week 2
Certolizumab (Cimzia)	Every 2 or 4 weeks	Week 3 or 5
Rituximab (Rituxan)	2 doses 2 weeks apart Every 4–6 months	Month 7
Tocilizumab (Actemra)	Every week (SQ) or every 4 weeks (IV)	Week 2 Week 5
Anakinra (Kineret)	Daily	Day 2
Secukinumab (Cosentyx)	Every 4 weeks	Week 5
Ustekinumb (Stelara)	Every 12 weeks	Week 13
Belimumab (Benlysta)	Every 4 weeks	Week 5
Tofacitinib (Xeljanz) STOP this medication 7 days prior to surgery	Daily or twice daily	7 days after last dose
Severe SLE-specific medications: Continue these medications in the perioperative period	*Dosing interval*	*Continue/withhold*
Mycophenolate mofetil	Twice daily	Continue
Azathioprine	Daily or twice daily	Continue

(continued)

Table 30.5 (continued)

Cyclosporine	Twice daily	Continue
Tacrolimus	Twice daily (IV and PO)	Continue
Not severe SLE: Discontinue these medications 1 week prior to surgery	*Dosing interval*	*Continue/withhold*
Mycophenolate mofetil	Twice daily	Withhold
Azathioprine	Daily or twice daily	Withhold
Cyclosporine	Twice daily	Withhold
Tacrolimus	Twice daily (IV and PO)	Withhold

From Goodman et al. [48] with permission Elsevier
DMARDS Disease-modifying antirheumatic drugs, *SQ* Subcutaneous, *IV* Intravenous, *SLE* Systemic lupus erythematosus, *PO* per os (oral)

malities including renal or liver dysfunction. Continuation or discontinuation (whether temporary or permanent) of immunosuppressant medications requires careful consideration of the specific lupus patient, weighing the risk/benefit of disease flare against surgical or procedure-associated risks such as infection and healing time. This can be facilitated with an open dialogue among the care providers including the rheumatologist.

True/False Questions

1. (a) SLE affects males and females equally
   (b) Pericarditis is the commonest cardiac manifestation of SLE
   (c) Lupus nephritis is a rare complication of SLE
   (d) Post-intubation subglottic stenosis has been described in SLE patients after brief periods of intubation
   (e) Hematologic abnormalities in SLE affect all three blood cell types
2. (a) Patients with any disease activity are usually prescribed chloroquine or hydroxychloroquine unless contraindicated
   (b) Hydroxychloroquine can cause cardiotoxicity
   (c) Hydroxychloroquine should be discontinued perioperatively
   (d) Biologic agents should be stopped before surgery and not resumed for a minimum of 2 weeks postoperatively
   (e) Corticosteroid medication always requires perioperative surgical stress dosing

References

1. Lawrence RC, Helmick CG, Arnett FC, Deyo RA, Felson DT, Giannini EH, et al. Estimates of the prevalence of arthritis and selected musculoskeletal disorders in the United States. Arthritis Rheum. 1998;41(5):778–99.
2. Chakravarty EF, Bush TM, Manzi S, Clarke AE, Ward MM. Prevalence of adult systemic lupus erythematosus in California and Pennsylvania in 2000: estimates obtained using hospitalization data. Arthritis Rheum. 2007;56(6):2092–4.
3. D'Cruz DP. Systemic lupus erythematosus. BMJ. 2006;332(7546):890–4.
4. Wallace D, Gladman D. Clinical manifestations and diagnosis of systemic lupus erythematosus in adults. In: Post TW, editor. UpToDate. Waltham; 2020.
5. Hochberg MC. Updating the American College of Rheumatology revised criteria for the classification of systemic lupus erythematosus. Arthritis Rheum. 1997;40(9):1725.
6. Tan EM, Cohen AS, Fries JF, Masi AT, McShane DJ, Rothfield NF, et al. The 1982 revised criteria for the classification of systemic lupus erythematosus. Arthritis Rheum. 1982;25(11):1271–7.
7. Petri M, Orbai AM, Alarcon GS, Gordon C, Merrill JT, Fortin PR, et al. Derivation and validation of the Systemic Lupus International Collaborating Clinics classification criteria for systemic lupus erythematosus. Arthritis Rheum. 2012;64(8):2677–86.
8. Assan F, Seror R, Mariette X, Nocturne G. New 2019 SLE EULAR/ACR classification criteria are valuable for distinguishing patients with SLE from patients with pSS. Ann Rheum Dis. 2019:annrheumdis-2019-216222. https://doi.org/10.1136/annrheumdis-2019-216222. Epub ahead of print.
9. Ben-Menachem E. Review article: systemic lupus erythematosus: a review for anesthesiologists. Anesth Analg. 2010;111(3):665–76. https://doi.org/10.1213/ANE.0b013e3181e8138e.
10. Zeller CB, Appenzeller S. Cardiovascular disease in systemic lupus erythematosus: the role of traditional and lupus related risk factors. Curr Cardiol Rev. 2008;4(2):116–22.
11. Manzi S, Meilahn EN, Rairie JE, Conte CG, Medsger TA Jr, Jansen-McWilliams L, et al. Age-specific incidence rates of myocardial infarction and angina in women with systemic lupus erythematosus: comparison with the Framingham Study. Am J Epidemiol. 1997;145(5):408–15.
12. Moder KG, Miller TD, Tazelaar HD. Cardiac involvement in systemic lupus erythematosus. Mayo Clin Proc. 1999;74(3):275–84.
13. Imazio M. Acute pericarditis: treatment and prognosis. In: Post TW, editor. UpToDate. Waltham; 2020.
14. Roldan CA, Shively BK, Crawford MH. An echocardiographic study of valvular heart disease associated with systemic lupus erythematosus. N Engl J Med. 1996;335(19):1424–30.
15. Seferovic PM, Ristic AD, Maksimovic R, Simeunovic DS, Ristic GG, Radovanovic G, et al. Cardiac arrhythmias and conduction disturbances in autoimmune rheumatic diseases. Rheumatology (Oxford). 2006;45(Suppl 4):iv39–42.
16. Barile-Fabris L, Hernandez-Cabrera MF, Barragan-Garfias JA. Vasculitis in systemic lupus erythematosus. Curr Rheumatol Rep. 2014;16(9):440.
17. Cervera R, Khamashta MA, Font J, Sebastiani GD, Gil A, Lavilla P, et al. Morbidity and mortality in systemic lupus erythematosus during a 10-year period: a comparison of early and late manifestations in a cohort of 1,000 patients. Medicine (Baltimore). 2003;82(5):299–308.
18. Smilowitz NR, Katz G, Buyon JP, Clancy RM, Berger JS. Systemic lupus erythematosus and the risk of perioperative major adverse cardiovascular events. J Thromb Thrombolysis. 2018;45(1):13–7.
19. Mathis KW, Taylor EB, Ryan MJ. Anti-CD3 antibody therapy attenuates the progression of hypertension in female mice with systemic lupus erythematosus. Pharmacol Res. 2017;120:252–7.
20. Taylor EB, Ryan MJ. Understanding mechanisms of hypertension in systemic lupus erythematosus. Version 2. Ther Adv Cardiovasc Dis. 2016;11(1):20–32.
21. Singh S, Saxena R. Lupus nephritis. Am J Med Sci. 2009;337(6):451–60.
22. Danila MI, Pons-Estel GJ, Zhang J, Vila LM, Reveille JD, Alarcon GS. Renal damage is the most important predictor of mortality within the damage index: data from LUMINA LXIV, a multiethnic US cohort. Rheumatology (Oxford). 2009;48(5):542–5.

23. Swigris JJ, Fischer A, Gillis J, Meehan RT, Brown KK. Pulmonary and thrombotic manifestations of systemic lupus erythematosus. Chest. 2008;133(1):271–80.
24. Bertoli AM, Vila LM, Apte M, Fessler BJ, Bastian HM, Reveille JD, et al. Systemic lupus erythematosus in a multiethnic US Cohort LUMINA XLVIII: factors predictive of pulmonary damage. Lupus. 2007;16(6):410–7.
25. Karim MY, Miranda LC, Tench CM, Gordon PA, D'Cruz DP, Khamashta MA, et al. Presentation and prognosis of the shrinking lung syndrome in systemic lupus erythematosus. Semin Arthritis Rheum. 2002;31(5):289–98.
26. Warrington KJ, Moder KG, Brutinel WM. The shrinking lungs syndrome in systemic lupus erythematosus. Mayo Clin Proc. 2000;75(5):467–72.
27. Langford CA, Van Waes C. Upper airway obstruction in the rheumatic diseases. Rheum Dis Clin N Am. 1997;23(2):345–63.
28. Smith GA, Ward PH, Berci G. Laryngeal lupus erythematosus. J Laryngol Otol. 1978;92(1):67–73.
29. Raj R, Murin S, Matthay RA, Wiedemann HP. Systemic lupus erythematosus in the intensive care unit. Crit Care Clin. 2002;18(4):781–803.
30. Teitel AD, MacKenzie CR, Stern R, Paget SA. Laryngeal involvement in systemic lupus erythematosus. Semin Arthritis Rheum. 1992;22(3):203–14.
31. Sultan SM, Begum S, Isenberg DA. Prevalence, patterns of disease and outcome in patients with systemic lupus erythematosus who develop severe haematological problems. Rheumatology (Oxford). 2003;42(2):230–4.
32. Greenberg BM. The neurologic manifestations of systemic lupus erythematosus. Neurologist. 2009;15(3):115–21.
33. Mok CC. Investigations and management of gastrointestinal and hepatic manifestations of systemic lupus erythematosus. Best Pract Res Clin Rheumatol. 2005;19(5):741–66.
34. Runyon BA, LaBrecque DR, Anuras S. The spectrum of liver disease in systemic lupus erythematosus. Report of 33 histologically-proved cases and review of the literature. Am J Med. 1980;69(2):187–94.
35. Hallegua DS, Venuturupalli S. Gastrointestinal and hepatic manifestations. In: Wallace DJ, Hahn BH, editors. Dubois' lupus erythematosus and related syndromes. 8th ed. Philadelphia: Elsevier; 2013. p. 422.
36. Sultan SM, Ioannou Y, Isenberg DA. A review of gastrointestinal manifestations of systemic lupus erythematosus. Rheumatology (Oxford). 1999;38(10):917–32.
37. Lapadula G, Muolo P, Semeraro F, Covelli M, Brindicci D, Cuccorese G, et al. Esophageal motility disorders in the rheumatic diseases: a review of 150 patients. Clin Exp Rheumatol. 1994;12(5):515–21.
38. Sarabi ZS, Chang E, Bobba R, Ibanez D, Gladman D, Urowitz M, et al. Incidence rates of arterial and venous thrombosis after diagnosis of systemic lupus erythematosus. Arthritis Rheum. 2005;53(4):609–12.
39. Cervera R, Piette JC, Font J, Khamashta MA, Shoenfeld Y, Camps MT, et al. Antiphospholipid syndrome: clinical and immunologic manifestations and patterns of disease expression in a cohort of 1,000 patients. Arthritis Rheum. 2002;46(4):1019–27.
40. Love PE, Santoro SA. Antiphospholipid antibodies: anticardiolipin and the lupus anticoagulant in systemic lupus erythematosus (SLE) and in non-SLE disorders. Prevalence and clinical significance. Ann Intern Med. 1990;112(9):682–98.
41. Marschall K. Skin and musculoskeletal diseases. In: Hines R, Marschall K, editors. Stoelting's Anesthesia and co-existing disease. 7th ed. Philadelphia: Elsevier; 2017.
42. Cronin ME. Musculoskeletal manifestations of systemic lupus erythematosus. Rheum Dis Clin N Am. 1988;14(1):99–116.
43. Klemp P, Meyers OL, Keyzer C. Atlanto-axial subluxation in systemic lupus erythematosus: a case report. S Afr Med J. 1977;52(8):331–2.
44. Babini SM, Cocco JA, Babini JC, de la Sota M, Arturi A, Marcos JC. Atlantoaxial subluxation in systemic lupus erythematosus: further evidence of tendinous alterations. J Rheumatol. 1990;17(2):173–7.
45. Wallace D. Overview of the management and prognosis of systemic lupus erythematosus in adults. In: Post TW, editor. UpToDate. Waltham; 2020.
46. Gladman D, Ginzler E, Goldsmith C, Fortin P, Liang M, Urowitz M, et al. The development and initial validation of the Systemic Lupus International Collaborating Clinics/American College of Rheumatology damage index for systemic lupus erythematosus. Arthritis Rheum. 1996;39(3):363–9.
47. Wijeysundera D, Finlayson E. Preoperative evaluation. In: Gropper M, editor. Miller's anesthesia. Philadelphia: Elsevier; 2020.
48. Goodman SM, Springer B, Guyatt G, Abdel MP, Dasa V, George M, et al. 2017 American College of Rheumatology/American Association of Hip and Knee Surgeons guideline for the perioperative management of antirheumatic medication in patients with rheumatic diseases undergoing elective Total hip or Total knee arthroplasty. J Arthroplast. 2017;32(9):2628–38.

31 Duchenne Muscular Dystrophy

Derek Dillane

A 30-year-old male patient with Duchenne muscular dystrophy was admitted with a diagnosis of amiodarone-induced thyrotoxicosis. A preoperative opinion was sought on the grounds that total thyroidectomy was being considered as a treatment option. The patient had dilated cardiomyopathy with multiple previous episodes of ventricular tachycardia requiring implantable cardioverter defibrillator (ICD) with cardiac resynchronization therapy (CRT). He had restrictive lung disease requiring nightly bilevel positive airway pressure (BiPAP) and occasional daytime use. In addition, he had previously had a posterior cerebral artery stroke.

Medications: Carvedilol 25 mg twice daily; sacubitril/valsartan, spironolactone 12.5 mg daily; furosemide 20 mg twice daily; omeprazole, methimazole 10 mg 4 times daily; deflazacort 18 mg daily; hydrocortisone 25 mg daily; and prednisone 10 mg daily.

Physical Examination: The patient was wheelchair dependent. Blood pressure 96/60, heart rate 94, respiratory rate 19, SpO_2 99% on 3 L oxygen. A murmur consistent with mitral regurgitation was noted in addition to a displaced apex beat. Peripheral edema was present bilaterally in the ankles and feet. Lungs were clear to auscultation.

Investigations: Laboratory values revealed a hemoglobin 74 g/L, platelet count 235 × 10^9 /L, WBC count 5.4 × 10^9 /L, Na 132 mmol/L, K 4.5 mmol/L, creatinine 50 µmol/L, estimated glomerular filtration rate 138 mL/min/1.73m², free thyroxine (T4) 46.5 pmol/L (9.0–23.0 pmol/L), INR 1.0, and PTT 32.

Chest radiograph and electrocardiogram and can be seen in Figs. 31.1 and 31.2. *Pulmonary function test (PFT) results are shown in* Fig. 31.3. *Echocardiography revealed a severely dilated left ventricle with severely reduced systolic function as demonstrated by an ejection fraction of 19%. Right ventricle was normal in size and function. Moderate mitral regurgitation was noted, and the other valves were structurally and functionally normal.*

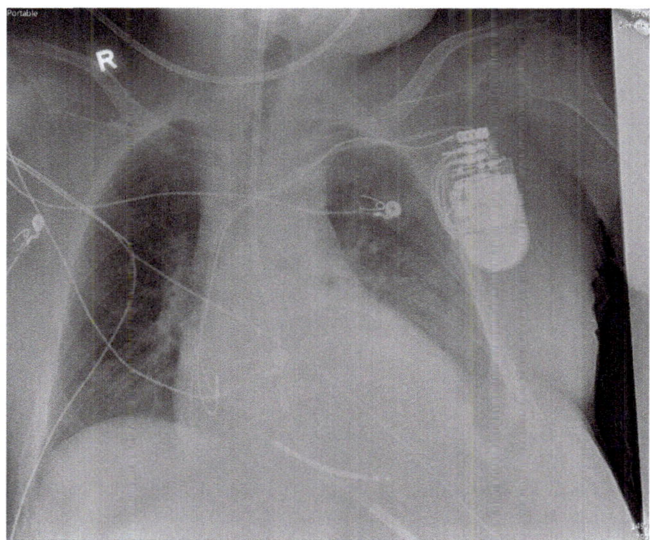

Fig. 31.1 Chest radiograph with enlarged cardiac silhouette, underinflated lungs, left lower lobe atelectasis, small left basal pleural effusion, and no evidence of pulmonary edema. The tip of a central venous line is seen in the superior vena cava/right atrium. The implantable cardioverter defibrillator device and leads are seen in the left hemithorax

What Is Duchenne Muscular Dystrophy?

The muscular dystrophies are a group of inherited progressive myopathies resulting in increasing muscle weakness over time. Duchenne muscular dystrophy (DMD) is the most common muscular dystrophy. It is also the most severe [1]. Onset of symptoms usually occurs between 2 and 5 years of age. It is transmitted via an X-linked recessive inheritance with an incidence of approximately 1/5000 live male births [2]. It is caused by a mutation in the dystrophin gene. Dystrophin is a protein found in skeletal, smooth, and cardiac muscles as well as the brain. It plays a vital role in stabilizing muscle cell membrane

D. Dillane (✉)
Department of Anesthesiology & Pain Medicine, University of Alberta, Edmonton, AB, Canada

D. Dillane, B. A. Finegan (eds.), *Preoperative Assessment*, https://doi.org/10.1007/978-3-030-58842-7_31

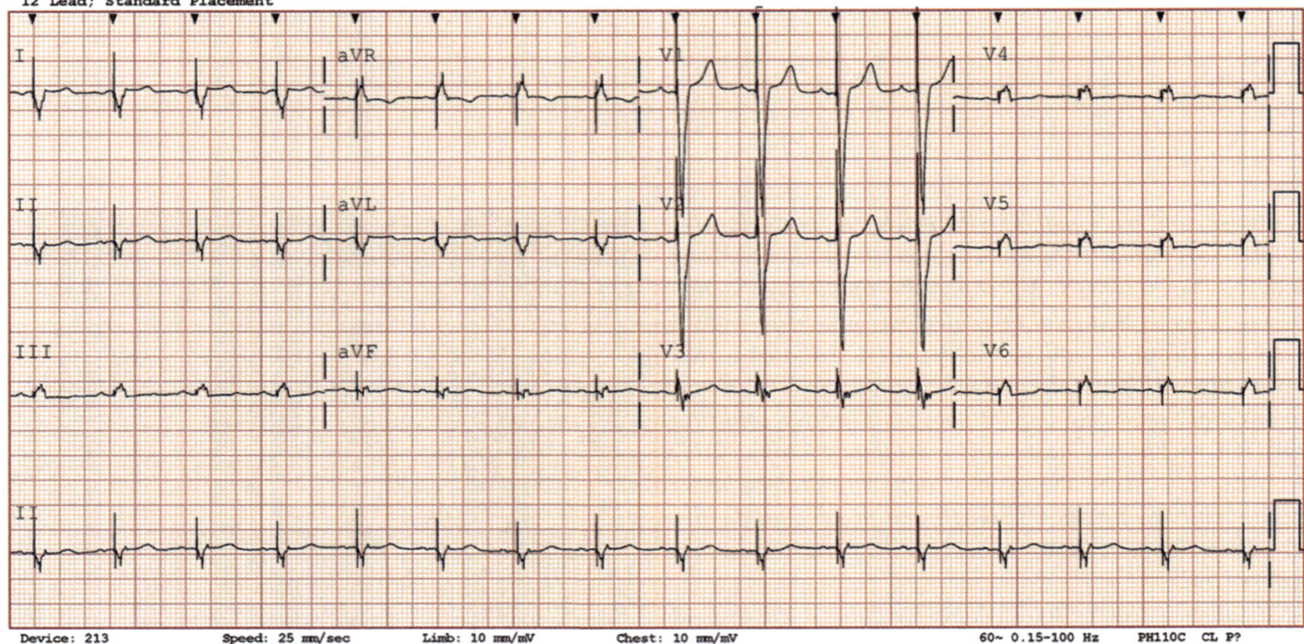

Fig. 31.2 Electrocardiograph with atrial-sensed ventricular-paced rhythm

(sarcolemma) integrity, particularly during contraction and relaxation [3]. Muscle weakness associated with DMD involves the lower more than the upper limbs and proximal more than distal muscle groups. Becker muscular dystrophy is also caused by a mutation in the dystrophin gene, but its clinical course is milder, and onset of symptoms is later. A third intermediate phenotype occurs that is between Duchenne and Becker with respect to clinical course. Finally, DMD-associated dilated cardiomyopathy is a disease subtype characterized by cardiac involvement with minimal or no skeletal muscle disease [1]. Females are usually asymptomatic carriers of the muscular dystrophies, but clinical manifestations in the form of muscle weakness or cardiomyopathy have been found in approximately 20% of carriers of Duchenne and Becker muscular dystrophy [4].

What Complications Can Be Expected Perioperatively in the Patient with Duchenne Muscular Dystrophy?

- Hyperkalemic cardiac arrest and rhabdomyolysis may occur because of the unstable sarcolemma. Succinylcholine should be avoided.
- There is an increased incidence of malignant hyperthermia (MH) even though the risk for an MH mutation is no higher than for the general population. Dantrolene should be readily available. The use of triggering agents is controversial. Volatile anesthetics have been known to cause hypermetabolic reactions in myopathic patients [3]. Total intravenous anesthesia (TIVA) with propofol is a popular choice in these patients, not only in reducing the risk of rhabdomyolysis, but in facilitating neurophysiological monitoring [5]. On the other hand, there have been concerns regarding the association of prolonged propofol infusion with rhabdomyolysis resulting from disruption of mitochondrial fatty acid oxidation seen in a pediatric ICU setting [5].
- Dilated cardiomyopathy and associated hemodynamic instability. Lack of dystrophin in the myocardium results in excess intracellular calcium. This activates proteases, which degrade contractile proteins leading to myocardial cell death and fibrosis [3].
- Congestive cardiac failure. All DMD patients will eventually develop a clinically apparent cardiomyopathy. It remains clinically latent until the later stages of the disease due to the non-ambulatory condition of most patients.

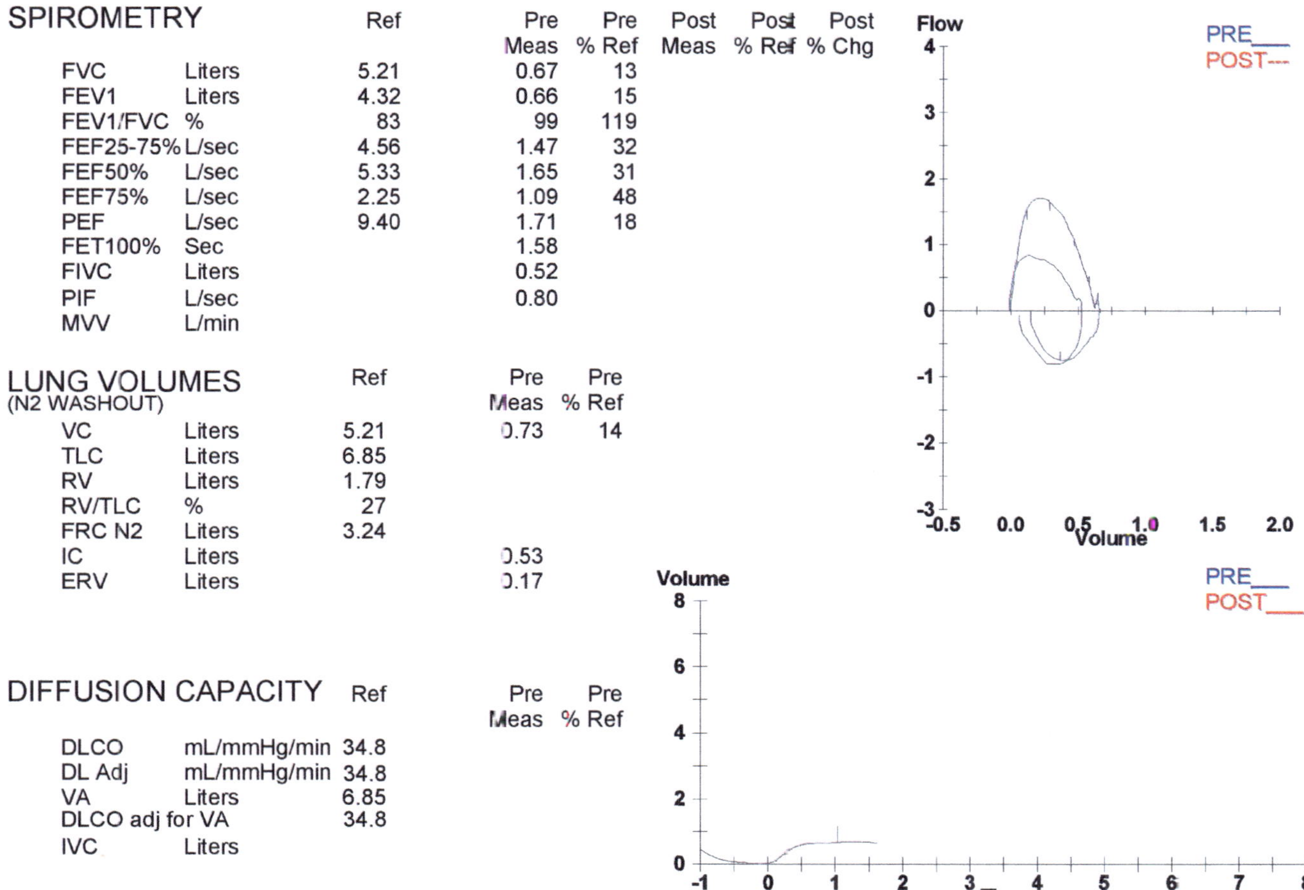

SPIROMETRY		Ref	Pre Meas	Pre % Ref	Post Meas	Post % Ref	Post % Chg
FVC	Liters	5.21	0.67	13			
FEV1	Liters	4.32	0.66	15			
FEV1/FVC	%	83	99	119			
FEF25-75%	L/sec	4.56	1.47	32			
FEF50%	L/sec	5.33	1.65	31			
FEF75%	L/sec	2.25	1.09	48			
PEF	L/sec	9.40	1.71	18			
FET100%	Sec		1.58				
FIVC	Liters		0.52				
PIF	L/sec		0.80				
MVV	L/min						

LUNG VOLUMES (N2 WASHOUT)		Ref	Pre Meas	Pre % Ref
VC	Liters	5.21	0.73	14
TLC	Liters	6.85		
RV	Liters	1.79		
RV/TLC	%	27		
FRC N2	Liters	3.24		
IC	Liters		0.53	
ERV	Liters		0.17	

DIFFUSION CAPACITY		Ref	Pre Meas	Pre % Ref
DLCO	mL/mmHg/min	34.8		
DL Adj	mL/mmHg/min	34.8		
VA	Liters	6.85		
DLCO adj for VA		34.8		
IVC	Liters			

Fig. 31.3 Spirometry, lung volumes, and diffusion capacity as part of pulmonary function testing. Minimum flow criteria were not met for flow-volume loops. Overall effort was suboptimal, and the patient was unable to remain off BiPAP long enough for diffusion capacity for carbon monoxide (DLCO) and nitrogen washout testing

- Arrhythmias, particularly persistent sinus tachycardia. Atrial fibrillation or flutter can accompany cor pulmonale and dilated cardiomyopathy [6].
- Progressive weakness of the diaphragm, intercostal and accessory muscles of respiration result in a restrictive respiratory defect eventually leading to respiratory failure. Non-depolarizing muscle relaxants have a prolonged duration of action in this population. Residual neuromuscular blockade increases the risk of respiratory complications.
- Upper airway obstruction.
- Recurrent aspiration and poor cough reflex predispose to frequent episodes of pneumonia.
- Difficulty weaning from mechanical ventilation.
- Atelectasis.
- Pulmonary hypertension and right heart failure secondary to nocturnal hypoventilation and obstructive sleep apnea.

How Should the Patient with Duchenne Muscular Dystrophy Be Evaluated Preoperatively?

Preoperative assessment requires a multidisciplinary approach that includes team members from anesthesiology, surgery, pulmonology, and cardiology. A useful starting place for the evaluating anesthesiologist is patient classification into one of three groups based on disease progression: ambulatory, early non-ambulatory, and late non-ambulatory [7].

Cardiac Evaluation

Evolving neuromuscular and respiratory therapies have changed the natural history of DMD to the extent that the current leading cause of death is cardiomyopathy. There is no relationship between the timing or severity of cardiac and skeletal muscle disease [3]. Although approximately 50–70% of all muscular dystrophy patients are thought to have a cardiac abnormality, it is subclinical in most. A clinically significant cardiac abnormality is present in only 10% of muscular dystrophy patients [8].

- *History:* Most patients have no symptoms of heart failure. Signs and symptoms of heart failure are often subtle or atypical, e.g., worsening fatigue, weight loss, anorexia, vomiting, abdominal pain, and insomnia. The New York Heart Association (NYHA) classification is not suitable in this population due to its reliance on physical activity as a discriminator.
- *Physical examination:* Vital signs including weight, heart rate, and blood pressure are measured. Resting sinus tachycardia is frequently seen, even in the absence of ventricular dysfunction [5]. Hypotension is common in the non-ambulatory stages. This is very often a precursor of significant intraoperative hypotension. Physical findings of note in cardiomyopathy include jugular venous distension, displaced apex beat, and presence of S3/4 gallop [3].
- *Investigations:* DMD patients typically visit a cardiologist annually during the ambulatory and early non-ambulatory stages and more frequently in the late non-ambulatory stage, at the discretion of the cardiologist [7]. Recommended annual investigations for DMD patients include electrocardiogram (ECG) and echocardiogram or cardiac magnetic resonance imaging (MRI). 24-hour Holter monitoring may be indicated if an arrhythmia is seen on ECG or the patient provides a history suggestive of arrhythmias. The main preoperative cardiac findings of note on non-invasive imaging are presence or degree of myocardial fibrosis, left ventricular enlargement, and left ventricular dysfunction. Cardiac MRI with gadolinium enhancement is particularly suitable for characterizing myocardial fibrosis, one of the earliest findings in cardiac involvement in DMD [9]. It is the cardiac imaging modality of choice for many cardiologists for DMD. Echocardiography may demonstrate mitral valve prolapse or posterobasilar hypokinesis in a thin-walled left ventricle [8]. A stress echocardiogram may be required to unmask the latent cardiac failure associated with DMD [8].

Pulmonary Evaluation

PFTs are useful in determining the need for postoperative ventilation. The American College of Chest Physicians (ACCP) Consensus on Preoperative Pulmonary Evaluation of DMD Patients is a useful guide in this regard (Table 31.1) [10]. It recommends preoperative assessment of oxygenation, lung volumes, and cough strength. Patients with ambulatory DMD typically undergo annual forced vital capacity (FVC) measurement, tests of cough strength, and sleep studies, while those who have progressed to non-ambulatory DMD have twice yearly pulmonary investigations [7].

Table 31.1 Preoperative pulmonary evaluation of Duchenne muscular dystrophy patients from the American College of Chest Physicians

Assessment	Monitoring level	Recommendation/evaluation
Oxygenation	$SpO_2 < 95\%$ on room air by pulse oximetry	Requires measurement of $PaCO_2$
Lung volumes	FVC in seated, upright position <50% of predicted	Increased risk of perioperative respiratory complications
	<30% of predicted	High risk of perioperative respiratory complications
Cough strength	MEP < 60 cm H_2O PCF < 270 L/min	Preoperative training in assisted cough devices

From Birnkrant et al. [10] with permission Elsevier

SpO_2 oxygen saturation, *FVC* forced vital capacity; *$PaCO_2$* arterial carbon dioxide tension, *MEP* maximum expiratory pressure, *PCF* peak cough flow

- Pulse oximetry in room air should be measured, and if <95%, a blood gas analysis is warranted.
- Measure maximum inspiratory pressure (MIP), maximum expiratory pressure (MEP), and peak cough flow (PCF). Patients with PCF < 270 L/min or MEP < 60 cm H_2O should be considered for preoperative training in mechanically assisted cough.
- Patients with an FVC < 50% of predicted should receive preoperative training with non-invasive positive pressure ventilation (NIPPV) to facilitate extubation [3]. Strong consideration should be given to extubation directly to NIPPV for both groups of patients, but especially for those with an FVC < 30% predicted.

Airway Evaluation

Patients with muscular dystrophy have potential for airway involvement, and a thorough airway examination is warranted preoperatively. Difficult laryngoscopy was noted in 3.4% of cases in a retrospective review of 91 DMD patients undergoing 232 general anesthetics for orthopedic surgery [11]. This may be related to skeletal muscle involvement or fibrosis of the masseter and neck muscles limiting movement.

Evaluation of Myopathy

Creatine kinase (CK) can provide an indication of the severity of myopathy. Serum CK peaks at the age of 2 years in patients with DMD when it may be 10–20 times the upper normal limit. It then decreases by 25% per year approaching the normal range as muscle is replaced by fat and fibrosis [1].

Gastrointestinal and Nutritional Evaluation

Electrolyte disturbances can precipitate arrhythmias—we know from the foregoing that DMD patients have a pre-existent predisposition to rhythm disturbances. Patients are assessed annually by a dietician nutritionist for monitoring of weight, height, dysphagia, gastroesophageal reflux (not uncommon in muscular dystrophy due to bulbar dysfunction), fluid and nutrient imbalance, and bone density [12]. The aim of these visits is to prevent obesity and malnutrition. The patient's nutritionist should be consulted preoperatively, time permitting.

Endocrine Evaluation

From a perioperative perspective, the most relevant endocrine complication of DMD and its treatment is adrenal insufficiency. This is due to suppression of the hypothalamic-pituitary-adrenal axis by exogenous glucocorticoid therapy. Surgical stress dosing may be required for the patient at risk of secondary adrenal insufficiency due to exogenous glucocorticoid therapy. A recent review on this subject suggests that patients taking prednisone 5 mg daily or less for any period of time do not need steroid stress dose administration [13]. As this patient was taking in excess of this amount, he would require surgical stress dosing if proceeding to surgery. A detailed approach to surgical stress dosing technique is provided in Chap. 19.

What Can Be Ascertained from This Patient's PFTs?

A restrictive pattern of pulmonary disease is present as evidenced by the low FVC. At less than 13% of predicted, this patient is considered very high risk for prolonged postoperative ventilation. Full PFT testing with diffusion capacity for carbon monoxide (DLCO) is indicated when a restrictive pattern is present. However, due to the low volumes attained and the patient's BiPAP dependence, lung volume and DLCO measurement were not attempted. We know that there is no element of obstruction in this disease pattern as the FEV1/FVC pattern is normal. An obstructive defect is present when FEV1/FVC is less than 70%.

What Is the Significance of This Patient Being on BiPAP?

There is evidence that nocturnal non-invasive ventilation (NIV) increases long-term survival. A retrospective review of 197 patients with DMD showed that the chances of survival to 25 years of age increased from 12% to 53% with nocturnal NIV [14].

Are DMD Patients at Increased Risk of Stroke?

Though epidemiological data are scarce, ischemic stroke in DMD has been described in a small number of patients [15]. The most likely underlying cause of thromboembolic stroke in this population is dilated cardiomyopathy.

What Options Are Available for Optimization of the Patient with DMD?

- Consensus guidelines recommend initiation of an angiotensin converting enzyme (ACE) inhibitor or angiotensin receptor blocker at 10 years of age [7, 9]. Preliminary long-term survival evidence suggests that ACE inhibitors may slow disease progression when left ventricular ejection fraction (LVEF) is normal at the beginning of therapy [16].
- Beta blockade may have a role to play in improving left ventricular function in DMD cardiomyopathy [17]. Beta blockers are usually started after ACE inhibitors for management of left ventricular dysfunction or tachycardia.
- Preoperative respiratory optimization includes lung volume recruitment, manual and mechanically assisted cough techniques, nocturnal ventilation, and assisted daytime ventilation. Patients should receive training in assisted coughing and NIV techniques to aid postoperative recovery.
- Patients in whom NIV is unsuccessful may require a tracheostomy to facilitate invasive ventilation [1].
- Glucocorticoids are the cornerstone of pharmacologic treatment and have been shown to improve motor function, strength, and pulmonary function; reduce the risk of scoliosis; and prolong independent ambulation [18]. Deflazacort is a commonly prescribed glucocorticoid in the treatment of DMD [19]. It is unclear if it offers any benefits over prednisone.

- In DMD patients with heart failure, benefit of ICD outweighs risk when ejection fraction <35%.
- Use of antiarrhythmic agents for atrial and ventricular arrhythmias follows that for heart failure management and arrhythmia management (see Chaps. 5 and 6).

The patient was admitted to ICU for medical management and optimization of his thyroid disease. Although thyroidectomy was considered, it was not felt to be an imminently necessary procedure. Over the course of 10 days, he responded well to medical therapy and thus avoided surgery.

True-False Questions

1. (a) Duchenne muscular dystrophy (DMD) is the commonest of the muscular dystrophies
   (b) Onset of DMD is usually in the second decade of life
   (c) DMD is an X-linked disorder that affects the gene responsible for dystrophin production
   (d) Females are asymptomatic carriers who never exhibit clinical manifestations of the disease
   (e) DMD affects skeletal, smooth, and cardiac muscles
2. (a) Heart failure resulting from dilated cardiomyopathy is the commonest cause of death in DMD
   (b) Most patients with DMD have clinically significant cardiac disease
   (c) Patients with FVC > 50% are unlikely to require prolonged postoperative ventilation
   (d) Patients with dilated cardiomyopathy should be administered an ACE inhibitor as first-line therapy
   (e) The use of glucocorticoids in ambulatory patients has been shown to prolong ambulation

References

1. Darras B. Duchenne and Becker muscular dystrophy: clinical features and diagnosis. In: Post TW, editor. UpToDate. Waltham: 2020.
2. Verhaart IE, Aartsma-Rus A. Therapeutic developments for Duchenne muscular dystropy. Nat Rev Neurol. 2019;15(7):373–86.
3. Urban M. Muscle diseases. In: Fleisher L, editor. Anesthesia and uncommon diseases. 6th ed. Philadelphia: Elsevier; 2012. p. 296–318.
4. Hoogerwaard EM, Bakker E, Ippel PF, Oosterwijk JC, Majoor-Krakauer DF, Leschot NJ, et al. Signs and symptoms of Duchenne muscular dystrophy and Becker muscular dystrophy among carriers in The Netherlands: a cohort study. Lancet. 1999;353(9170):2116–9.
5. Cripe LH, Tobias JD. Cardiac considerations in the operative management of the patient with Duchenne or Becker muscular dystrophy. Paediatr Anaesth. 2013;23(9):777–84.
6. Rajdev A, Groh WJ. Arrhythmias in the muscular dystrophies. Card Electrophysiol Clin. 2015;7(2):303–8.
7. Birnkrant DJ, Bushby K, Bann CM, Alman BA, Apkon SD, Blackwell A, et al. Diagnosis and management of Duchenne muscular dystrophy, part 2: respiratory, cardiac, bone health, and orthopaedic management. Lancet Neurol. 2018;17(4):347–61.
8. Zhou J, Bose D, Allen PD, Pessah IN. Malignant hyperthermia and muscle-related disorders. In: Miller RD, editor. Miller's anesthesia. 8th ed. Philadelphia: Saunders; 2015. p. 1287–314.
9. McNally EM, Kaltman JR, Benson DW, Canter CE, Cripe LH, Duan D, et al. Contemporary cardiac issues in Duchenne muscular dystrophy. Working Group of the National Heart, Lung, and Blood Institute in collaboration with Parent Project Muscular Dystrophy. Circulation. 2015;131(18):1590–8.
10. Birnkrant DJ, Panitch HB, Benditt JO, Boitano LJ, Carter ER, Cwik VA, et al. American College of Chest Physicians consensus statement on the respiratory and related management of patients with Duchenne muscular dystrophy undergoing anesthesia or sedation. Chest. 2007;132(6):1977–86. https://doi.org/10.1378/chest.07-0458.
11. Muenster T, Mueller C, Forst J, Huber H, Schmitt HJ. Anaesthetic management in patients with Duchenne muscular dystrophy undergoing orthopaedic surgery: a review of 232 cases. Eur J Anaesthesiol. 2012;29(10):489–94.
12. Birnkrant DJ, Bushby K, Bann CM, Apkon SD, Blackwell A, Brumbaugh D, et al. Diagnosis and management of Duchenne muscular dystrophy, part 1: diagnosis, and neuromuscular, rehabilitation, endocrine, and gastrointestinal and nutritional management. Lancet Neurol. 2018;17(3):251–67.
13. Liu MM, Reidy AB, Saatee S, Collard CD. Perioperative steroid management: approaches based on current evidence. Anesthesiology. 2017;127(1):166–72.
14. Eagle M, Baudouin SV, Chandler C, Giddings DR, Bullock R, Bushby K. Survival in Duchenne muscular dystrophy: improvements in life expectancy since 1967 and the impact of home nocturnal ventilation. Neuromuscul Disord. 2002;12(10):926–9.
15. Winterholler M, Hollander C, Kerling F, Weber I, Dittrich S, Turk M, et al. Stroke in Duchenne muscular dystrophy: a retrospective longitudinal study in 54 patients. Stroke. 2016;47(8):2123–6.
16. Duboc D, Meune C, Pierre B, Wahbi K, Eymard B, Toutain A, et al. Perindopril preventive treatment on mortality in Duchenne muscular dystrophy: 10 years' follow-up. Am Heart J. 2007;154(3):596–602.
17. Viollet L, Thrush PT, Flanigan KM, Mendell JR, Allen HD. Effects of angiotensin-converting enzyme inhibitors and/or beta blockers on the cardiomyopathy in Duchenne muscular dystrophy. Am J Cardiol. 2012;110(1):98–102.
18. Darras B. Duchenne and Becker muscular dystrophy: glucocorticoid and disease-modifying treatment. In: Post TW, editor. UpToDate. Waltham; 2020.
19. McAdam LC, Mayo AL, Alman BA, Biggar WD. The Canadian experience with long-term deflazacort treatment in Duchenne muscular dystrophy. Acta Myol. 2012;31(1):16–20.

Part IX

Neurological

Myasthenia Gravis

32

Lora B. Pencheva

A 64-year-old female presented to the preassessment clinic 1 week prior to a sigmoid colon resection for bowel cancer. She had been diagnosed with seronegative myasthenia gravis (MG) over a decade prior to this visit.

She had recently seen her neurologist due to worsening oculobulbar weakness with diplopia, shortness of breath, paradoxical vocal cord movement, stridor, globus sensation, and dysphagia. She was started on prednisone 20 mg daily but did not receive intravenous immunoglobulin (IVIG) or plasma exchange due to religious beliefs; she was a Jehovah's Witness. She reported a return to her baseline condition following commencement of prednisone. She had no history of ICU admission or intubation because of myasthenic crisis.

She had a background history of controlled hypertension, morbid obesity, sleep apnea for which she used CPAP, and chronic back pain.

She had previously undergone a tubal ligation, hysterectomy, and breast reduction. All of these procedures were performed prior to diagnosis of MG.

Medications: ASA 81 mg daily, alendronate 70 mg weekly, amlodipine 5 mg daily, azathioprine 150 mg daily, candesartan 8 mg daily, clonidine 100mcg twice daily, duloxetine 60 mg daily, gabapentin 300 mg twice daily, hydromorphone 6 mg po twice daily, hyoscine butylbromide 10 mg daily, pantoprazole 40 mg daily, prednisone 20 mg daily, pyridostigmine slow release 180 mg nightly, pyridostigmine immediate release 120 mg four times per day.

Physical Examination: Blood pressure 121/68, pulse 84, temperature 36.2 °C, oxygen saturation (SpO_2) 94%, respiratory rate 18 bpm, height 1.52 m, weight 99.8 kg, body mass index (BMI) 43.

Respiratory and cardiovascular examinations were normal.

Airway Mallampati score II, thyromental distance (TMD) > 6 cm; full neck extension, upper denture.

Investigations: Acetylcholine receptor (AChR) antibody testing and muscle-specific tyrosine kinase (MuSK) antibody testing were both negative.

Electromyography (EMG) and Nerve Conduction Studies Bilateral carpal tunnel syndrome. Single fiber EMG abnormal jitter 16% of the time, resulting in a non-definitive diagnosis but possibility of myasthenia gravis.

Laboratory investigations and ECG at this visit to the preadmission clinic were normal. Results from pulmonary function testing, performed shortly after the visit, can be seen in Fig 32.1.

What Is Myasthenia Gravis?

Myasthenia gravis (MG) is an autoimmune disorder affecting the postsynaptic membrane of the neuromuscular junction of skeletal muscle. Autoantibodies against the α-subunit of the nicotinic acetylcholine receptor nAChR (muscle type only) cause receptor destruction and transmission failure, resulting in skeletal muscle weakness and fatiguability. The nAChR of the autonomic and central nervous systems are spared.

The incidence of MG varies between 0.25 and 2 per 100,000 with increasing frequency among those older than 60 years. Women are more likely to be diagnosed in the 30–40-year-old age group, whereas men are more often diagnosed from 60 years onwards [1].

L. B. Pencheva (✉)
Department of Anaesthesia & Pain Medicine, Middlemore Hospital, Auckland, New Zealand

D. Dillane, B. A. Finegan (eds.), *Preoperative Assessment*, https://doi.org/10.1007/978-3-030-58842-7_32

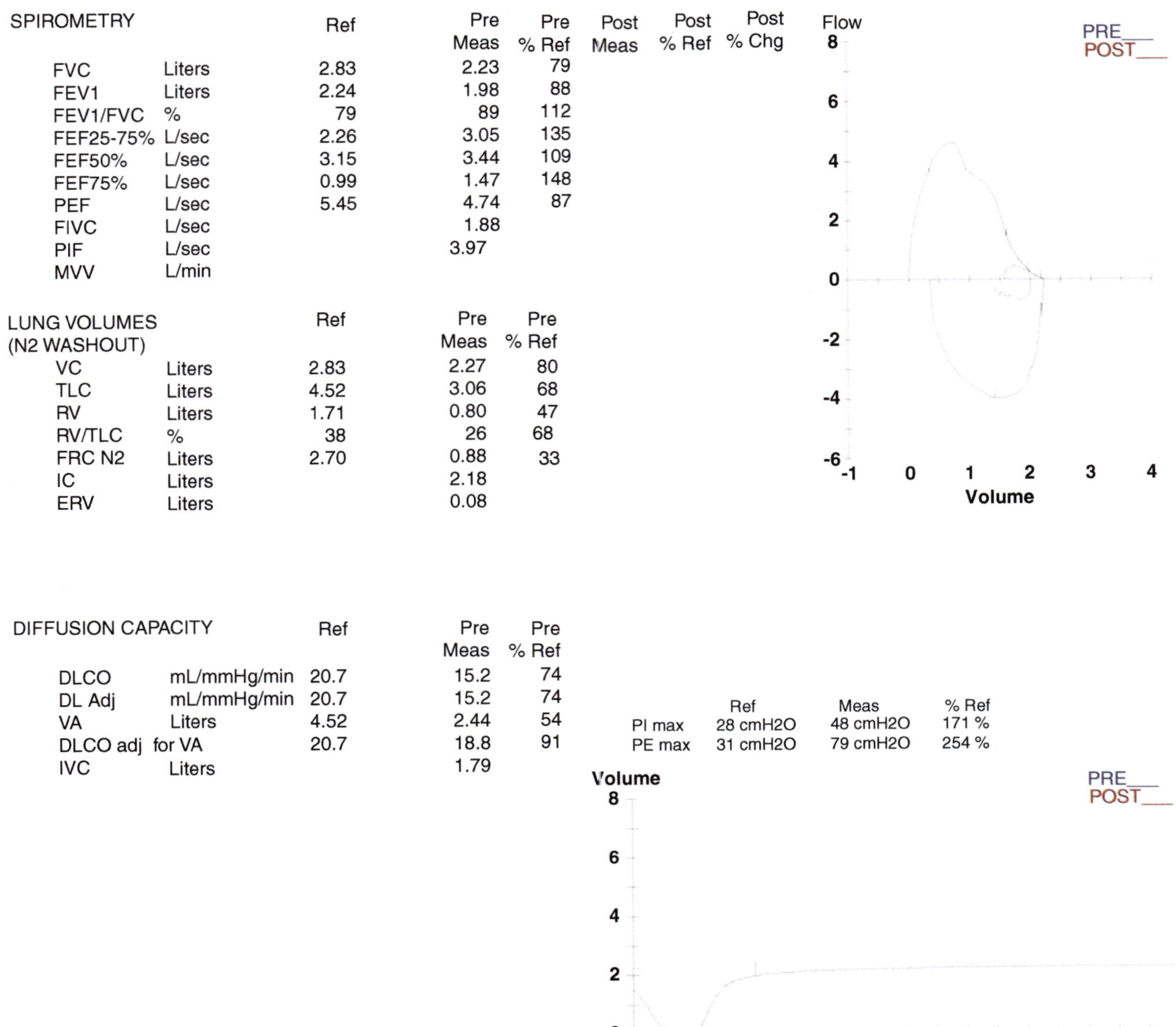

SPIROMETRY		Ref	Pre Meas	Pre % Ref	Post Meas	Post % Ref	Post % Chg
FVC	Liters	2.83	2.23	79			
FEV1	Liters	2.24	1.98	88			
FEV1/FVC	%	79	89	112			
FEF25-75%	L/sec	2.26	3.05	135			
FEF50%	L/sec	3.15	3.44	109			
FEF75%	L/sec	0.99	1.47	148			
PEF	L/sec	5.45	4.74	87			
FIVC	L/sec		1.88				
PIF	L/sec		3.97				
MVV	L/min						

LUNG VOLUMES (N2 WASHOUT)		Ref	Pre Meas	Pre % Ref
VC	Liters	2.83	2.27	80
TLC	Liters	4.52	3.06	68
RV	Liters	1.71	0.80	47
RV/TLC	%	38	26	68
FRC N2	Liters	2.70	0.88	33
IC	Liters		2.18	
ERV	Liters		0.08	

DIFFUSION CAPACITY		Ref	Pre Meas	Pre % Ref
DLCO	mL/mmHg/min	20.7	15.2	74
DL Adj	mL/mmHg/min	20.7	15.2	74
VA	Liters	4.52	2.44	54
DLCO adj	for VA	20.7	18.8	91
IVC	Liters		1.79	

	Ref	Meas	% Ref
PI max	28 cmH2O	48 cmH2O	171 %
PE max	31 cmH2O	79 cmH2O	254 %

Fig. 32.1 Pulmonary function test results

What Is Seronegative Myasthenia Gravis?

Patients who have undetectable levels of antibodies against nAChR are said to be seronegative. Ten percent of all MG patients are seronegative. These patients may have nAChR antibodies that are not detected because of insufficient test sensitivity [2].

What Are MuSK Antibodies?

In a subset of MG patients without nAChR antibodies, muscle-specific tyrosine kinease (MuSK) antibodies are detected. MuSK plays a crucial role in post-synaptic differentiation and clustering of nAChRs at the neuromuscular junction. Patients with MuSK MG are predominantly women with prominent oculobulbar weakness and dysarthria. Patients with MuSK antibodies may be resistant to treatment with anticholinesterases [3, 4].

How Does MG Present?

Early symptoms are oculobulbar and include fluctuating weakness and fatiguability of the ocular muscles and muscles supplied by the lower cranial nerves (VII-XII). Ophthalmoparesis, diplopia, and ptosis occur in 50% of patients. Dysarthria and dysphagia follow in 15% of patients. These may present with slurred nasal speech or may complain of a choking sensation, and pose an aspiration risk [5]. This is followed by generalized disease with fatigue spreading to the upper limbs and hands. The lower limbs tend to be less affected. Wheelchair use due to weakness is uncommon. Symptoms typically worsen at the end of the day, with heat, surgery, and emotional stress.

How Is MG Diagnosed?

1. History and physical examination are central to diagnosis, especially examination of the cranial nerves. Ptosis upon sustained upward gaze is a characteristic finding.
2. Antibody testing is performed routinely. Antibodies against nAChR and MuSK are both specific and sensitive for the detection of MG.
3. The Tensilon test was used in the past to confirm diagnosis. Edrophonium chloride was administered intravenously – a short-lived (10 min) improvement confirmed the diagnosis [6]. It has been replaced by antibody testing and is largely of historical interest.
4. Neurophysiology. Routine neurophysiological testing usually yields normal results. Specific testing includes the following:
    - Repetitive nerve stimulation, which has low sensitivity (70%) for the diagnosis of MG and can be even lower if disease is limited to the ocular muscles alone [7]
    - Single fiber electromyography, which has increased sensitivity of up to 100% but is not specific and is greatly operator dependent [8, 9]

What Conditions Are Associated with MG?

MG can be associated with other autoimmune conditions:

- Hyperthyroidism
- Pernicious anemia
- Polymyositis
- Rheumatoid arthritis
- Sarcoidosis
- Sjogren syndrome
- Systemic lupus erythematosus
- Ulcerative colitis
- Therapy with interferons, D-penicillamine, and bone marrow transplantation can also cause MG [10]

What Is the Role of the Thymus in the Pathogenesis of Myasthenia Gravis?

About 75% of patients with MG have abnormal histopathology of the thymus. Of these, 85% have thymic hyperplasia and 15% have thymoma [11]. Thymectomy aids symptom control and plays a preventative role in rate and severity of attacks in patients with and without thymoma [12, 13].

How Is Disease Severity in MG Graded?

A number of disease progression and severity scores can be utilized, e.g., Manual Muscle Testing (MMT) (Fig. 32.2), the modified Osserman and Genkins classification (Table 32.1) and Quantitative Myasthenia Gravis (QMG) scoring may be used in the preoperative period to establish a baseline [14, 15].

Can Aspiration Risk Be Predicted?

In a study investigating factors which were predictive of aspiration in MG, several bedside clinical tests including a self-directed questionnaire and a bedside clinical neurological assessment were useful aids in predicting the presence of aspiration [16]. This study also found that patients with a Modified Osserman and Genkins classification IIb or III were more likely to aspirate compared to those with lower grade disease. Patients with dysphagia and more severe MG are more likely to aspirate. Video fluoroscopic swallowing evaluation may be prudent prior to major elective surgery for patients at risk [16].

How is MG Treated?

1. Symptomatic treatment is with anticholinesterase agents, e.g., pyridostigmine. Most patients are on a combination of short-acting and slow-release agents. An intravenous formulation is available with the following conversion ratio: 1 mg IV = 30 mg PO.
2. Immunosuppressive therapy with steroids is used when pyridostigmine alone does not control symptoms. Azathioprine is the most commonly prescribed steroid-sparing agent. It is frequently prescribed in addition to prednisone because the combination results in greater efficacy with fewer complications than prednisone monotherapy [2]. Patients on long-term steroid treatment are at

Fig. 32.2 Manual muscle testing work sheet. Developed and introduced by Sanders et al. in 2003. MG-MMT score varies from 0 to 120. It is best used for assessing disease progression, rather than disease severity. (From Sanders et al. [14] with permission John Wiley)

Manual muscle testing (MMT) work sheet

	Right	Left	Sum
Lid ptosis	_____	_____	_____
Diplopia	_____	_____	_____
Eye closure	_____	_____	_____
Cheek puff	_____	_____	_____
Tongue protrusion	_____	_____	_____
Jaw closure	_____	_____	_____
Neck flexion	_____	_____	_____
Neck extension	_____	_____	_____
Shoulder abduction (deltoid)	_____	_____	_____
Elbow flexion (biceps)	_____	_____	_____
Elbow extension (triceps)	_____	_____	_____
Wrist extension	_____	_____	_____
Grip	_____	_____	_____
Hip flexion (iliopsoas)	_____	_____	_____
Knee extension (quadriceps)	_____	_____	_____
Knee flexion (hamstring)	_____	_____	_____
Ankle dorsiflexion (tibialis anterior +)	_____	_____	_____
Ankle plantar flexion	_____	_____	_____
TOTAL			

Note: Score each funciton as follows: 0, normal; 1, 25% weak/mild impairment; 2, 50% weak/moderate impairment; 3, 75% weak/severe impairment; 4, paralyzed/unable to do.
In addition, record any conditions other than MG causing weakness in any of these muscles.

risk of hypothalamic-pituitary axis suppression. Surgical stress dosing is discussed in detail in Chap. 19. Patients taking any dose of glucocorticoid for less than 3 weeks, or those taking prednisone 5 mg daily for any period of time are not candidates for stress dosing [17].

3. Rapid, immunomodulating treatments, e.g., plasmapheresis and intravenous immunoglobulin (IVIG) may be required for acute exacerbations. Plasmapheresis or plasma exchange acts by removing circulating anti-AChR antibodies and immune complexes. It is used to treat myasthenic crisis or to optimize the unstable myasthenic patient prior to surgery. It brings about a quick improvement in symptoms (1–7 days), but the effect does not last beyond 2 months. Plasmapheresis has been described in patients who are Jehovah's Witness followers. In these cases, albumin has been used in place of plasma [18]. IVIG is pooled from thousands of donors. The therapeutic mechanism is unclear. It has a similar onset, offset, and efficacy as plasmapheresis [19]. Its use is determined by availability and familiarity.
4. Thymectomy is indicated for patients with thymoma and those with non-thymomatous generalized MG. It improves symptoms and reduces the requirement for immunosuppressant therapy and the complications related to it. It can also be considered in patients with seronegative MG who have failed to respond to standard treatment or are treatment intolerant [20].

What Is a Myasthenic Crisis?

A myasthenic crisis is a potentially fatal condition due to the rapid deterioration of neuromuscular function. It is associated with respiratory compromise due to ventilatory muscle insufficiency and/or weakness of the upper airway muscles. Myasthenic crisis may occur at least once in the lifetime of up to 20% of patients with generalized MG [21].

Table 32.1 Modified Osserman and Genkins classification [21, 22]

Stage		Symptoms	Likelihood of myasthenic crisis
I	Ocular	Involvement restricted to the extraocular muscles	Low risk
IIa	Mild chronic generalized	Generalized weakness without respiratory muscle involvement	Low risk
IIb	Moderate chronic generalized	More severe generalized involvement, bulbar symptoms, and relative sparing of respiratory muscles	Increased risk
III	Acute fulminating	Rapid onset (<6 months) and respiratory muscle involvement	High risk
IV	Late severe	Progressive severity after >2 years of milder disease	High risk

Myasthenic crisis can be triggered by infection, emotional or physical stress, medication changes (especially tapering of immunosuppression), and electrolyte disturbances. It can be helpful to perform risk stratification preoperatively and to discuss the risk of myasthenic crisis with the patient. The Modified Osserman and Genkins classification can be used for risk assessment (Table 32.1) [21, 22]. In addition to the foregoing, a pyridostigmine dose >750 mg/day has been associated with increased likelihood of myasthenic crisis [23]. Extubation may be delayed if weakness persists at the end of surgery, and the patient may need to be transferred to ICU for ventilation. Plasmapheresis or IVIG treatment may be required.

What Measures Can Be Taken Preoperatively to Ensure That the Patient with MG Is Optimized for Anesthesia and Surgery?

1. Pulmonary function tests should be performed to determine a baseline, to establish criteria for extubation, and to determine the need for postoperative ventilation.
2. Liaise with the treating neurologist in the unstable or non-responding patient for consideration of more complex preoperative therapies, e.g., intravenous immunoglobulin, plasma exchange, or pulse steroid therapy [24].
3. Plan for postoperative disposition, e.g., ICU referral.
4. Assess aspiration risk of patients with dysphagia who may need further evaluation with video fluoroscopic assessment. This may help to establish the need for rapid sequence induction.

What Recommendations Regarding Preoperative Management of MG Medications Should Be Provided to the Patient?

1. Continue anticholinesterases, including on the morning of surgery, to avoid preoperative respiratory/bulbar symptoms [25].
2. Long-term immunosuppressants can be withheld on the day of surgery, e.g., azathioprine, but the normal steroid dose must be taken if the patient is on a regular glucocorticoid regimen.

What Is the Optimal Time for Elective Surgery?

Elective procedures should be performed during a period of myasthenic stability. The patient should be taking the lowest possible dose of steroid that maintains symptom control. Surgery should be scheduled early in the day when muscle strength is better.

The Patient Wants to Know If She Can Have an Epidural for Postoperative Analgesia. What Do You Tell Her?

Neuraxial anesthesia may reduce and even eliminate the need for muscle relaxants for abdominal surgery in MG patients. Epidural analgesia has been used successfully for laparotomy, as a sole anesthetic for laparoscopic cholecystectomy, and even for thymectomy [26, 27]. Case reports are emerging of its safe use for a multitude of indications, including in obstetric patients [28].

Epidural analgesia needs to be carefully titrated. A high epidural may compromise respiratory function by affecting intercostal muscle function, decrease forced vital capacity (FVC), and (forced expiratory volume) FEV_1, and may necessitate mechanical ventilation. In addition, high volume local anesthetic may decrease the sensitivity of the post-junctional membrane to acetylcholine. Ester local anesthetics should be avoided, as anticholinesterases may impair their hydrolysis [29]. Spinal anesthesia has been successfully used for emergency laparotomy, inguinal hernia repair, and transurethral ureterolithotripsy procedures [30–32].

Preoperative pulmonary function tests showed reduced vital capacity (VC), total lung capacity (TLC), and residual volume (RV). In patients with MG, VC is reduced because of inspiratory and expiratory muscle weakness. Spirometry in MG patients typically shows a restrictive ventilatory defect with reasonably well-preserved forced expiratory flow rates. Patients with restrictive lung disease tend towards proportional reduction in FEV_1 *and FVC with a normal or increased* FEV_1/FVC*. The severity of this patient's PFT abnormality is mild when categorized according to the American Thoracic Society Grades for Severity of a Pulmonary Function Test* (Table 32.2) [33, 34].

The patient was a Modified Osserman and Genkins class IIb, which placed her at increased for myasthenic crisis and aspiration. She was asked to take her pyridostigmine slow release as usual on the night before surgery and to take her normal dose of immediate release pyridostigmine on the morning of surgery. She held the azathioprine but was instructed to take her prednisone as normal. She received hydrocortisone 100 mg IV at induction as a surgical stress dose (Table 32.3) [17].

She did not require a muscle relaxant for intubation. If rapid sequence induction was deemed necessary, a higher dose of succinylcholine (1.5–2 mg/kg) would have been required. This is possibly due to the reduced number of ACh receptors at the neuromuscular junction. Onset of succinylcholine is slower and the effect may be prolonged due to concurrent therapy with cholinesterase inhibitors, which hinders its clearance [34]. *Non-depolarizing muscle relaxants (NMDRs) should be avoided or titrated slowly because of extreme sensitivity and unpredictable effects. The response to NDMR can be variable even among patients with only ocular symptoms or those in remission. Monitoring with quantitative train-of-four testing is recommended when NMDRs are used. Reversal with neostigmine should be avoided, as this can precipitate a cholinergic crisis, which can be difficult to distinguish from myasthenic crisis. This is a manifestation of its muscarinic effects, including nausea, vomiting, abdominal cramps, diarrhea, miosis, lacrimation, bronchospasm, increased bronchial secretions, diaphoresis, and bradycardia* [10]. *Sugammadex has been suggested as the optimal reversal agent when rocuronium or vecuronium is used, as it does not have muscarinic effects. One case series reports successful block reversal with 2–4 mg/kg, depending on block intensity* [35].

Table 32.2 Severity of any spirometry abnormality based on the forced expiratory volume in 1 second (FEV_1)

Degree of severity	FEV_1 (% predicted)
Mild	>70
Moderate	60–69
Moderately severe	50–59
Severe	35–49
Very severe	<35

From Pellegrino et al. [34] with permission of the © ERS 2020: *European Respiratory Journal* 2005 26: 948–968; DOI: https://doi.org/10.1183/09031936.05.00035205

Table 32.3 Surgical stress by procedure and recommended steroid dosing

Surgery type	Endogenous cortisol secretion rate	Examples	Recommended steroid dosing
Superficial	8–10 mg per day (baseline)	Dental surgery Biopsy	Usual daily dose
Minor	50 mg per day	Inguinal hernia repair Colonoscopy Uterine curettage Hand surgery	Usual daily dose *plus* Hydrocortisone 50 mg IV before incision Hydrocortisone 25 mg IV every 8 h × 24 h Then usual daily dose
Moderate	75–150 mg per day	Lower extremity revascularization Total joint replacement Cholecystectomy Colon resection Abdominal hysterectomy	Usual daily dose *plus* Hydrocortisone 50 mg IV before incision Hydrocortisone 25 mg IV every 8 h × 24 h Then usual daily dose
Major	75–150 mg per day	Esophagectomy Total proctocolectomy Major cardiac/vascular Hepaticojejunostomy Delivery Trauma	Usual daily dose *plus* Hydrocortisone 100 mg IV before incision Followed by continuous IV infusion of 200 mg of hydrocortisone more than 24 h *or* Hydrocortisone 50 mg IV every 8 h × 24 h Tape dose by half per day until usual daily dose reached *plus* Continuous IV fluids with 5% dextrose and 0.2–0.45% NaCl (based on degree of hypoglycemia)

From Liu et al. [17] from Wolters Kluwer with permission

True/False Questions

1. (a) Myasthenia gravis is an autoimmune disorder affecting the presynaptic membrane of the neuromuscular junction
   (b) Ten percent of MG patients are seronegative for antibodies
   (c) Early symptoms of MG include diplopia and ptosis
   (d) The Tensilon test is routinely performed to confirm diagnosis
   (e) Symptoms of MG are usually worse in the morning
2. (a) Anticholinesterase agents should be discontinued 1 week before surgery
   (b) A myasthenic crisis is caused by ventilatory muscle insufficiency or weakness of the upper airway muscles
   (c) Stage 1 of the Modified Osserman and Genkins classification signifies the most severe disease
   (d) The Manual Muscle Testing score is best used for assessing disease progression rather than severity
   (e) Succinylcholine is contraindicated in MG patients

References

1. Vincent A, Palace J, Hilton-Jones D. Myasthenia gravis. Lancet. 2001;357(9274):2122–8.
2. Gilhus NE. Myasthenia gravis. N Engl J Med. 2016;375(26):2570–81.
3. Deymeer F, Gungor-Tuncer O, Yilmaz V, Parman Y, Serdaroglu P, Ozdemir C, et al. Clinical comparison of anti-MuSK- vs anti-AChR-positive and seronegative myasthenia gravis. Neurology. 2007;68(8):609–11.
4. Pasnoor M, Wolfe GI, Nations S, Trivedi J, Barohn RJ, Herbelin L, et al. Clinical findings in MuSK-antibody positive myasthenia gravis: a U.S. experience. Muscle Nerve. 2010;41(3):370–4.
5. Meriggioli MN, Sanders DB. Advances in the diagnosis of neuromuscular junction disorders. Am J Phys Med Rehabil. 2005;84(8):627–38.
6. Grob D, Arsura EL, Brunner NG, Namba T. The course of myasthenia gravis and therapies affecting outcome. Ann N Y Acad Sci. 1987;505:472–99.
7. Palace J, Vincent A, Beeson D. Myasthenia gravis: diagnostic and management dilemmas. Curr Opin Neurol. 2001;14(5):583–9.
8. AAEM Quality Assurance Committee. American Association of Electrodiagnostic Medicine. Literature review of the usefulness of repetitive nerve stimulation and single fiber EMG in the electrodiagnostic evaluation of patients with suspected myasthenia gravis or Lambert-Eaton myasthenic syndrome. Muscle Nerve. 2001;24(9):1239–47.
9. Padua L, Stalberg E, LoMonaco M, Evoli A, Batocchi A, Tonali P. SFEMG in ocular myasthenia gravis diagnosis. Clin Neurophysiol. 2000;111(7):1203–7.
10. Urban MK. Muscle diseases. In: Fleisher LA, editor. Anesthesia and uncommon diseases. Philadelphia: Elsevier; 2012. p. 313–5.
11. Castleman B. The pathology of the thymus gland in myasthenia gravis. Ann N Y Acad Sci. 1966;135(1):496–505.
12. Wolfe G, Kaminski H, Aban IB, Minisman G, Kuo H, et al. Randomized trial of thymectomy in myasthenia gravis. N Engl J Med. 2016;375(6):511–22.
13. Soleimani A, Moayyeri A, Akhondzadeh S, Sadatsafavi M, Shalmani HT, Soltanzadeh A. Frequency of myasthenic crisis in relation to thymectomy in generalized myasthenia gravis: a 17-year experience. BMC Neurol. 2004;4(12):1–6.
14. Sanders DB, Tucker-Lipscomb B, Massey JM. A simple manual muscle test for myasthenia gravis: validation and comparison with the QMG score. Ann N Y Acad Sci. 2003;998:440–4.
15. Barohn RJ, Herbelin L. The quantitative myasthenia gravis (QMG) test. Dallas: Myasthenia Gravis Foundation of America; 2000.
16. Koopman WJ, Wiebe S, Colton-Hudson A, Moosa T, Smith D, Bach D, et al. Prediction of aspiration in myasthenia gravis. Muscle Nerve. 2004;29(2):256–60.
17. Liu MM, Reidy AB, Saatee S, Collard CD. Perioperative steroid management: approaches based on current evidence. Anesthesiology. 2017;127(1):166–72. https://anesthesiology.pubs.asahq.org/article.aspx?articleid=2626031.
18. George JN, Sandler SA, Stankiewicz J. Management of thrombotic thrombocytopenic purpura without plasma exchange the Jehovah's Witness experience. Blood Adv. 2017;1(24):2161–5.
19. Gajdos P, Chevret S, Toyka KV. Intravenous immunoglobulin for myasthenia gravis. Cochrane Database Syst Rev. 2012;12(12):CD002277.
20. Cataneo AJM, Felisberto G Jr, Cataneo DC. Thymectomy in nonthymomatous myasthenia gravis – systematic review and meta-analysis. Orphanet J Rare Dis. 2018;13(1):99.
21. Osserman KE, Kornfeld P, Cohen E, Genkins G, Mendelow H, Goldberg H, Windsley H, Kaplan LI. Studies in myasthenia gravis; review of two hundred eighty-two cases at the Mount Sinai Hospital, New York City. AMA Arch Intern Med. 1958;102(1):72–81.
22. Osserman KE, Genkins G. Studies in myasthenia gravis: review of a twenty-year experience in over 1200 patients. Mt Sinai J Med. 1971;38(6):497–537.
23. Leventhal SR, Orkin FK, Hirsh RA. Prediction of the need for postoperative mechanical ventilation in myasthenia gravis. Anesthesiology. 1980;53(1):26–30.
24. Abel M, Eisenkraft JB. Anesthetic implications of myasthenia gravis. Mt Sinai J Med. 2002;69(1–2):31–7.
25. Tripathi M, Kaushik S, Dubey P. The effect of use of pyridostigmine and requirement of vecuronium in patients with myasthenia gravis. J Postgrad Med. 2003;49(4):311–4; discussion 314-5.
26. Altiparmak B, Sahan L, Demirbilek S. Thoracic epidural anesthesia for severe myasthenia gravis patient undergoing laparoscopic cholecystectomy (case report). Med Sci. 2017;6(1):117–9.
27. Saito Y, Sakura S, Takatori T, Kosaka Y. Epidural anesthesia in a patient with myasthenia gravis. Acta Anaesthesiol Scand. 1993;37(5):513–5.
28. Hopkins AN, Alshaeri T, Akst SA, Berger JS. Neurologic disease with pregnancy and considerations for the obstetric anesthesiologist. Semin Perinatol. 2014;38(6):359–69.
29. Nahguib M, Lien CA. Pharmacology of muscle relaxants and their antagonists. In: Miller RD, editor. Miller's anesthesia. 7th ed. Philadelphia: Churchill Livingstone/Elsevier; 2010. p. 859–911.
30. Rodríguez MA, Mencía TP, Alvarez FV, Báez YL, Pérez GM, García AL. Low-dose spinal anesthesia for urgent laparotomy in severe myasthenia gravis. Saudi J Anaesth. 2013;7(1):90–2.

31. Kocum A, Sener M, Bozdogan N, Turkoz A, Arslan G. Spinal anesthesia for inguinal hernia repair in 8-year-old child with myasthenia gravis. Pediatr Anaesth. 2007;17(12):1220–1.
32. Inoue S, Shiomi T, Furuya H. Bradycardia during spinal anaesthesia for transurethral ureterolithotripsy. Anaesth Intensive Care. 2001;29(5):556–7.
33. Eisenkraft JB, Book WJ, Mann SM, Papatestas AE, Hubbard M. Resistance to succinylcholine in myasthenia gravis: a dose-response study. Anesthesiology. 1988;69(5):760–3.
34. Pellegrino R, Viegi G, Brusasco V, Crapo RO, Burgos F, Casaburi R, et al. Interpretative strategies for lung function tests. Eur Respir J. 2005;26(5):948–68.
35. de Boer H, Shields M, Booij L. Reversal of neuromuscular blockade with sugammadex in patients with myasthenia gravis: a case series of 21 patients and review of the literature. Eur J Anaesthesiol. 2014;31(12):715–21.

33 Ischemic Stroke

Susan Halliday

A 59-year-old female presented for preoperative optimization prior to laparoscopic cholecystectomy for subacute cholecystitis. Six weeks before this, she had been diagnosed with gallstone pancreatitis. An endoscopic retrograde cholangiopancreatography with sphincterotomy was performed at this time after which the patient reported visual disturbances and was noted to have fluctuating confusion. Brain imaging subsequently demonstrated a small left occipital infarct. The patient was thereafter commenced on ramipril, aspirin, and rosuvastatin.

Prior to this episode of gallstone pancreatitis, the patient was otherwise healthy. She led an active lifestyle easily achieving six METS. She was an ex-smoker for approximately 15 years.

Physical Examination: Oxygen saturation on room air was 98%, blood pressure was 138/76, and heart rate was 83.

Investigations: Laboratory values demonstrated hemoglobin 124 g/l, platelet count 168 × 10^9 /L, white cell count 13.4 × 10^9 /L, Na 139 mmol/L, K 4.2 mmol/L, and creatinine 85 umol/L. The INR was 1.1 and PTT 34 s.

The ECG was unremarkable showing sinus rhythm. The echocardiogram performed following the stroke showed normal right and left ventricular function. There were no valvular abnormalities. There was no evidence of a cardiac source of embolism, atrial septal defect, or patent foramen ovale. The only abnormality noted was a mildly elevated right ventricular systolic pressure of 35–40 mmHg. Holter ambulatory electrocardiography did not identify any arrhythmias.

S. Halliday (✉)
Department of Anesthesiology & Pain Medicine, University of Alberta Hospital, Edmonton, AB, Canada
e-mail: halliday@ualberta.ca

What Complications Is the Patient with Prior Ischemic Stroke Subject to in the Perioperative Period?

- Ischemic stroke
- Acute myocardial infarction
- Cardiovascular death
- Bleeding secondary to antithrombotic or antiplatelet agents when continued perioperatively

What Evidence Is There That the Patient with a History of Ischemic Stroke Is at Increased Perioperative Risk for a Repeat Ischemic Stroke?

- The largest study to date to evaluate the association between recent ischemic stroke and perioperative complications found a strong time-dependent relationship between prior ischemic stroke and adverse postoperative outcome [1]. This was a retrospective cohort study of nearly half a million noncardiac procedures. Perioperative stroke occurred in 11.9% of patients with a history of ischemic stroke if surgery was performed within the first 3 months of the cerebrovascular event compared to a 0.1% perioperative stroke rate in those without a history of stroke [1]. This risk decreased as the interval from stroke to surgery increased, stabilizing at approximately 9 months, although still higher at this time point than in those patients with no history of stroke. The risk was the same regardless of whether the surgery was low, intermediate, or high risk. The authors of this large cohort study suggested that patients with a history of recent ischemic stroke should be considered at increased perioperative risk until 9 months have elapsed since the event.

D. Dillane, B. A. Finegan (eds.), *Preoperative Assessment*, https://doi.org/10.1007/978-3-030-58842-7_33

- In an analysis of 47,750 patients undergoing noncarotid major vascular surgery, a history of cerebrovascular disease (history of stroke with or without residual deficit, TIA, or preoperative hemiplegia) was found to be the risk factor most strongly associated with postoperative stroke [2].

What Other Factors Are Known to Increase the Risk of Perioperative Stroke?

Analysis of 523,059 noncardiac, non-neurologic patients in the American College of Surgeons National Surgical Quality Improvement Program (ACS NSQIP®) database showed additional independent predictors for perioperative stroke: age ≥ 62 years, hypertension requiring therapy, myocardial infarction within 6 months of surgery, acute renal failure, pre-existing dialysis, COPD, and current tobacco use [3].

Does Beta-Blockade Increase the Risk of Perioperative Stroke?

According to the Perioperative Ischemic Evaluation (POISE) trial, introduction of metoprolol in the immediate preoperative period reduced cardiac death and nonfatal myocardial infarction/cardiac arrest [4]. However, the incidence of all-cause mortality and stroke increased. Subsequent retrospective studies have looked at patients on chronic beta-blocker therapy. In a large retrospective study, continued use of metoprolol preoperatively in noncardiac surgery was associated with a fourfold increase in perioperative stroke [5]. There was a significantly higher incidence of stroke in patients taking preoperative metoprolol compared with those taking atenolol [5]. A single-center cohort study of 44,092 consecutive patients demonstrated that perioperative metoprolol and atenolol were both associated with an increased risk of perioperative stroke when compared to the more β_1-specific bisoprolol [6]. A recent Cochrane review concluded that in noncardiac surgery, the evidence shows an increase in death and a potential increase in stroke rate with the use of beta-blockers [7]. Overall, the evidence was deemed to be low to moderate in quality, not allowing definitive conclusions to be established. Knowing the risks associated with acute beta-blocker withdrawal, current practice is to continue beta-blockade in the perioperative period in those patients on established therapy. De novo initiation of beta-blockade preoperatively is not recommended.

What Is the Precise Definition of Perioperative Stroke?

Perioperative stroke includes any stroke, whether embolic, thrombotic, or hemorrhagic, occurring intra-operatively or within 30 days of surgery, that results in motor, sensory, or cognitive dysfunction that persists for ≥24 hours. The majority of perioperative strokes are ischemic in nature and associated with systemic atherosclerosis [8, 9].

What Is the Risk of Perioperative Stroke in the General Population?

The overall risk of clinically apparent perioperative stroke for noncardiac, non-neurological surgery ranges from 0.1% to 0.8% [3]. The incidence varies for type of surgery and presence of associated risk factors. Data from the ACS NSQIP database found that, when cardiac and neurological surgical procedures were excluded, the overall incidence of perioperative stroke to be 0.1% [3]. Another investigation using ACS NSQIP data found that patients undergoing noncarotid major vascular surgery had a 0.6% incidence of perioperative stroke [2].

Is Perioperative Stroke Always Clinically Obvious?

Covert perioperative strokes have no clinical symptoms or signs but are evident on magnetic resonance imaging of the brain. A prospective cohort study of patients undergoing elective noncardiac surgery found that 7% of patients had a perioperative covert stroke [10]. Given the lack of clinical signs, these may be erroneously mistaken for insignificant events. However, in this study, 42% of patients with a covert stroke experienced cognitive decline at 1 year following surgery compared to 29% of those in the control group. Increased postoperative delirium and overt stroke or transient ischemic attacks at 1 year were also associated with presence of perioperative covert stroke.

What Are the Consequences of a Perioperative Stroke?

The occurrence of a perioperative stroke has significant effects on morbidity and mortality. The ACS NSQIP review of noncardiac non-neurological procedures demonstrated that perioperative stroke caused significant morbidity and mortality and was associated with an eightfold increase in mortality within 30 days [3]. Review of noncarotid major vascular surgeries from the ACS NSQIP database found that perioperative stroke was associated with a threefold increase in 30-day mortality as well as increased length of hospital stay [2]. More recently in a retrospective analysis of 4,264,963 surgical procedures identified from the Nationwide Inpatient Sample (NIS) over an 11-year period, perioperative stroke was an independent predictor of 30-day in-hospital morbidity and mortality. It was also an independent predictor of length of hospital stay beyond 14 days, cardiovascular and pulmonary complications as well as in-hospital mortality [11].

What Is the Optimal Time Interval Between Ischemic Stroke and Surgery?

As highlighted in the large cohort study from Jørgensen et al. outlined above, the first 3 months following the cerebrovascular event pose the greatest risk for further stroke in the perioperative period [1]. At 9 months post event, the risk appears to have stabilized but is still higher than for those with no prior history of ischemic stroke. The recently published consensus statement from the Society for Neuroscience in Anesthesiology and Critical Care (SNACC) supports considering delaying elective surgery for 9 months after the stroke event [12].

How Should Patients with a History of Stroke or Transient Ischemic Attack Be Evaluated Preoperatively?

It is standard practice following a nondisabling stroke or transient ischemic attack for patients to be evaluated by a physician with stroke expertise [13]. Investigations undertaken as part of this assessment which should be reviewed preoperatively include brain imaging with noninvasive vascular imaging, laboratory tests including screening for diabetes and dyslipidemia, and a 12-lead ECG. Holter ECG monitoring and an echocardiography may have been undertaken if a cardiac embolic mechanism was suspected. Review of these findings, if available, is helpful in determining the mechanism and extent of injury.

For patients with a remote history of stroke and who have been stable for many years, a discussion of recurrent stroke risk is appropriate and should be documented.

Patients who have had a stroke within the previous 9 months should be fully informed of risk, with the timing and urgency of the elective procedure the subject of multidisciplinary consensus.

Thorough preoperative evaluation will enable risk factors for perioperative stroke to be identified and optimized within the given time frame, e.g., hypertension, hyperlipidemia, myocardial ischemia, renal impairment, diabetes, COPD, and smoking [3, 14].

What Is the Optimal Blood Pressure Target in the Ischemic Stroke Patient?

Hypertension is the single most important modifiable risk factor for stroke. The American Heart Association currently recommends a target blood pressure below 140/90 mmHg in previously untreated hypertensive patients who suffer a stroke/TIA, while a systolic blood pressure target of <130 mmHg may be reasonable in adults who have suffered a lacunar stroke [15]. Medical management of hypertension is discussed in greater detail in Chap. 4.

Should Aspirin Be Held Perioperatively in the Patient with a History of Stroke or Transient Ischemic Attack?

The decision to stop or continue aspirin in the perioperative period depends on the indication for aspirin, the risk of thromboembolism, the proposed surgery, and its associated risk of postoperative bleeding. Previous concerns regarding the preoperative cessation of aspirin were based on concerns about the prothrombotic effect of surgery and the rebound procoagulant response to abrupt termination of therapy. The POISE-2 trial, however, found that perioperative aspirin administration did not affect the primary outcomes of death or myocardial infarction after noncardiac surgery [16]. There was no difference in the incidence of stroke: 0.3% in the aspirin treatment group versus 0.4% in the placebo group ($p = 0.62$). On the other hand, major bleeding occurred in 4.6% of the aspirin group versus 3.8% of the treatment group ($p = 0.04$). Currently, there is no evidence to support the continuation of perioperative aspirin to reduce perioperative stroke in noncardiac surgery. Present guidelines recommend discontinuing aspirin 7–10 days prior to elective or nonurgent noncardiac surgery, except in patients with recent coronary stenting or those undergoing carotid endarterectomy [17]. Perioperative guidelines for aspirin in patients undergoing carotid endarterectomy are outlined in Chap. 10.

How Is Perioperative Anticoagulation Managed in Patients with Atrial Fibrillation Being Treated with a Direct Oral Anticoagulant After Ischemic Stroke?

Direct (non-vitamin K) oral anticoagulants (DOACs) are preferred over warfarin for nonvalvular atrial fibrillation [18]. A pragmatic approach to perioperative DOAC interruption takes account of surgical bleeding risk (Table 33.1) [19–21], renal function, and DOAC type [22].

Table 33.1 Risk stratification for procedural bleed risk as suggested by the ISTH Guidance Statement and BRIDGE Trial [19, 20]

High bleeding risk procedures[a] (30-day risk of major bleed >2%)	Major surgery with extensive tissue injury
	Cancer surgery, especially solid tumor resection
	Major orthopedic surgery, including shoulder replacement surgery
	Reconstructive plastic surgery
	Urologic or gastrointestinal surgery, especially anastomosis surgery
	Transurethral prostate resection, bladder resection, or tumor ablation
	Nephrectomy, kidney biopsy
	Colonic polyp resection
	Bowel resection
	Percutaneous endoscopic gastrostomy (PEG) placement, endoscopic retrograde cholangiopancreatography (ERCP)
	Surgery in highly vascular organs (kidneys, liver, spleen)
	Cardiac, intracranial, or spinal surgery
	Any major operation (procedure duration >45 min)
	Neuraxial anesthesia
Low/moderate bleeding risk procedures[c] (30-day risk of major bleed 0–2%)	Arthroscopy
	Cutaneous/lymph node biopsies
	Foot/hand surgery
	Coronary angiography[d]
	Gastrointestinal endoscopy ± biopsy
	Colonoscopy ± biopsy
	Abdominal hysterectomy
	Laparoscopic cholecystectomy
	Abdominal hernia repair
	Hemorrhoidal surgery
	Bronchoscopy ± biopsy
	Epidural injections
Minimal bleeding risk procedures[e] (30-d risk of major bleed ~0%)	Minor dermatologic procedures (excision of basal and squamous cell skin cancers, actinic keratoses, and premalignant or cancerous skin nevi)
	Ophthalmological (cataract) procedures
	Minor dental procedures (dental extractions, restorations, prosthetics, endodontics), dental cleanings, fillings
	Pacemaker or cardioverter-defibrillator device implantation

From Spyropoulos et al. [21], with permission John Wiley & Sons © 2019 International Society on Thrombosis and Haemostasis

[a]No residual anticoagulant effect at time of procedure (i.e., 4–5 drug half-life interruption preprocedure)

[b]Includes spinal and epidural anesthesia, consider not only absolute major bleed (MB) event rate but catastrophic consequences of a MB

[c]Some residual anticoagulant effect allowed (i.e., 2–3 drug half-life interruption preprocedure)

[d]Radial approach may be considered minimal bleed risk compared to femoral approach

[e]Procedure can be safely done under full-dose anticoagulation (may consider holding direct oral anticoagulant (DOAC) dose day of procedure to avoid peak anticoagulant

Patients with creatinine clearance greater than 50 ml/min should have DOACs held for 2 days before surgery with a high risk of bleeding and for 1 day before surgery with a low bleeding risk. Patients with a creatinine clearance of 30–50 ml/min and having surgery with a high bleeding risk should have dabigatran held for 4 days before surgery and anti Xa inhibitors, e.g., rivaroxaban, apixaban, and edoxaban held for 2 days. Patients with a creatinine clearance of 30–50 ml/min and having surgery with a low bleeding risk should have dabigatran held for 2 days before surgery and anti Xa inhibitors held for 1 day. The difference can be accounted for by the longer half-life of dabigatran, i.e., up to 18 hours with normal renal function and up to 23 hours with reduced creatinine clearance. Timing of DOAC interruption corresponds to three to four half-lives for surgical procedures with low bleeding risk and four to five half-lives for high bleeding risk procedures. Bridging with low molecular weight heparin (LMWH) is not required in most cases due to the much more rapid offset and onset times for DOACs compared with warfarin. Furthermore, an observational study of patients with atrial fibrillation being treated with dabigatran showed significantly more major bleeding in the group who were bridged with LMWH perioperatively compared to those who did not receive bridging therapy, and there was not a significant difference in thromboembolic events [23].

How Is Anticoagulation with Warfarin Managed Perioperatively?

Warfarin is the anticoagulant of choice in patients with a mechanical heart valve and moderate to severe mitral stenosis [18]. The bleeding risk for the surgical procedure should first be decided and the need for bridging therapy evaluated. Patient stratification for thromboembolic risk adapted from the American College of Chest Physicians Clinical Practice Guidelines is shown in Table 33.2 [21, 24, 25]. If warfarin is indicated for atrial fibrillation, the need for heparin bridging therapy will be dependent on the $CHADS_2$ score (see Chap. 6 on atrial fibrillation).

Where cessation of warfarin therapy is deemed appropriate, it should be omitted for 5 days preoperatively. If bridging therapy with subcutaneous low molecular weight heparin or intravenous unfractionated heparin is indicated, this should be commenced on the third preoperative day. The last dose of subcutaneous low molecular weight heparin should be administered on the morning of the day before surgery. Only half of the daily dose should be administered.

Table 33.2 Risk stratification for patient-specific periprocedural thromboembolism adapted from American College of Chest Physicians (ACCP) Guidelines [24, 25]

Risk category	Mechanical heart valve	Atrial fibrillation	Venous thromboembolism
High (>10%/year risk of ATE or >10%/month risk of VTE)	Any mechanical mitral valve Caged ball or tilting disc valve in mitral/aortic position Recent (<3 months) stroke or TIA	$CHADS_2$ score of 5 or 6 CHA2DS$_2$VASc score of 7 or more Recent (<3 months) stroke or TIA Rheumatic valvular heart disease	Deficiency of protein C, protein S, or antithrombin Antiphospholipid antibodies Multiple thrombophilias Associated with vena caval filter (Active cancer)[a]
Moderate (4–10%/year risk of ATE or 4–10%/month risk of VTE)	Bileaflet AVR with major risk factors for stroke[b]	$CHADS_2$ score of 3 or 4 CHA_2DS_2VASc score of 5 or 6	VTE within past 3–12 months Recurrent VTE Nonsevere thrombophilia Active cancer or recent history of cancer[c]
Low (<4%/year risk of ATE or <2%/month risk of VTE)	Bileaflet AVR without major risk factors for stroke[b]	$CHADS_2$ score of 0–2 (and no prior stroke or TIA) CHA_2DS_2VASc score of 1–4	VTE more than 12 months ago

From Spyropoulos et al [21], with permission John Wiley & Sons © 2019 International Society on Thrombosis and Haemostasis

ATE Arterial thromboembolism, *TIA* Transient ischemic attack

[a]Consider pancreatic cancer, myeloproliferative disorders, brain tumor, gastric cancer

[b]Atrial fibrillation, prior stroke or transient ischemic attack, hypertension, diabetes, congestive heart failure, age > 75 years

[c]Within 5 years if history of cancer, excluding non-melanoma skin cancer

Should the Patient's Ramipril Be Continued Perioperatively?

Angiotensin-converting enzyme inhibitors and angiotensin II receptor blockers should be held on the day of surgery due to their well-documented association with perioperative hypotension [26].

Should Statin Therapy Be Continued Perioperatively?

The use of statins in primary and secondary prevention of stroke is irrefutable. Statin therapy is therefore started or recommenced following all ischemic strokes or TIAs. Benefits of perioperative statin therapy in patients undergoing carotid endarterectomy include reduced in-hospital mortality, stroke, and long-term protection against MI [27, 28]. The discontinuation of statin therapy has been shown to increase risk of myocardial infarction following major vascular surgery [29]. The VISION study, a large international, prospective, cohort study in patients undergoing noncardiac surgery, demonstrated that preoperative statin therapy was independently associated with a lower risk of cardiovascular outcomes at 30 days. The relative risk of stroke at 30 days was 0.83 in patients being treated with a statin [30]. Although there are no large randomized trials, it seems prudent, in light of what has been shown, to continue statin therapy throughout the perioperative period including on the day of surgery for those patients already established on therapy.

The patient had been commenced on ramipril after her stroke and was consistently meeting BP targets for a nondiabetic patient. Aspirin was being used as a first-line agent for long-term secondary prevention of stroke. Other antiplatelet agents and combinations may be seen, e.g., clopidogrel or aspirin plus dipyridamole. However, aspirin alone was probably a reasonable choice when the stroke was not cardioembolic in nature. Even though the patient was 7 months from the optimal time between ischemic stroke and surgery, the need to address the underlying pathology in this instance was somewhat exigent. Aspirin was held 1 week before surgery, ramipril was held on the day of surgery and the patient was asked to continue taking rosuvastatin throughout the perioperative period. The surgery proceeded uneventfully 2 weeks after this preoperative visit.

True/False Questions

1. (a) The risk of repeat perioperative ischemic stroke is highest when surgery is performed within the first 3 months after the index stroke event.
   (b) The risk of repeat perioperative ischemic stroke returns to normal 9 months after an ischemic stroke.
   (c) A previous history of stroke is the risk factor most commonly associated with postoperative ischemic stroke.
   (d) Beta-blockade medication should be discontinued preoperatively due to its positive association with postoperative stroke.
   (e) A perioperative stroke is defined as any stroke occurring within 1 week of surgery.
2. (a) Based on current best evidence, it is recommended that an interval of at least 9 months should elapse between ischemic stroke and elective surgery.
   (b) Aspirin should be continued throughout the perioperative period for most noncardiac surgeries.

(c) Patients having carotid endarterectomy should be advised to continue aspirin therapy up to and including the day of surgery.
(d) Covert perioperative stroke is commoner than clinically evident perioperative stroke.
(e) The risk of perioperative clinically evident stroke for noncardiac, non-neurological surgery ranges from 0.1 to 0.8%.

References

1. Jorgensen ME, Torp-Pedersen C, Gislason GH, Jensen PF, Berger SM, Christiansen CB, et al. Time elapsed after ischemic stroke and risk of adverse cardiovascular events and mortality following elective noncardiac surgery. JAMA. 2014;312(3):269–77.
2. Sharifpour M, Moore LE, Shanks AM, Didier TJ, Kheterpal S, Mashour GA. Incidence, predictors, and outcomes of perioperative stroke in noncarotid major vascular surgery. Anesth Analg. 2013;116(2):424–34.
3. Mashour GA, Shanks AM, Kheterpal S. Perioperative stroke and associated mortality after noncardiac, nonneurologic surgery. Anesthesiology. 2011;114(6):1289–96.
4. Group PS, Devereaux PJ, Yang H, Yusuf S, Guyatt G, Leslie K, et al. Effects of extended-release metoprolol succinate in patients undergoing non-cardiac surgery (POISE trial): a randomised controlled trial. Lancet. 2008;371(9627):1839–47.
5. Mashour GA, Sharifpour M, Freundlich RE, Tremper KK, Shanks A, Nallamothu BK, et al. Perioperative metoprolol and risk of stroke after noncardiac surgery. Anesthesiology. 2013;119(6):1340–6.
6. Ashes C, Judelman S, Wijeysundera DN, Tait G, Mazer CD, Hare GM, et al. Selective beta1-antagonism with bisoprolol is associated with fewer postoperative strokes than atenolol or metoprolol: a single-center cohort study of 44,092 consecutive patients. Anesthesiology. 2013;119(4):777–87.
7. Blessberger H. Influence of beta-blockers on perioperative adverse events. Cochrane Database Syst Rev. 2018;3.
8. Kam PC, Calcroft RM. Peri-operative stroke in general surgical patients. Anaesthesia. 1997;52(9):879–83.
9. Selim M. Perioperative stroke. N Engl J Med. 2007;356(7):706–13.
10. Neuro VI. Perioperative covert stroke in patients undergoing non-cardiac surgery (NeuroVISION): a prospective cohort study. Lancet. 2019;394(10203):1022–9.
11. Lewis DJ, Al-Ghazawi SS, Al-Robaidi KA, Thirumala PD. Perioperative stroke associated in-hospital morbidity and in-hospital mortality in common non-vascular non-neurological surgery. J Clin Neurosci. 2019;67:32–9.
12. Vlisides PE, Moore LE, Whalin MK, Robicsek SA, Gelb AW, Lele AV, et al. Perioperative care of patients at high risk for stroke during or after non-cardiac, non-neurologic surgery: 2020 guidelines from the Society of Neuroscience in Anesthesiology and Critical Care. J Neurosurg Anesthesiol. 2020;32(3):210–26.
13. Boulanger JM, Lindsay MP, Gubitz G, Smith EE, Stotts G, Foley N, et al. Canadian stroke best practice recommendations for acute stroke management: prehospital, emergency department, and acute inpatient stroke care, 6th edition, update 2018. Int J Stroke. 2018;13(9):949–84.
14. O'Donnell MJ, Chin SL, Rangarajan S, Xavier D, Liu L, Zhang H, et al. Global and regional effects of potentially modifiable risk factors associated with acute stroke in 32 countries (INTERSTROKE): a case-control study. Lancet. 2016;388(10046):761–75.
15. Whelton PK, Carey RM, Aronow WS, Casey DE, Dennison Himmelfarb C, DePalma SM, et al. 2017 ACC/AHA/AAPA/ABC/ACPM/AGS/APhA/ASH/ASPC/NMA/PACN guideline for the prevention, detection, evaluation, and management of high blood pressure in adults: executive summary: a report of the American College of Cardiology/American Heart Association task force on clinical practice guidelines. J Am Coll Cardiol. 2018;71:2199–269.
16. Devereaux PJ, Mrkobrada M, Sessler DI, Leslie K, Alonso-Coello P, Kurz A, et al. Aspirin in patients undergoing noncardiac surgery. N Engl J Med. 2014;370(16):1494–503.
17. Thrombosis Canada. Perioperative management of antiplatelet therapy. 2019. Available from:https://thrombosiscanada.ca/clinicalguides/.
18. January CT, Wann LS, Calkins H, Chen LY, Cigarroa JE, Cleveland JC Jr, et al. 2019 AHA/ACC/HRS focused update of the 2014 AHA/ACC/HRS guideline for the management of patients with Atrial fibrillation: a report of the American College of Cardiology/American Heart Association task force on clinical practice guidelines and the Heart Rhythm Society in collaboration with the Society of Thoracic Surgeons. Circulation. 2019;140(2):e125–e51.
19. Spyropoulos AC, Al-Badri A, Sherwood MW, et al. Periprocedural management of patients receiving a vitamin K antagonist or a direct oral anticoagulant requiring an elective procedure or surgery. J Thromb Haemost. 2016;14:875–85.
20. Douketis JD, Spyropoulos AC, Kaatz S, et al. Perioperative bridging anticoagulation in patients with atrial fibrillation. N Engl J Med. 2015;373:823–33.
21. Spyropoulos AC, Brohi K, Caprini J, Samama CM, Siegal D, Tafur A, et al. Scientific and Standardization Committee Communication: guidance document on the periprocedural management of patients on chronic oral anticoagulant therapy: recommendations for standardized reporting of procedural/surgical bleed risk and patient-specific thromboembolic risk. J Thromb Haemost. 2019;17(11):1966–72. https://doi.org/10.1111/jth.14598.
22. Tafur A, Douketis J. Perioperative management of anticoagulant and antiplatelet therapy. Heart. 2018;104(17):1461–7.
23. Douketis JD, Healey JS, Brueckmann M, Eikelboom JW, Ezekowitz MD, Fraessdorf M, et al. Perioperative bridging anticoagulation during dabigatran or warfarin interruption among patients who had an elective surgery or procedure. Substudy of the RE-LY trial. Thromb Haemost. 2015;113(3):625–32.
24. Douketis JD, Spyropoulos AC, Spencer FA, et al. Perioperative management of antithrombotic therapy: antithrombotic therapy and prevention of thrombosis, 9th ed: American College of Chest Physicians evidence-based clinical practice guidelines. Chest. 2012;141:e326S–50S.
25. Douketis JD, Berger PB, Dunn AS, et al. The perioperative management of antithrombotic therapy: American College of Chest Physicians evidence-based clinical practice guidelines (8th edition). Chest. 2008;133:299S–339S.
26. Hollmann C, Fernandes NL, Biccard BM. A systematic review of outcomes associated with withholding or continuing angiotensin-converting enzyme inhibitors and angiotensin receptor blockers before noncardiac surgery. Anesth Analg. 2018;127(3):678–87.
27. Arinze N, Farber A, Sachs T, Patts G, Kalish J, Kuhnen A, et al. The effect of statin use and intensity on stroke and myocardial infarction after carotid endarterectomy. J Vasc Surg. 2018;68(5):1398–405.
28. Kennedy J, Quan H, Buchan AM, Ghali WA, Feasby TE. Statins are associated with better outcomes after carotid endarterectomy in symptomatic patients. Stroke. 2005;36(10):2072–6.
29. Schouten O, Hoeks SE, Welten GM, Davignon J, Kastelein JJ, Vidakovic R, et al. Effect of statin withdrawal on frequency of cardiac events after vascular surgery. Am J Cardiol. 2007;100(2):316–20.
30. Berwanger O, Le Manach Y, Suzumura EA, Biccard B, Srinathan SK, Szczeklik W, et al. Association between pre-operative statin use and major cardiovascular complications among patients undergoing non-cardiac surgery: the VISION study. Eur Heart J. 2016;37(2):177–85.

Parkinson Disease

34

Barry A. Finegan

A 69-year-old man with Parkinson disease (PD) presented for preoperative evaluation. PD had diagnosed 21 years previously after investigation of tremor. He had a bilateral globus pallidus interna deep brain stimulator (DBS) system implanted 5 years previously. He had recently noticed a gradual increase in motor complications, including freezing and dyskinesia. He presented for replacement of a depleted implanted pulse generator. Comorbidities included benign prostatic hypertrophy, urinary incontinence, gastroesophageal reflux disease, postural hypotension, osteoarthritis, and hypothyroidism.

Medications: Carbidopa/levodopa/entacapone (Stalevo) 37.5/150/200 mg and carbidopa/levodopa (Sinemet) 25/100 mg six times a day); amantadine 100 mg OD; selegiline 5 mg BID; levothyroxine 50 µg OD; tamsulosin 0.4 mg OD; dutasteride 0.5 mg OD; and clonidine 0.025 mg OD.

Physical examination: Revealed normal vital signs; airway, cardiovascular, and respiratory examinations were unremarkable. He had good tone and no lead pipe rigidity. He had a blank expression and mild drooling. He was mobile with reduced arm swing and a shuffling gait. He was cognitively intact.

Investigations: His laboratory data were unremarkable, and his electrocardiogram (ECG) (obtained with his pulse generator off) revealed sinus rhythm with a QTc of 390 mm and normal tracings.

What Is PD?

PD is a neurodegenerative disorder characterized by the progressive loss of dopaminergic neurons in the substantia nigra pars compacta (SNpc) [1]. It is a complex multifaceted disease with a prolonged prodromal period (up to 14 years). During the prodromal period, symptoms of sleep dysfunction, anosmia, constipation, and depression predominate. The appearance of the motor symptoms of tremor, bradykinesia, rigidity and impaired posture, balance, and gait herald the onset of classic PD. While early onset can occur, advanced age and male sex are key risk factors for developing PD.

There are two major clinical presentations: a tremor-dominant form with minimal involvement of other motor faculties, or a non-tremor-dominant variant that is associated with significant bradykinesia, rigidity, postural instability, and gait issues. The disease has a prolonged and progressive course.

Exacerbation of non-motor symptoms and signs occurs in the advanced stages of the disease. These include urinary frequency, incontinence, fatigue, orthostatic hypotension, and cognitive impairment/dementia.

Are Patients with PD More at Risk Than the General Population of Perioperative Morbidity and Mortality?

Patients with PD are more likely to be admitted to hospital, have a prolonged length of stay, and suffer greater morbidity and mortality during hospitalization than matched controls [2]. The major reasons for admission are treatment of pneumonia, motor decline, urinary tract infection and hip fracture. During hospitalization, patients with PD are five times as likely to suffer from delirium, three times as likely to suffer adverse drug events and syncope, and twice as likely to fall and have GI complications than other patients [3]. PD is a dynamic illness where life-threating events can acutely occur within minutes, particularly if timing of medications is altered or inappropriate drugs administered [4]. Personalized and responsive tailored management is key to minimizing adverse outcomes [5].

B. A. Finegan (✉)
Department of Anesthesiology & Pain Medicine, University of Alberta, Edmonton, AB, Canada
e-mail: bfinegan@ualberta.ca

D. Dillane, B. A. Finegan (eds.), *Preoperative Assessment*, https://doi.org/10.1007/978-3-030-58842-7_34

What Drugs Are Used to Treat the Motor Symptoms of PD?

Dopamine Replacement Therapy

Levodopa is the most commonly prescribed drug for PD. The half-life of levodopa is only 1–2 hours. It is taken orally, absorbed, and converted in the brain by the remaining dopaminergic neurons to dopamine (by the time motor symptoms develop in PD, it is estimated that there is a 60% loss of dopaminergic neurons in the SNpc).

Levodopa undergoes extensive first-pass metabolism (95%) in the gut. It is converted to dopamine through a process of decarboxylation by aromatic L-amino acid decarboxylase (AADC) as well as methylation by catechol-O-methyltransferase (COMT).

Levodopa is coadministered with inhibitors of these enzyme systems thereby reducing peripheral conversion of levodopa. The inhibitors do not cross the blood-brain barrier allowing free conversion of levodopa to dopamine in the brain. This combination strategy facilitates a reduction in the dose of levodopa and and the associated side effects of excess peripheral dopamine (vasoconstriction, dysrhythmias, and nausea).

Carbidopa inhibits AADC peripherally and is available in combination with levodopa (Sinemet; Merck & Co., Whitehouse Station NJ, USA or Parcopa; Azur Pharma, Philadelphia PA, USA).

Levodopa is also available combined with benserazide (Madopar; Hoffman La Roche,Basle, Switzerland or Prolopa; Hoffmann-La Roche, Mississauga, Ontario, Canada), the latter also an AADC inhibitor.

Entacapone (Comtan; Novartis, East Hanover NJ, USA) inhibits COMT and is often prescribed to enhance the duration of the levodopa effect.

A combination formulation of carbidopa, levodopa, and entacapone (Stalevo; Novartis, East Hanover NJ, USA) is commonly used. Regardless of the specific formulation, dosing must be individualized to optimize motor function as the clinical response is variable and alters over the course of the disease.

Dopamine Agonists

Dopamine agonists (DAs) are synthetic drugs that directly act on the dopamine receptor, typically have a longer duration of action than levodopa, and may be associated with less motor fluctuations (a decline in the usual benefit from a dose of levodopa). They are frequently used as monotherapy in younger patients (<60 years) or in combination with levodopa in advanced PD to treat motor fluctuations and dyskinesia. DA therapy is associated with an increased incidence of impulse control issues and psychiatric disturbances, which limit their utility [6]. In addition, dopamine agonist withdrawal syndrome (DAWS) can occur if DAs are discontinued. It is associated with anxiety, apathy, diaphoresis, orthostatic hypotension, agitation, and altered motor function. Treatment of DAWS is difficult and may be prolonged [7].

The following DAs are available in North America: bromocriptine, pramipexole, ropinirole, rotigotine (delivered transdermally via patch), and apomorphine (injectable).

Apomorphine is derived from morphine but has no opioid agonist effect. It is an effective drug to manage akinesia or "off" episodes (when levodopa is not working optimally, and symptoms return) [8]. If administered subcutaneously, it has a rapid onset of action (6–14 min) and relatively short duration of action (30–60 min). It is associated with postural hypotension and nausea. The latter should be managed by domperidone (Motilium; Janssen-Cilag Pty Ltd., North Ryde, Australia), a DA with a predominantly peripheral mechanism of action that crosses the blood-brain barrier in very limited quantities and seldom causes extrapyramidal effects or alteration of movement status in patients with PD. The use of ondansetron is contraindicated in patients taking apomorphine, as severe hypotension has been reported with this combination.

Apomorphine has been successfully used to manage PD in patients undergoing DBS insertion—oral PD medications are withdrawn and subcutaneous apomorphine infusion simultaneously initiated 3 days prior to surgery. Termination of the infusion temporarily facilitates awake trial stimulation of the DBS system. This approach may reduce the risk of neurologic and respiratory issues during DBS surgery [9].

Monoamine Oxidase-B Inhibitors

These are selective inhibitors of monoamine oxidase-B (MAO-B), an enzyme that catabolizes dopamine in the brain and prevents reuptake of dopamine; they prolong the effect of dopamine and consequently decrease off-time in PD. Commonly used MAO-B inhibitors include selegiline, rasagiline, and safinamide. These drugs in recommended doses are selective for MAO-B but in supratherapeutic doses may lose selectivity and inhibit MAO-A, the enzyme for metabolizing serotonin. This possibility raised theoretical concerns about the use of SSRIs to treat depression, a common issue in PD patients taking MAO-B inhibitors. A combination of MAO-B inhibitors and SSRIs can result in increased serotonergic effects leading to serotonin syndrome (fever, hallucinations, tachycardia, and GI symptoms). These worries have not been borne out by clinical data [10]. Meperidine, methadone, propoxyphene, and tramadol all modestly inhibit serotonin reuptake and are contraindicated in patients on MAO-B treatment.

Amantadine

Amantadine is a noncompetitive *N*-methyl-D-aspartate (NMDA) receptor antagonist and has been approved as a treatment for dyskinesia in patients with PD receiving levodopa management. Presynaptically, it acts by enhancing release of dopamine and inhibiting reuptake and, postsynaptically, by upregulating dopamine D_2 receptors. As abrupt cessation can result in acute delirium and hallucinations, amantadine should be restarted as soon as practical postoperatively.

What About the Non-motor Effects of PD?

It is vital to recognize that PD is not just a motor disease. A comprehensive review of this less recognized aspect of the disease is helpful to review [11]. Briefly, the symptoms may be grouped into the following: neuropsychiatric, autonomic, gastrointestinal, sensory, and sleep issues including vivid dreams, insomnia, and excessive daytime sleepiness. Some of these symptoms are improved by dopamine augmentation, others not. The PD patient may be on a plethora of medications sequentially added in an attempt to manage these issues [12].

What Are the Issues with Levodopa for the Patient Scheduled to Undergo Surgery?

A delay in usual levodopa or combination dose timing can result in significant consequences. These include exacerbation of symptoms, immobility, respiratory difficulties, and aspiration of gastric contents.

Abrupt withdrawal of levodopa can, on rare occasions, precipitate Parkinson-hyperpyrexia syndrome, a state of rigidity, fever, dysautonomia, and/or mental status alteration mimicking a septic state. It has been described in the perioperative period in a patient in whom the DBS pulse generator battery system became depleted [13]. This is a neurological emergency requiring urgent re-institution of levodopa therapy.

The preoperative evaluation should detail the patient's usual schedule of levodopa dosing, and if oral intake cannot be sustained and/or gastrointestinal absorption will be compromised postoperatively, alternatives to oral levodopa must be initiated. One option is to use an carbidopa/levodopa enteral suspension (Duopa; AbbVie, North Chicago, IL, USA) delivered via a percutaneous endoscopic gastrostomy (PEG) with jejunal extension tube (J-PEG) that has recently been approved [13]. This formulation, delivered directly into the duodenum, has the theoretical advantage of overcoming the delayed gastric emptying that occurs in advanced PD. The suspension may have a role in patients undergoing surgery where postoperative ileus is anticipated, but no studies have investigated this approach to management.

Describe a General Approach to the Perioperative Management of Medications Used to Control the Symptoms of PD

1. A complete listing of all PD-related drugs and the timing of same should be detailed.
2. Schedule the patient as the first case to optimize timing of medications.
3. All PD medications should be continued according to the patient's individualized schedule until the time of induction.
4. Let the patient self-medicate his/her PD drugs pre- and postoperatively if possible.
5. If ileus is likely postoperatively or the planned procedure >3 hours in duration, involve a physician with specialist knowledge of PD regarding intraoperative and postoperative management.

Are There Any Issues in Preoperative Assessment Specifically Related to the Presence of a DBS System in This Patient?

An active DBS system will render analysis of an ECG difficult due to interference. Request the patient to bring the remote DBS patient programmer (Fig. 34.1) to the clinic so that therapy can be temporarily discontinued during the ECG exam. Prolonged QTc is not uncommon in patients with PD [14] and should be assessed preoperatively, as many drugs used during the course of anesthesia can exacerbate QTc prolongation [15].

If This Patient Was Scheduled to Undergo a Bowel Resection, What Other Management Steps Should Be Considered?

Levodopa alone or in combination with other agents (as in this patient) remains the mainstay of PD therapy. If poor absorption of oral medications is anticipated (postoperative ileus), monotherapy with a DA that can be delivered subcutaneously/transdermally (apomorphine or rotigotine) should be considered. In these circumstances, involvement of a neurologist/movement disorders specialist in perioperative management is indicated.

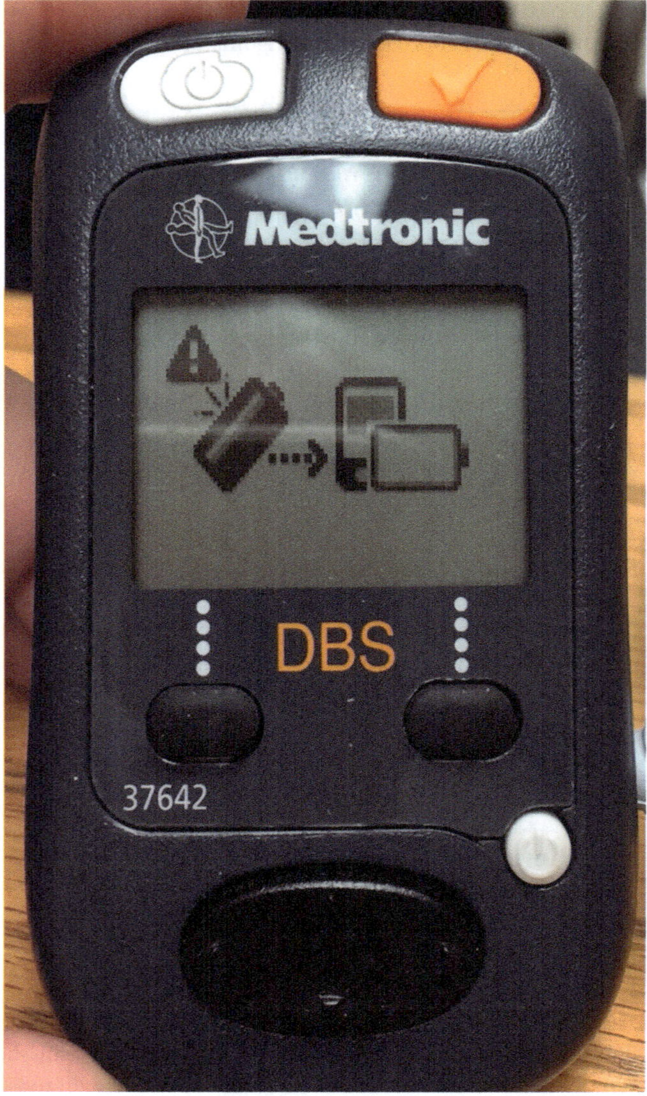

Fig. 34.1 Remote deep brain stimulator (DBS) patient programmer (Medtronic, Minneapolis, MN, USA)

On close questioning, the patient indicated that his PD medications were still effective. Onset time for relief of symptoms was 30 min after oral administration, but this time could be shortened if he chewed the pills. He indicated that recently he took up to three extra doses of Sinemet during the day to control his dyskinesia. He had infrequent "freezing" episodes and none within the last 2 weeks. No alteration of his medications appeared warranted.

He underwent uneventful surgery under general anesthesia as the first case of the day and managed his own medications as soon as he recovered from anesthesia. He was discharged on the day after the procedure without incident.

True/False Questions

1. Patients with PD
   (a) Are more likely to have complications following surgery than matched controls
   (b) Should have their levodopa held on the day of surgery to avoid hypertension
   (c) Have no major issues with cessation of levodopa for up to 12 hours
   (d) Not uncommonly have delirium after surgery
   (e) Who develop Parkinson-hyperpyrexia syndrome are usually asymptomatic
2. A PD patient scheduled for surgery should
   (a) Be scheduled as the first case of the day
   (b) Be let self-medicate if at all possible
   (c) Be very unlikely to have a prolonged QTc on his ECG
   (d) Be prescribed amantadine for pain control routinely
   (e) Be given tramadol for pain if on MAO-B inhibitor therapy

References

1. Kalia LV, Lang AE. Parkinson's disease. Lancet. 2015;386(9996):896–912.
2. Low V, Ben-Shlomo Y, Coward E, Fletcher S, Walker R, Clarke CE. Measuring the burden and mortality of hospitalisation in Parkinson's disease: a cross-sectional analysis of the English Hospital Episodes Statistics database 2009–2013. Parkinsonism Relat Disord. 2015;21(5):449–54.
3. Lubomski M, Rushworth RL, Tisch S. Hospitalisation and comorbidities in Parkinson's disease: a large Australian retrospective study. J Neurol Neurosurg Psychiatry. 2015;86(3):324–9.
4. Institute for Safe Medical Practices. Delayed administration and contraindicated drugs place hospitalized Parkinson's disease patients at risk. 12 Mar 2015. https://www.ismp.org/resources/delayed-administration-and-contraindicated-drugs-place-hospitalized-parkinsons-disease. Accessed 26 May 2020.
5. Okun MS. Management of Parkinson disease in 2017: personalized approaches for patient-specific needs. JAMA. 2017;318(9):791–2.
6. Antonini A, Moro E, Godeiro C, Reichmann H. Medical and surgical management of advanced Parkinson's disease. Mov Disord. 2018;33(6):900–8.
7. Nirenberg MJ. Dopamine agonist withdrawal syndrome: implications for patient care. Drugs Aging. 2013;30(8):587–92.
8. Fox SH, Katzenschlager R, Lim SY, Barton B, de Bie RMA, Seppi K, et al. Movement Disorder Society Evidence-Based Medicine Committee. International Parkinson and Movement Disorder Society evidence-based medicine review: update on treatments for the motor symptoms of Parkinson's disease. Mov Disord. 2018;33(8):1248–66.
9. Slotty PJ, Wille C, Kinfe TM, Vesper J. Continuous perioperative apomorphine in deep brain stimulation surgery for Parkinson's disease. Br J Neurosurg. 2014;28(3):378–82.

10. Robakis D, Fahn S. Defining the role of the monoamine oxidase-b inhibitors for Parkinson's disease. CNS Drugs. 2015;29(5):433–41.
11. Lee HM, Seong-Beam K. Many faces of Parkinson's disease: non-motor symptoms of Parkinson's disease. J Mov Disord. 2015;8(2):92–7.
12. McLean G, Hindle JV, Guthrie B, Mecer SW. Co-morbidity and polypharmacy in Parkinson's disease: insights from a large Scottish primary care database. BMC Neurol. 2017;17:126.
13. AbbVie. DUOPA (carbidopy and levodopa) enteral suspenction. Initial U.S. Approval: 1975. Reference 3680433. 03-B053 Revised Jan 2015. https://www.accessdata.fda.gov/drugsatfda_docs/label/2015/203952s000lbl.pdf.
14. Cunnington AL, Hood K, White L. Outcomes of screening Parkinson's patients for QTc prolongation. Parkinsonism Relat Disord. 2013;19(11):1000–3.
15. Ashes C, Roscoe A. Transesophageal echocardiography in thoracic anesthesia: pulmonary hypertension and right ventricular function. Curr Opin Anaesthesiol. 2015;28(1):38–44.

Multiple Sclerosis

35

Derek Dillane

A 49-year-old female patient with an 11-year history of multiple sclerosis (MS) is scheduled for ankle fusion surgery. She had permanent foot drop secondary to MS. Her initial symptoms included painful left-sided loss of vision and diplopia in addition to balance difficulties. With disease progression, she developed urinary retention requiring self-catheterization, lower limb weakness with frequent reliance on a wheelchair, and movement-induced muscle spasms of the lower limbs. Bowel function was normal; there was no history of seizures or cognitive decline and no difficulties with speech, swallowing, or respiration. She had no other medical comorbidities.
Medications: Interferon beta, baclofen, venlafaxine, and gabapentin.
Laboratory investigations: Chest radiograph, and ECG were normal.

What Is Multiple Sclerosis?

MS is a chronic immune-mediated inflammatory disease causing focal or multifocal demyelination of axons within the central nervous system. It follows one of two courses: relapsing-remitting or progressive.

The majority of cases (approximately 90%) are relapsing-remitting, which is characterized by relapses separated by periods of recovery, either full or incomplete. There is little or no disease progression during remission. However, residual disability may persist and accumulate after a relapse [1].

Progressive MS may be primary progressive or secondary progressive. Primary progressive MS is characterized by a progressive deterioration of neurological disability from disease onset. Secondary progressive disease starts as relapsing-remitting MS before becoming progressive [1, 2]. Most cases of relapsing-remitting MS evolve into a secondary progressive pattern over time.

What Are the Epidemiological Features of MS?

- Prevalence varies with country and population. It is more prevalent in northern Europe, Canada, the northern United States, south-east Australia, and New Zealand. Prevalence in these geographical areas varies between 100 and 400 per 100,000.
- It is more common in females; approximately 75% of people with MS are female [3].
- Typical age of onset is 25–45 years, but it can occasionally be diagnosed in the eighth decade of life.
- The cause of MS is unknown. Current thinking points towards a genetic predisposition combined with environmental triggers. More than 200 gene variants have been associated with MS. People with a first-degree relative with MS have a 2–4% risk of developing the condition compared with the 0.1–0.4% risk in the general population.
- In addition to temperate latitude, environmental risk factors that may be trigger agents include smoking, obesity, and Epstein-Barr virus mononucleosis.

How Is MS Diagnosed?

- Clinical diagnosis is supported by MRI and CSF findings
- Clinical features suggestive of MS are outlined in Table 35.1 [2, 4].
- The McDonald criteria are a set of clinical, radiological, and laboratory diagnostic guidelines for diagnosis of MS.

D. Dillane (✉)
Department of Anesthesiology & Pain Medicine, University of Alberta, Edmonton, AB, Canada

D. Dillane, B. A. Finegan (eds.), *Preoperative Assessment*, https://doi.org/10.1007/978-3-030-58842-7_35

Table 35.1 Clinical features of multiple sclerosis [2–4]

Visual disturbances	Almost always unilateral, painful partial or complete visual loss or painful eye movements due to optic neuritis
Sensory deficits	Paresthesia, numbness, or tingling of extremities; facial numbness
Motor deficits	Lesions in descending motor pathways cause progressive weakness that may lead to paraplegia. Upper limbs involved less frequently.
Cerebellar involvement	Tremor, gait imbalance, slurred speech
Spasticity of extremities	A common feature, associated with exaggerated deep tendon reflexes
Fatigue	–
Pain	Another common feature reported in up to 63% of MS patients [4]. Manifest as headache, back pain, neuropathic extremity pain, painful spasms, and trigeminal neuralgia. Lhermitte sign, a transient sensation akin to an electric shock down the spine to the extremities on neck flexion is frequently, though not exclusively, associated with MS [2].
Cognitive impairment	–
Neurogenic bladder and bowel dysfunction	–

These criteria can be used to diagnose both relapsing-remitting at the first clinical attack or primary progressive MS [5].

- Lesions separated in space (radiographically) and time are essential elements of the McDonald criteria.
- MRI features used to diagnose MS include one or more lesions, representing demyelinated plaques, disseminated in space in regions susceptible to demyelination, e.g., periventricular white matter, cerebral cortex, cerebellum, or spinal cord.
- CSF analysis for presence of oligoclonal bands can be used to confirm the diagnosis if there are doubts regarding dissemination in space and time.

What Drugs Are Used for Management of MS?

Pharmacological therapy for MS is non-curative. However, MS patients may be on a variety of agents for (a) symptom control; (b) treatment of acute exacerbations; (c) reduction of relapse frequency, duration, and accumulation of brain lesions for patients with relapsing remitting disease; and d) treatment of progressive MS. A general approach to these drug categories and specific agents is outlined in Table 35.2 [6, 7].

For How Long Are Disease-Modifying Agents Continued in Patients with Relapsing-Remitting MS?

If the disease remains stable and there are no side effects or safety concerns, these agents can be continued indefinitely [6].

What Are the Perioperative Implications of Drugs Used for Treatment of MS?

Disease-modifying drugs have numerous associated side effects that may have perioperative implications. These are summarized in Table 35.3 [2, 6].

Should Disease-Modifying Medications Be Continued Perioperatively?

In the presence of complications associated with disease-modifying agents, it is best to make this decision with a neurologist. Outside of the perioperative sphere, there are a number of reports of the appearance of new symptoms or deterioration of existing disease after discontinuing treatment [8, 9]. A common feature of these reports is the occurrence of relapses after discontinuation of disease-modifying agents in the presence of high disease activity. Therefore, the decision to temporarily discontinue MS medications in the perioperative period is dependent on the presence and potential perioperative impact of drug complications. If stopped, these medications should be restarted as soon as possible.

What Complications is the Patient with MS Subject to in the Perioperative Period?

- Perioperative stress associated with anesthesia and surgery may lead to disease exacerbation in the form of relapse occurrence or exacerbation of symptoms. There is no clear evidence of a link between perioperative stress and disease exacerbation, but it is prudent to counsel the patient with regard to the possibility of such an occur-

Table 35.2 Pharmacological management of multiple sclerosis [6, 7]

Treatment category	Goal of treatment	Drug
Disease modifying therapy for relapsing-remitting MS	Decreased relapse rate Decrease rate of accumulation of brain lesions on MRI	*Infusion therapy* for very active disease: Natalizumab every 4 weeks *Subcutaneous or intramuscular injection therapy*: Interferon beta alternate days to once weekly Glatiramer acetate 3 times per week *Oral therapy*: Dimethyl fumarate twice daily Fingolimod daily
Treatment of primary progressive MS	Reduce disability progression	Ocrelizumab
Treatment of secondary progressive MS	Reduce disability progression	Siponimod Cladribine Continue disease modifying therapy used in relapsing remitting phase Low dose methotrexate
Symptom control		Anticholinergic and antimuscarinic agents for bladder muscle overactivity Alpha-1-blockade, e.g. Terazocin. Tamsulosin for failure to empty bladder SSRI, e.g., escitalopram, sertraline for depression, anxiety Fluoxetine or bupropion for fatigue and depression Dalfampridine for gait impairment Carbamazepine for paroxysmal sensory and motor symptoms Baclofen for spasticity
Treatment of acute exacerbations	Accelerate time to recovery. Does not improve long-term recovery or reduce risk of future relapses.	Glucocorticoids: High dose intravenous methylprednisolone for 3 days followed by low dose oral prednisone for 11 days.

SSRI Selective serotonin reuptake inhibitor

Table 35.3 Complications associated with disease-modifying agents of multiple sclerosis with perioperative implications [2, 5]

Interferon beta	Leukopenia, thrombocytopenia, anemia, asymptomatic liver dysfunction
Glatiramer acetate	Hepatotoxicity
Natalizumab	Bronchitis, bronchospasm, bradycardia, hepatotoxicity, multifocal leukoencephalopathy
Dimethyl fumarate	Liver injury, lymphocytopenia
Fingolimod	Cardiac conduction abnormalities, cardiomyopathy, bradycardia, atrioventricular (AV) conduction block
Mitoxantrone	Cardiac toxicity to such an extent it is used only as a last resort for MS treatment
Siponimod	Hypertension, bradycardia, liver toxicity

rence. Of course, the unpredictable nature of remission and relapse makes it difficult to definitively associate perioperative deterioration with events related to the surgical procedure rather than to a natural progression of the disease state.

- Hyperthermia is frequently cited as being a trigger for perioperative exacerbation of symptoms. This may be due to a complete conduction block in demyelinated axons after a period of heat exposure [2]. An elevation in temperature of as little as 1 °C has been associated with disease exacerbation [10]. Continuous temperature monitoring and control of hyperthermia are strongly recommended through the appropriate deployment of cooling devices, cooled fluid administration, ambient temperature control, and antipyretic and antibiotic administration.
- Response to non-depolarizing neuromuscular relaxants can be unpredictable. Resistance to the effects of these agents may be due to an increase in the number of postjunctional receptors. Increased sensitivity and a resultant prolonged response may be caused by decreased skeletal muscle mass [2, 10]. Of greater concern, arguably, is the response of the MS patient to depolarizing muscle relaxants. Use of succinylcholine can lead to life-threatening hyperkalemia secondary to an upregulation of skeletal muscle nicotinic acetylcholine receptors. The hyperkalemic risk has been associated with acute exacerbations of MS and progressive disease [11, 12]. Succinylcholine should be avoided in MS patients if at all possible, while non-depolarizing muscle relaxants should be titrated using a peripheral nerve stimulator in a non-affected or least affected extremity [2]. Rocuronium with sugammadex reversal has been posited as a safe alternative [13]. The reversal of rocuronium by sugammadex is not affected by MS.
- Respiratory dysfunction may be present secondary to cervical or thoracic lesions and subsequent respiratory muscle weakness and diaphragmatic paralysis, or derangements in the response of the respiratory center to carbon dioxide

homeostasis. The net effect may be hypoventilation and atelectasis. These issues can be compounded by residual neuromuscular blockade as discussed above.
- Obstructive sleep apnea due to either MS lesions of the respiratory center, obesity, or drug side effects, e.g., GABA-B receptor agonist activity of baclofen [2].
- Hemodynamic instability resulting from autonomic nervous system involvement. This is manifest as profound hypotension with reduced response to fluid bolus or vasopressor administration.

What Are the Objectives of Preoperative Evaluation?

- From the history and physical examination, identify MS type, presence of acute exacerbation, history of relapse occurrence, current medications, and degree of neurological impairment.
- Determine the degree of respiratory dysfunction from clinical assessment and spirometry. Respiratory dysfunction is common even in the early stages of MS, especially during relapse [14]. Patients with severe MS can have profound respiratory dysfunction and should be evaluated for the presence of respiratory infection. Elective procedures may need to be postponed until this has been appropriately treated.
- Patients with severe MS who exhibit signs of severe weakness, respiratory distress, and swallowing abnormalities will likely need high dependency or intensive postoperative care and respiratory support.
- Assess for autonomic nervous system involvement; is there a history of orthostatic hypotension, bladder, or bowel dysfunction; gastroparesis; sexual dysfunction; arrhythmias; or vasovagal episodes?
- Evaluate cardiac function to detect cardiotoxic effects of the drugs being used for treatment of MS.
- Abrupt baclofen withdrawal can lead to seizures and hallucinations. There is no intravenous form—it can be transitioned to diazepam over a 2-week period.

Is There Evidence for Preferred Anesthetic Agents When Administering General Anesthesia to an MS Patient?

There is no evidence that any inhalational or intravenous technique or agent is preferential. The safe use of propofol, etomidate, fentanyl, remifentanil, sevoflurane, and desflurane has been described [15–17].

Should Premedication Be Prescribed for This Patient?

Preoperative administration of a benzodiazepine may be beneficial in reducing stress, a known trigger for disease exacerbation [2]. Midazolam has been linked with reduction of core body temperature through a mechanism that involves inhibition of tonic thermoregulatory vasoconstriction [18]. Premedication should be used with caution in the presence of respiratory compromise.

Is Neuraxial Anesthesia Contraindicated in This Patient?

This is controversial—there is no definitive answer. The successful and safe use of subarachnoid blockade has been described in case reports without prolongation of block or neurologic complications [19, 20]. Conversely, a deterioration (frequently transient) in neurological symptoms or unmasking of MS symptoms has also been described after spinal anesthesia [21]. In theory, demyelinated nerves are more susceptible to the toxic effects of local anesthetics. Another source of concern in this regard is the integrity of the blood-brain barrier, which may be disrupted in MS patients. At this juncture, there is no clear cause-effect relationship between spinal anesthesia and MS deterioration. Epidural anesthesia is considered a safer option to spinal anesthesia due to the lower concentration of local anesthetic entering the subarachnoid space—the concentration of local anesthetic in the white matter of the spinal cord is three to four times higher following spinal compared with epidural anesthesia [22]. Repeat dosing via an epidural catheter may decrease the size of this protective effect. On balance, if after a thorough conversation with the patient spinal anesthesia is deemed preferential, consider using a lower dose and concentration of local anesthetic or performing an epidural.

Is Insertion of a Popliteal Sciatic Nerve Block Catheter Contraindicated?

MS is a disease of the central nervous system. However, some patients also have demyelination of peripheral nerves. There is no consensus on the incidence of peripheral involvement, and the few studies that have investigated the phenomenon are too small to allow derivation of any meaningful conclusion, [23–25]. A case of severe brachial plexopathy (with incomplete reversal) after ultrasound-guided single-shot interscalene brachial plexus blockade has been reported. The authors opine that the decision to perform a peripheral nerve block in a patient with MS should be based on the perceived benefits of avoiding opioid-based analgesia or general anesthesia. It is also worth adding that the quality of a peripheral block for analgesia is likely to be superior to that provided by opioid-based analgesia, thus going a considerable way toward reducing unwanted perioperative stress.

The patient proceeded to have ankle fusion surgery performed under general anesthesia. She received a successful popliteal sciatic continuous block for postoperative analgesia without neurological sequelae.

True-False Questions

1. (a) Multiple sclerosis is primarily a disease of the peripheral nervous system.
   (b) Most MS cases belong to the relapsing-remitting disease category.
   (c) Optic neuritis is a common presenting sign of MS.
   (d) Disease-modifying agents are continued indefinitely in MS unless intolerable complications develop.
   (e) Glatiramer acetate is frequently used as a first-line disease-modifying agent for relapsing-remitting MS.
2. (a) Spinal anesthesia is absolutely contraindicated in MS.
   (b) Epidural anesthesia is likely safer than spinal anesthesia in MS.
   (c) There is no risk associated with peripheral nerve blockade in the MS patient.
   (d) Baclofen can be safely stopped on the morning of surgery.
   (e) Response to non-depolarizing muscle relaxants can be unpredictable in MS.

References

1. Olek MJ, Howard J. Clinical presentation, course, and prognosis of multiple sclerosis in adults. In: Post TW, editor. UpToDate. Waltham: UpToDate; 2020.
2. Makris A, Piperopoulos A, Karmaniolou I. Multiple sclerosis: basic knowledge and new insights in perioperative management. J Anesth. 2014;28(2):267–78.
3. Reich DS, Lucchinetti CF, Calabresi PA. Multiple sclerosis. N Engl J Med. 2018;378(2):169–80.
4. Foley PL, Vesterinen HM, Laird BJ, Sena ES, Colvin LA, Chandran S, et al. Prevalence and natural history of pain in adults with multiple sclerosis: systematic review and meta-analysis. Pain. 2013;154(5):632–42.
5. Thompson AJ, Banwell BL, Barkhof F, Carroll WM, Coetzee T, Comi G, et al. Diagnosis of multiple sclerosis: 2017 revisions of the McDonald criteria. Lancet Neurol. 2018;17(2):162–73.
6. Olek MJ, Mowry E. Disease-modifying treatment of relapsing-remitting multiple sclerosis in adults. In: Post TW, editor. UpToDate. Waltham: UpToDate; 2020.
7. Goodin DS. Glucocorticoid treatment of multiple sclerosis. Handb Clin Neurol. 2014;122:455–64.
8. Havla JB, Pellkofer HL, Meinl I, Gerdes LA, Hohlfeld R, Kumpfel T. Rebound of disease activity after withdrawal of fingolimod (FTY720) treatment. Arch Neurol. 2012;69(2) 262–4.
9. O'Connor PW, Goodman A, Kappos L, Lublin FD, Miller DH, Polman C, et al. Disease activity return during natalizumab treatment interruption in patients with multiple sclerosis. Neurology. 2011;76(22):1858–65.
10. Pasternak J, Lanier W. Diseases affecting the brain. In: Hines RL, Marschall KE, editors. Stoelting's anesthesia and co-existing disease. 7th ed. Philadelphia: Elsevier; 2018. p. 296–8.
11. Cooperman LH. Succinylcholine-induced hyperkalemia in neuromuscular disease. JAMA. 1970;213(11):1867–71
12. Kytta J, Rosenberg PH. Anaesthesia for patients with multiple sclerosis. Ann Chir Gynaecol. 1984;73(5):299–303.
13. Carron M, Ieppariello G. Benefit of sugammadex in a morbidly obese patient with multiple sclerosis and severe respiratory dysfunction. J Clin Anesth. 2019;52:119–20.
14. Turakhia P, Barrick B, Berman J. Patients with neuromuscular disorder. Med Clin North Am. 2013;97(6):1015–32.
15. Hedstrom AK, Hillert J, Olsson T, Alfredsson L. Exposure to anaesthetic agents does not affect multiple sclerosis risk. Eur J Neurol. 2013;20(5):735–9.
16. Acar A, Nuri Deniz M, Erhan E, Ugur G. Anesthetic technique in a patient with multiple sclerosis scheduled for laparoscopic nephrectomy for a renal tumor: a case report. Anesth Pain Med. 2013;2(3):138–40.
17. Sahin L, Korkmaz HF, Sahin M, Aydin T, Toker S, Gulcan E. Desflurane anaesthesia in a patient with multiple sclerosis in total hip replacement. Arch Med Sci. 2010;6(6):984–56.
18. Honarmand A, Safavi MR. Comparison of prophylactic use of midazolam, ketamine, and ketamine plus midazolam for prevention of shivering during regional anaesthesia: a randomized double-blind placebo controlled trial. Br J Anaesth. 2008;101(4):557–62.
19. Bouchard P, Caillet JB, Monnet F, Banssillon V. Spinal anesthesia and multiple sclerosis. Ann Fr Anesth Reanim. 1984;3(3):194–8. [*Article in French*].
20. Martucci G, Di Lorenzo A, Polito F, Acampa L. A 12-month follow-up for neurological complication after subarachnoid anesthesia in a parturient affected by multiple sclerosis. Eur Rev Med Pharmacol Sci. 2011 15(4):458–60.
21. Bornemann-Cimenti H, Sivro N, Toft F, Halb L, Sandner-Kiesling A. Neuraxial anesthesia in patients with multiple sclerosis - a systematic review. Rev Bras Anestesiol. 2017;67(4) 404–10. [*Article in Portuguese*].
22. Warren TM, Datta S, Ostheimer GW. Lumbar epidural anesthesia in a patient with multiple sclerosis. Anesth Analg. 1982;61(12):1022–3.
23. Neal JM, Barrington MJ, Brull R, Hadzic A, Hebl JR, Horlocker TT, et al. The second ASRA practice advisory on neurologic complications associated with regional anesthesia and pain medicine: executive summary 2015. Reg Anesth Pain Med. 2015;40(5):401–30.
24. Pogorzelski R, Baniukiewicz E, Drozdowski W. Subclinical lesions of peripheral nervous system in multiple sclerosis patients. Neurol Neurochir Pol. 2004;38(4):257–64. [*Article in Polish*].
25. Misawa S, Kuwabara S, Mori M, Hayakawa S, Sawai S, Hattori T. Peripheral nerve demyelination in multiple sclerosis. Clin Neurophysiol. 2008;119(8):1829–33.

Intracranial Mass

36

Michael J. Jacka

A 42-year-old man presented to the anesthesia preassessment clinic 1 day before craniotomy for resection of an intracranial mass. He had a concurrent seizure disorder. The seizures began 4–5 months before presentation. A CT scan and subsequent MRI confirmed and delineated a mass in the right temporal lobe that was noted to be spiculated and associated with vasogenic edema. His neurologist had prescribed carbamezapine for seizure control 1 month prior to the clinic visit. Dexamethasone was initiated when the decision was made to proceed to surgery. The seizures had not recurred, and the patient had no neurologic impairment. The neurosurgeon requested general anesthesia for frozen section biopsy of the mass and subsequent complete resection at the same craniotomy surgery.

He was an otherwise well person with a good exercise tolerance. Surgical history was remarkable for a distant appendectomy.

He was a nonsmoker, did not use cannabis or illicit drugs but drank alcohol occasionally.

Medications included acetaminophen on occasion, taken for headaches. He has no drug allergies.

Physical examination was unremarkable.

Laboratory investigations including complete blood count and chemistry were normal.

What Is a Seizure?

A seizure involves involuntary muscle contraction due to an unregulated focus of electrical activity in the brain. A seizure may be generalized (consciousness is lost) or focal (consciousness preserved).

What Is Status Epilepticus?

This definition has varied, but it usually involves a generalized seizure lasting 30 minutes. Since this is impractical and assertive treatment should be initiated sooner than that, a more common definition is a single seizure of 5 minutes duration or two ictal events within 5 minutes without complete recovery between events. Status epilepticus is a serious emergency as it is associated with high mortality in the range of 10% or higher, although this includes the mortality associated with the underlying condition. The severe metabolic acidemia that occurs during status epilepticus often results in brain injury.

What Causes Seizures?

A seizure is due to an unregulated focus of electrical activity in the brain. Seizures are typically differentiated as being due to structural or non-structural causes. Examples of structural causes include brain tumors (more common with primary than secondary tumors), traumatic head injury, infection, hemorrhage, and ischemic stroke. Examples of non-structural causes include drug and medication use, and severe metabolic disturbances, e.g., hypoglycemia and hyponatremia.

What Medications Are Commonly Used to Control Seizures in Patients with Brain Tumors?

Monotherapy with the lowest effective dose of a first-line anticonvulsant medication should be commenced after a first seizure. Levetiracetam and topiramate are frequently chosen due to their minimal effect on hepatic enzymes and subsequently are associated with fewer drug interactions. This is especially germane in patients receiving chemotherapeutic agents. Valproate is also frequently used as an anticonvulsant in patients with brain tumors. Even though it is a strong

M. J. Jacka (✉)
Department of Anesthesiology & Pain Medicine/Department of Critical Care, University of Alberta, Edmonton, AB, Canada
e-mail: mjacka@ualberta.ca

D. Dillane, B. A. Finegan (eds.), *Preoperative Assessment*, https://doi.org/10.1007/978-3-030-58842-7_36

inhibitor of hepatic enzymes, there are few known adverse drug interactions between valproate and chemotherapeutic agents [1]. However, there is a dose-dependent risk of thrombocytopenia with valproate use.

Phenytoin has historically been used and remains the mainstay for the management of status epilepticus. Benzodiazepines are commonly used for acute management. Barbiturates, propofol, and volatile anesthetic agents are used for refractory situations that are resistant to the foregoing therapies.

Which Antiseizure Medications Induce Hepatic Metabolism?

Induction of hepatic metabolism is a common effect of anticonvulsants and is associated with multiple drug consequences. The most general effect is a reduction in the measured effectiveness of a drug and a consequent increase in the dose necessary to produce the desired effect. For example, phenytoin classically induces hepatic metabolism. The effect of other drugs that are hepatically metabolized will be changed when phenytoin is used. Such drugs that are affected this way include coumadin, most other anticonvulsants, many antibiotics, oral contraceptives, and several narcotics, among others.

Barbiturates, phenytoin, and carbamazepine are commonly associated with hepatic enzyme induction. These drugs are occasionally added to control seizures when first-line medications that are less potent enzyme inducers have not controlled seizures successfully.

Is There a Role for Glucocorticoids in the Management of Patients with an Intracranial Mass?

Peritumoral cerebral edema may cause severe headaches and dizziness, can contribute to increased intracranial pressure, and can make surgical resection of the tumor more difficult. High-dose dexamethasone has long been used to reduce this cerebral edema. However, there are few prospective studies that support this use of dexamethasone. The long-term side effects of steroid use, e.g., immunosuppression, truncal obesity, myopathy, hyperglycemia, fluid retention, and mood changes, necessitate that glucocorticoids be used only for patients with peritumoral edema who are symptomatic [2].

Is Premedication Contraindicated?

The principal factor when deciding whether to prescribe premedication for the patient with an intracranial mass is the presence and/or severity of raised ICP. Sedating premedication can conceal changes in mental status that may be indicative of worsening raised ICP. Moreover, sedation-induced depression of respiratory drive and associated hypercarbia will lead to vasodilatation and amplification of increased ICP [3]. Small doses of a benzodiazepine premedication can be used with caution in patients who are asymptomatic for raised ICP. Otherwise, it is best to wait until the patient is fully monitored prior to administering sedative premedication.

What Is Intracranial Hypertension?

Intracranial pressure (ICP) refers to the pressure within the head. Normally, the pressure within the head is atmospheric at rest in the supine position but is less than zero with deep inspiration or with standing. With positive pressure ventilation, some of the pressure within the thorax is transmitted to other body parts, including the head.

Pathology in the head, whether due to tumors, bleeds, or infection, often increases the ICP as does positive pressure ventilation. Concern occurs when the pressure in the brain is high enough that arterial blood flow into the head is reduced, leading to brain injury. The positive pressure of mechanical ventilation may also be sufficient when added to the intracranial process to produce the same effect on ICP. Pressures within the head that are greater than 20 cm of water are generally the danger point at which blood flow into the brain is reduced unless the blood pressure is artificially elevated using vasopressors.

Does the Patient Require a Preoperative Electroencephalogram (EEG)?

Once an intracranial mass has been diagnosed on neuroimaging, preoperative EEG will not change management and is not necessary. Intraoperative EEG, on the other hand, is frequently used to detect ischemia and seizure activity, and this has implications for how anesthesia is conducted.

Does the Patient Require Preoperative Consultation with a Neurologist?

This is not necessary. However, a baseline neurologic assessment should be performed at the preoperative visit to include recording of neurological deficits and appraisal of signs and symptoms of raised ICP.

How Can the Risk of Venous Air Embolism Be Modified Preoperatively?

Preoperative echocardiography can be conducted if the risk of venous air embolism is high, e.g., sitting position or for surgery close to the venous sinuses. It may be prudent to avoid the sitting position for patients with an intracardiac shunt, e.g., patent foramen ovale, atrial septal defect, or ventricular septal defect [4].

Are Seizures Commonly Associated with a Brain Mass?

Yes. Brain masses are commonly associated with a seizure disorder, more so with lower grade neoplasms than with the higher grades. On the other hand, most seizure disorders are not associated with a brain mass.

Of the brain masses associated with a seizure disorder, seizures are much more common with primary brain neoplasms than with brain metastases from other sources.

What Are the Anesthetic Options for Craniotomy?

Surgery may require a responsive patient for a careful resection during an "awake" craniotomy. An awake craniotomy is frequently chosen when cortical mapping is to be performed for a tumor sited close to functionally eloquent cortex, e.g., primary sensory and motor cortex, Broca and Wernicke areas, and the primary visual and auditory cortex. More commonly, general anesthesia is requested

An "awake" craniotomy requires a cooperative patient and is generally done to facilitate very precise resection of brain tissue. Sedation may not be necessary, but if used, options include dexmedetomidine or remifentanil as well as propofol.

General anesthesia for craniotomy can be done using volatile or intravenous-based techniques. The craniotomy itself is seldom as painful as major joint or visceral surgery, and narcotics can be used judiciously. Blood loss is always possible and can easily involve a blood volume or more – reliable intravenous access is essential. Monitoring of blood pressure is commonly done continuously with an in situ arterial access.

What Additional Preoperative Preparation Is Necessary for the Patient Scheduled for Awake Craniotomy?

Patient selection is critical. The patient needs to be motivated and understand what is expected of them during the procedure. Patients with anxiety disorder, confusion, or severe claustrophobia are not suitable. Those with anticipated difficult airway or at risk of airway compromise are also not good candidates.

Are Intraoperative Mannitol and Hypertonic Saline Required?

No. Both mannitol and hypertonic saline are options that may facilitate surgical exposure. Both medications are osmotic diuretics and function by reducing total body water from all cells. They are commonly used as aids in brain surgery because the brain is part of the vessel-rich group of organs and will preferentially shrink promptly after the osmotic diuretic is given.

Both mannitol and hypertonic saline can cause flux in sodium levels and serum osmolarity that can interfere with electrical conduction in the heart and the brain, although this is usually only seen in extreme situations.

Is Intraoperative Hyperventilation Required?

No. Carbon dioxide is a vasodilator, and the relationship between carbon dioxide and cerebral blood flow is linear between partial pressures of 25 and 60-mm Hg. Lower partial pressure of carbon dioxide reduces the cerebral blood flow and may also facilitate surgical exposure. However, this also reduces the blood flow globally to all body tissues and is not recommended for extended periods.

The Surgeon Decides to Do the Craniotomy Under MRI Guidance. How Does This Affect Anesthetic Management?

Certain centers have the capacity for intraoperative MRI. This is a complex undertaking for the anesthesiologist. All monitors, infusion devices, and anesthetic equipment must be MR safe, i.e., not ferromagnetic [5]. Anything within the MRI suite that becomes magnetized may become a projectile and represents a hazard for both people and equipment. Of note, cellular telephones, credit cards, and computers can be erased by the magnetic field of the MRI and cannot be taken into the MRI suite. Finally, the MRI itself is very noisy when in operation, and precautions should be taken to protect the ears of staff and patients using soft snug earplugs.

True/False Questions

1. (a) Phenytoin is the commonest first-line anticonvulsant medication for seizure control in the patient with an intracranial mass.
   (b) Phenytoin is a mainstay in the management of status epilepticus.
   (c) Levetiracetam is a first-line antiseizure medication in patients with intracranial mass due to its minimal effect on hepatic enzyme metabolism.
   (d) Dexamethasone is used to reduce peritumoral cerebral edema regardless of symptom profile.
   (e) Sedative premedication is contraindicated in patients with signs of raised ICP.
2. (a) Preoperative EEG is a prerequisite in the preoperative workup for craniotomy for intracranial mass resection.
   (b) Presence of intracardiac shunt is a relative contraindication for a sitting position craniotomy.
   (c) Intracranial masses are commonly associated with seizure disorder.
   (d) Seizures are more common with primary brain neoplasms than with brain metastases.
   (e) Pathologic intracranial hypertension is present at a pressure ≥15 mm Hg.

References

1. Englot DJ, Chang EF, Vecht CJ. Epilepsy and brain tumors. Handb Clin Neurol. 2016;134:267–85.
2. Lee EQ, Wen PY. Corticosteroids for peritumoral edema: time to overcome our addiction? Neuro-Oncology. 2016;18(9):1191–2.
3. Bodner N. Intracranial mass, intracranial pressure, venous air embolism, and autoregulation. 2nd ed. London: Churchill Livingstone; 1995.
4. Paisansathan C, Ozcan MS. Anesthesia for craniotomy. In: Post TW, editor. UpToDate. Waltham: UpToDate; 2020.
5. Reddy U, White M, Wilson S. Anaesthesia for magnetic resonance imaging. Contin Educ Anaesth Crit Care Pain. 2012;12(3):140–4.

Part X

Hematological

37 Easy Bruising

Barry A. Finegan

The patient was a 70-year-old moderately obese female presenting for elective cholecystectomy. She had experienced right upper quadrant pain intermittently over the 3 years prior to presentation, which was associated with the intake of fatty food. An ultrasound of the abdomen demonstrated the presence of fatty liver disease and multiple stones in her gallbladder. Systems review was non-contributory apart from a 35-year smoking history (10 cigarettes/day), moderate alcohol intake (she admitted to five standard drinks/week), and mild lower back pain.

However, in response to the screening question, "Any bleeding issues?" she indicated that she had experienced "easy bruising" over the last week. On further questioning, she mentioned that she had noticed gingival bleeding on teeth brushing in the last month but denied any incidents of hematuria or melena. There was no family history of bleeding disorders. She had three uneventful vaginal births without excessive bleeding and had never been transfused. She denied any menorrhagia in the past or any postmenopausal uterine bleeding. She had never undergone surgery before or had any admissions to hospital. Past medical history was essentially negative apart from mild depression and hypothyroidism. Medications: Trandolapril 2 mg and L-thyroxine (1.2 µg/kg), daily. She was adamant that she did not take herbal medications, analgesics, or anticoagulant drugs.

Physical Examination: The patient was hemodynamically stable. Physical examination was otherwise unremarkable except for the presence of areas of multiple (>10) purpuric lesions (8–10 mm in diameter) on her lower limbs, a palpable tender mass overlying her left calf compatible with a hematoma. There was no evidence of a compartment syndrome. There was evidence of oral cavity bleeding on removal of a dental plate. She was not able to recollect any trauma that might have caused these lesions and had only become aware of them 2 days before the clinic visit.

Investigations: A complete blood count (CBC) performed 4 weeks prior to the clinic visit revealed a hemoglobin value of 112 g/L; mean corpuscular volume (MCV) 84 fL, and platelet count of 248 × 10⁹/L. The remaining components of the CBC were within normal limits. Prothrombin time (PT), activated partial prothrombin time (APTT), electrolytes, and renal and liver function tests on file from 4 months previously were normal. A stat CBC, peripheral blood smear, PT, APTT, and fibrinogen were requested.

What Is a Practical Approach to the Patient Presenting in the Preoperative Clinic with a History of Apparently Clinically Significant Coagulation Disorder?

An excellent schema on how to assess such a patient has been outlined by Harrison et al. [1].

Key facets of the history include the following:

- Clarifying the patient's definition of what exactly they mean by a bruise?
- Is the bruising acute or longstanding?
- Do they have photographs of past lesions?
- Have they noticed petechiae or purpura with the bruises?
- Are the bruises spontaneous or associated with trauma?
- Family history of bleeding?
- What is the age of the patient?
- What medications/herbal products is the patient taking?
- What is the diet and state of nutrition of the patient?
- Are there risk factors for liver disease?

The examination should include assessing the following:

- The size, number, and location of bruises
- Signs of poor nutrition – cachexia and brittle hair
- Signs of liver disease – jaundice, hepatomegaly, and ascites

B. A. Finegan (✉)
Department of Anesthesiology & Pain Medicine, University of Alberta, Edmonton, AB, Canada
e-mail: bfinegan@ualberta.ca

D. Dillane, B. A. Finegan (eds.), *Preoperative Assessment*, https://doi.org/10.1007/978-3-030-58842-7_37

Screening baseline investigations should include the following:

- CBC, blood smear, coagulation screen, and renal and liver function tests

The patient should be requested to complete the International Society on Thrombosis and Hemostasis Bleeding Assessment Tool (ISTH-BAT). This tool is available at https://bleedingscore.certe.nl/. The ISTH-BAT records the presence and severity of bleeding symptoms in 14 situations, e.g., epistaxis, hematuria, and dental extraction, and has been validated as a useful screening and structured tool to assist in determining who should undergo further testing for Von Willebrand disease (VWD), the most common inherited disorder of coagulation [2]. There is limited evidence that the ISTH-BAT is abnormal in those with congenital defects in platelet function [3]. A "normal" ISTH-BAT cut-off is 3 for males and 5 for females [4].

What Is the Basic Sequence of Events When the Hemostatic System Is Activated?

Primary hemostasis involves vasospasm at the site of injury, exposure of subendothelial collagen on vascular disruption, platelet adhesion mediated by von Willebrand factor (VWF), and activation and aggregation of platelets leading to plug development.

Secondary hemostasis occurs simultaneously and involves activation of the coagulation cascade and subsequent fibrin clot formation.

How May Bleeding Disorders Be Broadly Classified?

Primary hemostatic defects – decreased platelet number or impaired platelet function, and VWF deficiency.

Secondary hemostatic defects – coagulation factor defects.

What Does the PT and APTT Assess?

The PT and APTT are non-specific tests for secondary hemostatic defects.

The PT assesses the extrinsic and final common pathway of the coagulation system.

The extrinsic pathway is initiated by release of tissue factor (TF), a transmembrane receptor for factor VII/VIIa (FVII/VIIa). TF is constitutively expressed by subendothelial tissue but is separated from circulating FVII by an intact endothelium. TF is expressed in relative abundance in the brain, lung, uterus, testis, and heart [5]. Breach of the endothelium by trauma or other injury allows TF to initiate immediate activation of the extrinsic system.

The APTT assesses the intrinsic and final common pathways of the coagulation system.

The intrinsic pathway is initiated by trauma within the vascular system via activated platelets, exposed endothelium, and other initiators. It involves FXII, XI, IX, X, and VIII among other factors.

How Should Prolonged PT and APTT Results Be Interpreted?

An excellent approach to this question has been outlined by Kamal et al. [6].

1. Are the values artifactually elevated?
   (a) A high hematocrit reduces the volume of plasma collected resulting in a relative increase in the volume of citrate anticoagulant in the collecting tube. When the plasma is added to the clotting test reagents, the excess citrate causes an artifactual increase in clotting time. This can occur if the hematocrit is >55%. Advise the laboratory of this condition so the tubes containing the appropriate calibrated amount of anticoagulant can be used.
   (b) Plasma turbidity present in lipemic, hemolyzed, or icteric plasma can interfere with photo-optical clot systems. Manual visualization of clot formation overcomes this artifactual error.
2. Is the patient receiving anticoagulants?
   (a) Coumadin
   (b) Xa and thrombin inhibitors
   (c) Heparin (including low molecular weight heparin, which can prolong the APTT)
   (d) Herbal products
3. Is the prolongation due to systemic disease?
   (a) Liver
   (b) Auto-immune
   (c) Disseminated intravascular coagulation (DIC)
   (d) Fibrinolysis
   (e) Other

A reasonable approach, in the absence of the above, is to repeat the tests and request a mixing study. If the prolonged values are confirmed, the mixing study helps assess if the patient has a factor deficiency or has a factor-inhibiting antibody. It is very helpful in determining the next steps in assessing the exact cause of the coagulation abnormality.

What Is a Mixing Study?

The test involves mixing an equal volume of the patient's plasma with pooled normal plasma and repeating the PT and APTT immediately.

Correction of the values to normal is suggestive of a factor deficiency.

No correction or partial correction suggests the presence of a coagulation inhibitor.

Who Should Have Surgery Deferred and/or Be Referred to a Hematologist for Further Evaluation and Management?

1. Abnormal coagulation studies warrant further investigation and/or referral if not readily explainable based on coexisting disease, medication use, known presence of an inhibitor, or past history.
2. Any individual who appears to have a previously undiagnosed clinically significant bleeding disorder should be investigated prior to surgery. Using the ISTH-BAT can be helpful in making this decision.
3. Concerning findings on history and especially physical examination, even in the absence of definitive laboratory findings, should prompt postponement and referral for specialist evaluation.

What Can Cause Isolated APTT Prolongation But Is Not Associated with Bleeding?

The APTT test involves the addition, among other substances, of phospholipid to the plasma sample of the patient. The presence of lupus anticoagulant (LAC), an antiphospholipid antibody, in the sample will interfere with the added phospholipid and cause prolongation of the APTT (act as an inhibitor). No correction or partial correction of values is seen when a mixing study is performed. Patients who have LAC antibodies are at increased risk of thrombosis, as they bind to endothelial cells, monocytes, and platelets and can cause activation of the coagulation system.

What Condition Causes Easy Dermal Bruising in the Elderly in the Face of Normal Coagulation Studies?

Older individuals are susceptible to actinic purpura, a condition that arises secondary to loss of collagen, thinning of the dermis, and reduced connective tissue support for vessels and capillaries. This form of bruising is commonly seen on the dorsum of the hands and extensor areas of the hands and shins. It is benign and usually resolves within 3 weeks of a traumatic event.

How Common and Concerning Is Easy Bruising Preoperatively?

"Easy bruising" and other events suggestive of a bleeding disorder (epistaxis, menorrhagia, bleeding after tooth extraction or surgery) are commonly reported, and any one of these events may occur in >25% of the general population [7]. Screening for bleeding disorders prior to surgery using a bleeding assessment tool (BAT) is recommended by the European Society of Anesthesiology with referral to a hematologist if any inherited bleeding disorders are suspected [8].

Vries et al. [9] screened over 35,000 patients with a BAT-like questionnaire over 3 years at a single site and uncovered many patients reporting bleeding symptoms (≈10% of the sample). In the small subset of this group who underwent comprehensive coagulation testing, including factor assays and platelet function analysis, minor hemostatic abnormalities were detected in 8.8%, a value less than that noted in the group denying bleeding symptoms (10.5%). Only one patient in the "bleeding symptoms" group was referred to a hematologist, as there was concern that the patient had clinically significant bleeding.

From these data, we can conclude that "easy bruising" is very commonly reported and of doubtful, if any, clinical significance. Nevertheless, as the case described demonstrates, there are occasional circumstances where "easy bruising" is indicative of a serious underlying abnormality. In the vast majority of cases, elimination of a significant cause can be achieved from history alone obviating the need for extensive workup.

The patient's ISTH-BAT score was 6. The results of the laboratory tests were as follows: Hemoglobin 7.9 g/dL and platelet count 387 × 10^9/L. The other components of the CBC were normal. Blood smear showed normocytic and normochromic RBCs, morphologically normal white cells and platelets; fibrinogen levels were within normal limits. The PT was PT 11 s and APTT 79.4 s.

Surgery was postponed, a mixing study was requested, and the patient was referred for immediate evaluation by hematology. She was urgently admitted under this service; the mixing study did not correct the prolonged APTT. Factor assays revealed reduced FVIII activity and the presence of FVIII inhibitors in the patient's serum. Given these assay data, the negative family history of coagulation/bleeding disorders and recent onset of the condition, a diagnosis of acquired hemophilia A (AHA) was made.

AHA is very rare disease that tends to occur in elderly patients and has a high morbidity and mortality from hemorrhagic-related complications. Most cases are idio-

pathic. It is a hematological emergency that results from the spontaneous production of IgG autoantibodies targeting endogenous FVIII. It can recur even after initial successful inhibitor eradication. A comprehensive outline of the management of AHA has recently been published [10].

It was decided that replacement or bypass therapy was not indicated acutely. The patient was treated with oral prednisone and cyclophosphamide to facilitate inhibitor eradication. On follow up 4 months later, FVIII levels were normalized and her FVIII inhibitor assay was negative. Surgery proceeded uneventfully thereafter without any perioperative bleeding issues. She has remained under the care of a hematologist and undergoes periodic assessment to ensure no recurrence of her condition.

True/False Questions

1. Which of the following results in a prolonged APTT?
   (a) Factor VIII deficiency
   (b) Lupus anticoagulant positive plasma
   (c) Xa inhibitor medications
   (d) Platelet dysfunction
   (e) Disseminated intravascular coagulation
2. "Easy bruising" reported by a patient is a condition
   (a) where a BAT-like questionnaire is helpful
   (b) where a VIII assay is helpful
   (c) that is usually benign
   (d) commonly associated with abnormal coagulation studies
   (e) where lupus anticoagulant is usually positive

References

1. Harrison LB, Nash MJ, Fitzmaurice D, Thachil J. Investigating easy bruising in an adult. BMJ. 2017;356:j251.
2. O'Brien SH. Bleeding scores: are they really useful? Hematology Am Soc Hematol Educ Program. 2012;2012:152–6.
3. Adler M, Kaufmann J, Alberio L, Nagler M. Diagnostic utility of the ISTH bleeding assessment tool in patients with suspected platelet function disorders. J Thromb Haemost. 2019;17(7):1104–12.
4. Elbatarny M, Mollah S, Grabell J, Bae S, Deforest M, Tuttle A, et al. Normal range of bleeding scores for the ISTH-BAT: adult and pediatric data from the merging project. Haemophilia. 2014;20(6):831–5.
5. MacKman N. The role of tissue factor and factor VIIa in hemostasis. Anesth Analg. 2009;108(5):1447–52.
6. Kamal AH, Tefferi A, Pruthi RK. How to interpret and pursue an abnormal prothrombin time, activated partial thromboplastin time, and bleeding time in adults. Mayo Clin Proc. 2007;82(7):864–73.
7. Sadler JE. Von Willebrand disease type 1: a diagnosis in search of a disease. Blood. 2003;101(6):2089–93.
8. Kozek-Langenecker SA, Ahmed AB, Afshari A, Albaladejo P, Aldecoa C, Barauskas G. Management of severe perioperative bleeding: guidelines from the European Society of Anaesthesiology: first update 2016. Eur J Anaesthesiol. 2017;34(6):332–95.
9. Vries MJ, van der Meijden PE, Kuiper GJ, Nelemans PJ, Wetzels RJ, van Oerle RG, et al. Preoperative screening for bleeding disorders: a comprehensive laboratory assessment of clinical practice. Res Pract Thromb Haemost. 2018;2(4):767–77.
10. Kruse-Jarres R, Kempton CL, Baudo F, Collins PW, Knoebl P, Leissinger CA, et al. Acquired hemophilia A: updated review of evidence and treatment guidance. Am J Hematol. 2017;92(7):695–705. Review

Thrombocytopenia

38

Barry A. Finegan

A 25-year-old male was scheduled to undergo splenectomy. Two months previously, he presented to the emergency room of his local hospital complaining of the recent development of a rash on his limbs. The rash had appeared spontaneously 3 weeks before this visit. The patient stated he was well and not fatigued. He had taken no medications or street drugs in the last 6 months. His alcohol intake was moderate (5 standard drinks per week). Review of systems was non-contributory. He denied any bleeding episodes. Examination of his upper and lower limbs revealed the presence of small rounded spots, approximately 1–2 mm in size (Fig. 38.1). *There was no evidence of ecchymoses. Physical examination was otherwise normal. Specifically, there was no evidence of hepatosplenomegaly or lymphadenopathy. A complete blood count (CBC) was obtained, which revealed a platelet count of 8 × 10⁹/L. A repeat CBC confirmed the initial value. A peripheral blood smear was normal. There were no dysplastic changes or abnormal circulating cells noted on the smear. His CBC 6 months previously was normal. A presumptive diagnosis of autoimmune idiopathic thrombocytopenic purpura (ITP) was made and high-dose steroid therapy initiated.*

The patient was initially treated with high-dose dexamethasone (40 mg/day for 4 days × 2 cycles). He was vaccinated for pneumococcus, haemophilus, and meningococcus. He had an excellent initial response to treatment but relapsed some weeks after therapy. A second course of steroid treatment was initiated, and intravenous immunoglobulin was administered. Despite an early response, the patient did not stay in remission. He did not wish to consider management with a thrombopoietin-receptor agonist, and a laparoscopic splenectomy was scheduled. In the week before surgery, a tapered dose of steroids was administered. His platelet count at the time of assessment was 80 × 10⁹/L. He had no evidence of petechia, hematoma, or recent bleeding.

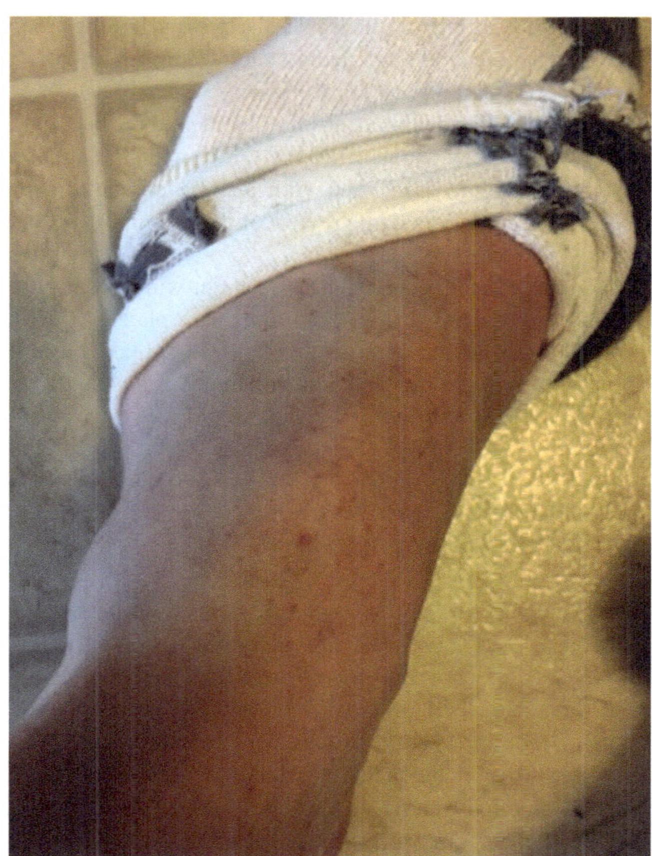

Fig. 38.1 Petechia present on the upper limb of a 25-year-old male at time of presentation with ITP, 2 months before subsequent splenectomy

What Is Thrombocytopenia?

An individual with a platelet count of <150 × 10⁹/L is considered thrombocytopenic.

B. A. Finegan (✉)
Department of Anesthesiology & Pain Medicine, University of Alberta, Edmonton, AB, Canada
e-mail: bfinegan@ualberta.ca

D. Dillane, B. A. Finegan (eds.), *Preoperative Assessment*, https://doi.org/10.1007/978-3-030-58842-7_38

How Should an Incidental Preoperative Finding of Recent Onset (<3 Months) Thrombocytopenia Be Approached?

A rational approach to the incidental finding of recent-onset thrombocytopenia has been outlined by Bradbury and Murray [1].

An unexpected low platelet count should be confirmed by a repeat CBC and trigger an assessment of a blood smear to exclude clumping or the presence of giant platelets.

Outside a surgical setting, individuals with platelet counts of 100–150 × 10^9/L without features suggestive of systemic disease may be subject to observation and follow-up with another CBC in 6 weeks. It would seem reasonable in the preoperative setting to follow a similar approach if the procedure is scheduled in the immediate future. Inform the patient, document the finding, and proceed with surgery.

For individuals with recent-onset incidental thrombocytopenia with platelet counts <100 × 10^9/L or with undiagnosed thrombocytopenia associated with anemia or neutropenia, postponing surgery pending review of the patient by a hematologist is warranted.

Urgent referral is indicated in a patient with recent-onset incidental thrombocytopenia and a platelet count ≤50,000 × 10^9/L. An emergent referral should take place if, in addition, signs of petechia or bruising are present, or the patient presents with active bleeding.

What Are the Common Causes of Thrombocytopenia?

Thrombocytopenia occurs because of impaired production, increased destruction/consumption, or abnormal distribution of platelets, or a combination of these factors [1, 2].

Common causes of *impaired production* include bone marrow failure or suppression, recent chemotherapy, infection, nutritional deficiencies (B_{12} and folate), congenital conditions, myelodysplastic syndrome, and neoplastic bone marrow infiltration.

Increased destruction/consumption states include sepsis, autoimmune syndromes (e.g., systemic lupus erythematosus, sarcoid), drug-induced (e.g., quinine, NSAIDs), heparin-induced, immune mediated purpura, mechanical (mechanical heart valves or extracorporeal support devices), disseminated intravascular coagulation (DIC), and preeclampsia.

Sequestration/combination factors include chronic alcohol intake, liver disease, pulmonary emboli, portal hypertension, splenomegaly, and dilutional states.

Isolated thrombocytopenia in an asymptomatic patient with a normal blood smear in the absence of factors such as those listed above is usually ITP. It is a diagnosis of exclusion and can occur at any stage of life, including childhood.

Dysplastic causes are more common in older patients. Dysplasia is not always malignant but may proceed to malignancy. Bruising, petechia, and bleeding episodes in association with thrombocytopenia are concerning, as are symptoms of night sweats, fevers, and weight loss, which suggest a malignant cause. Any form of cancer may be associated with thrombocytopenia.

Thrombocytopenia may indicate the presence of HIV, hepatitis, or other still occult infection.

Drug-induced thrombocytopenia is relatively common [3]. Typically, this occurs within 1 week of drug initiation and will resolve within a week of stopping the implicated medication.

Drugs used in the perioperative period such as vancomycin and piperacillin are well-recognized triggers of drug-induced thrombocytopenia. Anesthetic agents have not been found to cause thrombocytopenia.

Heparin-induced thrombocytopenia (HIT) should always be considered in those who have recently been hospitalized or undergone invasive investigations. HIT occurs as a consequence of the development of antibodies to complexes of heparin and platelet factor 4 (PF4).

PF4 is a positively charged platelet protein released when platelets are activated. PF4 inhibits endothelial antithrombin, thereby promoting thrombosis.

Administered therapeutic heparin displaces PF4 from its endothelial binding sites and forms immunogenic PF4/heparin complexes. Development of HIT antibodies in response to heparin infusions is not uncommon (up to 50% of patients develop them following cardiopulmonary bypass) [4].

Only a small percentage of those exposed to heparin suffer the clinical features of HIT, thrombocytopenia, and thrombosis occurring in temporal association with heparin administration.

The thrombocytopenia usually occurs within 5–14 days after the provoking heparin dose. If heparin-PF4 antibodies are already present in the circulation (heparin exposure in the last 100 days in susceptible individuals), rapid-onset HIT can occur and thrombocytopenia may become apparent with 24 hours of the new provoking heparin dose.

Unfractionated heparin is more immunogenic than low molecular weight heparin.

Chronic alcohol intake is associated with thrombocytopenia, but platelet values are usually >50 × 10^9/L; with cessation, values rebound rapidly (within days).

Thrombocytopenia is a relatively early indicator of portal hypertension.

What Is the Usual Course of ITP?

ITP results from a combination of the development of antiplatelet antibodies, impaired megakaryocytopoiesis, and T-cell destruction of platelets [5]. Newly diagnosed ITP is treated with steroids. Prednisone 1 mg/kg for 2–4 weeks was the standard therapy, but recent studies suggest that high-dose dexamethasone pulse treatment may be a more effective approach [6]. Relapse is common despite steroid therapy, and in these circumstances rituximab and intravenous immune globulin (IVIg) are treatment options. Continued relapse calls for second-line therapy—it is in these circumstances that splenectomy is considered, as this procedure has a long-term complete restoration of normal platelet values of ~70%. An alternative option now available is chronic treatment with a thrombopoietin receptor agonist (TPO-RA). Romiplostim and eltrombopag are TPO-RAs currently approved by the US Food and Drug Administration (FDA) for management of chronic ITP. Studies are lacking on the efficacy and long-term effects of these agents [5].

Platelet Counts and Neuraxial Anesthesia—Is There a Consensus on What Are "Safe" Values?

A recent combined guideline from the Association of Anaesthetists of Great Britain & Ireland, The Obstetric Anaesthetists' Association, and Regional Anesthesia UK provides some nuanced suggestions about the management of neuraxial block in obstetric patients with low platelet counts arising as a consequence of pre-eclampsia and ITP [7]. On a continuum of risk ranging from normal through increased, high, and very high, their assessment is seen in Table 38.1.

A report from the Multicenter Perioperative Outcomes Group in the United States, using their national database from 14 major medical centers, assessed the risk of epidural hematoma in parturients undergoing neuraxial anesthesia and analgesia [8]. They identified 573 patients with a platelet count of <100 × 10⁹/L who had epidural or spinal anesthesia. The risk of hematoma was 11%, 3%, and 0.2% in those with counts ≤49 × 10⁹/L, 50–69 × 10⁹/L, and 70–100 × 10⁹/L, respectively. The authors caution that there are insufficient data to have confidence in the risk estimates for platelet counts <70 × 10⁹/L. The evidence on this topic is poor. It seems clear that the risk of hematoma development after lumbar puncture or neuraxial block in the thrombocytopenic patient is influenced by the underlying etiology of the thrombocytopenic state. Definitive guidance awaits further large population-based studies.

Table 38.1 Relative risks related to neuraxial blocks in obstetric patients with abnormalities of coagulation [7]. The risk is primarily related to spinal hematoma and cord compression

	Platelet count			
	Normal risk	Increased risk	High risk	Very high risk
Pre-eclampsia	100 × 10^9/L within 6 h of block	75–100 × 10^9/L Stable and normal coagulation tests	75–100 × 10^9/L Decreasing and normal coagulation tests	<75 × 10^9/L or HELLP syndrome or abnormal coagulation tests
ITP	>75 × 10^9/L within 24 hrs of block	50–75 × 10^9/L	20–50 × 10^9/L	<20 × 10^9/L

HELLP syndrome Hemolysis, elevated liver enzymes low platelet count

When Is Prophylactic Platelet Transfusion Prior to Surgery Appropriate in the Thrombocytopenic Patient?

There are no robust data to support the practice of prophylactic platelet transfusion except in the setting of acute leukemia [9]. There is emerging evidence that prophylactic platelet transfusions are of little value in reducing transfusion rates and bleeding complications prior to surgery or other invasive procedures [10, 11]. A reasonable approach would be to ensure platelets are readily available, if required, in patients with platelet counts ≤50 × 10⁹/L scheduled to undergo a major surgical procedure.

How Does the Platelet Count Relate to Bleeding Risk?

The platelet count is a relatively imprecise indicator of bleeding risk unless the count is very low. Recent data from a study of oncology patients receiving chemotherapy found that counts ≤5 × 10⁹/L were a hallmark of great hemorrhagic risk relative to those with counts ≥81 × 10⁹/L [12].

Patients with platelet counts >50 × 10⁹/L are usually asymptomatic. Those with counts ≤30 × 10⁹/L are susceptible to trauma-induced bleeding, while patients with counts <10 × 10⁹/L are at risk of "spontaneous" bleeding, may have petechiae, present with epistaxis or a major organ-related bleeding episode [13].

The patient underwent laparoscopic splenectomy without any complications 2 days after his preoperative assessment. Blood loss was minimal, and platelets were not transfused. Two months after surgery, his platelet count was 201 × 10⁹/L.

True/False Questions

1. Thrombocytopenia
   (a) is not present if the platelet count is ≤125 × 10⁹/L
   (b) is common in sepsis
   (c) can arise as a consequence of the use of NSAIDs

(d) is a relatively common finding in patients with alcohol use disorder
(e) may be an indicator of portal hypertension

2. ITP
   (a) occurs because of activation of platelet factor 4
   (b) is frequently associated with heparin administration
   (c) does not recur once successfully treated
   (d) can present as a medical emergency
   (e) splenectomy can be a very effective intervention

References

1. Bradbury C, Murray J. Investigating an incidental finding of thrombocytopenia. BMJ. 2013;346:f11.
2. Gauer RL, Braun MM. Thrombocytopenia. Am Fam Phisician. 2012;85(6):612–22.
3. George JN, Aster RH. Drug-induced thrombocytopenia: pathogenesis, evaluation, and management. Hematology Am Soc Hematol Educ Program. 2009:153-8. doi: 10.1182/asheducation-2009.1.153. PMID: 20008194; PMCID: PMC4413903. George JN, Aster RH. Drug-induced thrombocytopenia: pathogenesis, evaluation, and management. Hematology Am Soc Hematol Educ Program. 2009:153-8. doi: 10.1182/asheducation-2009.1.153. PMID: 20008194; PMCID: PMC4413903.
4. Arepally GM. Heparin-induced thrombocytopenia. Blood. 2017;129:2864–72.
5. Lambert MP, Gernsheimer TB. Clinical updates in adult immune thrombocytopenia. Blood. 2017;129(21):2829–35.
6. Wei Y, Ji XB, Wang YW, Wang JX, Yang EQ, Wang ZC, et al. High-dose dexamethasone vs prednisone for treatment of adult immune thrombocytopenia: a prospective multicenter randomized trial. Blood. 2016;127(3):296–303. quiz 370
7. Harrop-Griffiths W, Cook T, Gill H, Hill D, Ingram M, Makris M, et al. Regional anaesthesia and patients with abnormalities of coagulation: the Association of Anaesthetists of Great Britain & Ireland the Obstetric Anaesthetists' Association Regional Anaesthesia UK. Anaesthesia. 2013;68(9):966–72.
8. Lee LO, Bateman BT, Kheterpal S, Klumpner TT, Housey M, Aziz MF, Multicenter Perioperative Outcomes Group Investigators, et al. Risk of epidural hematoma after neuraxial techniques in thrombocytopenic parturients a report from the Multicenter Perioperative Outcomes Group. Anesthesiology. 2017;126(6):1053–64.
9. Blumberg N, Cholette JM, Schmidt AE, Phipps RP, Spinelli SL, Heal JM, et al. Management of platelet disorders and platelet transfusions in icu patients. Transfus Med Rev. 2017;31(4):252–7.
10. Warner MA, Jia Q, Clifford L, Wilson G, Brown MJ, Hanson AC, et al. Preoperative platelet transfusions and perioperative red blood cell requirements in patients with thrombocytopenia undergoing noncardiac surgery. Transfusion. 2016;56(3):682–90.
11. Warner MA, Woodrum D, Hanson A, Schroeder DR, Wilson G, Kor DJ. Preprocedural platelet transfusion for patients with thrombocytopenia undergoing interventional radiology procedures is not associated with reduced bleeding complications. Transfusion. 2017;57(4):890–8.
12. Uhl L, Assmann SF, Hamza TH, Harrison RW, Gernsheimer T, Slichter SJ. Laboratory predictors of bleeding and the effect of platelet and RBC transfusions on bleeding outcomes in the PLADO trial. Blood. 2017;130(1):1247–58.
13. Ho-Tin-Noé B, Jadoui S. Spontaneous bleeding in thrombocytopenia: is it really spontaneous? Transfus Clin Biol. 2018;25(3):210–6.

Long-Term Anticoagulation

39

Derek Dillane

A 76-year-old female patient presented for preoperative optimization prior to repeat right parietal craniotomy for resection of a glioblastoma. A right-sided temporoparietal tumor had initially been resected 3 years prior to this visit. She developed a right lower limb deep venous thrombosis (DVT) on two occasions after previous operative procedures and subsequently was on long-term anticoagulation with warfarin. She had a background history of hypertension. Additionally, she had postsurgical spine syndrome having previously undergone a lumbar microdiscectomy and L1–5 vertebroplasties on separate occasions.
Medications: Lorazepam, hydromorphone 3 mg q 3 hours, fentanyl patch 100 mcg/h, warfarin 3 mg OD (INR target range 2.0–3.0), valsartan, furosemide, diclofenac/misoprostol, nortriptyline, and denosumab.
Physical examination was normal.
Laboratory investigations did not reveal any abnormalities apart from an INR of 3.5.

What Potential Complications Is the Patient with a History of Venous Thromboembolism (VTE) Subject to in the Perioperative Period?

Depending on whether long-term anticoagulation is temporarily held over the perioperative period or continued, the main risks relate to VTE and bleeding. The likelihood of either occurrence must be evaluated for each patient and surgical procedure. On the basis of this evaluation, anticoagulation will be continued or held. If held, a further decision is required regarding the implementation of bridging therapy and timing of re-introduction of long-term anticoagulation after surgery.

D. Dillane (✉)
Department of Anesthesiology & Pain Medicine, University of Alberta, Edmonton, AB, Canada

What Are the Main Risk Factors for Development of Perioperative Thromboembolism?

The three principal predisposing factors are atrial fibrillation, presence of a mechanical heart valve, and previous VTE. In the United States, over six million patients with one or more of these conditions take long-term thromboprophylaxis [1, 2]. Other predisposing factors for which patients may be on long-term anticoagulation therapy include hereditary thrombophilia (e.g., protein C and protein S deficiency) and certain specific causes of cerebrovascular and peripheral arterial disease.

How Is the Thromboembolic Risk Associated with Atrial Fibrillation Estimated?

This is determined by whether or not the atrial fibrillation (AF) is valvular in nature.

Valvular AF refers to patients in AF with moderate to severe mitral stenosis or a mechanical mitral valve prosthesis [3]. The further increase in risk of VTE (in addition to that arising from AF) in the patient with mitral stenosis or a mechanical heart valve results from conditions of low flow in the left atrium in the case of mitral stenosis and the thrombophilic properties of mechanical heart valves [4].

Valvular AF is considered an indication for long-term anticoagulation with warfarin. Patients with moderate to severe mitral stenosis and AF have been largely excluded from randomized controlled trials on the efficacy and safety of direct oral anticoagulants (DOACs) for long-term anticoagulation. Subsequently, there is insufficient evidence at this time to treat these patients with DOACs [3]. DOACs are contraindicated in patients with mechanical heart valves. This recommendation is based on the observed increase in ischemic stroke rate and bleeding complications in patients receiving dabigatran compared with warfarin in the RE-ALIGN trial [5].

D. Dillane, B. A. Finegan (eds.), *Preoperative Assessment*, https://doi.org/10.1007/978-3-030-58842-7_39

Non-valvular AF, the most common medical indication for chronic anticoagulation, occurs in the absence of moderate to severe mitral stenosis or a mechanical heart valve [3]. Non-valvular AF can occur in the presence of other valvular disorders (e.g., mitral regurgitation, aortic stenosis).

Thromboembolic risk for the non-valvular AF patient is calculated using the CHA_2DS_2-Vasc score [6]. A CHA_2DS_2-Vasc score of 2 or more in men and 3 or more in women requires oral anticoagulation.

What Factors Determine Thromboembolic Risk in Patients with a Mechanical Heart Valve?

The American College of Chest Physicians (ACCP) stratifies risk for perioperative thromboembolism according to the type and location of mechanical heart valve [7–9]. The presence of other cardiac risk factors must also be taken into consideration (e.g., atrial fibrillation, previous transient ischemic attack or stroke, hypertension, cardiac failure, and diabetes [10]). Patients with a bileaflet aortic valve prosthesis without previous stroke or atrial fibrillation have the lowest annual thromboembolic risk (<4%). Patients with a mitral valve prosthesis, or stroke or transient ischemic attack (TIA) within 3 months of surgery have the highest risk (>10%) (Table 39.1) [7, 8].

Table 39.1 Risk stratification for perioperative thromboembolism in patients with a mechanical heart valve or history of VTE

Risk category	Mechanical heart valve	VTE
High (>10%/year risk of ATE or >10%/month risk of VTE)	Any mechanical mitral valve Caged ball or tilting disc valve in mitral/aortic position Recent (<3 months) stroke or TIA	Recent (within 3 months) VTE Severe thrombophilia, e.g., protein C deficiency, protein S deficiency, antithrombin deficiency, antiphospholipid antibodies
Moderate (4–10%/year risk of ATE or 4–10%/month risk of VTE)	Bileaflet AVR with major risk factors for stroke[a]	VTE within past 3–12 months Recurrent VTE Nonsevere thrombophilia, e.g., heterozygous factor V Leiden Active cancer or recent history of cancer
Low (<4%/year risk of ATE or <2%/month risk of VTE)	Bileaflet AVR without major risk factors for stroke[a]	VTE more than 12 months ago

Adapted from American College of Chest Physicians suggested risk stratification for patient-specific periprocedural thromboembolism [7] (From Spyropoulos et al. [8], with permission John Wiley & Sons © 2019 International Society on Thrombosis and Haemostasis)

ATE Arterial thromboembolism, *TIA* Transient ischemic attack

[a]Atrial fibrillation, prior stroke or transient ischemic attack, hypertension, diabetes, congestive heart failure, age > 75 years

Do Patients with a Nonmechanical or Bioprosthetic Valve Require Chronic Anticoagulation?

Patients with tissue/bioprosthetic valves do not require long-term anticoagulation for the valve itself, as the risk of thrombosis or thromboembolism is low (0.2% per year) [11]. It is common for patients who have recently had a bioprosthetic valve implanted to be on short-term anticoagulation with warfarin for 3–6 months until the sewing ring has endothelialized. Long-term aspirin therapy is commonly prescribed for patients with a bioprosthetic valve [10]. Elective surgery should be postponed, if possible, for 3–6 months after bioprosthetic valve implantation [9]. If surgery must proceed, warfarin can be stopped without bridging and reinstituted postoperatively when the risk of bleeding has abated [9, 10].

How Is the Risk of Recurrent Venous Thromboembolism Estimated in Patients with a History of Prior VTE?

This risk can be stratified into high, moderate, and low categories. It is largely dependent on how recent the thromboembolic event is, in addition to the presence of other predisposing factors such as inherited thrombophilia, malignancy, or chronic heart failure (see Table 39.1) [7, 8]. Risk of recurrent VTE is clearly highest within the first 3 months of the index event. Therefore, surgery should be delayed, if possible, until after this 3-month period.

For What Period of Time Is Long-Term Anticoagulation Required in a Patient Who Has Had a VTE?

Patients diagnosed with VTE receive long-term anticoagulation for a minimum of 3 months. Beyond this, a decision is made according to the patient's specific risk factors, i.e., was the VTE provoked or unprovoked? Were risk factors transient or long term? Extending long-term anticoagulation beyond 3 months to as long as 6 or 12 months is not routinely considered other than in the presence of a persistent risk factor. Therefore, it is unusual for a patient with a remote history of VTE to be on long-term anticoagulation.

Which Patient Populations May Benefit from Indefinite Anticoagulation After VTE?

The decision to institute indefinite long-term anticoagulation is based on the risk of recurrence of VTE versus anticoagulation-related bleeding events. Consent of a fully informed patient is essential given the lifestyle choice inherent in such therapy. Indefinite anticoagulation is considered in patients with unprovoked proximal DVT, symptomatic pulmonary embolus, recurrent unprovoked DVT, or active malignancy. For patients with an inherited thrombophilia, the decision to continue with long-term thromboprophylaxis is frequently based on whether the DVT was provoked.

What Are the First-Line Agents for Long-Term Anticoagulation after VTE?

In the absence of severe renal insufficiency, factor Xa inhibitors (e.g., apixaban, rivaroxaban) and direct thrombin inhibitors (e.g., dabigatran) are the first-choice oral anticoagulant agents. As these newer oral agents are renally excreted, they are avoided in severe renal insufficiency, whereby warfarin becomes the agent of choice. For patients with mild to moderate renal impairment, i.e., creatinine clearance ≥30 ml/minute, dose adjustments are necessary.

How Is the Risk of Procedural Bleeding Estimated?

The risk of bleeding is calculated for each individual case based on surgical invasiveness, consequences of bleeding, patient comorbidities and medical history, antithrombotic medications, previous individual or family history of postoperative bleeding, individual anatomy and pathology, in addition to the experience of the surgical team. Several tools have been developed to estimate bleeding risk in anticoagulated AF patients [12]. The HAS-BLED score (hypertension, abnormal hepatic and renal function, stroke, bleeding tendency, labile INR, age ≥ 65 years, concomitant use of antiplatelet agents, and excess alcohol use) is an example which is relatively easy to use and provides a 1-year risk of major bleeding [13].

Which Patients Are Considered Candidates for Perioperative Bridging?

Bridging with heparin is considered in patients who have a high perioperative risk of VTE if anticoagulation is discontinued. This serves to minimize the risk of VTE associated with discontinuation of long-term anticoagulation and bleeding associated with continuing it. It is generally reserved for patients on long-term anticoagulation with warfarin. The rapid onset of action and predictable half-lives of factor Xa inhibitors and direct thrombin inhibitors usually precludes the routine use of perioperative bridging therapy.

Table 39.2 Summary of recommended perioperative anticoagulation management strategies

Category	High bleeding risk procedure	Low bleeding risk procedure
High thromboembolic risk		
Warfarin	Give last dose 6 days before operation, bridge with LMWH or UFH, resume 24 h postoperatively	Give last dose 6 d before operation, bridge with LMWH or UFH, resume 24 h postoperatively
DOAC	Give last dose 3 days before operation,[a] resume 2 to 3 days postoperatively	Give last dose 2 days before operation,[a] resume 24 h postoperatively
Intermediate thromboembolic risk		
Warfarin	Give last dose 6 days before operation, determine need for bridging by clinician judgment and current evidence, resume 24 h postoperatively	Give last dose 6 days before operation, determine need for bridging by clinician judgment and current evidence, resume 24 h postoperatively
DOAC	Give last dose 3 days before operation,[a] resume 2 to 3 days postoperatively	Give last dose 2 days before operation,[a] resume 24 h postoperatively
Low thromboembolic risk		
Warfarin	Give last dose 6 days before operation, bridging not recommended, resume 24 h postoperatively	Give last dose 6 days before operation, bridging not recommended, resume 24 h postoperatively
DOAC	Give last dose 3 days before operation,[a] resume 2 to 3 days postoperatively	Give last dose 2 days before operation,[a] resume 24 h postoperatively

From Hornor et al. [9] with permission

DOAC direct oral anticoagulant, *LMWH* low-molecular-weight heparin, *UFH* unfractionated heparin

[a]In patients with CrCl<50 mL/min on dabigatran, the last dose should be given 3 days before the procedure for low bleeding surgery, and 4 to 5 days before the procedure for high bleeding risk operation

Describe the Common Approaches to Perioperative Anticoagulation Management in the Presence of Varying Thromboembolic and Bleeding Risks?

A comprehensive overview of the most commonly used approaches is outlined in Table 39.2 [9].

What Are the Indications for Placement of a Temporary Vena Cava Filter?

Temporary vena cava filter placement may be indicated for patients with a recent VTE, i.e., in the past month, who require interruption of anticoagulation for an urgent surgical procedure. In general, use of vena cava filters is recommended only when surgery cannot be postponed [2]. Other indications for IVC filter placement include anticoagulation failure, hemodynamic instability, mobile thrombus, and iliocaval DVT [14]. IVC filter use is not without complication, e.g., IVC thrombosis has been associated with their use [15].

Even though there was no evidence of recurrent VTE in the history of the patient presented here, the persistent nature of the malignancy was deemed to be of sufficient risk to warrant indefinite anticoagulation. There was no definite strong indication for utilization of warfarin for long-term anticoagulation other than physician preference.

The surgery was stratified as high risk for bleeding and the patient was guided to discontinue warfarin therapy 6 days before surgery. The patient was deemed to be high risk for perioperative VTE based on her history of recurrent DVT and active cancer. The perioperative team elected not to bridge this patient due to concerns regarding the timing of resumption of bridging postoperatively. Rather, she had a temporary IVC filter placed when warfarin was stopped preoperatively. Deployment of an IVC filter in this case may appear incongruent in light of published recommendations. However, the risk of perioperative recurrence of VTE was judged to be high enough for the period of disruption of anticoagulation to warrant its temporary use.

True/False Questions

1. (a) Non-valvular atrial fibrillation is the commonest indication for long-term thromboprophylaxis.
   (b) Non-valvular atrial fibrillation can occur in the presence of aortic stenosis.
   (c) Thromboembolic risk for the non-valvular AF patient is calculated using the CHA_2DS_2-VASc score.
   (d) Patients with bioprosthetic valves require long-term anticoagulation.
   (e) Patients with a mechanical mitral valve prosthesis have an annual risk of thromboembolism of over 10%.
2. (a) Elective surgery should be delayed for at least 3 months after occurrence of VTE.
   (b) Occurrence of VTE more than 1 year prior to surgery has a low annual risk (<5%) of VTE recurrence.
   (c) Long-term anticoagulation for at least 1 year is required in most patients who have had a VTE.
   (d) Factor Xa inhibitors are ideal agents in patients with renal failure.
   (e) Temporary vena cava filter is recommended in all major surgery patients who have had a VTE in the past 6 months.

References

1. Roger VL, Go AS, Lloyd-Jones DM, Benjamin EJ, Berry JD, Borden WB, et al. Heart disease and stroke statistics–2012 update: a report from the American Heart Association. Circulation. 2012;125(1):e2–e220.
2. Baron TH, Kamath PS, McBane RD. Management of antithrombotic therapy in patients undergoing invasive procedures. N Engl J Med. 2013;368(22):2113–24.
3. January CT, Wann LS, Calkins H, Chen LY, Cigarroa JE, Cleveland JC Jr, et al. 2019 AHA/ACC/HRS focused update of the 2014 AHA/ACC/HRS guideline for the Management of Patients with Atrial Fibrillation: a report of the American College of Cardiology/American Heart Association task force on clinical practice guidelines and the Heart Rhythm Society. J Am Coll Cardiol. 2019;74(1):104–32. Erratum in: J Am Coll Cardiol. 2019;74(4):599
4. Fauchier L, Philippart R, Clementy N, Bourguignon T, Angoulvant D, Ivanes F, et al. How to define valvular atrial fibrillation? Arch Cardiovasc Dis. 2015;108(10):530–9.
5. Eikelboom JW, Connolly SJ, Brueckmann M, Granger CB, Kappetein AP, Mack MJ, et al. Dabigatran versus warfarin in patients with mechanical heart valves. N Engl J Med. 2013;369(13):1206–14.
6. Lip GY, Nieuwlaat R, Pisters R, Lane DA, Crijns HJ. Refining clinical risk stratification for predicting stroke and thromboembolism in atrial fibrillation using a novel risk factor-based approach: the euro heart survey on atrial fibrillation. Chest. 2010;137(2):263–72.
7. Douketis JD, Spyropoulos AC, Spencer FA, Mayr M, Jaffer AK, Eckman MH, et al. Perioperative management of antithrombotic therapy: antithrombotic therapy and prevention of thrombosis, 9th ed: American College of Chest Physicians Evidence-Based Clinical Practice Guidelines. Chest. 2012;141(2 Suppl):e326S–e50S.
8. Spyropoulos AC, Brohi K, Caprini J, Samama CM, Siegal D, Tafur A, et al. Scientific and standardization committee communication: guidance document on the periprocedural management of patients on chronic oral anticoagulant therapy: recommendations for standardized reporting of procedural/surgical bleed risk and patient-specific thromboembolic risk. J Thromb Haemost. 2019;17(11):1966–72.
9. Hornor MA, Duane TM, Ehlers AP, Jensen EH, Brown PS Jr, Pohl D, et al. American College of Surgeons' guidelines for the perioperative management of antithrombotic medication. J Am Coll Surg. 2018;227(5):521–36 e1. https://doi.org/10.1016/j.jamcollsurg.2018.08.183.
10. Whitlock RP, Sun JC, Fremes SE, Rubens FD, Teoh KH. Antithrombotic and thrombolytic therapy for valvular disease: antithrombotic therapy and prevention of thrombosis, 9th ed: American College of Chest Physicians Evidence-Based Clinical Practice Guidelines. Chest. 2012;141(2 Suppl):e576S–600S.
11. Thrombosis Canada. Mechanical and bioprosthetic heart valves: Anticoagulant Therapy 2017. Available from: http://thrombosiscanada.ca/wp-content/uploads/2017/01/35.-Mechanical-and-Bioprosthetic-Heart-Valves-2017Jan22-FINAL.pdf.
12. Apostolakis S, Lane DA, Guo Y, Buller H, Lip GY. Performance of the HEMORR(2)HAGES, ATRIA, and HAS-BLED bleeding risk-prediction scores in patients with atrial fibrillation undergoing anticoagulation: the AMADEUS (evaluating the use of SR34006

compared to warfarin or acenocoumarol in patients with atrial fibrillation) study. J Am Coll Cardiol. 2012;60(9):861–7.
13. Lip GY. Implications of the CHA(2)DS(2)-VASc and HAS-BLED scores for thromboprophylaxis in atrial fibrillation. Am J Med. 2011;124(2):111–4.
14. Weinberg I. Appropriate use of inferior vena cava filters 31 Oct 2016. American College of Cardiology Expert Analysis. Available from: https://www.acc.org/latest-in-cardiology/articles/2016/10/31/09/28/appropriate-use-of-inferior-vena-cava-filters?w_nav=TI.
15. Weinberg I, Abtahian F, Debiasi R, Cefalo P, Mackay C, Hawkins BM, et al. Effect of delayed inferior vena cava filter retrieval after early initiation of anticoagulation. Am J Cardiol. 2014;113(2):389–94.

Venous Thromboembolic Disease

40

Barry A. Finegan

A 22-year-old man scheduled to undergo bladder augmentation for management of urinary incontinence secondary to neurogenic bladder presented in the preoperative assessment clinic 2 weeks prior to the proposed surgery. His aunt was in attendance. He was born with a meningomyelocele and was largely confined to a wheelchair due to lower limb spasticity. He had undergone multiple surgical procedures as a child and young adult without incident. He had a history of latex allergy.

His last operative procedure was a cystoscopy under general anesthesia performed 6 months previously. When questioned as to how this surgery had proceeded, he indicated that there were no issues with the surgery itself, but that 2 weeks after the operation he had developed pain and swelling in his left leg. He visited the local emergency room and was given a diagnosis of cellulitis and treated with antibiotics. A referral was made to an infectious disease (ID) specialist. The ID specialist ordered a duplex ultrasound as he suspected the patient was suffering from a deep venous thrombosis (DVT) in view of his family history (mother died suddenly of a pulmonary embolus), the presence of provoking factors prior to the event and the findings on examination. The ultrasound revealed a DVT in the left common femoral and popliteal veins. Rivaroxaban therapy was initiated. Subsequent investigation revealed that the patient was homozygous for Factor V Leiden. The calf pain and swelling resolved with time.

Physical examination during preoperative assessment was unremarkable apart from the obvious signs of bilateral lower limb weakness and spasticity. There was no evidence of leg edema or erythema.

The patient was still being treated with rivaroxaban at the time of the clinic visit. Routine laboratory values were within normal limits, his PT was at the upper limit of normal.

The patient requested guidance on his rivaroxaban therapy perioperatively and inquired as to whether he should continue it in the future.

What Is a Deep Venous Thrombosis (DVT)?

A DVT occurs when a clot forms in a deep vein. DVTs most commonly occur in the deep veins of the lower limb (especially in the calf veins) but can also occur in deep veins of the upper limb and viscera. The pathophysiology of a DVT involves hemodynamic alterations (stasis/decreased venous flow), endothelial injury/dysfunction, and hypercoagulability. A DVT is one of a range of venous thromboembolic (VTE) diseases from superficial thrombophlebitis to pulmonary embolus.

What Are the Symptoms/Signs of a DVT and How Is It Diagnosed?

DVTs are frequently asymptomatic and the classic symptom of lower limb pain associated with signs of leg edema and erythema are non-specific and may be associated with multiple other conditions [1].

Early diagnosis and treatment of a DVT is essential to avoid the complications of pulmonary embolism, post-thrombotic syndrome, recurrent DVT, and death.

The mainstay of diagnosis of DVT in outpatients is to initially use the validated clinical prediction rule – the Wells score (Table 40.1) [2].

Thereafter, those with "High Probability" should proceed directly to imaging, usually duplex ultrasound of the limb, to determine if a DVT is present. In the "Moderate and Low Probability" groups, high sensitivity D-dimer testing is indicated. A normal value for D-dimer is reassuring and the diagnosis of a DVT is very unlikely. An abnormal D-dimer value in those with a "Moderate/Low Probability" score is an indication for diagnostic imaging. Caution should be exercised

B. A. Finegan (✉)
Department of Anesthesiology & Pain Medicine, University of Alberta, Edmonton, AB, Canada
e-mail: bfinegan@ualberta.ca

D. Dillane, B. A. Finegan (eds.), *Preoperative Assessment*, https://doi.org/10.1007/978-3-030-58842-7_40

Table 40.1 Wells clinical criteria for probability of DVT [2]

Clinical variable	Score
Active cancer—Treatment ongoing or within previous 6 months or in palliative state	1
Paralysis, paresis, or recent plaster immobilization of the lower extremities	1
Recently bedridden for 3 days or more, or major surgery within the previous 12 weeks requiring general or regional anesthesia	1
Entire leg swelling	1
Calf swelling at least 3 cm larger than that on the asymptomatic leg (measured 10 cm below the tibial tuberosity)[a]	1
Pitting edema confined to the symptomatic leg	1
Collateral superficial veins (non-varicose)	1
Previously documented DVT	1
Alternative diagnosis at least as likely as DVT	−2

Scoring: ≥3 High Probability; 1–2 Moderate Probability, and if 0 or <0 Low Probability

[a]If symptoms in both legs, use the more symptomatic leg

in interpreting D-dimer values in the elderly, those with cancer and hospitalized patients as false positive results may be seen in these groups.

In hospitalized patients where a DVT is suspected, diagnostic imaging is the appropriate initial investigation.

As noted from the foregoing our patient should have, at the time of his initial presentation to the emergency room, undergone clinical predictive scoring and D-dimer measurement or diagnostic imaging thereafter as appropriate.

What Is the Incidence of Venous Thrombosis?

The incidence of DVT in young individuals is very low (<1/10,000 persons/year) but rises markedly with age (>4/1000 persons/year in those over 75 years).

What Are the Risk Factors for a DVT?

A thromboembolic event, such as a DVT, can be considered provoked or unprovoked by risk factors [3].

A provoking event can be transient or persistent.

Examples of *provoking transient major* risk factors for a DVT include any of the following occurring within 3 months of diagnosis of a DVT: surgery under general anesthesia greater than 30 minutes in duration, being confined to bed for at least 3 days duration, or undergoing a Caesarean section.

Examples of *provoking transient minor* risk factors for a DVT include estrogen therapy, surgery with general anesthesia <30 minutes in duration, being pregnant, prolonged air travel, and having a leg injury with reduced mobility for at least 3 days.

Provoking persistent risks factors for a DVT include active cancer, hereditary thrombophilia, advanced age, and ongoing inflammatory bowel disease. VTE events (including DVT) and bleeding associated with the treatment/prophylaxis of same are thought to be the second most common cause of death in cancer patients. The cumulative incidence of diagnosed VTE events in patients with malignancy ranges from 1% to 8% depending on the stage and type of cancer [4].

In general, patients whose DVT is associated with a provoking transient risk factor are less likely to suffer recurrence of a DVT, whereas those with a persistent provoking factor, particularly active cancer, are at much greater risk of recurrence of a VTE event.

Furthermore, those with persistent risk factors who are then exposed to a transient risk factor (major or minor) are at higher risk of an initial or recurrent thromboembolic event than those without persistent risk factors.

What Are the Clinical Characteristics Suggestive of Thrombophilia During a Thromboembolic Episode?

The following scenarios are suggestive of inherited thrombophilia: Thromboembolic event in the presence of minor provoking factors in an individual <50 years of age, an event in a first-degree family member at a young age, multiple events at a young age, and/or at unusual sites (visceral veins) [5].

What Is the Most Common Inherited Thrombophilia Disorder?

Factor V Leiden mutation is the most prevalent inherited thrombophilia. The heterozygous condition is present in ~5% of Caucasians overall but is especially prevalent among those of Northern European extraction (10–15%). Hispanic, African American, and Asian individuals have a lower prevalence. Homozygous Factor V Leiden is present in about 1:5000 of the North American/European Caucasian population.

How Does Factor V Leiden Alter Coagulation?

Under normal circumstances, when Protein C is activated after binding with thrombin (Activated Protein C) it proteolytically inactivates Factor Va and Factor VIIIa thereby downregulating the coagulation cascade. Factor V Leiden is resistant to the effect of Activated Protein C. Those with the heterozygous Factor V Leiden mutation have an up to fivefold increased risk of venous thromboembolism, while those with the homozygous mutation have up to an 80-fold higher risk that those without the mutation [6].

If One Suspects a Patient May Have Inherited Thrombophilia, What Is the Best Course of Action to Follow?

Testing for thrombophilia is relatively common in North America but is fraught with issues related to when and whom to screen, which assays to use, and how to deal with the consequences of test results [7]. Referral to a hematologist with expertise in inherited coagulation disorders is indicated.

How Long Should a Direct Oral Anticoagulant (DOAC) Be Taken for Following an Isolated Provoked Transient Thromboembolic Event?

Current guidelines suggest that if a patient has been prescribed a DOAC following a diagnosis of a first-time DVT that has occurred after a provoking transient event, the therapy should be continued for at least 3 months [3].

In this case, where the patient has an underlying provoking persistent risk factor, there is lack of clarity about long-term management. A discussion of the risk-benefits of long-term prophylactic anticoagulant management is best left to a hematologist with experience in inherited coagulation disorders.

How Should This patient's DOAC Be Managed During the Perioperative Period?

The suggested approach for every patient on a DOAC is to: (1) estimate risk of thromboembolism, (2) estimate the risk of bleeding, (3) determine the time of DOAC interruption, and (4) decide if bridging is indicated.

In this case, the risk of both thromboembolism and bleeding during the surgery was considered moderate. The drug was interrupted for a period of 48 hours prior to the procedure and resumed 48 hours after the procedure The patient was referred to a hematologist after the procedure. The hematologist discussed with the patient the pros and cons of lifetime treatment with DOACs in view of his provoking persistent risk factors. The decision of the patient was not to take long-term prophylactic DOAC treatment.

True/False Questions

1. In the case of a DVT
   (a) Calf tenderness, swelling, and erythema are diagnostic.
   (b) Asymptomatic cases are rare.
   (c) Duplex ultrasound is appropriate if estimated risk is moderate to high.
   (d) An elevated D-dimer level is diagnostic particularly in older patients.
   (e) Using a clinical predictive score, such as the Wells, can be very helpful.
2. Factor V Leiden is an inherited disorder of coagulation:
   (a) That results in increased risk of hemorrhage during surgery.
   (b) Can be treated successfully by a platelet transfusion prior to major surgery.
   (c) Alters the responsiveness of Factor V to the modulating influence of Activated Protein C
   (d) That is the most common cause of a VTE event.
   (e) Which when present in a heterozygous manner, carries no elevated risk of VTE.

References

1. Olaf M, Cooney R. Deep venous thrombosis. Emer Med Clin North Am. 2017:35(4):743–70.
2. Wells PS, Owen C, Doucette S, Fergusson D, Tran H. Does this patient have deep vein thrombosis? JAMA. 2006;295(2):199–207.
3. Kearon C, Ageno W, Cannegieter SC, Cosmi B, Geersing GJ, Kyrle PA, Subcommittees on Control of Anticoagulation, and Predictive and Diagnostic Variables in Thrombotic Disease. Categorization of patients as having provoked or unprovoked venous thromboembolism: guidance from the SSC of ISTH. J Thromb Haemost. 2016;14(7):1480–3.
4. Frere C, Farge D. Clinical practice guidelines for prophylaxis of venous thomboembolism in cancer patients. Thromb Haemost. 2016;116(4):618–25.
5. Connors JM. Thrombophilia testing and venous thrombosis. New Engl J Med. 2017;377(12):1177–87.
6. Favaloro EJ, McDonald D. Futility of testing for factor V Leiden. Blood Transfus. 2012;10(3):260–3.
7. Favaloro EJ, McDonald D, Lippi G. Laboratory investigation of thrombophilia: the good, the bad, and the ugly. Semin Thromb Hemost. 2009;35(7):695–710.

Anemia

41

Barry A. Finegan

A 28-year-old male presented for assessment prior to repair of an abdominal incisional hernia. Two years previously, he had a left hepatic lobectomy for suspected hepatic adenoma, which was thought to be related to prior anabolic steroid abuse. He was also noted to have mild gastroesophageal reflux disease, insomnia, a mildly decreased Duke Activity Status index for an individual his age, and mild fatigue on exertion. He admitted to occasional cocaine and daily cannabis use.

Medications: Temazepam and pantoprazole.

Physical Examination: Vital signs were stable with no evidence of cardio-respiratory decompensation.

Investigations: Review of his laboratory data from 6 months previously revealed hemoglobin (Hb) of 92 g/L and a mean corpuscular volume (MCV) of 61 fL. His liver enzymes and creatinine were within normal limits. MRI of his abdomen was scheduled on the day he was seen in the preoperative clinic. A STAT complete blood count (CBC), a peripheral blood smear (PBS), and ferritin were ordered.

The CBC and PBS data were as follows:

Hb 93 g/L; MCV 65 fL; mean cell hemoglobin concentration 220 g/L; red cell distribution width 23.7%; platelet count 711 × 10^9/L; and white blood cell count 11.4 × 10^9/L. The PBS demonstrated an increase in polychromasia and thrombocytosis.

A ferritin, iron level, and total iron binding capacity (TIBC) were ordered: ferritin 3 ug/L (normal 12–300), iron 7 umol/L (normal 8–30), and TIBC 62 umol/L (normal 40–80).

Further questioning revealed a diet with apparently adequate iron intake and no history suggestive of active bleeding. The patient was diagnosed with iron deficiency anemia (IDA). The surgery was postponed so that iron treatment could be initiated, and the results of the pending MRI obtained and reviewed.

The MRI demonstrated the presence of 12 hepatic lesions of varying sizes situated throughout the residual hepatic lobe. The largest was a subcapsular lesion situated high within liver segment VIII, which measured up to 6.2 cm in diameter. Several smaller lesions had considerably increased in size since the last MRI, 11 months previously. Contrast enhancement with gadolinium demonstrated homogenous avid arterial enhancement. The spleen was noted to be mildly enlarged. No other pathology was noted. The lesions were felt to be consistent with hepatic adenomas and, given the expanding nature of the lesions, gave considerable cause for concern.

What Is Anemia?

Anemia is a reduction from "normal" in the absolute number of red blood cells (RBCs). In clinical practice, anemia is diagnosed based on Hb or hematocrit (HCT) values that are below "normal." There are controversies about what exactly constitutes "normal" values, as Hb and HCT values can be influenced by many factors, including, but not limited to, altitude of domicile, smoking status, hydration, race, age, gender, pregnancy, and disease state. Using the World Health Organization (WHO) criteria for anemia offers a simple, if imperfect, guide for the practitioner [1]. After due consideration of the context of the reported value, entertaining the diagnosis of anemia is appropriate where the Hb values are as follows: <130 g/L in adult male, <120 g/L in adult females and <110 g/L in pregnant females.

What Is the Prevalence of Anemia Prior to Elective Surgery and Is It Associated with Adverse Outcome?

Preoperative anemia is a marker for increased morbidity and mortality in elective cardiac and non-cardiac surgery. An analysis of 3500 consecutive patients undergoing cardiac

B. A. Finegan (✉)
Department of Anesthesiology & Pain Medicine, University of Alberta, Edmonton, AB, Canada

D. Dillane, B. A. Finegan (eds.), *Preoperative Assessment*, https://doi.org/10.1007/978-3-030-58842-7_41

surgery found an overall prevalence of preoperative anemia of 26% (defined as Hb < 125 g/L) [2]. After exclusion of those with Hg < 95 g/L, patients with renal failure and those undergoing emergency surgery, risk-adjusted odds of a severe adverse outcome (composite of in-hospital death, stroke, or acute kidney injury) doubled in those with preoperative anemia. Anemia is present in up to 30% of patients presenting for major elective non-cardiac surgery requiring an overnight stay in hospital [3]. The analysis of the American College of Surgeons National Surgical Quality Improvement Program (NSQIP) data of over 225,000 patients presenting for non-cardiac surgery found that anemia (defined using WHO criteria) was present preoperatively in 30.4%, and even mild anemia was independently associated with an increased risk of 30-day morbidity and mortality.

What Is the Major Cause of Preoperative Anemia in Adults?

Iron deficiency anemia is estimated to affect 20% of the world's population, especially children and young women in low-income countries in Central and West Africa and South Asia where poor nutrition, cereal-based diets, and helminthic infection are key ethological factors [4]. In high-income countries, IDA is the most common form of anemia observed in patients presenting for surgery especially among the elderly [5]. Functional iron deficiency (FID), on the other hand, is a condition where there is insufficient iron incorporated into erythroid precursors despite the apparently adequate body iron stores. FID is the predominant mechanism of anemia in cancer patients where enhanced hepatic hepcidin production is frequently noted. Hepcidin is a hormone that inhibits iron absorption in the small intestine and the release of recycled iron from macrophages, thereby causing iron-restricted erythropoiesis and anemia.

Why Are FID/IDA So Common in Surgical Patients?

Daily iron requirements are approximately 25 mg/day, and up to 95% of this comes from recycling of heme iron by macrophage phagocytosis of senescent RBCs. Excess iron is toxic; consequently, nutritional iron absorption is tightly controlled, being limited to about 1–2 mg/day. This amount is equivalent to daily physiological losses due to normal GI tract cell turnover. It is not surprising, therefore, that any perturbation of iron homeostasis can result in deficiency and the potential for anemia.

In high-income countries, FID arises primarily because of dietary choices, malabsorption states, blood loss through menorrhagia, and gastrointestinal or urinary tract lesions. Specifically, drug-induced neutralization of gastric pH by proton pump inhibitors and/or H_2–receptor blockers can significantly reduce iron uptake and result in iron deficiency ± anemia [6]. This arises as plant-sourced iron is predominantly in the ferric form. Iron absorption occurs predominantly in the duodenum and proximal jejunum. Gastric acid lowers pH in the proximal duodenum, thereby enhancing the solubility and uptake of ferric iron. Any mechanism that impairs gastric acid production will reduce iron absorption. For similar reasons, patients who have undergone bariatric procedures are at particular risk if they have undergone *roux-en-Y* procedures, and more than 50% of this population have iron deficiency on follow-up [7].

What Other Types of Anemia Are Relatively Common in the Surgical Population?

Anemia of inflammation (AI), also known as anemia of chronic disease, is the most common form of anemia other than IDA observed in the surgical population. In AI, iron stores may be normal or increased. Almost any chronic condition can be associated with AI, including obesity; cancer; autoimmune conditions; infections; and chronic lung, heart, and kidney disease [8]. In AI:

1. Iron availability is restricted by inflammatory-mediated decreases in iron absorption across the duodenum and pathological retention of iron in macrophages, the key cellular element involved in the efficient recycling of iron from senescent erythrocytes.
2. Erythropoietin production/activity is reduced.
3. Erythrocyte survival is impaired by increased erythrocyte phagocytosis by macrophages and hemolysis.

B_{12} and folate deficiency anemia, manifest by a macrocytic profile, may arise as a consequence of drug use—for example proton pump inhibitors inhibit B_{12} and iron absorption; prolonged use is associated with anemia [6].

Myelodysplastic syndromes may manifest as anemia—a peripheral blood smear is very helpful in confirming this diagnosis.

The abovementioned conditions involve decreased RBC production, but perioperative anemia may arise because of increased hemolysis/destruction of RBCs or occult or overt blood loss.

What Can Be Deduced from Review of Values Shown on a CBC?

The CBC is an excellent diagnostic tool in the investigation of anemia. Tefferi et al. [9] outline a simple schema to follow in this endeavor and provide excellent diagnostic algorithms

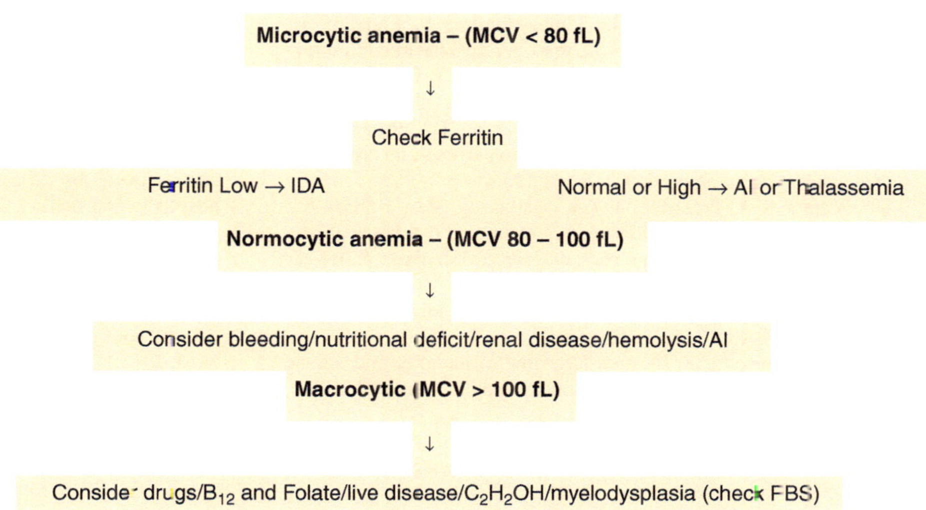

Fig. 41.1 Simple schema (as outlined by Tefferi et al. [9]) that uses mean corpuscular volume (MCV) and peripheral blood smear (PBS) data from a complete blood count to provide a diagnostic algorithm for anemia. (IDA = iron deficiency anemia; AI = anemia of inflammation)

depending on MCV and PBS data. In general, alterations in MCV data suggest possible diagnoses as outlined in Fig. 41.1.

What Is "Patient Blood Management"?

There is a clear relationship between preoperative anemia and the transfusion of blood products perioperatively. Transfusion of even one unit of RBCs is associated with increased morbidity [10]. Interventions directed at managing anemia perioperatively are effective in reducing transfusion rates, costs, length of stay, and in improving outcome [11]. These facts have led to the development of perioperative anemia clinics where the most common, simply treatable causes of perioperative anemia, FID and IDA, are managed prior to surgery [12]. This approach and adherence to restrictive transfusion practices constitute the pillars of a patient blood management program [13].

Is There a Relationship Between Hepatic Adenomatosis and IDA?

Hepatic adenomas are uncommon benign tumors that are associated with anabolic steroid use in males and oral contraceptive use in females. Hepatic adenomas are more common in individuals with glycogen storage disease or iron-overload disorders. They are usually solitary lesions that can undergo malignant transformation and occasionally cause fatal intraperitoneal or hepatic hemorrhage. Large tumors are usually excised to avoid these complications. IDA due to chronic intratumoral hemorrhage can present as the initial manifestation of multifocal hepatic adenomatosis, a rare but potentially fatal condition [14].

The patient was referred to the anemia clinic and underwent transfusion of 1 gram of ferric carboxymaltose. An urgent visit to a hepatobiliary surgeon was arranged and the patient subsequently underwent resection of liver segment VIII without incident.

True/False Questions

1. Anemia
   (a) Is uncommon in developed countries.
   (b) Is commonly caused by iron deficiency.
   (c) Can be precipitated by the chronic use of proton pump inhibitors.
   (d) If mild, is not associated with any adverse outcomes.
   (e) Prior bariatric surgery is a risk factor.
2. Normocytic (MCV 80–100 fL) anemia
   (a) Is never due to hemorrhage.
   (b) Can arise as a consequence of nutritional deficiency.
   (c) Can be associated with renal insufficiency.
   (d) Is not uncommon in hemolysis.
   (e) Is characteristic of excessive alcohol use.

References

1. Beutler E, Waalen J, Dc W. The definition of anemia: what is the lower limit of normal of the blood hemoglobin concentration? Blood. 2006;107(5):1747–50.
2. Karkouti K, Wijeysundera DN, Beattie WS, Reducing Bleeding in Cardiac Surgery (RBC) Investigators. Risk associated with preoperative anemia in cardiac surgery: a multicenter cohort study. Circulation. 2008;117(4):478–84.
3. Musallam KM, Tamim HM, Richards T, Spahn DR, Rosendaal FR, Habbal A, et al. Preoperative anaemia and postoperative outcomes in non-cardiac surgery: a retrospective cohort study. Lancet. 2011;378(9800):1396–407.
4. Camaschella C. Iron-deficiency anemia. N Engl J Med. 2015;372(19):1832–43.

5. Muñoz M, Laso-Morales MJ, Gómez-Ramírez S, Cadellas M, Núñez-Matas MJ, García-Erce JA. Pre-operative haemoglobin levels and iron status in a large multicentre cohort of patients undergoing major elective surgery. Anaesthesia. 2017;72(7):826–34.
6. Lam JR, Schneider JL, Quesenberry CP, Corley DA. Proton pump inhibitor and histamine-2 receptor antagonist use and iron deficiency. Gastroenterology. 2017;152(4):821–9.
7. Obinwanne KM, Fredrickson KA, Mathiason MA, Kallies KJ, Farnen JP, Kothari SN. Incidence, treatment, and outcomes of iron deficiency after laparoscopic roux-en-Y gastric bypass: a 10-year analysis. J Am Coll Surg. 2014;218(2):246–52.
8. Weiss G, Ganz T, Goodnough LT. Anemia of inflammation. Blood. 2019;133(1):40–50.
9. Tefferi A, Hanson CA, Inwards DJ. How to interpret and pursue an abnormal complete blood cell count in adults. Mayo Clin Proc. 2005;80(7):923–36.
10. LaPar DJ, Hawkins RB, McMurry TL, Isbell JM, Rich JB, Speir A, et al. Investigators for the Virginia cardiac services quality initiative. Preoperative anemia versus blood transfusion: which is the culprit for worse outcomes in cardiac surgery? J Thorac Cardiovasc Surg. 2018;156(1):66–74.e2.
11. Leahy MF, Hofmann A, Towler S, Trentino KM, Burrows SA, Swain SG, et al. Improved outcomes and reduced costs associated with a health-system-wide patient blood management program: a retrospective observational study in four major adult tertiary-care hospitals. Transfusion. 2017;57(6):1347–58.
12. Steinbicker AU. Role of anesthesiologists in managing perioperative anemia. Curr Opin Anaesthesiol. 2019;32(1):64–71.
13. Sadana D, Pratzer A, Scher LJ, Saag HS, Adler N, Volpicelli FM, et al. Promoting high-value practice by reducing unnecessary transfusions with a patient blood management program. JAMA Intern Med. 2018;178(1):116–22.
14. Mota C, Carvalho AM, Fonseca V, Silva MT, Victorino RMM. Exuberant liver adenomatosis presenting with iron deficiency anemia. Clin Case Rep. 2017;5(5):574–7.

Sickle Cell Disease

42

Barry A. Finegan

A 20-year-old African American female, with a history of sickle cell disease (SCD) diagnosed at birth, was assessed preoperatively prior to planned elective cholecystectomy. She indicated that she had had two episodes of acute abdominal pain in the last month. There was concern that her symptoms were the harbinger of an impending vaso-occlusive crisis. However, subsequent ultrasound examination found a sonographic Murphy's sign, cholelithiasis, a thickened gall bladder wall (>3 mm), and a collection of pericholecystic fluid. A diagnosis of acute cholecystitis was made, and the patient was schedule for cholecystectomy.

Medications: Hydroxyurea, folic acid, and vitamin D.

The patient's genotype was Hb SS. She had been admitted to hospital several times as a child for management of pain crises related to her SCD and had undergone numerous transfusions. Four years prior to her current admission, she had an episode of acute chest syndrome (ACS) thought to be due to a mycoplasma infection. The episode was managed supportively without the need for ICU admission. Later in the same year, she had two moderate pain crises and she was initiated on hydroxyurea therapy (20 mg/kg/d). Pneumococcal and ongoing seasonal vaccinations were suggested. She had been compliant with these recommendations and had no severe pain events in the 4 years prior to this preoperative evaluation. She had good exercise tolerance and reported no serious SCD-related health issues other than cholelithiasis in the last year. She was under the care of a hematologist whom she visited on a routine basis.

Physical Examination: Vital signs were within normal limits and physical examination was normal apart from pale sclera and mild icterus. Oxygen saturation was 96%.

Investigations: Chest radiograph and ECG were normal.

How Common Is SCD in the United States?

The Centers for Disease Control and Prevention (CDC) estimates that between 70,000 and 100,000 Americans have SCD. One in every 365 African American children is born with SCD, and it occurs in one out of every 16,300 Hispanic American births [1].

What Is the Pathophysiology of SCD?

Mendelian inherited single gene mutation results in the production of hemoglobin (Hb) with abnormal β-globin chains termed sickle hemoglobin (HbS) instead of normal adult hemoglobin (HbA). Deoxygenation of HbS renders it insoluble, encourages polymerization and tubule formation with resultant red blood cell damage and dehydration (sickled cells). Sickled cells are prone to adhere to the endothelium and to undergo lysis [2]. Interaction between sickled cells, lytic components, adherent leukocytes, and a dysfunctional endothelium can cause vaso-occlusion and end-organ damage [3].

There are several SCD genotypes. The most common being Hb SS, which is the most severe form and is associated with the greatest complication rate. Hb SS along with the much less common Hb Sβ^0-thalassemia are the forms of SCD that are associated with anemia. Other forms of SCD include Hb Sβ^+-thalassemia, Hb SC, Hb SD, and Hb SO. Patients with sickle cell trait (Hb AS) have >60% Hb A and are usually totally asymptomatic but should avoid dehydration especially during intense exercise or in hypoxic environments.

B. A. Finegan (✉)
Department of Anesthesiology & Pain Medicine, University of Alberta, Edmonton, AB, Canada
e-mail: bfinegan@ualberta.ca

D. Dillane, B. A. Finegan (eds.), *Preoperative Assessment*, https://doi.org/10.1007/978-3-030-58842-7_42

What Acute Complications Can Occur in the SCD Patient That Require Evaluation and Treatment?

Vaso-occlusive events are usually manifest as a pain crisis related to the organ(s) affected. Their onset is unpredictable and frequently unheralded by any prodromal symptoms or precipitating event. Dehydration, exposure to hypoxic environments, and cold conditions can trigger a crisis. Bone pain is common and is due to marrow infarction. Similarly, abdominal pain may be the marker of liver and kidney ischemia and consequent acute on chronic functional impairment of these organs. There is marked variability in the occurrence of vaso-occlusive events among those with SCD. Some will suffer few, if any, episodes, while other patients may have multiple episodes annually. There is limited understanding of this anomalous pattern of disease manifestation.

Acute chest syndrome (ACS) is a particularly dangerous vaso-occlusive-related phenomenon. It is the leading cause of mortality in patients with SCD. Classically, patients present with fever, hypoxia, and pulmonary infiltrates on chest radiograph. ACS may be associated with *Mycoplasma pneumoniae* (children) or *Chlamydophilia pneumoniae* (adults) infection. Fat and pulmonary emboli related to microvascular occlusion may also precipitate ACS; this presentation is more common in adults and is associated with greater mortality than ACS in children. Acute respiratory failure can occur rapidly, and urgent admission and supportive management in an ICU or high-dependency unit is appropriate [4].

Severe infection per se is ongoing risk for all patients with SCD [5]. Vaccination against *Streptococcus pneumoniae* and *Haemophilus influenzae* type B is essential as is strict adherence to sterile precautions and prophylactic antibiotic regimes perioperatively.

Auto-splenectomy due to repeated episodes of splenic ischemia and consequent vulnerability to infection occurs in up to 90% of patients by the age of 5.

Acute stroke, usually ischemic in children and hemorrhagic in adults, can occur at any time and is frequently unnoticed.

Acute splenic sequestration of red blood cells results in acute volume depletion and, in most cases, is managed by emergency transfusion of blood. Recurrence is not unusual.

Acute anemia in SCD should always be investigated. Aplastic crisis must be considered, especially in children, when there is an unusual fall in Hb. Determining the absolute reticulocyte count allows one to assess if the anemia is due to decreased RBC production or arises form blood loss due to hemolysis or bleeding. A reduction in the reticulocytes count in the peripheral blood <1.0% (normal value: 0.5–2.5%) and an absolute reticulocyte count of <10,000/μL is indicative of aplasia. Due to the short half-life of SCD red cells (12–20 days), even a brief cessation in erythropoiesis will lead to the development of a severe life-threating anemia very rapidly. Aplastic anemia in children is usually caused by parvovirus B19. Isolation (to limit infection spread) and supportive therapy may be sufficient, but emergency management of the patient with SCD is essential.

What Are the Current Disease-Modifying Therapies Used in SCD?

Pain related to an acute vaso-occlusive event is the most common reason for a SCD patient to engage with the health system. Much attention has been directed to develop therapy to reduce the frequency of painful vaso-occlusive episodes.

Hydroxyurea is a mainstay of preventive treatment for SCD complications. Hydroxyurea causes myelosuppression but by mechanisms yet unknown induces the production of fetal hemoglobin (Hb F). Hb F interferes with the polymerization of Hb S and thus decreases vaso-occlusive events and other complications.

Crizanlizumab is a monoclonal antibody to the adhesion molecule P-selectin. Upregulation of P-selectin in SCD contributes to cell-cell interactions that are related to the genesis of vaso-occlusive events. Crizanlizumab reduces the incidence of pain crises and was approved by the FDA in 2019.

Voxelotor is a hemoglobin S polymerization inhibitor also approved by the FDA in 2019. It has been shown to increase Hb levels in SCD patients. Further safety and efficacy trials are ongoing.

L-Glutamine, a precursor of the antioxidant glutathione, is approved as a disease-modifying agent in SCD. It has been found to reduce the incidence of pain crises possibly by reducing RBC oxidative stress.

Scheduled blood transfusions are used in selected patients with difficult-to-treat recurrent pain crises. Transfusion can be used acutely in the treatment of SCD patients with acute stroke, transient ischemic attack, and organ failure. Prophylactic transfusion is used to reduce stroke incidence in children with SCD and to mitigate against the complications listed below.

Hematopoietic cell transplantation is a novel emerging potentially curative therapy, albeit with the attendant risks of graft-versus-host disease and other complications.

What Are Some of the Chronic Complications of SCD?

- Pulmonary hypertension
- Chronic restrictive lung disease
- Left ventricular diastolic dysfunction
- Cardiac iron overload
- Venous sinus thrombosis
- Functional asplenia and increased susceptibility to infection

- Renal impairment/failure
- Hepatic dysfunction/cholelithiasis
- Skin ulceration
- Avascular necrosis
- Ocular retinopathy

What Are the Key Issues to Elucidate During the Perioperative Evaluation of the Patient with SCD?

- Patient's genotype
- Past occurrence of vaso-occlusive events
- Symptoms of heart failure/pulmonary hypertension/renal failure
- Compliance with medical therapy
- Vaccination history
- Name and location of consulting hematologist

What Are the Laboratory Investigations That Should Be Ordered?

- Complete blood count.
- Electrolytes and creatinine.
- Coagulation screen.
- Group and cross match—indicate patient has SCD—request alloantibody screen.

Hydroxyurea may cause leukopenia, neutropenia, and thrombocytopenia.

In SCD, an elevated absolute reticulocyte count is to be expected as there is ongoing hemolysis.

If the absolute reticulocyte count is low, then the possibility of an imminent acute aplastic crisis should be considered (vide supra).

SCD causes multiple renal abnormalities that become more apparent with age.

Alloimmunization is relatively common in SCD patients. Transfused blood should be leukoreduced, and appropriate testing for extended phenotype matching performed.

What Should Be Considered Preoperatively to Mitigate the Occurrence of Adverse Perioperative Events?

Hematology and blood transfusion specialist engagement in care is mandatory.

Consider preoperative transfusion to increase Hb > 100 g/L. Transfusion to this Hb level appears to decrease the occurrence of complications, particularly ACS, following low or *medium* risk surgery including cholecystectomy. An ACS life-threatening event can occur suddenly and typically presents with symptoms of cough and dyspnea, signs of pulmonary congestion, and the presence of infiltrates on chest radiograph. The timeline to progression to respiratory failure can be very brief and appropriate monitoring, supportive treatment, and transfusion should be provided as indicated.

"Simple" transfusion implies just that transfusion to a target Hb. Many patients, particularly children with SCD, undergo "exchange transfusions" where sickle cells are replaced by normal donor cells. This form of transfusion reduces the volume of donor cells required and reduces the risk of iron overload but is expensive. Both simple and exchange transfusions have been shown to reduce the occurrence of stroke in pediatric patients with SCD. There are limited data available to review the relative merits of either transfusion approach prior to surgery. The 2014 *Evidence-Based Management of Sickle Cell Disease: Expert Panel Report by the National Heart, Lung and Blood Institute* recommends transfusing to a target of 100 g/L in children and adults prior to any consequential surgical procedure involving general anesthesia [6].

Admission the day prior to surgery is advisable to ensure stable physical status and appropriate hydration.

With regard to our patient, Hb was 72 g/L, hematocrit 25%, platelet count 475 × 10⁹/L, and absolute reticulocyte count 204,000/μL. Creatinine and electrolyte values were within normal limits. No alloantibodies were detected. The patient was seen by her hematologist and "simple" transfusion to a Hb > 100 g/L was recommended. Following the transfusion, the patient underwent a laparoscopic cholecystectomy without incident. She was admitted to the surgical stepdown unit for 48 hours where oximetry and enhanced nursing care was available for routine observation. She was subsequently discharged without incident.

True/False Questions

1. In SCD acute chest syndrome the following are diagnostic:
   (a) Chest pain on breathing
   (b) Cough
   (c) Hypoxia
   (d) New pulmonary infiltrates on chest radiograph
   (e) Fever
2. Transfusion therapy
   (a) is a mainstay of management of SCD
   (b) to achieve a Hb level above 10 g/L is recommended prior to all surgery under general anesthesia
   (c) exchange transfusion may reduce the risk of iron overload
   (d) requirement is not reduced by hydroxyurea therapy
   (e) should be avoided if the reticulocyte is low

References

1. Centers for Disease Control and Prevention. Sickle cell disease (SCD) [Internet]. [cited 16 Jun 2017]. https://www.cdc.gov/ncbddd/sicklecell/data.html.
2. Nath KA, Hebbel RP. Sickle cell disease: renal manifestations and mechanisms. Nat Rev Nephrol. 2015;11(3):161–71.
3. Piel FB, Steinberg MH, Rees DC. Sickle cell disease. N Engl J Med. 2017;376(16):1561–73.
4. Howard J, Hart N, Roberts-Harewood M, Cummins M, Awogbade M, Davis B. Guideline on the management of acute chest syndrome in sickle cell disease. Br J Haematol. 2015;169(4):492–505.
5. Sobota A, Sabharwal V, Fonebi G, Steinberg M. How we prevent and manage infection in sickle cell disease. Br J Haematol. 2015;170(6):757–67.
6. Yawn BP, Buchanan GR, Afenyi-Annan AN, Ballas SK, Jassell KL, James AH, et al. Management of sickle cell disease. Summary of the 2014 evidence-based report by expert panel members. JAMA. 2014;312(10):1033–48.

Part XI
Miscellaneous

The Pregnant Patient

43

Jalal A. Nanji

A 22-year-old, gravida 1, para 0 at 33 weeks' gestation presented to the endoscopy suite for repeat esophageal dilation. Because of long-standing achalasia and dysphagia, she had undergone esophagectomy with gastric pull-up 5 years previously but was having ongoing issues with an anastomotic stricture requiring repeated esophageal dilations, including earlier during this pregnancy. Given the severity of her dysphagia, her gastroenterologist felt that postponing the current esophageal dilation until after delivery was not advisable. She was otherwise healthy and took no medications other than prenatal vitamins and a proton-pump inhibitor. She had an allergy to latex and tree nuts.

Pre-procedure vital signs included a blood pressure of 108/66 and heart rate of 92 with regular rhythm, respiratory rate of 18, and SpO_2 of 98% on room air. Fetal heart rate monitoring before and after the procedure revealed a Category 1 tracing with good fetal heart rate variability. There was no evidence of preterm contractions on uterine tocodynamometry either before or after the procedure.

Her most recent pregnancy ultrasound revealed a biophysical profile of 6/8. There was marginal cord insertion in an otherwise normal placenta.

What Are the Important Physiologic Changes Associated with Pregnancy?

Pregnancy is characterized by an increase in alveolar ventilation, chronic respiratory alkalosis, and decreased functional residual capacity (FRC). The reduced FRC means that pregnant patients desaturate quickly and have less tolerance for apnea or positioning such as lithotomy or Trendelenburg before the onset of hypoxemia. Capillary engorgement caused by circulating progesterone may result in airway edema and difficulty with mask ventilation and endotracheal intubation. There is a decrease in systemic vascular resistance but a concomitant increase in heart rate and stroke volume that results in a large overall increase in cardiac output (50% at term). Aortocaval compression from the gravid uterus can lead to maternal hypotension, decreased uteroplacental perfusion, and increased risk of deep vein thrombosis in the supine position after 20 weeks of gestation; for this reason, patients in the second half of pregnancy should always be positioned tilted to the left or with the uterus displaced laterally. A disproportionate rise in plasma volume relative to red cell mass results in the "physiologic anemia of pregnancy," which is most pronounced in the second trimester.

How Should We Assess the Airway of a Pregnant Patient Prior to Non-obstetric Surgery?

The airway can be challenging in pregnant patients because of capillary engorgement, tissue friability, and edema. Elements of a standard airway examination are useful in pregnant patients; a combination of thyromental distance and upper lip bite test has recently been shown to be highly specific and sensitive for difficult intubation [1]

The Obstetric Anaesthetists' Association and the Difficult Airway Society in the UK have published a set of guidelines for the management of difficult and failed intubations in obstetrics. They emphasize the role of preoperative planning and communication, team decision-making, and the complexities of dealing with difficult airway scenarios when two patients (mother and fetus) need to be considered (Fig. 43.1) [2].

J. A. Nanji (✉)
University of Alberta Faculty of Medicine and Dentistry, Department of Anesthesiology and Pain Medicine, Royal Alexandra Hospital DTC OR, Edmonton, AB, Canada
e-mail: jnanji@ualberta.ca

D. Dillane, B. A. Finegan (eds.), *Preoperative Assessment*, https://doi.org/10.1007/978-3-030-58842-7_43

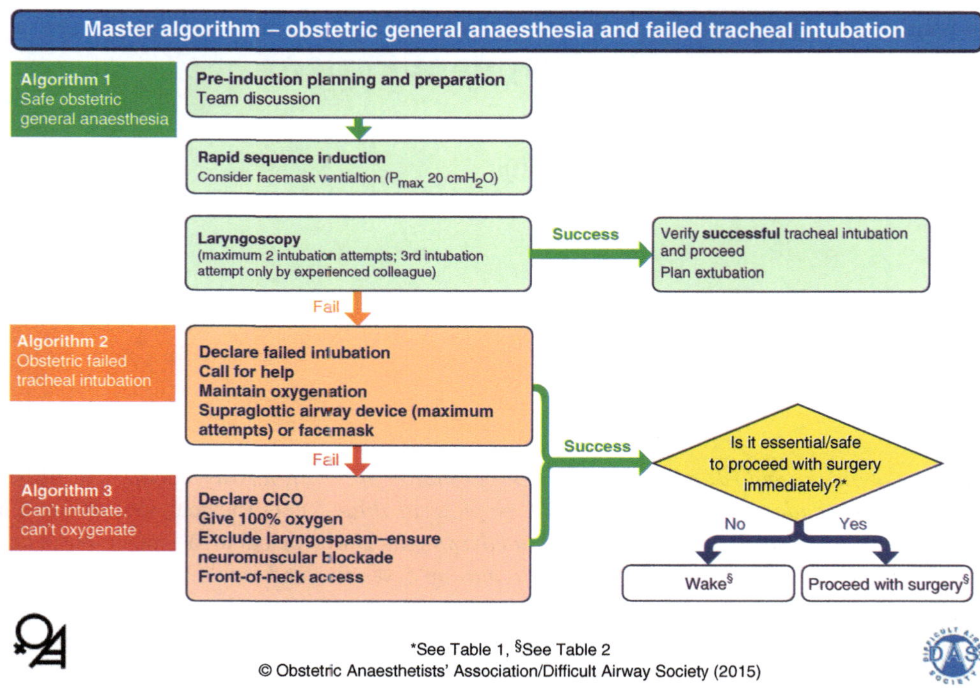

Fig. 43.1 Master algorithm—obstetric general anesthesia and failed tracheal intubation (From Mushambi et al. [2], with permission John Wiley and Sons, the Obstetric Anaesthetists' Association, and the Difficult Airway Society) (© Obstetric Anaesthetists' Association)

Why Are Pregnant Patients Considered at Risk of Aspiration Under Anesthesia?

Increased progesterone leads to decreased lower esophageal sphincter tone. Additionally, increased intraabdominal pressure from the gravid uterus predisposes pregnant patients to reflux of gastric contents and may lead to aspiration under general anesthesia. Gastric emptying, however, is not delayed in pregnant patients until they are in labor [3]. Rapid sequence induction of anesthesia should be performed whenever general anesthesia is employed in a pregnant patient. The combination of nonparticulate antacids and H2-blockers may be somewhat useful to mitigate risk by reducing intragastric pH [4].

Are Fasting Guidelines Different in the Pregnant Patient?

Despite the potential for increased aspiration risk after 20 weeks' gestation, no difference in fasting guidelines exists for pregnant undergoing non-obstetric surgery. Adherence to the recommendations of national societies such as those of the American Society of Anesthesiologists and Canadian Anesthesiologists' Society that clear fluids are permitted up to 2 hours prior to elective surgery, and that a light meal or a heavier meal be restricted to 6 and 8 hours prior to surgery, respectively, is prudent [5, 6]. Current guidelines further suggest that solid foods not be permitted for pregnant patients once active labor is established, and that individual institutions develop protocols with respect to clear fluid intake during labor [5].

What Are the Fetal Risks Associated with Non-obstetric Surgery During Pregnancy?

There are three major categories of risk to the unborn fetus, which can vary depending on when, during pregnancy, surgery and anesthesia are undertaken, namely, preterm labor, teratogenicity, and intrauterine asphyxia.

Can the Risk of Preterm Labor Be Mitigated?

Preterm labor is a theoretical risk with any procedure; it is possible that either direct mechanical irritation or inflammation caused by abdominopelvic procedures may increase this risk compared to procedures performed in other areas of the body. Unfortunately, there has been no proven benefit demonstrated with the use of tocolytic drugs (e.g., magnesium sulfate and terbutaline) to try and prevent preterm labor in a pregnant patient underdoing non-obstetric surgery [7].

What Role Do Glucocorticoids Play in Procedures Undertaken During Pregnancy?

Antenatal administration of glucocorticoids (e.g., dexamethasone or betamethasone) in select patients has been shown to improve neonatal morbidity and mortality related to preterm complications, e.g., respiratory distress syndrome, intracranial hemorrhage, and necrotizing enterocolitis. The American

College of Obstetricians and Gynecologists (ACOG) recommends a single course of corticosteroids for patients at risk of preterm delivery within 7 days who are between 24 0/7 and 33 6/7 weeks gestation and that it may be considered in late preterm patients (i.e., between 34 0/7 and 36 6/7 weeks). Suggested treatment consists of either two 12-mg doses of betamethasone given intramuscularly 24 hours apart or four 6-mg doses of dexamethasone administered intramuscularly every 12 hours [8].

Are Any Drugs Used in the Conduct of General Anesthesia Teratogenic?

Teratogenicity is most likely to occur in the first trimester, and the former US Food and Drug Administration (FDA) category "X" drugs are those that must absolutely be avoided during pregnancy. This classification, in use since 1979, was replaced in 2015 with a new, narrative system [9]. Importantly, no drugs used as part of anesthetic practice, including nitrous oxide (N2O), neuromuscular blocking agents, volatile anesthetics, induction drugs, or opioid analgesics, have been shown to be teratogenic in *clinically relevant concentrations in humans*. Nitrous oxide can affect DNA synthesis and has been shown to be teratogenic in animals after long exposures in high concentrations. Research in human subjects has been limited to case-control studies with many confounders, and the ACOG does not recommend avoidance of specific anesthetic drugs in pregnant patients if they are indicated [10].

Are Non-steroidal Anti-Inflammatory Drugs (NSAIDs) Safe During Pregnancy?

NSAIDs may be prescribed by a physician for tocolysis in preterm labor or for prevention of vascular complications from disorders such as pre-eclampsia. Alternatively, they may be self-administered by pregnant patients for common ailments such as joint pain or fevers and malaise. Fetal complications of maternal NSAID use may include premature closure of the ductus arteriosus, leading to persistent pulmonary hypertension of the newborn, necrotizing enterocolitis, and oligohydramnios. For these reasons, NSAIDs are best avoided after 30 weeks' gestation and used in the lowest doses for the shortest duration possible if maternal benefit outweighs fetal risk [11].

What Are the Risk Factors for Intrauterine Asphyxia?

The age-old directive to "avoid hypoxia and hypotension" is especially important when considering the pregnant patient undergoing non-obstetric surgery, as perfusion to the fetus through the placenta is highly dependent on these (and other factors). There is no autoregulation in the uteroplacental circulation, unlike in the brain. Blood flow is directly related to mean uterine perfusion pressure (and therefore maternal mean arterial pressure) and inversely related to the vascular resistance of uterine vessels. Support of maternal blood pressure with fluid administration or vasopressors is important to prevent uteroplacental insufficiency during the perioperative period. Direct acting α-agonists such as phenylephrine are safe and cause less neonatal acidosis than ephedrine; both are likely safe, however, during non-obstetric surgery during pregnancy. Finally, maternal hypoxemia leads to fetal hypoxemia and uterine vasoconstriction, which, if prolonged, can lead to irreversible brain damage or intrauterine death. Similarly, maternal hypercarbia can cause uterine vasoconstriction as well as fetal acidosis.

What Is a Biophysical Profile (BPP) and What Is the Significance of a BPP of 6/8?

A BPP is an antenatal test meant to evaluate fetal well-being. Fetal heart rate (FHR) monitoring (the nonstress test or NST) is combined with four unique ultrasound measurements (breathing, movement, muscle tone, and amniotic fluid level) to give a snapshot of fetal health. Each of the resulting five elements is given a score of 0 or 2. BPP scores of 8 or 10 are considered reassuring. Depending on many factors, including individual clinical circumstances and gestational age, scores of 6 or below may simply require repeat testing either the same or the next day, or in some cases a plan for delivery is required [12].

How Should We Assess Fetal Well-Being During Surgery?

The decision to use fetal monitoring must take into account the timing of the proposed procedure, access to the maternal abdomen, and the availability of personnel equipped to respond to an ominous fetal heart rate tracing should it occur. Decreased fetal heart rate variability may not always represent fetal distress, however, and can be seen with the administration of general anesthesia, maternal hypothermia, or drugs that affect the maternal cardiovascular system. The optimal choice of fetal monitoring is therefore a complex decision-making process. According to ACOG "Because of the difficulty of conducting large-scale randomized clinical trials in this population, there are no data to allow for specific recommendations. It is important for a physician to obtain an obstetric consultation before performing non-obstetric surgery and some invasive procedures (e.g., cardiac catheterization or colonoscopy) because obstetricians are uniquely qualified to discuss aspects of maternal physiology and anatomy that may affect intraoperative maternal–fetal well-being" [10].

For Which Non-obstetric Surgical Cases Should Fetal Monitoring Be Utilized?

The decision to use fetal monitoring should be individualized, and each case warrants a team approach for optimal safety of both mother and baby. Generally speaking, Doppler assessment of the FHR before and after the procedure is sufficient for previable fetuses. For fetuses that have passed the age of viability, FHR assessment and contraction monitoring (tocodynamometry) can be performed before and after the procedure to ensure fetal well-being and rule out preterm labor. *Intraoperative* monitoring is useful only if there is a possibility of intervention (i.e., emergency caesarean delivery) should fetal distress be encountered. This necessitates having access to the maternal abdomen, as well as the immediate availability of a physician capable of performing an emergency delivery [10].

How Are Fetal Heart Rate Tracings Categorized?

A three-tier classification scheme for FHR tracings was adopted in 2008, in which Category 1 tracings are those with no ominous features and are considered *normal*, Category 3 are fetal heart rate tracings thought to represent significant fetal compromise and are *abnormal*, and Category 2 being those that fall into neither of the other two categories and are therefore *indeterminate* [13]. A detailed review of FHR tracings is beyond the scope of this chapter, and the reader is encouraged to refer to numerous existing publications on this subject.

Is There Any Evidence That Obstetric or Neonatal Outcomes Are Worse When Non-obstetric Surgery Has Been Performed During Pregnancy?

Isolating the effects of anesthesia from the surgical procedure and the underlying surgical condition is difficult if not impossible. It has been estimated that 1–2% of pregnant patients will undergo procedures unrelated to pregnancy, and quantifying the risks associated with these procedures has proved elusive. Analysis of administrative data suggests that the risk of complications for both mother and fetus/newborn is low when surgery is performed during pregnancy and that it is relatively safe, especially with modern anesthetic and surgical techniques [14].

When Should Surgery Be Undertaken?

Traditional dogma, including the most recent Committee Opinion by ACOG [9], suggests that surgery be carried out in the second trimester if possible, as the risk of teratogenicity and miscarriage may be higher in the first trimester of pregnancy and risk of preterm labor highest closer to term. There has recently been a reappraisal of this time-honored teaching given the fact that maternal-fetal care, surgical technique, and diagnostic testing have all advanced since the initial studies examining this topic were performed [15]. Withholding surgery when indicated *because* a patient is pregnant may actually confer more risk to the patient due to the severity of the underlying surgical disease and is therefore unwarranted. This is important, as the overwhelming majority of procedures undertaken during pregnancy are not elective, and therefore being able to time them to coincide with the second trimester is often neither practical nor possible.

True/False Questions

1. Which factors are involved in the decision about whether or not to perform continuous intraoperative fetal monitoring during non-obstetric surgery during pregnancy?
   (a) Duration of procedure
   (b) Access to maternal abdomen
   (c) Immediate availability of physician capable of performing emergency delivery
   (d) Anesthetic technique (e.g., neuraxial vs. general)
   (e) Gestational age of fetus
2. Which anesthetic medication is absolutely contraindicated during pregnancy?
   (a) Nitrous oxide
   (b) Ketamine
   (c) Neostigmine
   (d) Fentanyl
   (e) None of the above

References

1. Yildirim I, Inal MT, Memis D, Turan FN. Determining the efficiency of different preoperative difficult intubation tests on patients undergoing caesarean section. Balkan Med J. 2017;34(5):436–43.
2. Mushambi MC, Kinsella SM, Popat M, Swales H, Ramaswamy KK, Winton AL, et al. Obstetric Anaesthetists' Association and difficult airway society guidelines for the management of difficult and failed tracheal intubation in obstetrics. Anaesthesia. 2015;70(11):1286–306.
3. Cheek TG, Baird E. Anesthesia for nonobstetric surgery: maternal and fetal considerations. Clin Obstet Gynecol. 2009;52(4):535–45.
4. Paranjothy S, Griffiths JD, Broughton HK, Gyte GM, Brown HC, Thomas J. Interventions at caesarean section for reducing the risk of aspiration pneumonitis. Cochrane Database Syst

Rev. 2010;1:CD004943. https://doi.org/10.1002/14651858.CD004943.pub3. Update in: Cochrane Database Syst Rev. 2014;2:CD004943. 6
5. Dobson G, Chong M, Chow L, Flexman A, Kurrek M, Laflamme C, et al. Guidelines to the practice of anesthesia – revised edition 2018. Can J Anaesth. 2018;65(1):76–104.
6. Practice Guidelines for Preoperative Fasting and the Use of Pharmacologic Agents to Reduce the Risk of Pulmonary Aspiration. Application to healthy patients undergoing elective procedures: an updated report by the American Society of Anesthesiologists Task Force on preoperative fasting and the use of pharmacologic agents to reduce the risk of pulmonary aspiration. Anesthesiology. 2017;126(3):376–93.
7. Webb MP, Helander EM, Meyn AR, Flynn T, Urman RD, Kaye AD. Preoperative assessment of the pregnant patient undergoing nonobstetric surgery. Anesthesiol Clin. 2018;36(4):627–37.
8. Committee on Obstetric P. Committee Opinion No. 713. Antenatal corticosteroid therapy for fetal maturation. Obstet Gynecol. 2017;130(2):e102–e9.
9. Mosley JF 2nd, Smith LL, Dezan MD. An overview of upcoming changes in pregnancy and lactation labeling information. Pharm Pract (Granada). 2015;13(2):605.
10. American College of Obstetrics and Gynecology. Nonobstetric Surgery During Pregnancy 2019. [April 2019]. Available from:https://www.acog.org/clinical/clinical-guidance/committee-opinion/articles/2019/04/nonobstetric-surgery-during-pregnancy. Accessed 31 May 2020.
11. Antonucci R, Zaffanello M, Puxeddu E, Porcella A, Cuzzolin L, Pilloni MD, et al. Use of non-steroidal anti-inflammatory drugs in pregnancy: impact on the fetus and newborn. Curr Drug Metab. 2012;13(4):474–90.
12. Oyelese Y, Vintzileos AM. The uses and limitations of the fetal biophysical profile. Clin Perinatol. 2011;38(1):47–64. v–vi
13. Macones GA, Hankins GD, Spong CY, Hauth J, Moore T. The 2008 National Institute of Child Health and Human Development workshop report on electronic fetal monitoring: update on definitions, interpretation, and research guidelines. Obstet Gynecol. 2008;112(3):661–6.
14. Balinskaite V, Bottle A, Sodhi V, Rivers A, Bennett PR, Brett SJ, et al. The risk of adverse pregnancy outcomes following nonobstetric surgery during pregnancy: estimates from a retrospective cohort study of 6.5 million pregnancies. Ann Surg. 2017 265(2):260–6.
15. Tolcher MC, Fisher WE, Clark SL. Nonobstetric surgery during pregnancy. Obstet Gynecol. 2018;132(2):395–403.

The Psychiatric Patient

44

Barry A. Finegan

A 59-year-old female with COPD presented for assessment prior to right total hip arthroplasty. She had a 30-year history of tobacco use but had recently quit. Past medical history was positive for mild sleep apnea, gastroesophageal reflux disease (GERD), hypertension, and cervical carcinoma for which she underwent a hysterectomy without incident. She had a longstanding diagnosis of bipolar disorder, which she indicated had been stable for 2 years. She reported two episodes of mania in the last 5 years, both of which required inpatient management, including brief courses of electroconvulsive therapy (ECT).

Medications: Tiotropium bromide 2.5 mg OD, fluticasone propionate/salmeterol 100 µg/50 µg BID, albuterol 100 µg PRN Q6H, lithium 600 mg BID, quetiapine 400 mg OD, and acetaminophen 500 mg QID.

The patient did not make eye contact during the initial stages of the interview. Although she was appropriately dressed, her clothes were somewhat unkempt and slightly soiled. She repeatedly twisted her fingers and exhibited an unsettled posture. Her speech was rapid, lilting, and loud. She appeared to be anxious and had some flight of ideas.

On being questioned as to her mood, she readily admitted that the last few weeks had been very difficult and that she felt "on the edge." Her husband was undergoing chemotherapy and now she was being scheduled for surgery. She indicated that earlier in the day she felt she was "going to lose it and start screaming." She seemed relieved to be able to express these feelings. She denied any suicidal ideation. She admitted that she had discontinued her lithium and quetiapine 2 months previously. She agreed that she needed some help, as she was becoming preoccupied with morbid thoughts and readily agreed to a surgical postponement and referral to her psychiatrist for assessment and management.

A Suggested Approach to the Patient with a Pre-existing Psychiatric Diagnosis

1. Perform a brief mental status examination.
2. Determine if the patient is stable or in need of referral for further psychiatric management prior to surgery.
3. Review current medications and assess for potential side effects, drug interactions, and consequences of withdrawal or interruption of these medications perioperatively.

What Are the Components of a Mental Status Examination (MSE)?

A Appearance and behavior
S Speech and motor activity
E Emotion (mood and affect)
P Perception
T Thought content and process
I Insight and judgment
C Cognition

Appropriate questions to ask any patient with a psychiatric history include the following:

- How is your mood?
- Have you felt sad/down recently?
- Have you felt in control lately?

While many components of the MSE are elicited through observation during a routine history and physical examination, assessing some aspects, including thoughts, perceptions, attitude, and insight, requires directed interrogation. Assessing cognition can be challenging. The Mini-Cog is a screening tool that is accessible in the public domain (https://mini-cog.com), simple to administer, and helpful in determining many aspects of cognition: attention, language, memory, orientation, and visuospatial proficiency. It is very

B. A. Finegan (✉)
Department of Anesthesiology & Pain Medicine, University of Alberta, Edmonton, AB, Canada
e-mail: bfinegan@ualberta.ca

D. Dillane, B. A. Finegan (eds.), *Preoperative Assessment*, https://doi.org/10.1007/978-3-030-58842-7_44

sensitive, in the absence of other acute mental health issues, in determining the presence of dementia [1].

What Is the Prevalence of Mental Illness in the Population?

The National Institute of Mental Health estimates that nearly one in five adults in the United States live with a mental illness, with 4.5% of the population suffering serious mental illness. The latter is defined as "a mental, behavioral, or emotional disorder resulting in serious functional impairment, which substantially interferes with or limits one or more major life activities" [2]. Up to 25% of those with serious mental illness remain untreated.

Is It Important to Identify Those with Decompensating Mental Illness Prior to Elective Surgery?

In general, many patients with serious mental illness have social and occupational challenges and engage in behavioral choices that contribute to poor physical health. These factors include inadequate diet, tobacco use, excess alcohol, and illicit drug intake. In consequence, the baseline risk for this patient group is elevated. However, it is clear that if patients with serious mental health issues require an intervention to manage their psychiatric illness during admission following elective surgery, their morbidity and mortality far exceed that of the general population [3]. These data underscore the need to identify, assess, and treat decompensated mental illness prior to an elective surgical procedure in a similar fashion as is routine for occult coronary and respiratory illness.

What Are the Potential Consent Issues in Patients with Decompensating Mental Illness Prior to Elective Surgery?

Individuals with an inadequately managed serious mental disorder may not have the capacity to legally provide informed consent to elective surgery. Consent requires that one both *understands* the information that is relevant to deciding and has the *capacity* to make such a decision. The decision to agree to a surgical procedure does not necessarily extend to consent to undergo an anesthetic [4]. Indeed, in elective surgery, the evolving and fluctuating nature of mental status in patients with unstable comorbidities may require reassessment of a previously obtained consent. Cognitive rather than psychotic or mood disorders are more likely to impair appropriate decision-making capacity [5].

It was clear in this case that the patient understood the risk and benefits of treatment, appreciated her clinical situation, was independently able to arrive at a reasonable decision, and communicate that decision. The latter are the four essential components of the decision-making capacity [4].

What Are the Classes of Drugs Currently Used to Manage Psychiatric Disorders and What Are the Issues to Be Aware of When Evaluating Patients Using These Medications?

This subject has recently been comprehensively reviewed [6, 7]. The major categories and issues of concern to the perioperative physician are outlined as follows:

1. Selective serotonin reuptake inhibitors [SSRIs] (citalopram; fluoxetine and others).
   Issues:
   (a) Fluoxetine inhibits the cytochrome P450—dose adjustment may be required of drugs metabolized by P450 system.
   (b) Serotonin syndrome can occur and presents with symptoms and signs including agitation, confusion, tachycardia, hypertension, dilated pupils, and muscle rigidity.
   (c) SSRIs decrease platelet serotonin content and are associated with an increased GI bleeding especially is co-prescribed with NSAIDs.
2. Tricyclic antidepressants (amitriptyline, imipramine, and others).
   Issues:
   (a) QRS, PR, and QTc prolongation due to the depletion of cardiac noradrenergic catecholamines.
   (b) There is an increased propensity to develop malignant dysrhythmias.
   (c) Exaggerated response to ephedrine due to increased postsynaptic norepinephrine content. The use of a direct-acting vasopressor drug, such as phenylephrine, is advisable.
   (d) Serotonin syndrome may occur.
3. Monoamine oxidase inhibitors (phenelzine, moclobemide, and others).
   Issues:
   (a) Exaggerated response to ephedrine. Use direct-acting vasopressor drugs (phenylephrine).
4. Mood stabilizers.
   Issues:
   (a) Lithium is approved for the treatment of manic episodes and for maintenance and as a relapse preventative strategy in bipolar disorder. Lithium has anti-suicidal and neuroprotective properties. The use of lithium has decreased somewhat in recent years due to concerns about its toxicity (vide infra) [8]. Blood level monitoring is recommended in view of its narrow therapeutic range (0.8–1.2 mmol/l measured 12 hours after last dose).

Issues:

(i) Side effects that can occur within the therapeutic range include hypothyroidism and diabetes insipidus.

(ii) Toxicity can be caused by excessive intake or decreased excretion of lithium is seen when levels of the drug exceed the therapeutic range. Symptoms of toxicity include tremor, lethargy, low muscle tone, restlessness, ataxia, and eventually coma.

(iii) Lithium is not metabolized but almost entirely excreted by the kidney. Renal impairment is a contraindication to the use of lithium. Dehydration increased plasma lithium levels.

(iv) Cardiac effects include reversible T wave changes and increase risk of Brugada syndrome in susceptible individuals.

(v) Increased sensitivity to anesthetic agents—decreases neurotransmitter release in the central and peripheral nervous systems.

(vi) NSAIDs may decrease excretion of lithium.

(vii) Nephrotoxic.

1. 20% will suffer a decline in renal function.
2. 20% will develop diabetes insipidus.

(viii) Consensus recommendation is not to discontinue preoperatively.

(b) Carbamazepine is an anticonvulsant used in the management of bipolar disorder, trigeminal neuralgia, and epilepsy.

Issues:

(i) Toxic epidermal necrolysis and Stevens-Johnson syndrome have been reported especially in individuals from Asia or of Asian ancestry.

(ii) Aplastic anemia and agranulocytosis have been reported.

(iii) Induces the P450 enzyme system and chronic treatment will enhance metabolism of benzodiazepines, opioids, and most volatile anesthetics.

(iv) Inappropriate antidiuretic hormone (ADH) syndrome can occur as carbamazepine stimulates the release of vasopressin. Hyponatremia should be investigated by assessing the serum and urine osmolality. Serum osmolality <280 mOsm/kg and a high urine osmolality >100 mOsm/kg is diagnostic of inappropriate ADH syndrome.

(c) Valproate is used to treat bipolar disorder, anxiety, epilepsy, and to prevent migraine.

Issues:

(i) Hepatoxicity especially in children under 2 years of age, usually occurs within the first 6 months of treatment.

(ii) Teratogenicity such as neural tube defects, careful consideration is required when used in female migraine patients.

(iii) Pancreatitis that can occur at any time during treatment (even years after commencement).

5. Antipsychotics.

(a) Typical (prochlorperazine, chlorpromazine, and others): act by blocking dopamine, histamine, and α1 adrenergic and cholinergic receptors.

Issues:

(i) Extra-pyramidal syndromes can occur.

(ii) Seizures (especially chlorpromazine).

(iii) Postural hypotension is not uncommon.

(iv) Neuroleptic malignant syndrome may occur; this is manifest by hyperthermia, rigidity, and autonomic dysfunction.

(b) Atypical (quetiapine, risperidone, and others): these block receptor subtypes of dopamine and less likely to have extra-pyramidal syndromes.

Issues:

(v) Seizures (especially quetiapine).

(vi) Neuroleptic malignant syndrome.

(vii) Postural hypotension.

(c) Patients being treated with clozapine for the management of treatment-resistant schizophrenia deserve special surveillance perioperatively. Although especially effective in managing this condition and reducing suicide rates, it is associated with the development of myocarditis and cardiomyopathy, usually within the first month of treatment [9]. Additionally, there is a risk of agranulocytosis after initiation of therapy.

How Should Psychiatric Patients Be Managed Preoperatively?

Patients should be maintained on their psychotropic medications perioperatively, mindful of drug side effects and interactions. The consequences of abrupt withdrawal of therapy can be very distressing for the patient and significantly exacerbate the underlying psychiatric state. In a brittle patient who is undergoing a procedure with an anticipated in-hospital admission of longer than 24 hours, requesting a psychiatric consultation during the hospital stay is appropriate and worthy of consideration.

The patient was restarted on lithium and quetiapine with rapid resolution of her hypomania. Surgery was rescheduled within 1 month of re-initiation of therapy and proceeded without incident.

True/False Questions

1. Mental illness is
   (a) Not common in the surgical population
   (b) Untreated in a significant minority of patients

  (c) Difficult to assess in the clinic
  (d) A consideration in the consent process
  (e) Not a factor in postoperative morbidity
2. In the psychiatric patient being assessed for surgery the following are appropriate:
  (a) A mood assessment by the patient and the physician
  (b) An inquiry regarding sadness/being down
  (c) Assessment of renal function in the patient on lithium
  (d) Assessing the ECG for QTc prolongation in a patient on tricyclic antidepressants
  (e) Discontinuing psychotropic medications preoperatively to avoid side effects

References

1. Norris L, Cobbs EL. Bedside cognitive assessment. Med J Aust. 2018;208:200–1.
2. National Institute of Mental Health (U.S. Department of Health and Human Services). Statistics. https://www.nimh.nih.gov/health/statistics/index.shtml. Accessed 18 Apr 2019.
3. McBride KE, Solomon MJ, Young JM, Steffens D, Lambert TJ, Glozier N, Bannon PG. Impact of serious mental illness on surgical patient outcomes. ANZ J Surg. 2018;88:673–7.
4. Marcucci C, Seagull FJ, Loreck D, Bourke DL, Sandson NB. Capacity to give surgical consent does not imply capacity to give anesthesia consent: implications for anesthesiologists. Anesth Analg. 2010;110(2):596–600.
5. Boettger S, Boettger S, Bergman M, Jenewein J. Assessment of decisional capacity: prevalence of medical illness and psychiatric comorbidities. Palliat Support Care. 2015;13(5):1275–81.
6. Kaye AD, Kline RJ, Thompson ER, Kaye AJ, Terracciano JA, Siddaiah HB, et al. Perioperative implications of common and newer psychotropic medications used in clinical practice. Best Pract Res Clin Anaesthesiol. 2018;32(2):187–202.
7. Peck T, Wong A, Norman E. Anaesthetic implications of psychoactive drugs. Contin Educ Anaesth Crit Care Pain. 2010;10(6):177–81.
8. Morsel AM, Morrens M, Sabbe B. An overview of the pharmacotherapy of bipolar 1 disorder. Expert Opin Pharmacother. 2018;19(3):203–22.
9. Bellissima BL, Tingle MD, Cicović A, Alawami M, Kenedi C. A systematic review of clozapine-induced myocarditis. Int J Cardiol. 2018;259:122–9.

The Obese Patient Undergoing Non-Bariatric Surgery

45

Derek Dillane

A 57-year-old female scheduled for right mastectomy presented for evaluation 10 days prior to surgery. On the referral letter, she was described as "super morbidly obese" with a weight of 151.5 kg and a BMI of 63.4. She had a history of hypertension, hypothyroidism, gastroesophageal reflux disease (GERD), and obstructive sleep apnea (OSA) for which she used a continuous positive airway pressure (CPAP) machine nightly. She had been diagnosed with type 2 diabetes 6 years previously.

Medications: Irbesartan, metformin, levothyroxine, dexlansoprazole, prometrium, and glucosamine.

Physical Examination: The patient appeared deconditioned, grossly overweight, and short of breath at rest. Blood pressure was 175/90. Heart sounds were distant, and breath sounds diminished. She was assigned a Mallampati Class III score, had a markedly decreased thyromental distance, decreased neck mobility, and was noted to have a large amount of adipose tissue in the hypoglossal space.

Investigations: Chest radiograph and electrocardiogram (ECG) can be seen in Figs. 45.1 and 45.2. *Echocardiography performed 2 years prior to this visit reported an ejection fraction of 55% with grade 1 diastolic dysfunction. The right ventricle was noted to be grossly normal in size with good ventricular function. Left and right atria were normal in size. Right ventricular systolic pressure (RVSP)/pulmonary artery systolic pressure (PASP) was 28 mmHg. A dipyridamole myocardial perfusion scan performed at the same time as the echocardiogram showed normal perfusion at rest and following stress. Myocardial perfusion single-photon emission computerized tomography (SPECT) was normal.*

What Is Super Morbid Obesity? How Is Obesity Defined and Classified?

Obesity is defined and classified according to body mass index (BMI), which is weight in kilograms divided by the height in meters squared (kg/m^2). The World Health Organization (WHO) and National Institutes of Health (NIH) have classified obesity according to BMI (Table 45.1) [1]. The terms "severe obesity" (BMI 35–39.9), "morbid obesity" (BMI 40–49.9), and "super morbid obesity" (BMI ≥ 50) are also in occasional use [2].

What Medical Comorbidities Can Be Seen in Patients with a High BMI?

- Cardiovascular disease
  - Hypertension, coronary artery disease, heart failure, hyperlipidemia, cerebrovascular disease, thromboembolic disease
- Respiratory
  - Obstructive sleep apnea, obesity hypoventilation syndrome, pulmonary hypertension
- Endocrine
  - Diabetes mellitus, hypothyroidism, metabolic syndrome
- Gastrointestinal
  - Hiatus hernia, GERD, non-alcoholic fatty liver disease

D. Dillane (✉)
Department of Anesthesiology & Pain Medicine, University of Alberta, Edmonton, AB, Canada

D. Dillane, B. A. Finegan (eds.), *Preoperative Assessment*, https://doi.org/10.1007/978-3-030-58842-7_45

Vent. rate	94	BPM	Normal sinus rhythm
PR interval	156	ms	Low voltage QRS
QRS duration	70	ms	Nonspecific T wave abnormality
QT/QTc	344/430	ms	Abnormal ECG
P-R-T axes	45 16	7	

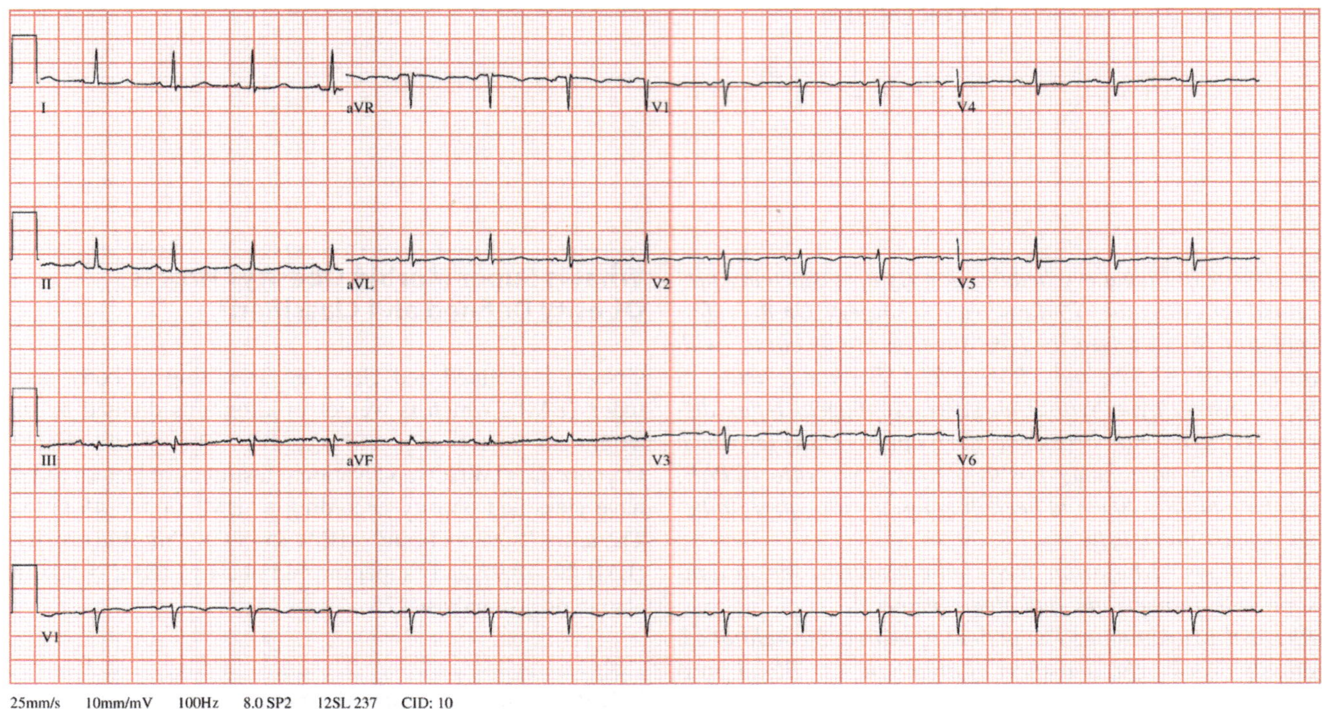

Fig. 45.1 Normal sinus rhythm. Low QRS voltage. Nonspecific T wave abnormality

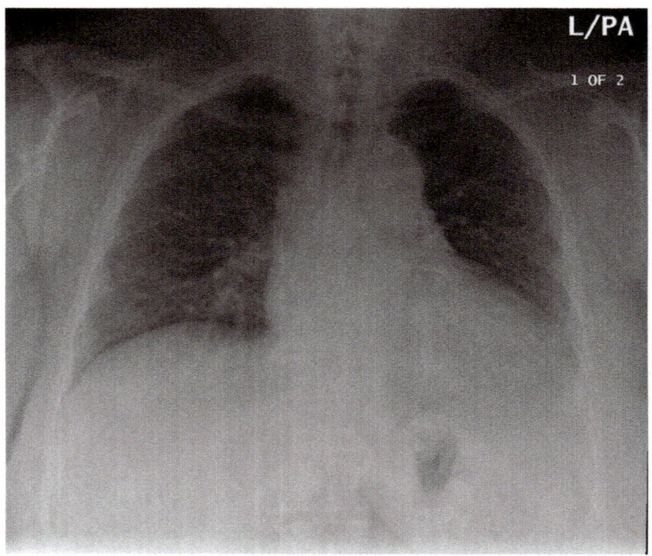

Fig. 45.2 Chest radiograph in full inspiration. The image quality is slightly limited by body habitus. Penetration is suboptimal, e.g., posterior ribs are difficult to see. Cardiomegaly is present—the left side of the heart is touching the left lateral chest wall, and the heart is over 50% of the diameter of the mediastinum. The diaphragm is raised on both sides

Table 45.1 Classification of obesity

Body mass index (BMI)	Classification
15–19.9	Underweight
20–24.9	Normal weight
25–29.9	Pre-obesity/overweight
30–34.9	Class I obesity
35–39.9	Class II obesity
≥40	Class III obesity

Adapted from the World Health Organization and the National Institutes of Health [1]

What Complications Is the Obese Patient Subject to in the Perioperative Period?

- Venous thromboembolism—obesity is an independent risk factor [3, 4]. Mechanical compression devices, early ambulation, and thromboprophylaxis with low molecular weight or unfractionated heparin are recommended by the American Society for Bariatric and Metabolic Surgery [5].
- Rhabdomyolysis.

- Wound infection—strong evidence exists for surgical site infection in obese patients undergoing a variety of orthopedic [6, 7] and non-orthopedic surgeries [8].
- Pulmonary aspiration secondary to GERD and/or the presence of a gastric band [9, 10].
- Atelectasis and pneumonia—found to be the two leading pulmonary complications following bariatric surgery in study of over 158,000 patients [11].
- Failed intubation.
- Postoperative cognitive decline.

What Physiological Changes Can Be Seen in the Respiratory System of the Obese Patient?

Respiratory mechanics are significantly altered in obesity. Reduction in chest wall compliance (secondary to increased chest wall mass) and lung compliance (secondary to the effects of increased intraabdominal pressure on the diaphragm) produces a restrictive pattern of lung impairment. Lung volumes are reduced, especially functional residual capacity (FRC), leading to de facto right-to-left shunting in dependent regions with ensuing rapid desaturation during apnea [12]. The increased resting metabolic rate of obesity leads to increased work of breathing and increased oxygen demands, resulting in rapid, shallow breathing.

What Is the Incidence of OSA in Obese Patients?

Severe OSA has been diagnosed in 10–20% patients with BMI > 35, and it may be undiagnosed in at least a further 10–20% [13]. Indeed, in a study of 1042 volunteers who underwent polysomnography, the incidence of moderate to severe OSA [apnea hypopnea index ≥15) was 11% in normal weight males, 21% in overweight males, and 63% in obese males [14].

How Is OSA Screened for in the Anesthesia Pre-admission Clinic?

The STOP-Bang screening questionnaire has been validated in several studies of surgical patients [15, 16] (Fig. 45.3). If positive, formal testing with overnight oximetry or polysomnography is appropriate in elective surgery when time permits. Polysomnography results will give an indication of severity of OSA. Risk of morbidity and mortality increases with increasing severity of OSA. CPAP is the usual mode of treatment for OSA. OSA patients who use CPAP should be questioned with regard to compliance with the device as well as device settings. It is normally set between 5 and 20 cm H_2O. A more comprehensive overview of OSA can be found in Chap. 13

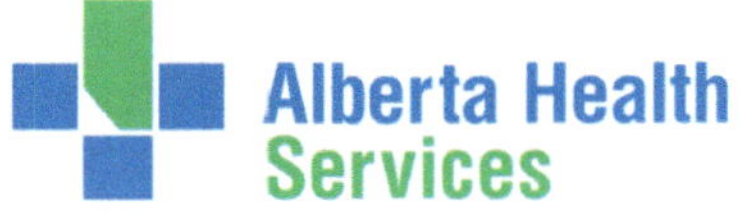

Patient Sticker

STOP-BANG Sleep Apnea Questionnaire
Chung F et al Anesthesiology 2008 and BJA 2012

STOP		
Do you SNORE loudly (louder than talking or loud enough to be heard through closed doors)?	Yes	No
Do you often feel TIRED, fatigued, or sleepy during daytime?	Yes	No
Has anyone OBSERVED you stop breathing during your sleep?	Yes	No
Do you have or are you being treated for high blood PRESSURE?	Yes	No
BANG	Yes	No
BMI more than 35kg/m2?	Yes	No
AGE over 50 years old?	Yes	No
NECK circumference > 16 inches (40cm)?	Yes	No
GENDER: Male?	Yes	No
TOTAL SCORE		

High risk of OSA: Yes 5 – 8; Intermediate risk of OSA: Yes 3 – 4; Low risk of OSA: Yes 0 – 2

Fig. 45.3 STOP-Bang questionnaire used at the authors' institution

What Is Obesity Hypoventilation Syndrome (OHS)?

OHS is a combination of daytime/awake hypoventilation and obesity which results in hypoxemia and hypercapnia. It is a diagnosis of exclusion made after other conditions known to be associated with hypoventilation have been ruled out. Patients with OHS have a significantly higher BMI compared to obese patients without hypercapnia [17]. In obese patients with OSA, the prevalence of OHS is estimated at 9–20% [18].

Why Do Obese Patients Get Pulmonary Hypertension?

This may be a consequence of untreated OSA, OHS, obesity-related heart failure, or chronic thromboembolic disease. OSA and OHS are independent risk factors for the development of pulmonary hypertension. Up to 20% of patients with OSA and as many as 50% of patients with OHS develop pulmonary hypertension [19].

Right Ventricular Systolic Pressure (RVSP) and Pulmonary Artery Systolic Pressure (PASP) Were Reported Together for our Patient. Is RVSP the Same as PASP?

RVSP is equal to PASP in the absence of right ventricular outflow tract obstruction [20]. Pulmonary hypertension and its diagnosis are explored in more detail in Chap. 8. Bearing in mind the limitations of echocardiography when compared with right heart catheterization for diagnosis of pulmonary hypertension, an echocardiography-derived PASP <40 mmHg is reassuring for ruling out the presence of pulmonary hypertension in the absence of other clinical or echocardiographic findings.

How Should Respiratory Function Be Assessed Preoperatively in the Obese Patient?

- If OSA is undiagnosed, use a validated screening tool, e.g., STOP-Bang score, and proceed to polysomnography or overnight oximetry if indicated.
- If OSA is diagnosed, assess compliance with CPAP treatment.
- Arterial blood gas (ABG) is useful for establishing baseline levels of hypoxemia and hypercapnia, if present. Moreover, a diagnosis of OHS is made using ABG on room air during wakefulness. $PaO_2 < 70$ mmHg and $PaCO_2 \geq 45$ mmHg indicate OHS [21]. Finally, serum $HCO_3 \geq 28$ mmol/L in the presence of a STOP-Bang score ≥ 3 increases the specificity of this screening tool to 85% for diagnosis of OSA [22].
- Chest radiograph may be useful if heart failure or risk factors are present.
- Spirometry and body plethysmography.
- Echocardiogram +/− right heart catheterization to assess for presence and severity of pulmonary hypertension.

What Perioperative Complications Is the Patient with OSA Subject To?

Several studies demonstrate a higher perioperative complication rate in the presence of OSA [23–25]. Indeed, untreated OSA can almost double (44% vs. 28%) the risk of postoperative cardiac and respiratory complications [26]. Complications reported across multiple studies include respiratory failure, opioid-exacerbated respiratory depression, aspiration pneumonia, emergency postoperative re-intubation, arrhythmia, myocardial infarction, confusion and delirium, unanticipated ICU admission, and prolonged duration of stay [26].

How Can the Obese Patient with OSA Be Optimized Preoperatively?

Compliance with CPAP use should be assessed. In a study of CPAP adherence of newly diagnosed OSA patients prior to elective surgery, only 25% were using their CPAP devices for ≥4.5 hours per night [27], the typical minimal number of hours of use thought to be of benefit. The systemic benefits of CPAP are well documented; when used as prescribed it has been shown to reduce postoperative blood pressure [28], cardiovascular complications [29], and length of stay [30]. Clinical improvement becomes significant after 3 months of CPAP therapy, and a shorter period may be beneficial [31].

Are Obese Patients More Difficult to Intubate? Are Any Airway Evaluation Techniques of Specific Value in This Patient Population?

This is controversial, and the evidence is not overwhelming for or against. The Fourth National Audit Project (NAP4) found airway problems to occur twice as commonly in obese and four times as commonly in morbidly obese patients compared with patients with BMI ≤ 30 [32]. However, "airway problems" do not equate to difficult intubation. Airway problems also included supraglottic airway-related problems, failed face mask ventilation, and extubation-related problems. The proportion of primary airway problems related to intubation was similar in obese and non-obese patients in this large audit. The primary airway problems which did occur more frequently in obese patients were related to supraglottic device placement and failed mask ventilation. Further evidence can be found in a retrospective study of almost 500,000 patients in four tertiary care centers which found that BMI ≥ 30 was an independent risk factor for difficult mask ventilation combined with difficult direct laryngoscopy, i.e., simultaneous occurrence [33].

Short neck, higher neck circumference, Mallampati score III or IV, and mandibular protrusion have been associated with difficult mask ventilation in obese patients [34]. Mallampati score III or IV, OSA, reduced cervical spine mobility, thyromental distance, and neck circumference have been identified as risk factors for difficult intubation in obese patients [35, 36]. A finding of note in all of these studies is that predictors of difficult intubation in obese patients are no different than those in non-obese patients.

What Physiological Changes Can Be Seen in the Cardiovascular System in the Presence of Obesity?

- Left ventricular failure: Increased total body weight promotes a larger circulating blood volume and cardiac output. This increase in cardiac output is generated by an elevation in stroke volume. The increased systolic workload leads to left ventricular (LV) hypertrophy, which progresses over time to LV dilatation and LV failure. LV diastolic dysfunction also develops, resulting in incomplete left atrial (LA) emptying, LA dilatation, and atrial fibrillation [37]. LVF in the presence of sleep apnea/obesity hyperventilation-induced pulmonary hypertension may be accompanied by right ventricular failure (RVF).
- Hypertension: The increased prevalence of primary hypertension in obesity is multifactorial in pathogenesis. Endothelial dysfunction and atherosclerosis in combination with pathological activation of the renin-angiotensin-aldosterone system and altered sodium metabolism have all been implicated [17].
- Coronary artery disease: Diabetes, dyslipidemia, hypertension, and a chronic inflammatory and prothrombotic state are risk factors for myocardial infarction in obesity.

What ECG Abnormalities Are Associated with Obesity?

Most ECG changes seen in obese patients result from altered cardiac morphology, although fatty infiltration of the conduction system can cause arrhythmias [37]. More commonly seen alterations include leftward shift of the P, QRS, and T wave axes (reversible with significant weight loss), alterations in P wave morphology, changes associated with left ventricular hypertrophy, low QRS voltage, T wave flattening in the inferolateral leads, and QT interval prolongation [38]. There have been several case reports of sudden death in obese individuals usually involving co-existent LVH and/or congestive cardiac failure [39, 40].

How Is the Obese Patient Assessed Preoperatively from a Cardiac Perspective?

- A focused history should assess for the presence of hypertension, hyperlipidemia, diabetes, symptoms of coronary artery disease, cardiac failure, and peripheral vascular disease, e.g., transient ischemic attacks (TIAs) or intermittent claudication.
- The Revised Cardiac Risk Index (RCRI) and the American College of Surgeons National Surgical Quality Improvement Program (NSQIP) risk model calculator can be useful in determining which patients require further investigation [41, 42].
- Typical symptomatology of coronary artery disease may not be available as a result of the patient's physical inactivity or immobility. If functional assessment, e.g., metabolic equivalent (MET) or Duke Activity Status Index (DASI) score [43], is not helpful or indicates poor functional capacity, a dobutamine stress echocardiogram or myocardial perfusion scan proceeding to angiography as appropriate should be performed where clinical suspicion is strong [44, 45].
- The decision to proceed to angiography after abnormal pharmacological stress testing depends on the patient's willingness to undergo a revascularization procedure (angiography and stenting or coronary artery bypass grafting), and the urgency of the elective surgery under consideration. The American College of Cardiology/American Heart Association Guideline on Perioperative Cardiovascular Evaluation and Management of Patients Undergoing Noncardiac Surgery can be a useful guide in this regard [46].
- For patients with heart failure who are clinically stable, resting preoperative echocardiography is not routinely recommended for cardiac risk estimation unless there is evidence of an undiagnosed severe obstructive abnormality, e.g., aortic stenosis, mitral stenosis, or severe pulmonary hypertension [47]. If echocardiography is indicated, a transthoracic approach may not provide adequate views.

Is the Management of Hypertension Any Different in Obese Versus Non-obese Patients?

In obese patients, ACE inhibitors and angiotensin II receptor blockers (ARBs) are the first line of treatment. This is based on the role of the renin-angiotensin-aldosterone system in the pathogenesis of hypertension in obesity. Moreover, ACE inhibitors and ARBs may be beneficial as a result of their ability to increase insulin sensitivity [48]. A thiazide or loop diuretic can be used as a second-line agent or in combination with an ACE inhibitor. Care must be taken with thiazides, as they may exacerbate insulin resistance and dyslipidemia [49]. Beta blockers, particularly of the non-vasodilating variety, e.g., metoprolol and atenolol, unless specifically indicated for treatment of atrial fibrillation, should be avoided due to their association with insulin resistance.

What Is Metabolic Syndrome?

In simple terms, it is the co-existence of multiple risk factors for type 2 diabetes and cardiovascular disease. At various times, it has also been called insulin resistance syndrome, syndrome X, and obesity dyslipidemia syndrome. Several definitions exist, the most common being that of the National Cholesterol Education Program, which says that metabolic syndrome requires three or more of the following criteria [50]:

(a) Abdominal obesity (waist circumference >102 cm in males and >88 cm in females)
(b) Glucose intolerance (fasting glucose ≥110 mg/dL)
(c) Hypertension (≥130 mmHg systolic and / or ≥85 mmHg diastolic)
(d) Hypertriglyceridemia ≥150 mg/dL
(e) HDL cholesterol <40 mg/dL in males and <50 mg/dL in females

The incidence of metabolic syndrome in the Bariatric Outcomes Longitudinal Database investigation of more than 158,000 bariatric surgery patients was 12.7%. It was an independent significant risk factor for postoperative pulmonary complications [11].

Is Awareness More Common in Obese Patients?

The Fifth National Audit (NAP5) into awareness under anesthesia found that obesity is associated with a higher risk of accidental awareness [51]. Several reasons were postulated, including inadequate drug dosing secondary to the altered pharmacokinetics seen in obesity, i.e., increased body fat content, blood volume, and cardiac output in combination with alterations in plasma protein binding. The association between obesity and difficult airway was also implicated, though evidence is lacking.

The possibility of performing this surgery under a regional anesthesia technique was proposed by the patient's surgical team. A paravertebral or epidural block would be required to provide surgical anesthesia for this patient. High thoracic neuraxial and paravertebral techniques require an advanced skill set even in non-obese individuals. The higher risk of failure was deemed not acceptable in this instance, and the option was not explored further. The need for urgent airway intervention after failed regional anesthesia is a concept also explored in NAP4 [32]. *Awake fiberoptic intubation in controlled circumstances was opted for and successfully executed. Regional anesthesia may have been an option as part of a multimodal analgesia approach with the aim of reducing opioid use and associated postoperative complications. The patient was admitted for overnight monitoring. Regarding suitability for ambulatory surgery, this decision must be made on a per case basis, taking into account comorbidities, severity of OSA, surgical risk, type of anesthesia delivered, and home support. Currently, there is insufficient evidence available to create guidelines for obese patients undergoing ambulatory surgery, a fact acknowledged by the Society for Ambulatory Anesthesia on Clinical Practice Guidelines* [52].

True/False Questions

1. (a) A patient classified as having super morbid obesity could also be said to have class II obesity.
   (b) There is strong evidence that obesity is an independent risk factor for the development of postoperative wound infection.
   (c) Pneumothorax resulting from positive pressure ventilation is a common perioperative complication.
   (d) Increased neck circumference has been identified as a predictor of difficult intubation in obese patients.
   (e) ACE inhibitors are contraindicated for the management of hypertension in obesity.
2. (a) The STOP-Bang questionnaire is not validated for use in obese patients.
   (b) Obesity hypoventilation syndrome by definition occurs in awake patients.
   (c) CPAP for OSA is not effective when used for less than 6.5 hours per night.
   (d) Untreated OSA has been shown to almost double the risk of postoperative pulmonary and cardiac complications.
   (e) Measurement of serum HCO3 ≥ 28 mmol/L in the presence of a STOP-Bang score ≥ 3 increases the specificity of this screening tool.

References

1. Clinical guidelines on the identification, evaluation, and treatment of overweight and obesity in adults—the evidence report. National Institutes of Health. Obes Res. 1998;6(Suppl 2):51S–209S.
2. Suter M, Calmes JM, Paroz A, Romy S, Giusti V. Results of Roux-en-Y gastric bypass in morbidly obese vs superobese patients: similar body weight loss, correction of comorbidities, and improvement of quality of life. Arch Surg. 2009;144(4):312–8. discussion 8

3. Vandiver JW, Ritz LI, Lalama JT. Chemical prophylaxis to prevent venous thromboembolism in morbid obesity: literature review and dosing recommendations. J Thromb Thrombolysis. 2016;41(3):475–81.
4. Gould MK, Garcia DA, Wren SM, Karanicolas PJ, Arcelus JI, Heit JA, et al. Prevention of VTE in nonorthopedic surgical patients: antithrombotic therapy and prevention of thrombosis, 9th ed: American College of Chest Physicians Evidence-Based Clinical Practice Guidelines. Chest. 2012;141(2 Suppl):e227S–e77S.
5. American Society for Metabolic and Bariatric Surgery Clinical Issues Committee. ASMBS updated position statement on prophylactic measures to reduce the risk of venous thromboembolism in bariatric surgery patients. Surg Obes Relat Dis. 2013;9(4):493–7.
6. Olsen LL, Moller AM, Brorson S, Hasselager RB, Sort R. The impact of lifestyle risk factors on the rate of infection after surgery for a fracture of the ankle. Bone Joint J. 2017;99-B(2):225–30.
7. Ward DT, Metz LN, Horst PK, Kim HT, Kuo AC. Complications of morbid obesity in total joint arthroplasty: risk stratification based on BMI. J Arthroplast. 2015;30(9 Suppl):42–6.
8. Thelwall S, Harrington P, Sheridan E, Lamagni T. Impact of obesity on the risk of wound infection following surgery: results from a nationwide prospective multicentre cohort study in England. Clin Microbiol Infect. 2015;21(11):1008 e1–8.
9. Kocian R, Spahn DR. Bronchial aspiration in patients after weight loss due to gastric banding. Anesth Analg. 2005;100(6):1856–7.
10. Jean J, Compere V, Fourdrinier V, Marguerite C, Auquit-Auckbur I, Milliez PY, et al. The risk of pulmonary aspiration in patients after weight loss due to bariatric surgery. Anesth Analg. 2008;107(4):1257–9.
11. Schumann R, Shikora SA, Sigl JC, Kelley SD. Association of metabolic syndrome and surgical factors with pulmonary adverse events, and longitudinal mortality in bariatric surgery. Br J Anaesth. 2015;114(1):83–90.
12. Jense HG, Dubin SA, Silverstein PI, O'Leary-Escolas U. Effect of obesity on safe duration of apnea in anesthetized humans. Anesth Analg. 1991;72(1):89–93.
13. Lang LH, Parekh K, Tsui BYK, Maze M. Perioperative management of the obese surgical patient. Br Med Bull. 2017;124(1):135–55.
14. Tufik S, Santos-Silva R, Taddei JA, Bittencourt LR. Obstructive sleep apnea syndrome in the Sao Paulo epidemiologic sleep study. Sleep Med. 2010;11(5):441–6.
15. Tan A, Yin JD, Tan LW, van Dam RM, Cheung YY, Lee CH. Predicting obstructive sleep apnea using the STOP-Bang questionnaire in the general population. Sleep Med. 2016;27-28:66–71.
16. Doshi V, Walia R, Jones K, Aston CE, Awab A. STOP-BANG questionnaire as a screening tool for diagnosis of obstructive sleep apnea by unattended portable monitoring sleep study. Springerplus. 2015;4:795.
17. Lukosiute A, Karmali A, Cousins JM. Anaesthetic preparation of obese patients: current status on optimal work-up. Curr Obes Rep. 2017;6(3):229–37.
18. Balachandran J, Masa J, Mokhlesi B. Obesity hypoventilation syndrome. Sleep Med Clin. 2014;9:341–7.
19. Friedman SE, Andrus BW. Obesity and pulmonary hypertension: a review of pathophysiologic mechanisms. J Obes. 2012;2012:505274.
20. Armstrong DW, Tsimiklis G, Matangi MF. Factors influencing the echocardiographic estimate of right ventricular systolic pressure in normal patients and clinically relevant ranges according to age. Can J Cardiol. 2010;26(2):e35–9.
21. Chau EH, Mokhlesi B, Chung F. Obesity hypoventilation syndrome and anesthesia. Sleep Med Clin. 2013;8(1):135–47.
22. Chung F, Chau E, Yang Y, Liao P, Hall R, Mokhlesi B. Serum bicarbonate level improves specificity of STOP-Bang screening for obstructive sleep apnea. Chest. 2013;143(5):1284–93.
23. Gupta RM, Parvizi J, Hanssen AD, Gay PC. Postoperative complications in patients with obstructive sleep apnea syndrome undergoing hip or knee replacement: a case-control study. Mayo Clin Proc. 2001;76(9):897–905.
24. Memtsoudis S, Liu SS, Ma Y, Chiu YL, Walz JM, Gaber-Baylis LK, et al. Perioperative pulmonary outcomes in patients with sleep apnea after noncardiac surgery. Anesth Analg. 2011;112(1):113–21.
25. Opperer M, Cozowicz C, Bugada D, Mokhlesi B, Kaw R, Auckley D, et al. Does obstructive sleep apnea influence perioperative outcome? A qualitative systematic review for the Society of Anesthesia and Sleep Medicine Task Force on preoperative preparation of patients with sleep-disordered breathing. Anesth Analg. 2016;122(5):1321–34.
26. Vasu TS, Grewal R, Doghramji K. Obstructive sleep apnea syndrome and perioperative complications: a systematic review of the literature. J Clin Sleep Med. 2012;8(2):199–207.
27. Guralnick AS, Pant M, Minhaj M, Sweitzer BJ, Mokhlesi B. CPAP adherence in patients with newly diagnosed obstructive sleep apnea prior to elective surgery. J Clin Sleep Med. 2012;8(5):501–6.
28. Gottlieb DJ, Punjabi NM, Mehra R, Patel SR, Quan SF, Babineau DC, et al. CPAP versus oxygen in obstructive sleep apnea. N Engl J Med. 2014;370(24):2276–85.
29. Mutter TC, Chateau D, Moffatt M, Ramsey C, Roos LL, Kryger M. A matched cohort study of postoperative outcomes in obstructive sleep apnea: could preoperative diagnosis and treatment prevent complications? Anesthesiology. 2014;121(4) 707–18.
30. Nagappa M, Mokhlesi B, Wong J, Wong DT, Kaw R, Chung F. The effects of continuous positive airway pressure on postoperative outcomes in obstructive sleep apnea patients undergoing surgery: a systematic review and meta-analysis. Anesth Analg. 2015;120(5):1013–23.
31. Xie X, Pan L, Ren D, Guo Y. Effects of continuous positive airway pressure on systemic inflammation in obstructive sleep apnea: a meta-analysis. Sleep Med. 2013;14:1139–50.
32. Cook T, Woodall N, Frerk C, editors. 4th National Audit Project of The Royal College of Anaesthetists and The Difficult Airway Society. Major complications of airway management in the United Kingdom. Report and findings March 2011: The Difficult Airway society; 2011. https://www.nationalauditprojects.org.uk/downloads/NAP4%20Full%20Report.pdf. Accessd 7 Jun 2020.
33. Kheterpal S, Healy D, Aziz MF, Shanks AM, Freundlich RE, Linton F, et al. Incidence, predictors, and outcome of difficult mask ventilation combined with difficult laryngoscopy: a report from the multicenter perioperative outcomes group. Anesthesiology. 2013;119(6):1360–9.
34. Leoni A, Arlati S, Ghisi D, Verwej M, Lugani D, Ghisi P, et al. Difficult mask ventilation in obese patients: analysis of predictive factors. Minerva Anestesiol. 2014;80(2):149–57.
35. Gonzalez H, Minville V, Delanoue K, Mazerolles M, Concina D, Fourcade O. The importance of increased neck circumference to intubation difficulties in obese patients. Anesth Analg. 2008;106(4):1132–6.
36. De Jong A, Molinari N, Pouzeratte Y, Verzilli D, Chanques G, Jung B, et al. Difficult intubation in obese patients: incidence, risk factors, and complications in the operating theatre and in intensive care units. Br J Anaesth. 2015;114(2):297–306.
37. Nelson G, Clayton R. Anaesthesia in the obese patient. Anaesth Intensive Care Med. 2017;18(10):472–6.
38. Fraley MA, Birchem JA, Senkottaiyan N, Alpert MA. Obesity and the electrocardiogram. Obes Rev. 2005;6(4):275–81.
39. Warnes CA, Roberts WC. The heart in massive (more than 300 pounds or 136 kilograms) obesity: analysis of 12 patients studied at necropsy. Am J Cardiol. 1984;54(8):1087–91.
40. Messerli FH, Nunez BD, Ventura HO, Snyder DW. Overweight and sudden death. Increased ventricular ectopy in cardiopathy of obesity. Arch Intern Med. 1987;147(10):1725–8.
41. Lee TH, Marcantonio ER, Mangione CM, Thomas EJ, Polanczyk CA, Cook EF, et al. Derivation and prospective validation of a sim-

ple index for prediction of cardiac risk of major noncardiac surgery. Circulation. 1999;100(10):1043–9.
42. Bilimoria KY, Liu Y, Paruch JL, Zhou L, Kmiecik TE, Ko CY, et al. Development and evaluation of the universal ACS NSQIP surgical risk calculator: a decision aid and informed consent tool for patients and surgeons. J Am Coll Surg. 2013;217(5):833–42.e1-3.
43. Wijeysundera DN, Pearse RM, Shulman MA, Abbott TEF, Torres E, Ambosta A, et al. Assessment of functional capacity before major non-cardiac surgery: an international, prospective cohort study. Lancet. 2018;391(10140):2631–40.
44. Poirier P, Alpert MA, Fleisher LA, Thompson PD, Sugerman HJ, Burke LE, et al. Cardiovascular evaluation and management of severely obese patients undergoing surgery: a science advisory from the American Heart Association. Circulation. 2009;120(1):86–95.
45. Shah BN, Senior R. Stress echocardiography in patients with morbid obesity. Echo Res Pract. 2016;3(2):R13–8.
46. Fleisher LA, Fleischmann KE, Auerbach AD, Barnason SA, Beckman JA, Bozkurt B, et al. 2014 ACC/AHA guideline on perioperative cardiovascular evaluation and management of patients undergoing noncardiac surgery: a report of the American College of Cardiology/American Heart Association Task Force on Practice Guidelines. Circulation. 2014;130(24):e278–333.
47. Duceppe E, Parlow J, MacDonald P, Lyons K, McMullen M, Srinathan S, et al. Canadian cardiovascular society guidelines on perioperative cardiac risk assessment and management for patients who undergo noncardiac surgery. Can J Cardiol. 2017;33(1):17–32.
48. Sharma AM, Pischon T, Engeli S, Scholze J. Choice of drug treatment for obesity-related hypertension: where is the evidence? J Hypertens. 2001;19(4):667–74.
49. Landsberg L, Aronne LJ, Beilin LJ, Burke V, Igel LI, Lloyd-Jones D, et al. Obesity-related hypertension: pathogenesis, cardiovascular risk, and treatment–a position paper of the the Obesity Society and the American Society of Hypertension. Obesity (Silver Spring). 2013;21(1):8–24.
50. National Cholesterol Education Program Expert Panel on Detection E, Treatment of High Blood Cholesterol in A, Third report of the National Cholesterol Education Program (NCEP) expert panel on detection, evaluation, and treatment of high blood cholesterol in adults (adult treatment panel III) final report. Circulation. 2002;106(25):3143–421.
51. Pandit JJ, Andrade J, Bogod DG, Hitchman JM, Jonker WR, Lucas N, et al. 5th National Audit Project (NAP5) on accidental awareness during general anaesthesia: summary of main findings and risk factors. Br J Anaesth. 2014;113(4):549–59.
52. Joshi GP, Ahmad S, Riad W, Eckert S, Chung F. Selection of obese patients undergoing ambulatory surgery: a systematic review of the literature. Anesth Analg. 2013;117(5):1082–91.

The Frail Patient

46

Barry A. Finegan and Rachel G. Khadaroo

A 90-year-old male presented with a cecal cancer. He was quite active with a Duke Activity Score of six. He was able to walk approximately 3 km a day. He did not smoke. He lived independently in a lodge where there are common meals, but he performed all of his activities of daily living. He had a past medical history of a prostatectomy, myocardial infarction 10 years before presentation with two drug-eluting stents inserted at that time, hypertension, hyperlipidemia, gastroesophageal reflux disease, thyroid disease, COPD, emphysema, and glaucoma.

Medications: Tamsulosin 0.4 mg po at HS, metoprolol 25 mg po BID, levothyroxine 35 mcg OD, atorvastatin 10 mg at HS, and ASA 81 mg, enteric coated, OD.

Investigations: His laboratory data were within normal limits except for his hemoglobin which was 80 g/L. His ECG showed evidence of a past inferior wall myocardial infarction. An MIBI showed no defined defects with an LVEF > 65%. An echocardiogram indicated normal systolic ventricular function, mild LV diastolic dysfunction, and no hemodynamically significant valvular disease. Abdominal CT confirmed the findings of a previous colonoscopy and demonstrated cecal cancer with no metastatic disease.

His surgeon was unsure if he should proceed to laparoscopic surgery and requested preoperative assessment and suggestions for optimization.

What Are the Physiological Changes Associated with Advanced Age?

This subject has recently been comprehensively reviewed by Young and Maguire [1]. With aging, cognitive function is decreased, independent of dementia, due to neuronal loss, reduced neuronal growth and synaptic dysfunction. These changes make the older patient more vulnerable to delirium. The impairment of sensory functions, especially vision and auditory capabilities, can present practical and cognitive challenges. Pulmonary function begins an inexorable decline in most individuals after the mid-30s. Structural reductions in elastic recoil, increased chest wall rigidity, and decreased respiratory muscle effort reduce effective lung volumes, and closing capacity reaches supine functional residual capacity by the mid-40s. Ventilation-perfusion mismatch is increased with age as the changes redistribute ventilation towards the less perfused apices of the lungs. Diffusion capacity also diminishes with age. The cardiovascular system undergoes a plethora of changes with aging [2]. One of the most consequential is the loss of elastin in the media of the vascular tree and its replacement by collagen and Ca^{++}. These alterations increase pulse wave velocity and augment systolic blood pressure, which in turn evokes compensatory changes in myocyte physiology, function, and structure, enhancing vulnerability to cardiac ischemia, infarction and failure. Baroreceptor and β-receptor function deteriorate impairing blood pressure stability, particularly under anesthesia or preload-reduced conditions. Temperature regulation is less effective, and basal metabolic rate is reduced with aging underscoring the need for assessment of nutritional status during preoperative assessment.

B. A. Finegan (✉)
Department of Anesthesiology & Pain Medicine, University of Alberta, Edmonton, AB, Canada
e-mail: bfinegan@ualberta.ca

R. G. Khadaroo
Department of Surgery, University of Alberta, Edmonton, AB, Canada

D. Dillane, B. A. Finegan (eds.), *Preoperative Assessment*, https://doi.org/10.1007/978-3-030-58842-7_46

How Does Aging Influence Medication Kinetics?

Body water content and muscle mass decrease up to 30% with age and fat content may increase by 30%, leading to altered volumes of drug distribution, in addition, glomerular filtration rate and liver blood flow decrease, as does enzymatic function, prolonging drug elimination half-lives [3]. Drug dynamics are also influenced by age-related decreases in receptor density, function, and signaling. In the case of anesthetic drugs, titration and reduction in the administered dose by up to 50% may be warranted.

It is now well established that older patients can be subject to underuse of appropriate drugs, overuse of inappropriate drugs, failure to recognize adverse drug events, polypharmacy (> five drugs/day), and failure to adjust drug dosing in the face of reduced renal function/lean body mass.

In the perioperative setting, renal function should be assessed as many drugs indicated in the management of age-related conditions are subject to renal elimination. These include sotalol, olmesartan, metformin, most antibiotics, lithium, rivaroxaban, and apixaban. All nonessential medications and supplements should be discontinued.

What Is Frailty?

There is no universally agreed definition of frailty, but it describes an increased risk of adverse outcome for individuals of the same chronological age [4]. Frailty indices relate deficit accumulation such as inability to perform routine physical tasks, recent weight loss, perceived mental status, co-existing disease, and impaired physical fitness to a vulnerability state that portends an adverse outcome in the face of even relatively minor stresses [5]. Frailty has also been described phenotypically where the presence of specific physical attributes such as self-reported exhaustion, unintentional weight loss, poor grip strength, and slowness on walking define, depending on how many are present, the degree of frailty [6]. Both these approaches have limitations [7], not the least being the role of weighting of individual deficits or physical attributes to risk outcome. Nevertheless, these measures of frailty offer a general framework for identifying a cohort who are greater risk from an otherwise relatively minor trespass.

How Can Frailty Be Identified in the Preoperative Clinic?

There are multiple scales available to assess aged individuals with the goal of identifying the frail subgroup. When studied in the surgical setting, most, if not all, appear to identify those patients most at risk for death. In an elegant review of this topic, McIsaac et al [8]. concluded that the Clinical Frailty Scale (CFS) is an instrument that seems reasonable to use in the busy preoperative setting. The CFS (Fig. 46.1) scores subjects from 1 (Very fit) to 9 (Terminally ill) with those scoring 5 (Mildly frail – needs help in high-order independent activities of daily living such as shopping, walking outside alone, meal preparation, and housework), or above, being described as being in varying degrees of frailty. The CFS score can be rapidly obtained and does not require any special training or equipment to administer.

Is Frailty Associated with Adverse Outcome Following Surgery?

There is a clear relationship between frailty and surgical morbidity and mortality [9].There is emerging data that subjecting frail or very frail patients to low stress (e.g., inguinal hernia repair) or moderate stress procedures (e.g., cholecystectomy) may result in 90-day mortality rates approaching 10% and 30%, respectively [10].

Can One Predict Which Individual Patient Is Most Likely to Die Using a Frailty Scale?

This is not a question that can be answered using frailty scales [11]. What is clear is that, even for those of identical chronological age, being *frail* as distinct from *not frail* carries with it a significant burden of morbidity and mortality after both elective and emergency surgery. Awareness and identification of frailty allows patients consider risk appropriately and can facilitate directed interventions to possibly improve outcome. For those undergoing surgical procedures who already have limited life expectancy, risk of death may not be as important as an improvement in the quality of remaining life promised by the surgical intervention [12]. Here too, identification of frailty, provides context and facilitates choice.

Are There Interventions That Can Ameliorate Adverse Outcomes of Surgery in the Elderly?

Encouragingly, there is emerging evidence that adapting proven models of geriatric care in medical patients to the surgical setting can result in a decrease in major complications and death even in emergency surgery [13]. This approach is built on the concept that patient co-location, interdisciplinary team care, mindfulness of geriatric physiology/pharmacodynamics, and focused rehabilitation can positively influence outcome. In addition, in the elective surgical population targeted interventions to improve physical performance, nutrition, and manage mental issues *prior* to surgery may offer promise in reducing morbidity and mortality in older patients [8].

Clinical Frailty Scale*

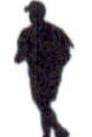
1 **Very Fit** – People who are robust, active, energetic and motivated. These people commonly exercise regularly. They are among the fittest for their age.

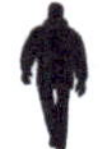
2 **Well** – People who have **no active disease symptoms** but are less fit than category 1. Often, they exercise or are very **active occasionally**, e.g. seasonally.

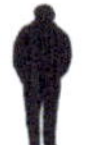
3 **Managing Well** – People whose **medical problems are well controlled**, but are **not regularly active** beyond routine walking.

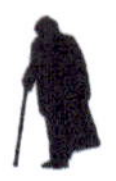
4 **Vulnerable** – While **not dependent** on others for daily help, often **symptoms limit activities.** A common complaint is being "slowed up", and/or being tired during the day.

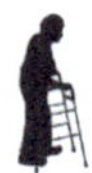
5 **Mildly Frail** – These people often have **more evident slowing,** and need help in **high order IADLs** (finances, transportation, heavy housework, medications). Typically, mild frailty progressively impairs shopping and walking outside alone, meal preparation and housework.

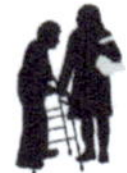
6 **Moderately Frail** – People need help with **all outside activities** and with **keeping house**. Inside, they often have problems with stairs and need **help with bathing** and might need minimal assistance (cuing, standby) with dressing.

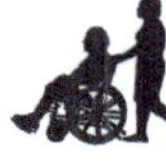
7 **Severely Frail** – **Completely dependent for personal care**, from whatever cause (physical or cognitive). Even so, they seem stable and not at high risk of dying (within ~ 6 months).

8 **Very Severely Frail** – Completely dependent, approaching the end of life. Typically, they could not recover even from a minor illness.

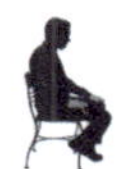
9. **Terminally Ill** - Approaching the end of life. This category applies to people with **a life expectancy <6 months**, who are **not otherwise evidently frail.**

Scoring frailty in people with dementia

The degree of frailty corresponds to the degree of dementia. Common **symptoms in mild dementia** include forgetting the details of a recent event, though still remembering the event itself, repeating the same question/story and social withdrawal.

In **moderate dementia**, recent memory is very impaired, even though they seemingly can remember their past life events well. They can do personal care with prompting.

In **severe dementia**, they cannot do personal care without help.

* 1. Canadian Study on Health & Aging, Revised 2008.
2. K. Rockwood et al. A global clinical measure of fitness and frailty in elderly people. CMAJ 2005;173:489-495.

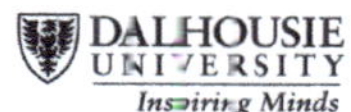

Fig. 46.1 Clinical Frailty Score developed by the AGMS Research Group (https://www.dal.ca/sites/gmr/our-tools/clinical-frailty-scale/cfs-guidance.html), (Courtesy of and with permission of Dalhousie University, Halifax, Nova Scotia, Canada)

What Are the Specific Issues That Should Be Addressed in the Preoperative Assessment of the Frail Patient?

Best practice recommendations regarding the perioperative care of the geriatric patient have been published by the American College of Surgeons and the American Geriatrics Society [14]. The following issues should be addressed during the preoperative visit:

(a) The treatment preferences of the patient and documentation of advanced directives
(b) Documentation of the proxy or surrogate decision maker
(c) Comprehensive discussion of risks and what responses are acceptable in the face of life-threatening problems
(d) Consider shortened clear fluid fasting (allow up to 2 hours preoperatively)
(e) Follow medication recommendations as discussed above
(f) Offer regional anesthesia techniques if feasible
(g) Develop a postoperative pain management plan using an opioid-sparing technique

The patient had made a living will and had delegated durable power of attorney to his son. He indicated that he did not want to be resuscitated beyond limited immediate measures should an emergency arise. He was willing to be treated in an intensive care unit but did not want extraordinary measures used to keep him alive. The patient scored 3 on the CFS – managing well – medical problems well controlled but rarely active beyond walking. As such, he was not considered frail. As he denied dyspnea on exertion, angina, or any symptoms of congestive heart failure and his cardiovascular examination was normal, no further cardiac investigations were ordered. He was seen by a geriatrician, and planned admission to a step-down unit followed by a stay in a postoperative geriatric surgical care ward was organized. He was booked for admission to a rehabilitation center after hospital discharge to facilitate his ongoing recovery. The acute pain service was consulted to assist in postoperative management and follow up. Continuous postoperative rectus sheath blockade was preferred to epidural analgesia, owing to the more favorable hemodynamic side-effect profile of the former. The surgeon was informed that the patient was a good candidate for elective surgery given the circumstances and that no further interventions were required. He was admitted to hospital the day before his procedure.

Surgery proceeded uneventfully, but his stay in hospital was moderately prolonged (11 days) before discharge to the rehabilitation center. He was not readmitted and was recovering well when last assessed 6 weeks after the procedure.

True/False Questions

1. The following are normal features of aging:
   (a) A decrease in cognitive function
   (b) Redistribution of ventilation to the base of the lungs
   (c) A decrease in pulse wave velocity due to replacement of elastin by collagen
   (d) Body water content decreases of up to 30%
   (e) An increase in β-receptor density
2. In patients older than 65 years of age
   (a) inability to perform routine physical tasks is a marker of frailty
   (b) a frailty assessment may be helpful in determining risk
   (c) if frailty is diagnosed then a CT should be performed to our rule a cerebral lesion
   (d) polypharmacy is not uncommon
   (e) renal function should be assessed before major surgery

References

1. Young F, Maguire S. Physiology of ageing. Anaesth Intensive Care Med. 2019;20(12):735–8.
2. Singam NSV, Fine C, Fleg JL. Cardiac changes associated with vascular aging. Clin Cardiol. 2020;43(2):92–8.
3. Thürmann PA. Pharmacodynamics and pharmacokinetics in older adults. Curr Opin Anaesthesiol. 2020;33(1):109–13.
4. Rockwood K, Howlett SE. Fifteen years of progress in understanding frailty and health in aging. BMC Med. 2018;16(1):1–4.
5. Searle SD, Mitnitski A, Gahbauer EA, Gill TM, Rockwood K. A standard procedure for creating a frailty index. BMC Geriatr. 2008;8:1–10.
6. Fried LP, Tangen CM, Walston J, Newman AB, Hirsch C, Gottdiener J, Cardiovascular Health Study Collaborative Research Group, et al. Frailty in older adults: evidence for a phenotype. J Gerontol A Biol Sci Med Sci. 2001;56(3):M146–56.
7. Chao YS, Wu HC, Wu CJ, Chen WC. Index or illusion: the case of frailty indices in the health and retirement study. PLoS One. 2018;13(7):e0197859.
8. McIsaac DI, MacDonald DB, Aucoin SD. Frailty for perioperative clinicians: a narrative review. Anesth Analg. 2020;130(6):1450–60.
9. Makary MA, Segev DL, Pronovost PJ, Syin D, Bandeen-Roche K, Patel P, et al. Frailty as a predictor of surgical outcomes in older patients. J Am Coll Surg. 2010;210(6):901–8.
10. Shinall MC Jr, Arya S, Youk A, Varley P, Shah R, Massarweh NN, et al. Association of preoperative patient frailty and operative stress with postoperative mortality. JAMA Surg. 2019;155(1):e194620.
11. McIsaac DI, Taljaard M, Bryson GL, Beaulé PE, Gagné S, Hamilton G, et al. Frailty as a predictor of death or new disability after surgery: a prospective cohort study. Ann Surg. 2020;271(2):283–9.
12. Shellito A, Russell MM, Rosenthal RA. Looking beyond mortality among older adults who are frail and considering surgical intervention. JAMA Surg. 2020;155(1):e194638.
13. Khadaroo RG, Warkentin LM, Wagg AS, Padwal RS, Clement F, Wang X, et al. Clinical effectiveness of the elder-friendly approaches to the surgical environment initiative in emergency general surgery. JAMA Surg. 2020;155(4):e196021.
14. Mohanty S, Rosenthal RA, Russell MM, Neuman MD, Ko CY, Esnaola NF. Optimal perioperative Management of the Geriatric Patient: a best practices guideline from the American College of Surgeons NSQIP and the American Geriatrics Society. J Am Coll Surg. 2016;222(5):930–47.

The Opioid-Tolerant Patient

47

Derek Dillane and Chris Douglas

A 21-year-old male patient was seen prior to total pancreatectomy and auto islet cell transplantation for intractable abdominal pain secondary to recurrent pancreatitis. He was noted to have hereditary pancreatitis due to a PRSS1 *mutation. He had a 10-year history of episodic abdominal pain that had been increasing in frequency and intensity in the year leading up to the current evaluation. He had a normal glucose tolerance test, and on his most recent surgical consultation, it was reported that he had no evidence of diarrhea, steatorrhea, or weight loss. Consequently, he was deemed to have normal exocrine and endocrine pancreatic function. He had been diagnosed with ulcerative colitis in the preceding year based on clinical findings and colonoscopy.*

Medications: Hydromorphone controlled release 15 mg twice daily, hydromorphone 2–4 mg q4 hours for breakthrough pain, mesalazine, dexlansoprazole, naproxen, gabapentin 300 mg twice daily, bupropion, and venlafaxine.

Physical Examination: Weight was 68.4 kg, height 1.73 m, HR was 90 and regular, and BP 128/88.

It had been previously noted that abdominal examination was not possible due to the presence of allodynia. Physical examination was otherwise unremarkable.

Investigations: Laboratory values revealed a hemoglobin 114 g/L, normal white blood cell count, albumin 22 g/L, lipase 185 U/L, hemoglobin A1C 5.8%, and C-reactive protein of 8.3 mg/L. Abdominal computed tomography and magnetic resonance imaging revealed normal pancreatic structure.

D. Dillane (✉)
Department of Anesthesiology & Pain Medicine, University of Alberta, Edmonton, AB, Canada

C. Douglas
Acute Pain Service, University of Alberta Hospital, Edmonton, AB, Canada

What Is Opioid Tolerance?

Tolerance to any drug is a decrease in pharmacological effect occurring after repeated administration. It may be a consequence of receptor desensitization, downregulation, or internalization. Tachyphylaxis can be thought of as the development of tolerance in a shorter time frame, possibly within hours, when patients are exposed to a high initial dose or repeated small doses [1]. The dose-response curve is shifted to the right, i.e., decreased potency can be overcome by increasing the dose of the drug (Fig. 47.1) [2].

What Is the Difference Between Opioid Tolerance and Opioid-Induced Hyperalgesia (OIH)?

OIH is a process that has been shown to occur where the administration of opioids can activate pronociceptive mechanisms in the central nervous system, resulting in a paradoxical increase in pain sensitivity with continued opioid administration (Fig. 47.2) [3].

Formerly thought to take months to develop (e.g., methadone maintenance patients), it is now known to occur over a matter of hours in certain situations, e.g., high-dose intraoperative remifentanil administration [4]. Remifentanil has been particularly implicated, but it is possible that OIH occurs with acute or chronic exposure, high or low doses, of any opioid or route of administration. Nociceptive sensitization is likely caused by neuroplastic changes in the central and peripheral nervous systems caused by opioid exposure, leading to paradoxical worsening of pain with increasing opioid doses. Both opioid tolerance and OIH require an increased dose to achieve an increase in effect. The difference is that in the long term, OIH is made worse by increasing opioid administration.

D. Dillane, B. A. Finegan (eds.), *Preoperative Assessment*, https://doi.org/10.1007/978-3-030-58842-7_47

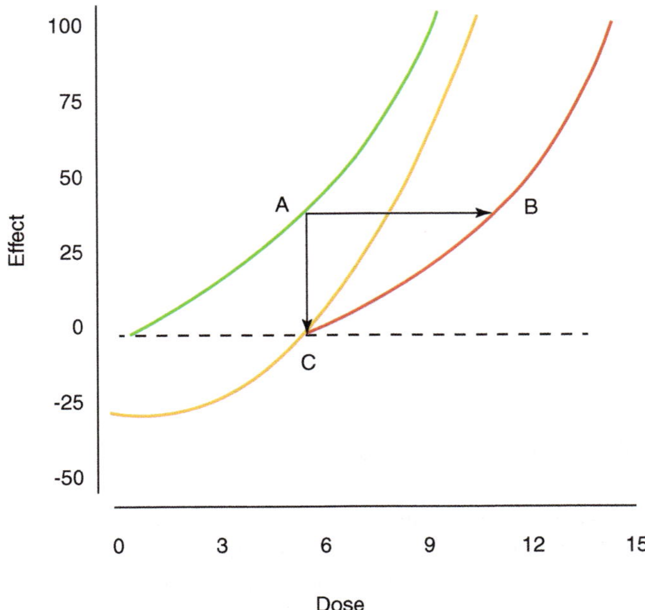

Fig. 47.1 The normal response to a dose of opioid is seen at point A. After tolerance is established, decreased drug potency is represented by a rightward shift of the dose-response relationship (A to B). Opioid-induced hyperalgesia and associated increased pain sensitivity are reflected by a downward shift of the dose-response curve. Both conditions require dose increases to achieve an increase in effect. The difference is that in the long term, opioid-induced hyperalgesia is made worse by increasing opioid administration

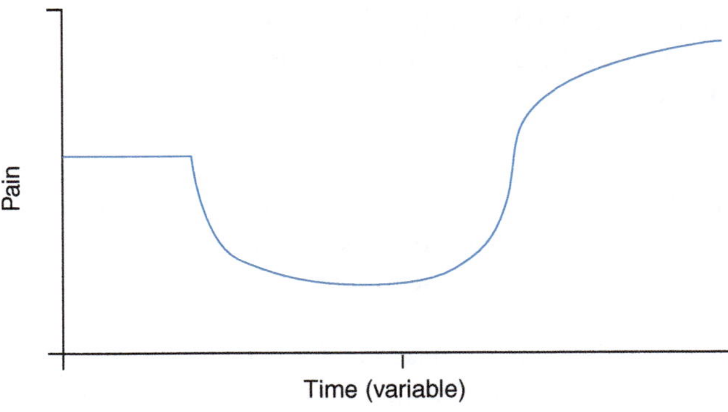

Fig. 47.2 Opioid-induced hyperalgesia is a paradoxical increase in pain sensitivity during continued opioid treatment. The timeline is variable. Previously thought to take many months to develop, it is now known to occur intraoperatively after relatively high doses of remifentanil. (Adapted from Colvin et al. [3], with permission Elsevier)

What Is the Significance of the Similarities Between Opioid Tolerance and OIH? Can a Definitive Diagnosis Be Made During Preoperative Evaluation?

The significance lies in how each condition is treated. Determining whether a patient is opioid tolerant or has OIH cannot be achieved with complete confidence, i.e., there are no definitive diagnostic criteria. However, increasing the dose of opioid is a simple measure that may be informative—the tolerant patient improves, while the OIH patient does not improve or worsens. Presence of allodynia and hyperalgesia, particularly widespread hyperalgesia, makes a diagnosis of OIH more likely. Quantitative sensory testing (a variety of tests can be used to test the response to light touch, vibration, pressure, and temperature) may be helpful. If the clinical picture clearly points towards opioid tolerance, the patient should be advised to continue taking their normal daily opioid dose up to and throughout the perioperative period. Conversely, a trial of opioid dose reduction could be utilized in the patient with clear diagnostic indicators of OIH.

How Are the Terms Addiction and Physical Dependence Defined?

Addiction is a chronic, relapsing neurobiological disease with genetic, psychosocial, and environmental factors influencing its development. It is characterized by compulsive drug seeking and use, impaired control over use, and continued use despite harm [5].

Physical dependence is a state of neuro-adaptation to a specific opioid characterized by a withdrawal syndrome produced by abrupt cessation, rapid dose reduction, decreasing plasma drug level, or administration of an antagonist [6].

How Should the Opioid-Tolerant Patient Be Evaluated Preoperatively?

An important component of the preoperative visit is to identify patients with opioid tolerance to facilitate establishing a comprehensive perioperative analgesia plan. A thorough history of opioid use is required, including specific agents, dose, frequency, and duration. The patient presented above was noted to require controlled release hydromorphone 15 mg twice daily and immediate release hydromorphone 2–4 mg as required every 4 hours for breakthrough pain. On further questioning, it emerged that he used 2 mg four times per day on average to control breakthrough pain. This amounts to hydromorphone 38 mg daily on average, his baseline daily requirement.

Clinical indicators of OIH may warrant further investigation at this juncture. At the very least, an enquiry should be made into the outcome of any recent increase in opioid dose. The acute perioperative pain service should be consulted or at least made aware of the patient. Patient education and reassurance with the aim of alleviating perioperative anxiety are likely as important as any other step at the preoperative phase. An analgesia treatment plan can be discussed with the patient and documented. This can include a written opioid agreement. It is helpful for both physician and patient to have a discussion regarding pain management expectations.

Clinical indicators of addiction should be sought, e.g., out-of-control opioid use, pain treatment plans unavailable, unclear reason for opioid use, illicit opioid use, impaired quality of life, or lack of concern regarding harmful effects of opioid use. Preoperative opioid misuse has been associated with increased morbidity and mortality after elective orthopedic surgery. Menendez et al. demonstrated a combined adverse risk incidence of 13% in postoperative patients with opioid-use disorder [7]. Pneumonia, respiratory failure, myocardial infarction, and renal failure were some of the complications seen. Therefore, referral to addiction services for evaluation and treatment may improve postoperative outcomes.

How Should the Patient Taking Oral Opioids Be Managed Preoperatively?

This patient population is at high risk for severe postoperative pain and is likely to benefit from advance analgesia planning. The patient should be advised to take their usual baseline opioid dose on the day of surgery. If oral administration is not possible, the oral opioid dose can be converted to a corresponding intravenous dose of the same agent (Table 47.1) [8, 9].

How Should the Patient Taking Transdermal Opioids Be Managed Preoperatively?

The most common transdermal preparations are fentanyl and buprenorphine. Buprenorphine use is addressed in the following section. Regardless of the specific agent, there is a risk of decreased absorption in complex surgeries involving large fluid shifts or skin temperature fluctuation, e.g., hypothermia and rewarming affects the kinetics of transdermal fentanyl. If this is expected, the fentanyl patch can be removed at induction. An equianalgesic dose of intravenous morphine or hydromorphone can then be used intraoperatively and for the first 24–48 postoperative hours via patient-controlled analgesia (PCA) such that the daily opioid requirements are met. If the surgery is of a less complex nature, the fentanyl patch can be maintained throughout the perioperative period.

Describe an Approach to Preoperative Evaluation and Management of the Patient Taking Buprenorphine

Buprenorphine is a partial mu opioid receptor agonist that has kappa antagonist properties. It is used for a variety of indications, including treatment of opioid addiction and acute and chronic pain. Perioperative management of patients taking buprenorphine is based on expert opinion and is largely inconsistent. It has previously been thought that

Table 47.1 An example of a practical guide to opioid conversion from the University of Alberta Multidisciplinary Pain

Drug	Parental dose (mg) equivalent to 10 mg IV morphine	Oral dose equivalent to 30 mg oral morphine	Bioavailability of oral dosage form	Dosing interval (h)
Morphine	10	30	0.3	3
Codeine	100	300	0.3	3
Diamorphine	8	12.5	0.4	3
Fentanyl	0.1	–	–	1
Hydromorphone (Dilaudid®; Abbott, North Chicago, IL, USA)	2	4–8	0.6	3
Meperidine (Demerol®; Sanofi Aventis, Bridgewater NJ, USA)	80	250	0.3	3
Methadone	2–10	2–10	1.0	8–12
Oxycodone (Percocet®; Endo Pharmaceuticals, Chadds Ford, PA, USA)/OcyContin®; Purdue Pharma, Stamford, CT, USA)	10	12	0.8	3
Sustained-release morphine (MS Contin®; Purdue Pharma, Stamford, CT, USA)	–	30	0.5	8–12

Adapted with permission from Saifee Rashiq, MD, Division of Pain Medicine, Department of Anesthesiology & Pain Medicine, University of Alberta, Edmonton, Alberta, Canada [9]

adequate perioperative analgesia cannot be achieved in the patient taking buprenorphine long term due to its opioid antagonist properties. This reasoning may not be entirely accurate. A recent systematic review of 18 studies (mostly comprised of case reports and series but with one controlled and four observational studies) concluded that there was no evidence against continuing buprenorphine use perioperatively, particularly when the dose ≤16 mg sublingually [10]. When the indication for buprenorphine use is addiction with a significant risk of relapse, a strong rationale for perioperative discontinuation should be present, supported by both the patient and the surgical team. Our practice is to continue buprenorphine perioperatively as a matter of routine.

How Should the Patient Taking Intrathecal Opioids Be Managed Preoperatively?

Intrathecal drug delivery systems for patients with malignant and chronic non-malignant pain or spasticity can be maintained during surgery for baseline opioid requirements. The intrathecal opioid dose should be recorded at the preoperative visit. The dose cannot be adjusted to treat acute postoperative pain, and supplemental multimodal analgesia should be used for this purpose. The intraoperative anesthetist and surgeon should be informed of the presence of an intrathecal drug delivery system, as it may interfere with the surgical field, or associated implanted electrodes may be subject to heating with the use of cautery [8]. Lumbar epidural anesthesia is not contraindicated but should be attempted with image guidance to avoid implanted components [11]. The perioperative analgesia plan should include non-opioid multimodal adjuncts, e.g., nonsteroidal anti-inflammatory drugs (NSAIDs), acetaminophen, ketamine, regional anesthesia techniques, and/or lidocaine infusion. Long-acting opioids should be avoided postoperatively. This includes PCA with a continuous basal rate, though PCA is not contraindicated. Continuous pulse oximetry should be utilized postoperatively. Communication with the chronic pain physician who attends to the patient is necessary both pre- and post-operatively.

How Should the Patient on Maintenance Methadone Be Managed Preoperatively?

Methadone is a synthetic opioid agonist used both for analgesia and withdrawal management in opioid-dependent patients. With an elimination half-life significantly longer than other opioids (8–59 hours; average 23 hours), it is administered once daily for opioid agonist therapy. Despite the fact that its effect on opioid withdrawal can last up to 48 hours, its analgesic effect is much shorter at approximately 6 hours [12]. Subsequently, the authors prefer to continue baseline methadone throughout the perioperative period, if possible, while using shorter acting opioids, e.g., morphine or hydromorphone as part of a comprehensive multimodal analgesia technique with an emphasis on the non-opioid component. Several factors can complicate perioperative analgesic management in the patient using methadone maintenance therapy. These patients are likely to have elements of both tolerance and OIH. They also develop cross-tolerance entailing higher and more frequent doses of other opioid analgesics [13, 14]. Finally, patients employing methadone for opioid agonist therapy are occasionally concerned about the risk of addiction relapse perioperatively when supplementary opioids are used to treat surgical pain. The evidence is sparse, but two small studies did not find evidence of relapse in patients on methadone maintenance therapy treated with additional opioids for surgery [15] and cancer-related pain [16].

What Opioid-Sparing Multimodal Analgesia Techniques Should Be Discussed with This Patient?

- Single shot or continuous neuraxial and peripheral nerve blockade
- Acetaminophen
- NSAIDs
- Ketamine
- Intravenous lidocaine
- Gabapentinoids
- Dexmedetomidine
- Psychosocial, e.g., relaxation, education, behavioral instruction
- Physiotherapy/exercise

What Is the Evidence in Favor of Opioid Rotation?

Opioid rotation (switching from one opioid to an equianalgesic dose of another) is commonly used in palliative care to improve analgesia and reduce the side effects related to one opioid. Most evidence for efficacy comes from expert opinion and case series [17], and there is very limited substantiation in the acute pain setting. Possible mechanisms include incomplete cross-tolerance and differing receptor activity. Rotation is performed by converting to an equivalent dose of a different opioid, using equivalency tables (see Table 47.1) and initially reducing the calculated dose by 30–50% to account for incomplete cross-tolerance.

Is There Any Evidence That Regional Anesthesia Techniques Are less Effective in Opioid-Tolerant Patients?

Practitioners of regional anesthesia are familiar with the concept of apparent decreased efficacy of neuraxial and peripheral nerve blockade among opioid-tolerant patients. The biopsychosocial model of pain is commonly held accountable, but there is emerging evidence that opioid-tolerant patients may also be less amenable to the effects of regional nerve blockade. Liu et al. demonstrated loss of lidocaine potency in the rat sciatic nerve in vitro after seven daily morphine injections [18]. Although analgesic efficacy to morphine recovered completely within days, the loss of lidocaine potency remained 35 days after the last morphine injection. Similarly, Vosoughian and colleagues describe shorter duration of spinal anesthesia in opium users (60 +/− 7 minutes vs. 83 +/− 10 minutes $p < 0.0001$) [19].

What Modifiable Preoperative Risk Factors Contribute to the Development of Chronic Postsurgical Pain?

Chronic postsurgical pain (CPSP) occurs in approximately 10% of patients who have surgery [20]. Several preoperative patient-specific risk factors are known to predispose towards the development of CPSP. Preoperative chronic pain and opioid use are notable red flags. These patients can be targeted for preoperative tapering of opioids if OIH is a significant contributory factor. Other modifiable risk factors include fear, obesity, preoperative use of benzodiazepines and antidepressants, smoking, alcohol, and illicit drug use. Education, psychological counseling, modification of addiction behavior, and weight loss programs may be initiated as part of an integrated multidisciplinary approach to prevention of CPSP. Even in the absence of modifiable risk factors, identification of patients who may benefit from perioperative monitoring, opioid restrictive strategies, and postoperative follow-up by a transitional pain service may prove beneficial.

The patient was counseled at length preoperatively, an analgesia plan was agreed upon that included a written opioid contract, and the Acute Pain Service was consulted. The patient was prescribed his normal morning dose of hydromorphone controlled release (15 mg). He was continued on his baseline opioid for the first 48 hours as a continuous infusion via *PCA administered hydromorphone. His baseline daily oral opioid requirement was calculated to be hydromorphone 38 mg. A conversion factor of 5:1 was used to calculate an equivalent intravenous dose of hydromorphone 7.6 mg IV, which was administered as a continuous infusion of 0.3 mg/h over 24 hours. A continuous ketamine infusion at 0.1 mg/kg/h was initiated after induction and maintained for 48 postoperative hours. Intravenous ketorolac and acetaminophen were also administered for the first 48 hours. Bilateral transversus abdominis plane catheters were inserted by the surgeon at the end of the case through which an infusion of 0.2% ropivacaine was infused for 72 hours after surgery. His maintenance dose of gabapentin 300 mg twice daily was continued when normal diet resumed.*

True/False Questions

1. (a) Pharmacological tolerance results in a rightward shift of the drug dose-effect curve.
   (b) Opioid-induced hyperalgesia results in a leftward shift of the drug dose-effect curve.
   (c) Opioid- induced hyperalgesia is usually treated by increasing the opioid dose.
   (d) Allodynia is a common sign in the opioid-tolerant patient.
   (e) Preoperative opioid misuse is associated with increased postoperative morbidity and mortality.
2. (a) Buprenorphine should never be continued throughout the perioperative period when the indication for use is opioid addiction.
   (b) Patients with intrathecal opioid delivery systems usually have the intrathecal opioid dose increased preoperatively to aid in the treatment of postoperative surgical pain.
   (c) Methadone is not an ideal opioid for management of postsurgical pain.
   (d) Transdermal preparations of fentanyl may be subject to altered absorption during complex surgeries involving large fluid shifts.
   (e) Lidocaine may have reduced potency for nerve blockade in opioid-tolerant patients.

References

1. Hayhurst CJ, Durieux ME. Differential opioid tolerance and opioid-induced hyperalgesia: a clinical reality. Anesthesiology. 2016;124(2):483–8.
2. Carroll IR, Angst MS, Clark JD. Management of perioperative pain in patients chronically consuming opioids. Reg Anesth Pain Med. 2004;29(6):576–91.
3. Colvin LA, Bull F, Hales TG. Perioperative opioid analgesia-when is enough too much? A review of opioid-induced tolerance and hyperalgesia. Lancet. 2019;393(10180):1558–68. https://doi.org/10.1016/S0140-6736(19)30430-1.
4. Fletcher D, Martinez V. Opioid-induced hyperalgesia in patients after surgery: a systematic review and a meta-analysis. Br J Anaesth. 2014;112(6):991–1004.
5. Heit HA. Addiction, physical dependence, and tolerance: precise definitions to help clinicians evaluate and treat chronic pain patients. J Pain Palliat Care Pharmacother. 2003;17(1):15–29.
6. Coluzzi F, Bifulco F, Cuomo A, Dauri M, Leonardi C, Melotti RM, et al. The challenge of perioperative pain management in opioid-tolerant patients. Ther Clin Risk Manag. 2017;13:1163–73.

7. Menendez ME, Ring D, Bateman BT. Preoperative opioid misuse is associated with increased morbidity and mortality after elective orthopaedic surgery. Clin Orthop Relat Res. 2015;473(7):2402–12.
8. Farrell C, McConaghy P. Perioperative management of patients taking treatment for chronic pain. BMJ. 2012;345:e4148.
9. Rashiq S. Opioid Conversion Guide [Available from: https://www.ualberta.ca/medicine/institutes-centres-groups/multidisciplinary-pain-clinic/for-healthcare-professionals/opioid-conversion-guide.
10. Goel A, Azargive S, Lamba W, Bordman J, Englesakis M, Srikandarajah S, et al. The perioperative patient on buprenorphine: a systematic review of perioperative management strategies and patient outcomes. Can J Anaesth. 2019;66(2):201–17.
11. Young A, Jaycox M, Lubenow T. Perioperative Management of Patients With Intrathecal Drug Delivery Systems. American Society of Regional Anesthesia and Pain Medicine. Advisories & Guidelines. Available from: https://www.asra.com/page/226/perioperative-management-of-patients-with-intrathecal-drug-delivery-systems.
12. Vadivelu N, Mitra S, Kaye AD, Urman RD. Perioperative analgesia and challenges in the drug-addicted and drug-dependent patient. Best Pract Res Clin Anaesthesiol. 2014;28(1):91–101.
13. Doverty M, Somogyi AA, White JM, Bochner F, Beare CH, Menelaou A, et al. Methadone maintenance patients are cross-tolerant to the antinociceptive effects of morphine. Pain. 2001;93(2):155–63.
14. Alford DP, Compton P, Samet JH. Acute pain management for patients receiving maintenance methadone or buprenorphine therapy. Ann Intern Med. 2006;144(2):127–34.
15. Kantor TG, Cantor R, Tom E. A study of hospitalized surgical patients on methadone maintenance. Drug Alcohol Depend. 1980;6(3):163–73.
16. Manfredi PL, Gonzales GR, Cheville AL, Kornick C, Payne R. Methadone analgesia in cancer pain patients on chronic methadone maintenance therapy. J Pain Symptom Manag. 2001;21(2):169–74.
17. Huxtable CA, Roberts LJ, Somogyi AA, MacIntyre PE. Acute pain management in opioid-tolerant patients: a growing challenge. Anaesth Intensive Care. 2011;39(5):804–23.
18. Liu Q, Gold MS. Opioid-induced loss of local anesthetic potency in the rat sciatic nerve. Anesthesiology. 2016;125(4):755–64.
19. Vosoughian M, Dabbagh A, Rajaei S, Maftuh H. The duration of spinal anesthesia with 5% lidocaine in chronic opium abusers compared with nonabusers. Anesth Analg. 2007;105(2):531–3.
20. Glare P, Aubrey KR, Myles PS. Transition from acute to chronic pain after surgery. Lancet. 2019;393(10180):1537–46.

Substance Abuse Disorder

48

Barry A. Finegan

A 32-year-old male was evaluated preoperatively prior to laparoscopic removal of accessory spleen tissue. He initially presented 14 months earlier with bleeding from his mouth and gums and a rash on his legs bilaterally. He denied any recent occurence of epistaxis, hematemesis, or melena. He indicated that he smoked heroin intermittently, used cannabis daily, and occasionally used methamphetamine. He denied intravenous drug use. He had been in a motor vehicle accident and had undergone splenectomy 8 years previously. On examination, there were lesions on his lips and gingiva that bled easily when touched. His platelet count was 1 × 10^9/L. His abdominal CT scan confirmed that he had indeed undergone splenectomy but also demonstrated multiple small modules in the splenic bed and on the liver surface. A diagnosis of idiopathic thrombocytopenic purpura (ITP) and splenosis was entertained. Bolus dexamethasone therapy (40 mg p.o. daily × 4 days) was initiated. He was not responsive to this treatment. Eltrombopag (50 mg p.o. daily) evoked an appropriate increase in his platelet count, and he was discharged home on this therapy. On this occasion, he was readmitted to hospital 2 days after discharge with an infected tattoo of the forearm. Enterococcus faecium and faecalis were cultured from his blood.

A relapse of ITP 2 months prior to the present visit was treated with rituximab. A technetium-99-labeled scan with heat-damaged red blood cells showed evidence of splenules in his pelvic area. He responded well to rituximab, and at discharge his platelet count was 30 × 10^9/L. A decision was made to electively operate to remove the residual splenules once his condition had stabilized.

At the time of his preadmission clinic visit, he was in full remission from his ITP. His platelet count was 345 × 10^9/L. He was on no prescription medications but did admit to continued polysubstance use, including occasional heroin and cocaine. He had snorted cocaine 3 weeks previously, had smoked cannabis the night before the clinic visit, and had taken a "hit" of methamphetamine 2 weeks before at a party. He admitted to three beers a day. Mental status exam was unremarkable. Serology for HIV and hepatitis was negative. A referral to a substance abuse program was declined. He was advised about the need not to engage in cocaine, methamphetamine, or excessive alcohol consumption before his surgical date, which was scheduled 2 weeks hence.

B. A. Finegan (✉)
Department of Anesthesiology & Pain Medicine, University of Alberta, Edmonton, AB, Canada
e-mail: bfinegan@ualberta.ca

What Is Splenosis?

Heterotopic transplantation of viable splenic tissue is termed "splenosis." This may occur particularly after traumatic splenic rupture but can also arise following elective splenic surgery [1]. The soft tissue nodules are usually located in the abdomen and pelvis but can on occasion be found elsewhere and be mistaken for cancerous lesions [2].

What Is Eltrombopag?

Eltrombopag is an oral agonist of the c-mpl receptor, the physiological target of thrombopoietin, and has been approved for the treatment of chronic ITP and aplastic anemia [3].

What Is the Prevalence of Drug Use in the Adolescent/Adult Population?

The Monitoring the Future study performed annually since 1975 by the University of Michigan's Institute for Social Research provides a contemporary snapshot of drug use among adolescents in the United States [4]. The sample size in 2017 was 43,700 students across the nation. *Annual* prevalence of any cannabis use was 10%, 26%, and 37% in grades 8, 10, and 12, respectively. *Daily* use was 1%, 3%, and 6%, respectively. *Annual* prevalence of use across all grades of amphetamine/stimulants ~7%; inhalants (glue, nail polish,

D. Dillane, B. A. Finegan (eds.), *Preoperative Assessment*, https://doi.org/10.1007/978-3-030-58842-7_48

solvents etc.) ~ 4%; LSD, cocaine, and 3,4-Methylenedioxy methamphetamine (MDMA) ~ 3%; narcotics other than heroin ~2%; methamphetamine ~1%; and heroin ~0.5%. In contrast, binge drinking (5+ drinks in a row at least once in the last 2 weeks) across all grades was reported by ~16% of adolescents surveyed.

The 2017 U.S. National Survey on Drug Use and Health prepared by the Substance Abuse and Mental Health Services Administration provides an insight into adult substance use and abuse in the United States [5]. Focusing on substance use/misuse in those aged 26 or older reveals the following estimates: *Past month* cannabis use 7.9%; *past month* misuse of psychotherapeutic drugs (defined as use in a way not directed by a doctor, use without a prescription, and use in supra-therapeutic amounts of tranquilizers, stimulants, and sedatives) $\leq$ 0.5%; and *past month* use of cocaine, inhalants, heroin, and methamphetamine $\leq$0.5%. Opioid misuse was more prevalent (3.8%); the most common opioids misused were hydrocodone and oxycodone. Binge drinking was reported by 25% of participants.

What Are the Key Issues to Address in the Preoperative Evaluation of a Substance-Using Patient?

Adolescent and adult patients should be questioned regarding drug and alcohol intake.

If a positive history is obtained, the nature, dose, frequency, method of administration, and time of last use should be elicited. Polysubstance use is very common, and the patient should be prompted to reveal all substances used within the last 3–6 months. Recent data suggest that methamphetamine use is increasing. It is being used as an opioid substitute, to manage the side effects of concurrent opioid use, and in some cases to provide a synergistic high [6]. Obtaining even a very remote history of illicit drug use (years ago) can be helpful, as it can prompt one to advise the patient to be screened for occult hepatitis/HIV.

Substance use is a marker for mental health issues. The appearance, behavior, speech, motor activity, mood, and cognitive status may provide clues to an uncontrolled psychiatric state and/or current intoxication or withdrawal.

If the patient is acutely intoxicated, a safety evaluation should be performed and further assessment postponed until the patient is in a sensate state. This decision should be communicated respectfully to the patient and, if feasible, an offer made to assist in referral to an appropriate addiction service.

Currently addicted users may not follow instructions and frequently put themselves at risk through inappropriate behavior. Admission the day prior to an elective procedure should be considered.

Acute/chronic excessive substance use has consequences for the entire organism. The cardiovascular (cardiomyopathy, endocarditis, and heart failure); pulmonary (COPD, fibrosis, pneumonia, pneumonitis, and edema); renal (impairment and failure) gastrointestinal (pancreatitis, hepatitis, and cirrhosis), and central nervous system (dementia, ischemic/hemorrhagic strokes, and traumatic brain injury) are all susceptible. Symptoms suggestive of decompensation should prompt a thorough assessment to see if improvement is possible prior to surgery. Acute/chronic viral or bacterial infections are commonplace as in our patient.

What Is Heroin?

Heroin is a semi-synthetic opioid (diacetylmorphine). Morphine is extracted from opium and through a complex chemical process (involving the use of acetic anhydride, chloroform, sodium carbonate, ether, and HCL) refined to heroin. Heroin is hydrolyzed to 6-monoacetylmorphine (6-MAM) in the body, and in turn is metabolized to morphine. 6-MAM is more lipid soluble than morphine and thus has a more rapid onset of cerebral effects.

What Is the Potency of Heroin Relative to Morphine, and What Are the Signs and Issues of Concern with Recent Use?

Heroin is approximately twice as potent as morphine. The initial response to heroin exposure is a sense euphoria followed rapidly by sedation and tranquility. Physical signs of recent use include decreased respiratory rate, bradycardia, miosis, pruritus, and perspiration. Daily heroin users will experience symptoms of withdrawal if they abstain from use for more than 6–12 hours. Consultation with an addiction specialist to develop a plan to avoid withdrawal postoperatively is prudent. Oral methadone or buprenorphine has been used successfully in this situation [7]. Chronic users will be tolerant to opioids, and adjustment of intraoperative and postoperative doses is appropriate.

What Is Cocaine and What Are the Signs and Issues of Concern with Recent Use?

Cocaine is extracted from the leaves of the coca plant. Among multiple effects, cocaine inhibits the reuptake of serotonin, epinephrine, norepinephrine, and dopamine peripherally and centrally. It is a potent Na^+ channel blocker. Cocaine exposure initially elicits an intense feeling of happiness or may provoke agitation and loss of contact with reality.

Physical signs of recent use include pyrexia, hypertension, tachycardia, dysrhythmias, myocardial ischemia, mydriasis, perspiration, seizures, and psychosis. Cocaine exerts its effects usually within 10 minutes of use, and effects last from 15 to 90 minutes. ECG findings of acute intoxication include Na^+ channel blockade-induced widening of the QRS complex (treated with sodium bicarbonate) and QTc prolongation associated with blockade of the K^+ rectifier channels.

There are many more recreational cocaine users than chronic users (> 4 times/month). It is imperative that all users are advised to desist from cocaine use in the immediate preoperative period, given the potentially catastrophic cardiovascular consequences of blocking neurotransmitter re-uptake and voltage-gated Na^+ channels during and immediately after surgery.

What Is Methamphetamine ("Ecstasy/Meth/Chalk/Ice/Glass") and What Are the Signs of Recent Use?

Methamphetamine is a synthetic stimulant that is an indirect agonist at dopamine, noradrenaline, and serotonin receptors [8]. Methamphetamine is smoked, sniffed, injected, and taken orally. The responses to low-/moderate-dose ingestion include arousal, euphoria, disinhibition, and positive mood. Physiologically dose-dependent hypertension, tachycardia, and pupillary dilatation are elicited by methamphetamine use. Violent, abusive, and incoherent behavior may occur. In overdose situations, hyperpyrexia, cardiac and renal failure, coma, and seizures have been observed. Chronic use of methamphetamine can result in the development of early onset coronary artery disease and/or cardiomyopathy. If the patient complains of chronic fatigue and/or dyspnea, obtaining an echocardiogram prior to surgery would be prudent.

It was decided to admit the patient to hospital on the night before surgery. At time of admission, he was coherent and did not appear to be under the influence of any illicit substances. The next morning, he arrived in the preoperative area of the OR in an agitated state and diaphoretic. He was complaining of severe central chest pain. When questioned, he admitted to snorting cocaine on two occasions that morning. On examination, his vital signs were abnormal: pulse 72/min; blood pressure 210/125; temperature 37.9 °C; respiratory rate 24/min; O_2 saturation 98% on room air; physical examination apart was otherwise unremarkable. A stat ECG was ordered and blood drawn to measure troponin.

The ECG findings were as shown in the Fig. 48.1. Based on the ECG findings of T wave inversion V2-V6, a provisional diagnosis of Wellens syndrome Type B (proximal stenosis/constriction of the left anterior descending coronary artery) was made. The patient was treated by the administration of aspirin 325 mg, sublingual nitroglycerine 0.4 mg, and IV diltiazem 10 mg. Midazolam 5 mg IV was administered as a sedative. With this therapy, the pain subsided and the ECG finding resolved.

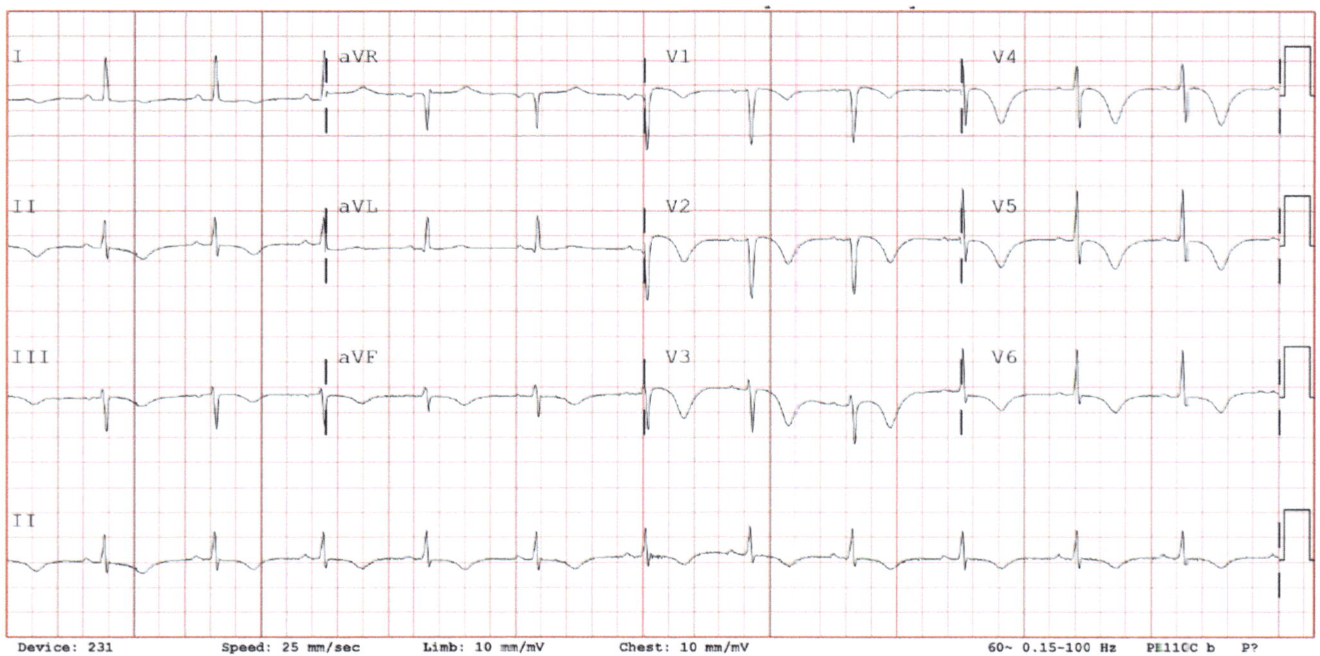

Fig. 48.1 Electrocardiogram finding in a 32-year-old male with a history of substance abuse shows T wave inversion V2-V6

Beta-blockers are relatively contraindicated in the face of acute cocaine-induced coronary vasoconstriction due to concerns about the consequences of unopposed alpha-adrenergic stimulation. Chest pain in the scenario described could also be a manifestation of acute aortic dissection. This is best ruled out by echocardiographic assessment.

The patient was admitted to the cardiac ICU for observation. There was no recurrence of the chest pain symptoms. The next morning, the patient discharged himself from the hospital against medical advice. He has since been lost to follow-up.

True/False Questions

1. In adults in North America
   (a) alcohol is the most common substance abused
   (b) cannabis use is infrequent
   (c) methamphetamine use is increasing
   (d) methamphetamine is commonly used with opioids
   (e) heroin use is uncommon
2. Cocaine
   (a) is a potent Na + channel blocker
   (b) inhibits reuptake of serotonin and dopamine
   (c) causes miosis of the pupil
   (d) is associated with Wellens syndrome
   (e) QTc shorting is an ECG sign of recent cocaine use

References

1. Tandon YK, Coppa CP, Purysko AS. Splenosis: a great mimicker of neoplastic disease. Abdom Radiol. 2018;43(11):3054–9.
2. Mpe M, Schauer C. Images in clinical medicine. Splenosis mimicking cancer. N Engl J Med. 2016;374(20):1965.
3. Cuker A. Transitioning patients with immune thrombocytopenia to second-line therapy: challenges and best practices. Am J Hematol. 2018;93(6):816–23.
4. Johnston LD, Miech RA, O'Malley PM, Bachman JG, Schulenberg JE, Patrick ME. Monitoring the future: national survey results on drug use: 1975–2017: overview, key findings on adolescent drug use. Ann Arbor: Institute for Social Research, The University of Michigan. https://eric.ed.gov/?id=ED589762. Accessed 9 Jun 2020
5. Substance Abuse and Mental Health Services Administration. Key substance use and mental health indicators in the United States: Results from the 2017 National Survey on Drug Use and Health (HHS Publication No. SMA 18–5068, NSDUH Series H-53). Rockville, MD: Center for Behavioral Health Statistics and Quality, Substance Abuse and Mental Health Services Administration; 2018. https://www.samhsa.gov/data/sites/default/files/cbhsq-reports/NSDUHFFR2017/NSDUHFFR2017.pdf. Accessed 9 Jun 2020.
6. Ellis MS, Kasper ZA, Cicero TJ. Twin epidemics: the surging rise of methamphetamine use in chronic opioid users. Drug Alcohol Depend. 2018;193:14–20.
7. Beaulieu P. Anesthetic implications of recreational drug use. Can J Anaesth. 2017;64(12):1236–64.
8. Cruickshank CC, Dyer KR. A review of the clinical pharmacology of methamphetamine. Addiction. 2009;104(7):1085–99.

Amyloidosis

49

Barry A. Finegan

A 61-year-old male scheduled for elective parathyroidectomy was referred for preoperative assessment. He was incidentally diagnosed with immunoglobulin light chain amyloidosis (AL) 7 years previously when being investigated for unexpected renal dysfunction, which evolved to end-stage renal failure requiring dialysis. In addition, he was found to have increased bone marrow plasma cells and was diagnosed with multiple myeloma. He underwent one cycle of successful treatment and was offered stem cell transplantation but refused this therapy. Remarkably, his condition stabilized, but in the months prior to his visit to the assessment clinic, he had complained of symptoms suggestive of right heart decompensation. His troponin levels were found to be chronically elevated. An MRI revealed biventricular volume increase with moderately decreased systolic function and findings suggestive of amyloid deposition in the myocardium. He was initiated on spironolactone with excellent symptomatic relief.

Systems review revealed a 40-year smoking history and a long-standing diagnosis of COPD. He was still an active smoker. He denied any symptoms of angina. His Duke Activity Score Index was five. He had long-standing hypothyroidism managed with replacement therapy. He indicated that he had been admitted to hospital 6 months previously with a bowel obstruction that resolved with conservative therapy. That episode was tentatively attributed to gastrointestinal amyloid-related ileus. There was no history of easy bruising or abnormal bleeding.

His dialysis schedule was twice a week. He was scheduled to undergo dialysis on the afternoon of his visit to the clinic.

Current medications included darbepoetin, levothyroxine, pantoprazole, spironolactone, inhaled fluticasone, and ipratropium.

Physical examination revealed an elevated resting pulse rate (94/min) with a low normal blood pressure (BP) (105/65). Resting oxygen saturation on room air was normal. He had bilateral mild ankle edema and mild crepitations audible in both bases. The jugular venous pressure was not elevated. Airway examination was normal.

Laboratory investigations revealed a hemoglobin of 102 g/L with a normal white blood cell count and electrolyte profile. His coagulation screen was normal. Thyroid-stimulating hormone was 5.9 mU/L. Intact parathyroid hormone was elevated at 52.8 pmol/L (reference range 1.6–6.9 pmol/L). Liver function tests were normal apart from a mild increase in gamma glutamyl transferase (the patient admitted to one bout of heavy alcohol use in the previous 7 days). B-natriuretic peptide (BNP) was markedly elevated at 1610 ng/L. Free Kapa and Lambda light chains were five times normal values, but his Kappa/Lambda ratio was normal. His ECG revealed atrial flutter with 2:1 block, left bundle block, and ST elevation related to his intraventricular conduction defect. His chest X-ray demonstrated small bilateral pleural effusions and mild pulmonary edema. A right internal jugular dialysis line was appropriately positioned.

What Is Amyloidosis?

Amyloidosis is the extracellular deposition of insoluble fibrils that form from circulating low molecular weight subunits of soluble precursor proteins. Fibrillogenesis is initiated by multiple processes, including heritable mutations and inflammatory, malignant, and chronic disease states [1]. Deposition of amyloid protein leads to tissue destruction and organ dysfunction. There are multiple subtypes of amyloidosis, depending on the precursor protein predominantly involved in fibril formation.

Amyloidosis is rare but the following are some recognized entities:

1. Amyloid light chain (AL) and, less commonly, immunoglobulin heavy chain (AH) amyloidosis arising from deposition of fibrils derived from immunoglobulin light

B. A. Finegan (✉)
Department of Anesthesiology & Pain Medicine, University of Alberta, Edmonton, AB, Canada
e-mail: bfinegan@ualberta.ca

D. Dillane, B. A. Finegan (eds.), *Preoperative Assessment*, https://doi.org/10.1007/978-3-030-58842-7_49

and heavy chain fragments, respectively. AL is the most commonly occurring form of amyloidosis. AL and AH are associated with clonal plasma cell dyscrasias, especially monoclonal gammopathy of undetermined significance (MUGUS) and multiple myeloma. Amyloid AL cardiomyopathy can progress rapidly after the onset of symptoms and carries a poor prognosis.

2. Amyloid A (AA) or acquired amyloid, arising from deposition of fibrils derived from serum amyloid A proteins, associated with chronic inflammatory disease states including rheumatoid arthritis and juvenile inflammatory arthritis, and intravenous drug abuse.
3. Amyloid transthyretin (ATTR), which is inherited due to mutations in the gene encoding transthyretin (a protein that transports thyroxine and retinol, previously called pre-albumin). This protein is produced by the liver, so liver transplantation may be recommended as therapy depending on the status of the patient.
4. Amyloid transthyretin wild type (ATTRwt), previously called senile amyloidosis, where non-mutated (normal) transthyretin forms fibrils that seem to be preferentially deposited in the heart. ATTRwt is responsible for transthyretin amyloid cardiomyopathy, an increasingly recognized entity in patients diagnosed with diastolic heart failure.
5. Dialysis-related or Aβ2M amyloidosis, where deposition of fibrils formed from β2 microglobulin (not filtered by the dialysis process), occurs primarily in synovium, joints and bone, causing severe arthralgia in patients undergoing dialysis. The symptoms are resolved with renal transplantation.

What Are the Common Manifestations of Amyloidosis?

Amyloid deposits can affect any organ system; in consequence, the presenting clinical features are variable and frequently nonspecific. Neuropathy is a frequent occurrence.

Renal and hepatic dysfunction are common and early features of AA and AL, but organ dysfunction related to plasma cell dyscrasias can occur in the absence of amyloid disease. In AL, most patients have renal dysfunction with nephrotic-range proteinuria (spot urine showing a protein to creatinine ratio of >3–3.5 mg protein/mg creatinine (300–350 mg/mmol).

Liver involvement is suggested by elevated alkaline phosphatase levels [2].

Cardiac amyloidosis is frequently observed in AL and ATTR/ATTRwt. In the latter, misfolded ATTR monomers aggregate to form amyloid fibrils that are found in the interstitial space of the myocardium, causing increased wall thickness and evoking conduction disorders and diastolic dysfunction. It has been estimated that ATTRwt is an etiological factor in up to 10% of older patients' heart failure. Given the emerging treatment options for ATTR-related cardiomyopathy, screening for ATTR/ATTRwt has been proposed in populations deemed at risk of the condition. Suggested red flag signs/symptoms of possible early stage ATTR/ATTRwt disease include a discrepancy between left ventricle thickness on echocardiography and QRS findings on ECG. A history of the combination of bilateral carpel tunnel syndrome, polyneuropathy, and atrioventricular block should prompt screening for ATTR/ATTRwt [3]. Echocardiography and 99mTc-labelled bisphosphonate scintigraphy (as used in bone scans) are both very helpful in screening and diagnosis of ATTR/ATTRwt cardiac amyloidosis. Specificity of scintigraphy in the diagnosis of ATTR cardiomyopathy approaches 100% in the absence of detectable monoclonal proteins or an abnormal serum free light chain ratio [3].

What Are the Treatment Options for Amyloid Disease?

The cornerstone of management is to reduce the production of precursor proteins.

1. Supportive therapy, and in the case of cardiomyopathy, salt restriction, diuretics, and pacemaker/ICD insertion to manage rhythm and conduction disorders.
2. In AL, therapy is guided by risk assessment and may involve chemotherapy/immunomodulation (cyclophosphamide, thalidomide, dexamethasone, and proteasome inhibitors, among other agents) to reduce or eliminate light chain precursors, stem cell transplant, and/or organ transplant [4].
3. In AA, tumor necrosis factor (TNF) inhibitors and interleukin-1 blockers have shown effectiveness in ameliorating progression of the disease.
4. In ATTR, multiple drugs are under investigation that suppress or stabilize transthyretin and appear to reduce mortality and hospitalization rates [5]. These include the recently approved tafamidis, which binds to transthyretin and prevents its dissassociation into monomers. Although effective in reducing the rate of hospitalization in patients with cardiomyopathy, its cost-effectiveness has been called into question [6].

What Are the Key Issues to Identify During the Preoperative Evaluation?

This has been concisely and comprehensively reviewed by Fleming et al. [7]

1. A high index of suspicion for the presence of the disease in patients who are at risk and may present with symptoms suggestive of organ failure, particularly cardiac decompensation.
2. In patients with an established diagnosis of amyloidosis assess:
   (a) Airway—macroglossia is common (20% of patients with AL); voice alteration, stridor, and odynophagia are suggestive of laryngeal involvement.
   (b) Cardiovascular system—conduction disorders, orthostatic hypotension, and diastolic heart failure may be present. Concerning features of impending severe decompensation include poor exercise performance, NYHA functional class ≥3, systolic BP < 100 mmHg, and elevated BNP and troponin levels.
   (c) Neurological system—neuropathy is common and should be documented especially prior to regional techniques.
   (d) Coagulation abnormalities including acquired factor X deficiency have been reported.
3. A clear disposition plan following surgery is indicated with a low threshold for admission to a monitored environment following surgical procedures, particularly in patients with poor functional status.

The patient was electively triaged to postoperative overnight monitoring in a stepdown unit. A brief episode of ventricular tachycardia that spontaneously converted was noted during his stay. The patient was assessed by cardiology who suggested that placement of an ICD might be appropriate. The patient declined this intervention. He was discharged home after 24 hours.

True/False Questions

1. Amyloidosis is a disease that
   (a) Is caused by the intracellular deposition of insoluble fibrils
   (b) Is frequently associated with renal impairment
   (c) Can occur as a consequence of renal dialysis
   (d) Can manifest as a neuropathy
   (e) Has no known effective treatment
2. In the preoperative assessment of a patient with amyloidosis
   (a) A history of carpel tunnel syndrome may be a feature
   (b) Airway issues may be noted due to macroglossia
   (c) Heart failure may be present
   (d) A bone scan should be performed
   (e) Coagulation abnormalities may be observed

References

1. Wechalekar AD, Gillmore JD, Hawkins PN. Systemic amyloidosis. Lancet. 2016;387(10038):2641–54.
2. Ryšavá R. AL amyloidosis: advances in diagnostics and treatment. Nephrol Dial Transplant. 2019;34(9):1460–6.
3. Witteles RM, Bokhari S, Damy T, Elliott PM, Falk RH, Fine NM, et al. Screening for transthyretin amyloid cardiomyopathy in everyday practice. JACC Heart Fail. 2019;7(8):709–16.
4. Manolis AS, Manolis AA, Manolis TA, Melita H. Cardiac amyloidosis: an underdiagnosed/underappreciated disease. Eur J Intern Med. 2019;67:1–13.
5. Quarta CC, Solomon SD. Stabilizing transthyretin to treat ATTR cardiomyopathy. N Engl J Med. 2018;379(11):1083–4.
6. Kazi DS, Bellows BK, Baron SJ, Shen C, Cohen DJ, Spertus JA, et al. Cost-effectiveness of tafamidis therapy for transthyretin amyloid cardiomyopathy. Circulation. 2020;141(15):1214–24.
7. Fleming I, Dubrey S, Williams B. Amyloidosis and anaesthesia. BJA Education. 2012;12(2):72–7.

True/False Answers

Chapter 2

1a. F
1b. T
1c. F
1d. F
1e. F
2a. F
2b. F
2c. T
2d. T
2e. T

Chapter 3

1a. F
1b. F
1c. T
1d. F
1e. F
2a. F
2b. F
2c. F
2d. F
2e. T

Chapter 4

1a. F
1b. F
1c. T
1d. F
1e. T
2a. T
2b. T
2c. F
2d. T
2e. T

Chapter 5

1a. T
1b. F
1c. T
1d. F
1e. T
2a. F
2b. F
2c. T
2d. F
2e. T

Chapter 6

1a. T
1b. F
1c. T
1d. F
1e. T
2a. T
2b. T
2c. T
2d. T
2e. F

Chapter 7

1a. F
1b. T
1c. F
1d. T
1e. T
2a. F
2b. T
2c. F
2d. F
2e. T

D. Dillane, B. A. Finegan (eds.), *Preoperative Assessment*, https://doi.org/10.1007/978-3-030-58842-7

Chapter 8

1a. T
1b. T
1c. F
1d. T
1e. T
2a. T
2b. T
2c. F
2d. T
2e. F

Chapter 9

1a. F
1b. F
1c. T
1d. T
1e. F
2a. F
2b. T
2c. T
2d. F
2e. F

Chapter 10

1a. T
1b. T
1c. F
1d. F
1e. F
2a. T
2b. F
2c. T
2d. F
2e. F

Chapter 11

1a. F
1b. F
1c. T
1d. T
1e. F
2a. F
2b. T
2c. T
2d. F
2e. T

Chapter 12

1a. T
1b. F
1c. T
1d. F
1e. T
2a. T
2b. F
2c. F
2d. T
2e. T

Chapter 13

1a. F
1b. F
1c. T
1d. T
1e. F
2a. T
2b. F
2c. F
2d. T
2e. F

Chapter 14

1a. T
1b. F
1c. T
1d. F
1e. F
2a. T
2b. T
2c. T
2d. T
2e. T

Chapter 15

1a. F
1b. T
1c. F
1d. F
1e. F
2a. T
2b. T
2c. F
2d. F
2e. T

Chapter 16

1a. F
1b. T
1c. F
1d. F
1e. F
2a. F
2b. F
2c. T
2d. T
2e. T

Chapter 17

1a. T
1b. F
1c. T
1d. F
1e. T
2a. F
2b. T
2c. F
2d. T
2e. F

Chapter 18

1a. F
1b. F
1c. T
1d. T
1e. T
2a. T
2b. F
2c. T
2d. F
2e. F

Chapter 19

1a. T
1b. T
1c. F
1d. T
1e. F
2a. F
2b. T
2c. T
2d. T
2e. F

Chapter 20

1a. F
1b. T
1c. T
1d. F
1e. T
2a. F
2b. T
2c. T
2d. F
2e. F

Chapter 21

1a. F
1b. F
1c. F
1d. T
1e. T
2a. F
2b. F
2c. T
2d. T
2e. F

Chapter 22

1a. F
1b. T
1c. T
1d. T
1e. F
2a. T
2b. F
2c. F
2d. T
2e. T

Chapter 23

1a. F
1b. T
1c. F
1d. F
1e. T
2a. T
2b. F
2c. F
2d. T
2e. T

Chapter 24

1a. F
1b. F
1c. T
1d. T
1e. F
2a. T
2b. F
2c. T
2d. F
2e. T

Chapter 25

1a. T
1b. F
1c. F
1d. T
1e. T
2a. T
2b. F
2c. F
2d. T
2e. T

Chapter 26

1a. T
1b. F
1c. T
1d. F
1e. T
2a. F
2b. F
2c. F
2d. T
2e. F

Chapter 27

1a. T
1b. F
1c. T
1d. F
1e. T
2a. F
2b. T
2c. T
2d. T
2e. F

Chapter 28

1a. T
1b. T
1c. F
1d. T
1e. T
2a. T
2b. F
2c. F
2d. T
2e. T

Chapter 29

1a. F
1b. T
1c. T
1d. F
1e. T
2a. F
2b. T
2c. T
2d. F
2e. F

Chapter 30

1a. F
1b. T
1c. F
1d. T
1e. T
2a. T
2b. T
2c. F
2d. T
2e. F

Chapter 31

1a. T
1b. F
1c. T
1d. F
1e. T
2a. T
2b. F
2c. T
2d. T
2e. T

Chapter 32

1a. F
1b. T
1c. T
1d. F
1e. F
2a. F
2b. T
2c. F
2d. T
2e. F

Chapter 33

1a. T
1b. F
1c. T
1d. F
1e. F
2a. T
2b. F
2c. T
2d. T
2e. T

Chapter 34

1a. T
1b. F
1c. F
1d. T
1e. F
2a. T
2b. T
2c. F
2d. F
2e. F

Chapter 35

1a. F
1b. T
1c. T
1d. T
1e. T
2a. F
2b. T
2c. F
2d. F
2e. T

Chapter 36

1a. F
1b. T
1c. T
1d. F
1e. T
2a. F
2b. T
2c. T
2d. T
2e. F

Chapter 37

1a. T
1b. T
1c. T
1d. F
1e. T
2a. T
2b. F
2c. T
2d. F
2e. F

Chapter 38

1a. F
1b. T
1c. T
1d. T
1e. T
2a. F
2b. F
2c. F
2d. T
2e. T

Chapter 39

1a. T
1b. T
1c. T
1d. F
1e. T
2a. T
2b. T
2c. F
2d. F
2e. F

Chapter 40

1a. F
1b. F
1c. T
1d. F
1e. T
2a. F
2b. F
2c. T
2d. F
2e. F

Chapter 41

1a. F
1b. T
1c. T
1d. F
1e. T
2a. F
2b. T
2c. T
2d. T
2e. F

Chapter 42

1a. T
1b. T
1c. T
1d. T
1e. T
2a. T
2b. T
2c. T
2d. F
2e. F

Chapter 43

1a. F
1b. T
1c. T
1d. F
1e. T
2a. F
2b. F
2c. F
2d. F
2e. T

Chapter 44

1a. F
1b. T
1c. F
1d. T
1e. F
2a. T
2b. T
2c. T
2d. T
2e. F

Chapter 45

1a. F
1b. T
1c. F
1d. T
1e. F
2a. F
2b. T
2c. F
2d. T
2e. T

Chapter 46

1a. T
1b. F
1c. F
1d. T
1e. F
2a. T
2b. T
2c. F
2d. T
2e. T

Chapter 47

1a. T
1b. F
1c. F
1d. F
1e. T
2a. F
2b. F
2c. T
2d. T
2e. T

Chapter 48

1a. T
1b. F
1c. T
1d. T
1e. T
2a. T
2b. T
2c. F
2d. T
2e. F

Chapter 49

1a. F
1b. T
1c. T
1d. T
1e. F
2a. T
2b. T
2c. T
2d. F
2e. T

Index

D. Dillane, B. A. Finegan (eds.), *Preoperative Assessment*, https://doi.org/10.1007/978-3-030-58842-7

B

C

N

O

GPSR Comp iance

The European Union's (EU) General Product Safety Regulation (GPSR) is a set of rules that requires consumer products to be safe and our obligations to ensure this.

If you have any concerns about our products, you can contact us on ProductSafety@springernature.com

In case Publisher is established outside the EU, the EU authorized representative is:

Springer Nature Customer Service Center GmbH
Europaplatz 3
69115 Heidelberg, Germany

Batch number: 10086230

Printed by Printforce, the Netherlands